Imaging in Pediatric Pulmonology

Robert H. Cleveland

Editor

Claire Langton

Associate Editor, Pathology

Andrew A. Colin

Associate Editor, Pediatric Pulmonology

Edward Y. Lee

Associate Editor, Imaging

Jeanne S. Chow

Assistant Editor, Imaging

Imaging in Pediatric Pulmonology

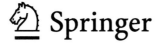 Springer

Editor
Robert H. Cleveland, MD
Professor
Department of Radiology
Harvard Medical School
Boston, MA, USA

Departments of Radiology and Medicine
Division of Respiratory Diseases
Children's Hospital Boston
Boston, MA, USA
Robert.Cleveland@childrens.harvard.edu

ISBN 978-1-4419-5871-6   e-ISBN 978-1-4419-5872-3
DOI 10.1007/978-1-4419-5872-3
Springer New York Dordrecht Heidelberg London

Library of Congress Control Number: 2011942783

Printed on acid-free paper

Springer is part of Springer Science+Business Media (www.springer.com)

Foreword

It is an honor and a privilege to be asked to write the foreword for *Imaging in Pediatric Pulmonology* edited by Dr. Robert H. Cleveland. It is the definitive reference for pediatric chest imaging.

Dr. Cleveland is a world renowned expert in pediatric pulmonary imaging. He has spent his academic career in Boston, having served as faculty at both Boston Children's Hospital as well as previously at Massachusetts General Hospital. He holds the appointment as Professor at Harvard Medical School. He has published multiple previous articles on pediatric pulmonary imaging. This textbook has been Dr. Cleveland's passion over the past several years and acts as an exclamation point to his esteemed career.

Dr. Cleveland has assembled an outstanding team of contributing authors. It includes international experts in chest imaging and the related pediatric pulmonary sciences. The organization of topics is appropriately by variable parameters. Some are organized by anatomic area: the table of contents covers topics of the lung, airway, pleura, mediastinum, and chest wall. Some chapters are organized by imaging finding, such as hyperlucency, cysts, or nodules. Some are organized by pathologic entitiy: cystic fibrosis and malignant medistinal masses, for example. Normal findings in the lung and airway are covered. Important subspecialty areas in pulmonary imaging are covered, such as imaging in lung transplantation and fetal imaging. Importantly, both commonly encountered pediatric problems, such as imaging in pneumonia, as well as uncommon topics, not easily found in many resources, such as hepatopulmonary fusion and horseshoe lung malformation, are covered.

The writing is excellent and impressively similar in style for a multiauthor textbook. The illustrations are plentiful and of high quality. I believe the combination of the topics covered and the quality of the writing and illustrations makes *Imaging in Pediatric Pulmonology* the definitive textbook in this area. Dr. Cleveland and his team are to be congratulated.

Orlando, FL, USA   Lane F. Donnelly, MD

Preface

This textbook came about as a result of my association with some very talented pediatric pulmonologists. Much of what I have learned about pediatric pulmonary diseases is the result of serving as the radiologist for the New England Pediatric Pulmonary Consortium for the past 30 years. There have been many conversations with both pediatric pulmonologists and pediatric radiologists and trainees about what is needed as a general reference source of pediatric pulmonary imaging. This book is an attempt to address those needs. Radiologists may find a new approach in the organization of the text. Clinicians hopefully will find a clinically "user-friendly" imaging resource.

The first section of the textbook is a series of algorithms for the most common clinical scenarios presenting to pediatric pulmonologists or pediatricians. The branch points in the algorithms serve as references to diseases discussed elsewhere in the book. There are also several chapters dedicated to specific topics, such as lung transplantation and fetal imaging.

Rather than assuming a priori knowledge or suspicion of the diagnosis, this text can lead the reader to a differential diagnosis based on clinical parameters and thus direct reading to the relevant diagnoses. If the readers know their topic of interest, the chapters are organized for easy access to a broad range of abnormalities.

There is an emphasis on plain film imaging as well as high technology imaging in this textbook. There are several reasons for this. Even in the current era of widespread use of CT, MR, SPECT, fusion imaging, etc., approximately 70% of the images acquired in pediatric centers are plain films. We also find ourselves in an era where reliance on ancillary data, such as imaging, is perceived to have caused deterioration in clinical skills [1, 2]. This has lead to an increased reliance on imaging in patient care. For most pediatric pulmonary issues, this begins with a plain film. In addition, with the heightened concern about radiation exposure, especially from CT, there is need to garner as much information with as little radiation exposure as possible. Even imaging within ALARA guidelines [3, 4], the best case is to avoid additional imaging, especially CT, if the answer is available elsewhere.

Finally, just as our colleagues have recognized deterioration in their clinical skills [1, 2], many radiologists who are trained in the pre-high-tech era are seeing a similar deterioration in plain film interpretive skills. This book will hopefully help us all to resharpen those skills and solidify our confidence in our use of those skills. There are many situations, however, in which the only avenue to the correct diagnosis is with advanced imaging or combinations of different imaging approaches. This is also covered in depth.

Boston, MA, USA   Robert H. Cleveland

References

1. Jauhar S. The demise of the physical exam. N Engl J Med. 2006;354:548–51.
2. Markel H. The stethoscope and the art of listening. N Engl J Med. 2006;354:551–3.
3. Society of Pediatric Radiology. The ALARA (as low as reasonably achievable) concept in pediatric CT intelligent dose reduction. Multidisciplinary conference organized by the Society of Pediatric Radiology, 18–19 August 2001. Pediatr Radiol. 2002;32:217–313.
4. Frush DP, Donnelly LF, Rosen NS. Computed tomography and radiation risks: what pediatric health care providers should know. Pediatrics. 2003;112:951–7.

Acknowledgments

This book would not have come into being without the convergence of several lucky events that I gratefully acknowledge.

First and foremost is the 30-year association I have enjoyed with the New England Pediatric Pulmonary Consortium. Since the group's founding, we have meet weekly at the Massachusetts General Hospital. As the radiologist in a group of extremely talented pediatric pulmonologists from across New England, I have had the pleasure of delving into the fine points of lung abnormalities, from the routine to the extraordinary. My pulmonary friends have taught me more physiology than I thought possible and helped me develop an appreciation of how this affects the images. I would like to especially mention two of these colleagues to whom I am most grateful for the early development of my interest in lung disease. Dr. Denise Strieder and Dr. Dan Shannon both have been brilliant physiologists, clinicians, and mentors.

It was during the early years of my career as a Pediatric Radiologist at the Massachusetts General Hospital that I gained the inspiration and techniques of navigating an academic medical career. My radiology colleagues were enthusiastic physicians who shared their knowledge and encouragement. During this Formative Period, I was fortunate to work with two very talented, Supportive Chairmen, Dr. Juan Taveras and Dr. Jim Thrall to whom I am much indebted for their leadership and guidance.

I have also had the pleasure to work with many talented, caring physicians and staff during my subsequent years at Children's Hospital Boston. The volume and breadth of clinical exposure has been extraordinary.

I am especially appreciative of the clinical and radiology colleagues who have provided chapters for this textbook. Special mention must be made of my Associate Editors. Two have been colleagues and friends for many years; without the significant input from Dr. Claire Langston and Dr. Andrew Colin, this text would not have been possible. For his boundless energy and enthusiasm, no words can adequately thank Dr. Ed Lee. The assistance provided by my Assistant Editor, Dr. MeiMei Chow, in image acquisition and writing several chapters, is much appreciated.

Finally, I want to thank my family and friends for all their support during the preparation of this book.

Boston, MA, USA   Bob Cleveland

Contents

Contributors

Ahmad I. Alomari, MD, MSc, FSIR Division of Vascular and Interventional Radiology, Children's Hospital Boston, Harvard Medical School, Boston, MA, USA

Debra Boyer, MD Department of Medicine, Pulmonary Division, Children's Hospital Boston and Harvard Medical School, Boston, MA, USA

Dorothy Bulas, MD Department of Diagnostic Imaging and Radiology, George Washington University Medical Center, Children's National Medical Center, Washington, DC, USA

Gulraiz Chaudry, MBChB, MRCP, FRCR Department of Radiology, Children's Hospital Boston, Harvard Medical School, Boston, MA, USA

Jeanne S. Chow, MD Department of Radiology, Harvard Medical School and Children's Hospital Boston, Boston, MA, USA

Ellen M. Chung, MD Department of Radiology and Radiological Sciences, Uniformed Services University of the Health Sciences, Bethesda, MD, USA

Robert H. Cleveland, MD Department of Radiology, Harvard Medical School, Boston, MA, USA

Departments of Radiology and Medicine, Division of Respiratory Diseases, Children's Hospital Boston, Boston, MA, USA

Anne Cameron Coates, MD Department of Pediatrics, Stanford School of Medicine/Lucille Packard Children's Hosptial at Stanford, Palo Alto, CA, USA

Andrew A. Colin, MD Miller School of Medicine, University of Miami, Miami, FL, USA

Veronica Donoghue, FRCR, FFR, RCSI Radiology Department, Children's University Hospital, Temple Street, Dublin, Ireland

Alexia Egloff, MD Department of Radiology, Pediatric Radiologist, Children's National Medical Center, Washington, DC, USA

Mary Shannon Fracchia, MD Pediatric Pulmonary Department, Massachusetts General Hospital, Harvard Medical School, Boston, MA, USA

Pradeep Govender, LRCP & SI, MB, BCh, BAO, FFRRCSI Division of Vascular and Interventional Radiology, Children's Hospital Boston, Harvard Medical School, Boston, MA, USA

Umakanth Khatwa, MD Division of Respiratory Diseases, Department of Medicine, Children's Hospital Boston, Boston, MA, USA

Jason E. Lang, MD Department of Pulmonology, Allergy and Immunology, Nemours Children's Clinic/Mayo Clinic College of Medicine, Jacksonville, FL, USA

Claire Langston, MD Department of Pathology, Texas Children's Hospital, Baylor College of Medicine, Houston, TX, USA

Edward Y. Lee, MD, MPH Division of Thoracic Imaging, Department of Radiology and Medicine, Pulmonary Division, Children's Hospital Boston, Harvard Medical School, Boston, MA, USA

Neil Mardis, DO Department of Radiology, University of Missouri-Kansas City School of Medicine, Kansas City, MO, USA

Benjamin A. Nelson, MD Department of Pediatrics, Harvard University/ Massachusetts General Hospital for Children, Boston, MA, USA

Kara Palm, MD Division of Respiratory Diseases, Children's Hospital Boston, Boston, MA, USA

Sanjay P. Prabhu, MBSS, FRCR Department of Radiology, Children's Hospital Boston and Harvard Medical School, Boston, MA, USA

Annabelle Quizon, MD Department of Pediatrics, Division of Pediatric Pulmonology, University of Miami/Miller School of Medicine, Batchelor Children's Research Institute, Miami, FL, USA

Shashi H. Ranganath, MD Department of Pediatric Radiology, Children's Hospital Boston, Harvard Medical School, Boston, MA, USA

Lawrence Rhein, MD Center for Healthy Infant Lung Development, Divisions of Newborn Medicine and Respiratory Diseases, Children's Hospital Boston, Boston, MA, USA

Dennis Rosen, MD Division of Respiratory Diseases, Harvard Medical School, Children's Hospital Boston, Boston, MA, USA

Efraim Sadot, MD Pediatric Intensive Care Unit, Department of Pediatric Pulmonology, Critical Care and Sleep Medicine, Dana Children's Hospital, Tel-Aviv Sourasky Medical Center, Tel-Aviv University, Tel-Aviv, Israel

Gregory S. Sawicki, MD, MPH Department of Pediatrics, Division of Respiratory Diseases, Children's Hospital Boston, Harvard Medical School, Boston, MA, USA

Dubhfeasa Maire Slattery, MD, PhD Department of Respiratory Medicine, Children's University Hospital, Temple Street, Dublin, Ireland

Gary Visner, DO Department of Medicine, Pulmonary Division, Children's Hospital Boston and Harvard Medical School, Boston, MA, USA

Meguru Watanabe, MD, PhD Department of Radiology, Children's Hospital Boston, Boston, MA, USA

Robert G. Zwerdling, MD Pediatric, Pulmonary, Asthma, Allergy, and Cystic Fibrosis Center, University of Massachusetts Memorial Medical Center, Worcester, MA, USA

Clinical Algorithms

Dennis Rosen, Jason E. Lang, and Andrew A. Colin

CONTENTS

1.1   Introduction

In medical practice, patients usually present without a known diagnosis. Physicians move from a set of signs and symptoms to the formation of a differential diagnosis to a final diagnosis. This introductory chapter provides seven clinical algorithms that encompass a large part of the spectrum of pediatric pulmonary practice. By navigating through the appropriate algorithm, reference to possible relevant diagnoses may be encountered which will provide direction to further reading in the textbook.

The algorithms are as follows:

- Chest pain
- Chronic cough
- Cyanosis/hypoxia
- Shortness of breath
- Airway bleeding
- Noisy breathing
- Tachypnea

1.2   Chest Pain

Jason E. Lang

See Fig. 1.1

Dennis Rosen, MD
Division of Respiratory Diseases, Children's Hospital Boston,
Harvard Medical School, Boston, MA, USA
e-mail: Dennis.Rosen@childrens.harvard.edu

Jason E. Lang, MD
Department of Pulmonology, Allergy and Immunology,
Nemours Children's Clinic/Mayo Clinic College of Medicine,
Jacksonville, FL, USA
e-mail: jelang@nemours.org

Andrew A. Colin, MD (✉)
Miller School of Medicine, University of Miami,
Miami, FL, USA
e-mail: AColin@med.miami.edu

R.H. Cleveland (ed.), *Imaging in Pediatric Pulmonology*,
DOI 10.1007/978-1-4419-5872-3_1, © Springer Science+Business Media, LLC 2012

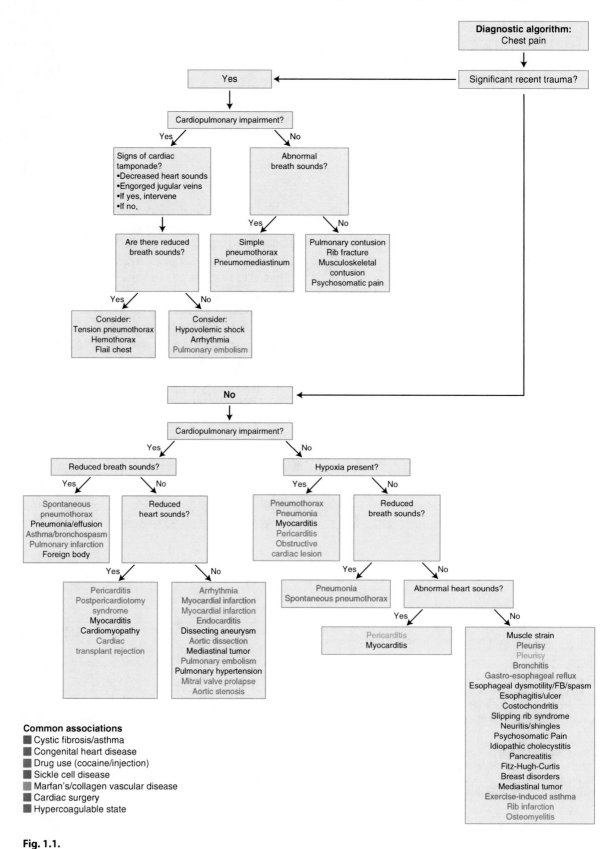

Fig. 1.1.

1.3 Chronic Cough

ANDREW A. COLIN

See Fig. 1.2

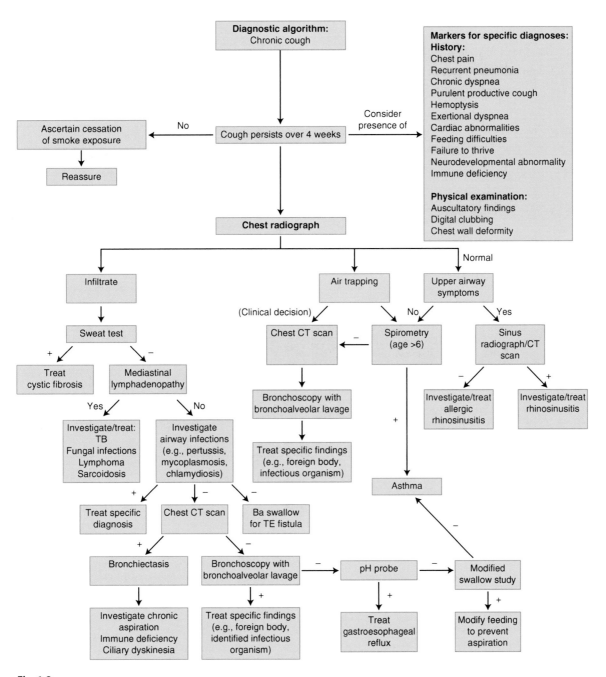

Fig. 1.2.

1.4   Cyanosis and Hypoxia

DENNIS ROSEN

Cyanosis is often associated with hypoxia, but the two do not always coexist (Fig. 1.3). *Acrocyanosis* is commonly associated with vasoconstriction, whereas *central cyanosis* is most often found in the perioral area and is reflective of at least 5 g/% of unsaturated hemoglobin. This can result from different causes, which will be reviewed systematically. In general, it is helpful to consider the causative mechanism of the cyanosis. These different mechanisms can include:

- Shunting of *blue* deoxygenated blood from the venous circulation to the arterial circulation, bypassing the alveolar capillary network
- Intrapulmonary shunting
- V/Q mismatching
- Inadequate ventilation
- Inadequate gas exchange at the level of the alveolus (diffusion defects)
- Inadequate bonding of O_2 to the red blood cells (hematologic causes)
- Inadequate perfusion

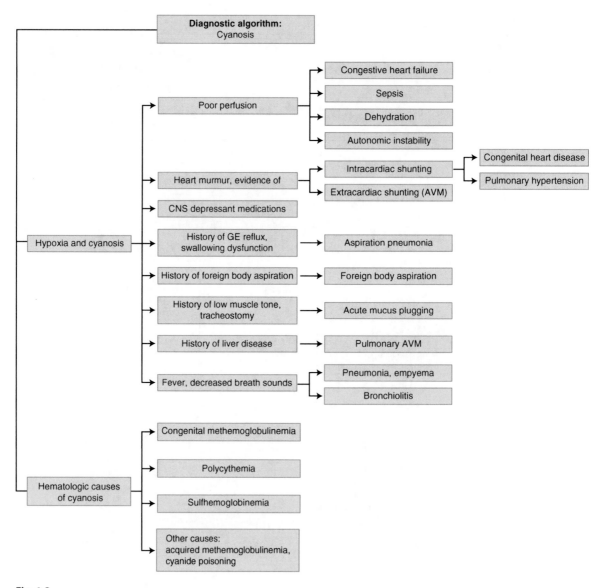

Fig. 1.3.

Shunting of blood can occur on many levels, primarily the heart, lung, periphery. Cardiac causes include cardiac malformation with right to left shunting, including primary heart lesions with right to left shunting (tetralogy of Fallot, transposition of great arteries, truncus arteriosus, pulmonic stenosis/atresia, aortic stenosis, Ebstein's anomaly, and hypoplastic left heart) and with lesions associated with pulmonary hypertension (either primary or secondary to increased pulmonary flow such as in Eisenmenger's syndrome), persistent fetal circulation, breath holding, and shunting through a patent foramen ovale.

Intrapulmonary shunting can occur with foreign body aspiration, in mucous plugging, atalectasis, in pneumonia with a large infiltrate, bronchiolitis, and pulmonary hemosiderosis. It is seen in cases of arteriovenous malformations (AVM), either primary, or in the setting of liver failure and the hepatopulmonary syndrome. It can also be seen in restrictive lesions such as pneumothorax, pleural effusion, pulmonary fibrosis, pulmonary hemosiderosis, meconium aspiration, and respiratory distress syndrome (RDS) in neonates.

V/Q mismatching is seen in pulmonary emboli, pulmonary hypertension, in hyperinflative states such as asthma and bronchiolitis, and congenital lobar emphysema.

Inadequate ventilation can result from restrictive defects such as pneumothorax, ribcage abnormalities, scoliosis, kyphosis, abdominal distention, and obesity; central control of breathing disorders such as congenital alveolar hypoventilation syndrome; and neuromuscular disease such as muscular dystrophy, Werdnig–Hoffman, diaphragmatic paralysis, polio, and Guillain Barré. Obstructive processes such as nasal obstruction, retropharyngeal abscesses, tonsillar hypertrophy, severe croup, laryngeal webs, foreign body aspiration, obstructive sleep apnea, and hypoventilation syndrome. CNS depressant medications can also inhibit the respiratory drive.

Diffusion defects are caused by interstitial processes such as interstitial lung disease (ILD), bronchopulmonary dysplasia (BPD), pulmonary edema, hypersensitivity pneumonitis, and adult respiratory distress syndrome (ARDS).

Hematologic causes of cyanosis include methemoglobinemia, either acquired (medication or nitrite ingestion) or congenital, polycythemia, and sulfahemoglobinemia. These are nonhypoxemic and can be distinguished by measurement of blood PaO_2 levels.

Poor perfusion leading to cyanosis can be cardiac in origin, stemming from congestive heart failure (primary, postischemia, secondary to myocarditis, arrhythmias, heart block, and pericarditis) or systemic, including shock, sepsis, autonomic instability, and drug-mediated.

1.5 Shortness of Breath

Jason E. Lang

See Fig. 1.4

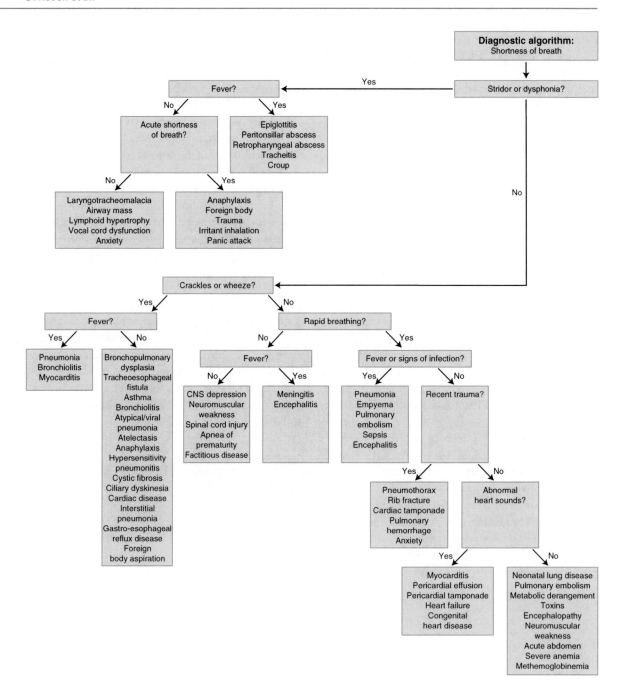

Fig. 1.4.

1.6 Airway Bleeding

Andrew A. Colin

See Fig. 1.5

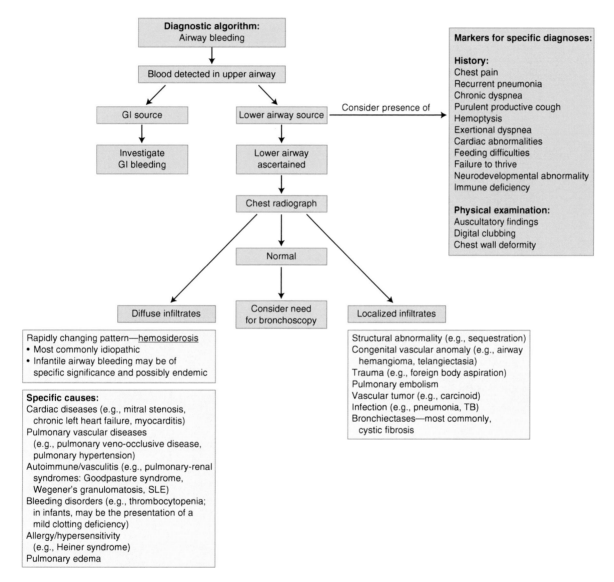

Fig. 1.5.

1.7   Noisy Breathing

Dennis Rosen

See Fig. 1.6a–c

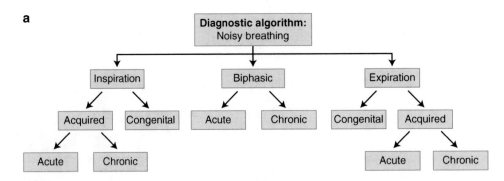

Fig. 1.6.

b

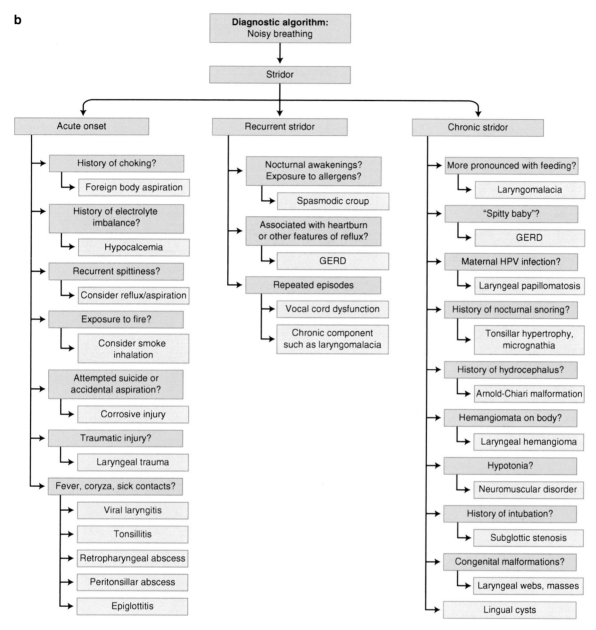

Fig. 1.6. (continued)

c

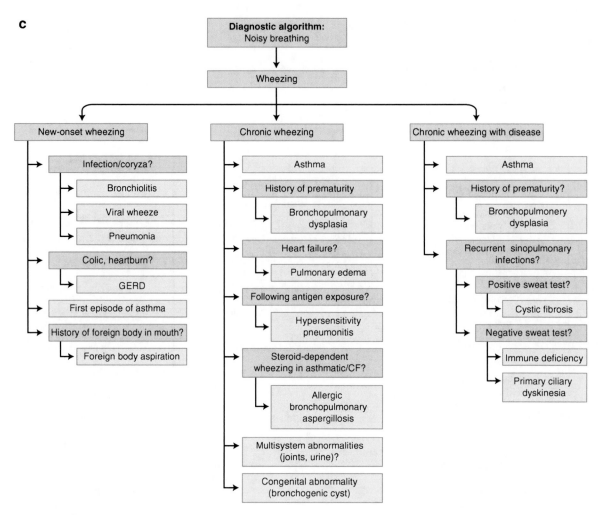

Fig. 1.6. (continued)

1.8 Tachypnea

DENNIS ROSEN

Tachypnea is defined as a respiratory rate above the age-appropriate range, measured while the child is at rest (Fig. 1.7). The emphasis on age appropriateness is important, as infants may have resting respiratory rates ranging 24–40 breaths per minute, whereas children over the age of 2 will generally have resting respiratory rates ranging between 12 and 20 breaths per minute. This stems from the relatively high chest wall compliance found in infants and toddlers, which decreases as children advance in age. Tachypnea is a sign of an underlying disorder and in most cases represents an attempt by the body to improve gas exchange. It is detrimental as it results in increased energy expenditure, thus diverting calories away from other tasks such as growth. It can result in metabolic derangements such as hyperventilation and respiratory alkalosis, and is difficult to sustain for a prolonged period of time because of progressive muscle fatigue. When caring for a child with tachypnea, it is important to identify the underlying cause and to treat it, so as to prevent progression to respiratory failure.

1.8.1 Causes of Tachypnea

There is a broad differential diagnosis for a child with tachypnea, which encompasses not only pulmonary causes, but also systemic, psychological, neurological, cardiac, and metabolic causes, which are for the most part beyond the purview of this book.

Psychological

Emotional stress or anxiety can provoke tachypnea, often accompanied by hyperventilation, sometimes resulting in metabolic alkalosis and tetany.

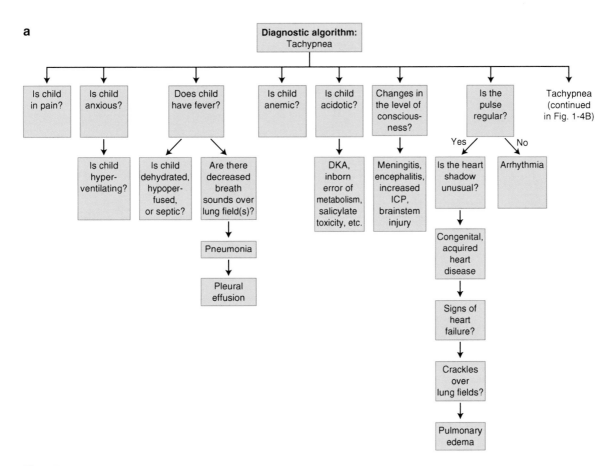

a

Fig. 1.7.

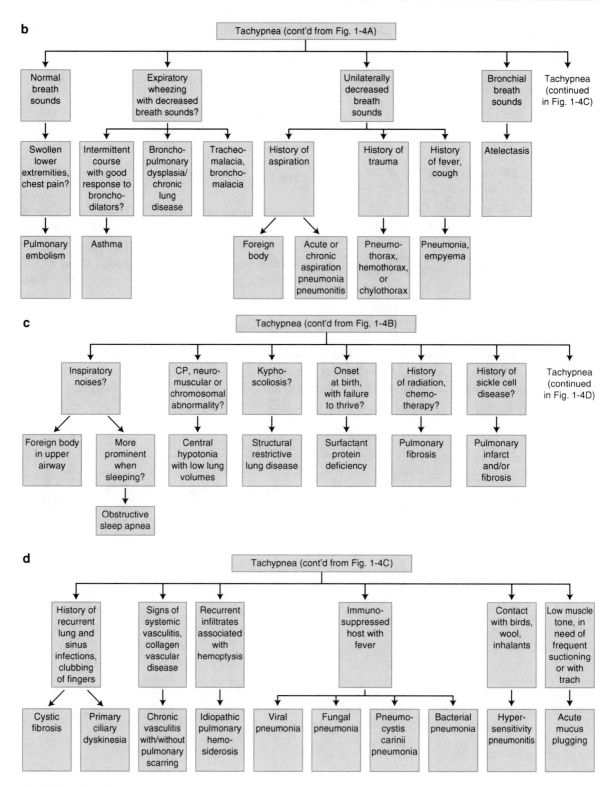

Fig. 1.7. (continued)

Systemic

Pain and fever are both nonpulmonary causes of tachypnea. Poor perfusion accompanied by hypotension (such as in the case of dehydration or sepsis) can also lead to this, both as a compensatory mechanism to correct developing metabolic acidosis and as an attempt to improve oxygen delivery to end organs and tissues.

Metabolic

Both hypoxia and hypercarbia can increase the respiratory drive. Hypoxia can result from a decrease in the partial pressure of inspired oxygen, such as occurring at high altitudes, or from one or more of many pulmonary processes, which will be discussed shortly. Even when the intake and transport of oxygen are normal, in severe anemia, one can have a decrease in oxygen delivery to end-organs and tissues, and subsequently an increased respiratory rate.

There are many inborn errors of metabolism which can also bring about an increased basal respiratory rate, including urea cycle defects, methylmalonic academia, and isovaleric academia, to name but a few.

Acquired metabolic acidosis can induce hyperventilation with tachypnea as an attempt to correct the acidosis by increasing the clearance of CO_2 from the body, as described earlier. Causes of this include diabetic ketoacidosis, lactic acidosis, uremia, salicylate poisoning, dehydration, and sepsis.

Cardiac

Heart failure can cause tachypnea, either secondary to fluid accumulation in the lungs, such as in the case of pulmonary edema, or because of poor perfusion due to myocardial dysfunction. The presence of an irregular, weak or rapid pulse, a murmur on physical exam, pulmonary edema, or an enlarged or abnormally shaped heart on chest X-ray should prompt a closer investigation of the heart and its function.

Neurological

Changes in intracranial pressure, encephalitis, and stroke are all recognized causes of tachypnea, and should be considered in the context of the child's illness and presentation.

Pulmonary

Many types of pulmonary disease result in tachypnea because of a decrease in the proportion of tidal volume taking part in active gas exchange. In order to maintain minute ventilation, the respiratory rate needs to be increased. This can occur in obstructive processes, with air trapping; in restrictive processes, when the vital capacity is reduced, with the dead space volume decreasing, remaining the same or increasing; and in diffusion defects, when the amount of oxygen with any given breath traversing the alveolar membrane decreases. In cases of V/Q mismatching, such as pulmonary embolus, where tachypnea is one of the most common presenting signs, this is a result of the increase in functional dead space. Tachypnea also occurs in shunting, when a portion of the blood flow through the lungs is not exposed to the inspired air, resulting in hypoxemia, which in turn triggers a heightened respiratory drive.

Obstructive Processes

Obstructive processes can be subdivided into upper and lower airway obstruction, which refer to the location of the obstruction relative to the thoracic inlet. Examples of upper airway obstruction include acute laryngitis, foreign body aspiration, laryngomalacia, and obstructive sleep apnea. Lower airway obstruction can result from acute processes such as acute aspiration, or asthma exacerbation, and from chronic processes such as cystic fibrosis, bronchiectasis, bronchomalacia, tracheomalacia, BPD, chronic lung disease of prematurity, and chronic aspiration.

Restrictive Lung Disease

Restrictive lung disease can result from physical restriction of the lungs' capacity to insufflate, such as occurring chronically with kyphoscoliosis, neuromuscular disease, central hypotonia (in Down's syndrome, Prader Willi syndrome, other chromosomal disorders, and cerebral palsy), meningomyelocele, and congenital chest wall abnormality. It can be the result of an acute process that leads to physical restriction of the lungs' capacity to insufflate, such as chest wall injury, pneumo/hemo/chylothorax, or pleural effusion. It can also be the result of fibrosis of the lungs that occurs during the recovery phase from acute lung injury, such as radiation or drug injury, or pulmonary infarction secondary to pulmonary vascular disease, such as occurring with sickle cell disease. Fibrosis can also be caused as the result of chronic inflammation, such as is caused by some collagen vascular diseases.

Reversible Shunting

Reversible shunting occurs with atalectasis, which can result from mucus plugging, foreign body aspiration, and asthma. It can also occur in lobar pneumonia and pulmonary hemosiderosis. Chronic shunting can occur on the cardiac level, or the pulmonary level, via AVMs, which can be either congenital or acquired, such as in the case of the hepatopulmonary syndrome.

Diffusion Defects

Diffusion defects, stemming from ILD, can be acute processes, such as in the case of infectious pneumonitis, caused by viruses, fungi, or PCP, hypersensitivity pneumonitis, or chronic aspiration. Acute ILD can also be caused by radiation or drug injury. Pulmonary edema, which can be caused by a number of mechanisms, such as cardiogenic, neurologic, or postobstructive, will also reduce diffusion capacity and thus lead to tachypnea.

Normal Growth and Physiology

2

Andrew A. Colin and Dennis Rosen

CONTENTS

2.1 Overview of Respiratory Physiology

Dennis Rosen and Andrew A. Colin

In analyzing a chest radiograph, it is important to have an understanding of some of the basic principles of respiratory physiology, and to appreciate how certain pathophysiological processes can cause distinct disease states, each with its own specific clinical signs and symptoms [1, 2]. These can be divided into broad categories, which include obstructive lung disorders, restrictive lung disorders, disorders of gas diffusion, shunts, and ventilation-perfusion abnormalities. The following is a short overview of the physiologic considerations of these complex disorders. For more detail, the reader is advised to refer to the references below.

2.1.1 Obstructive Disorders

Obstructive disorders affect the conducting airways, and result from increased resistance to airflow within the airways and/or increased compliance of the airways. These disorders can be diffuse or localized. They can be caused by the presence of congenitally narrowed bronchi, scarred bronchi (such as in post-infectious bronchiolitis obliterans), intraluminal lesions, debris, or secretions (such as in acute bronchiolitis); dynamic airway wall changes leading to increased resistance to airflow as seen with bronchoconstriction, or increased compliance as is seen in emphysema; and extraluminal compression by a blood vessel or mass. Depending upon which segment of the conducting airways the obstruction is located in, the mechanism involved, and its severity, different phases of the respiratory cycle can be affected. Extrathoracic obstruction primarily causes problems in the inspiratory phase (though the stridor, expiratory phase can be affected as well), and intrathoracic obstruction will cause predominantly expiratory abnormalities (though here too, the Wheezing, inspiratory phase can be affected). The underlying mechanism of this variable behavior is that during inspiration, negative intrathoracic pressure is generated by the inspiratory muscles, drawing air and the walls of the extrathoracic airways

Andrew A. Colin, MD (✉)
Miller School of Medicine, University of Miami,
Miami, FL, USA
e-mail: Acolin@med.miami.edu

R.H. Cleveland (ed.), *Imaging in Pediatric Pulmonology*,
DOI 10.1007/978-1-4419-5872-3_2, © Springer Science+Business Media, LLC 2012

inward while the intrathoracic airways expand. During expiration, positive pressure is generated within the chest, propelling air outward, causing the intrathoracic airways toward closure, and the extrathoracic airways to expand. When intrathoracic obstruction is significant enough to cause inhomogeneity of emptying in some or many parts of the lung, the chest radiograph shows hyperinflation and air trapping. Examples of common diffuse obstructive disorders include asthma, cystic fibrosis (CF), bronchiolitis obliterans, bronchiectasis, and bronchopulmonary dysplasia. A bronchial foreign body represents a localized obstructive defect. Spirometry, which measures airflow, can quantify the degree of obstruction and is the standard pulmonary function test.

2.1.2 Restrictive Lung Disorders

Restrictive lung disorders occur when the lungs are unable to inflate to normal volumes. They can occur with parenchymal abnormalities, such as interstitial lung disease (idiopathic or secondary to an underlying disorder, such as a surfactant protein deficiency). They can also be caused by a musculoskeletal or neuromuscular abnormality which prevents the chest wall from expanding to full capacity during a maximal inspiratory effort. Examples of this type of restrictive process include congenital myopathies and neuromuscular disorders (such as spinal muscular atrophy). Bony chest wall abnormalities (such as scoliosis and thoracic dysplasia) inhibit lung growth and expansion, as do intrathoracic processes (such as a diaphragmatic hernia, large pleural effusion, or tumor). The chest radiograph may show reduced lung volumes, albeit this may be difficult to pick up in the young child with a limited inspiratory effort. More obvious are distorted or bell-shaped chest walls, scoliosis, or an abnormally diffuse parenchymal process, depending upon the underlying disorder. Physiologic assessment of these disorders is made with lung and thoracic gas volumes measurement using plethysmography and helium dilution methods to quantify the degree of restriction, and measurement of maximal respiratory pressures to assess muscle weakness. With a few exceptions, these methods require patient cooperation and are therefore limited in the young child. While the regular chest radiograph has limited value for quantification of restriction, algorithms exist to assess lung volumes using chest computed tomography (CT) scans.

2.1.3 Gas Diffusion Disorders

Gas diffusion disorders affect the absorption of oxygen into the bloodstream with resulting hypoxemia. This typically occurs due to a structural abnormality or thickening of the alveolar wall through which the gas exchange between the alveolus and the adjacent capillary occurs, resulting in hampered gas exchange. This can be seen in disease states such as interstitial lung diseases and pulmonary edema. Gas diffusion disorders may present symptomatically with dyspnea upon exertion or at rest, tachypnea, and/or hypoxemia. The chest radiograph often shows an abnormally diffuse parenchymal process. Measurement of the diffusion capacity of the lung with carbon monoxide (DLCO) is diagnostic.

2.1.4 Shunt

Shunt occurs when there is perfusion of a portion of lung without concomitant ventilation of the same area. This results in unoxygenated blood returning to the heart and being pumped into the arterial blood stream, leading to hypoxemia. The hypoxemia caused by shunts does not typically respond to the administration of oxygen. This is because the blood that is being shunted does not come in contact with the supplemental oxygen, while the blood flowing through the normally perfused portions of the lung is already well saturated. Shunts can be seen with arteriovenous malformations, pneumonias, and acute atalectasis. The chest radiograph is frequently reflective of the underlying pathology; however, small vascular malformation in the lungs can be elusive to the standard chest radiograph and need more advanced radiologic methods such as chess CT or MRI imaging.

2.1.5 Ventilation-Perfusion Abnormalities

Ventilation-perfusion abnormalities (also known as V/Q mismatch) occur when there is ventilation of a portion of lung without its concomitant perfusion. They can occur in congenital disorders such as absent development of a pulmonary artery, or due to intra-vascular processes such as pulmonary emboli. The physiologic/clinical effect of these disorders is mild relative to shunt, in particular with the long-standing circumstances such as congenital vascular anomalies, often with absence or minor hypoxic effects. The common chest radiograph often is of limited diagnostic value. Thus, when a V/Q mismatch is suspected, a ventilation-perfusion scan may give the clue, and, in cases where a pulmonary embolus is suspected, a CT with IV contrast can be diagnostic.

Andrew A. Colin

2.2 Lung Development and Effects on Lung Physiology

For the pediatric radiologist, lung mechanics and in particular those related to changes in lung volume are of crucial significance. One has to keep in mind that the radiograph of the noncooperative young child is never obtained at the optimal full inflation typical for the older person who inhales to full lung capacity (thus, total lung capacity or TLC) and breath-holds. The lung volumes reflected in the pediatric radiograph (assuming quiet breathing) span a volume range from functional residual capacity (FRC) (the volume at end expiration) to peak of tidal volume (the volume at end inspiration). Thus, by definition, the volume of the normal pediatric radiograph is *always* well below the lung volume of the cooperative patient, with all the implications that this has on the quality of the radiograph. Obviously, the lower the lung volume, the less reliable is the interpretation of pathology.

2.2.1 Stages of Lung Development

Early growth and development of the human lung is a continuous process that is highly variable between individuals and has traditionally been divided into five stages [3]. The first is the embryonic phase (26 days to 6 weeks of gestational age [wGA]), followed by the pseudoglandular (6–16 wGA) stage. At the end of this stage, the major elements of the bronchial tree complete their branching. The third is the canalicular stage (16–28 wGA). In its later phase of this stage, the

prealveolar elements may allow infant survival. The saccular stage (28–36 wGA) is the one in which most premature infants are born, and is followed by the alveolar (36 wGA–term) phase, which continues into childhood. The saccular period, 28–36 wGA, is a transitional phase before full maturation of alveoli occurs. The primitive alveoli that become gradually more effective as gas exchangers have alveolar walls that are more compact and thicker than the final thin walls of alveoli; they also have an immature capillary structure. However, this partially developed structure is capable of carrying out a limited function of gas exchange that fully matures in the alveolar phase. Mature alveoli are not uniformly present until 36 wGA at which time the epithelium and interstitium decrease in thickness, air space walls proliferate, and the capillary network matures to its final single capillary network. Alveolar proliferation represents the predominant element of lung growth after birth. The alveolar proliferation rate is maximal in the first 2 years of life, and subsequently decelerates; however, it is not well established until what age alveolar proliferation is maintained.

The structural changes associated with the transition to mature alveoli through the alveolar stage, and the following alveolar proliferation, account for the subsequent gains in lung volume. Physiologically, these maturational changes not only affect gas exchange, but together with the changes in the chest wall that will be discussed below, have profound effects on the mechanical properties of the respiratory system, and as such on the radiographic characteristics that are affected by these structural and mechanical considerations.

2.2.2 Changes in Lung Volume During the Last Trimester of Gestation

Calculations by Langston et al. [3] revealed that total lung volume undergoes rapid changes during the last trimester of gestation. At 30 wGA, the lung volume is only 34% of the ultimate lung volume at mature birth, and at 34 weeks only reaches 47% of the final volume at maturity. In contrast, the air space walls decrease in thickness such that at 30 and 34 weeks, they are 164% (28 μm) and 135% (23 μm), respectively, relative to the ultimate wall thickness at mature birth (17 μm). In parallel, dramatic increases in air space surface area occur. Surface area increases from 1.0–2.0 m^2 at 30–32 wGA, to 3.0–4.0 m^2 at term.

These volume changes likely have direct mechanical implications in reducing the vulnerability caused by a low and unstable FRC. Maturation of the alveolar network improves parenchymal elastance and therefore airway tethering.

2.2.3 Functional Residual Capacity Tends to be Low and Unstable in Infancy

Maintenance of a stable and adequate FRC is important to secure effective gas exchange. FRC is determined by the balance between the opposing forces of the chest wall and lung and is thus a direct function of their respective mechanical properties. In early life, a compliant chest wall offers little outward recoil to the respiratory system and thus the elastic characteristics of the respiratory system approximate those of the lung. The lung is also more compliant (i.e., has less elastance) in premature and newborn infants. The lung becomes less compliant (i.e., increases in elastance) as it undergoes alveolization and the interstitial network becomes more intricately woven. (*Note*: interstitium here represents the alveolar wall; a different concept from the same term utilized in radiology). Compliance of the chest wall is extremely high in premature infants and undergoes rapid stiffening in late intrauterine life [4], but this stiffening (or decline in compliance) continues over the first 2 years of life [5]. Therefore, in early life (and more so in premature infants), the lung–chest wall equilibrium results in a mechanically determined FRC that is low relative to older children and adults.

Thus, the baseline FRC in the young infant tends to drive itself to low volumes because of the mechanical characteristics discussed above. To circumvent this limitation, infants, unlike older children, actively elevate their FRC. At least three mechanisms are involved in the protection of a high end-expiratory volume: (a) initiation of inspiration at an end-expiratory volume above that determined by the mechanical properties of the chest wall and lung [6]. The other two mechanisms modulate the expiratory flow; (b) use of laryngeal braking during tidal expiration [7], and (c) persistence of inspiratory muscle activity into the expiratory phase [8].

The age at which transition to an *adult* pattern and cessation of these protective mechanisms has not been established for all of them, but based on one study [9] they persist at least into late in the first year and into the second year of life. It is likely that for premature infant the transition may be delayed. Interference with these active protective mechanisms, such as apnea or sedation, immediately drives the system toward low lung volumes. Also to be kept in mind is that the infant's sleeping state, supine position, and REM sleep (predominant in infancy) all substantially reduce lung volumes [10].

2.2.4 Airway Tethering

An additional crucial mechanism that secures airway patency and thus adequate maintenance of FRC is airway tethering. Tethering is mediated through the elastic components in alveolar walls that surround bronchi. These elastic fibers are anchored to each other creating an extended mesh that exerts a circumferential pull on the intraparenchymal airways. This complex elastic network transmits tension from the pleural surface to individual bronchi; thus, tethering couples lung volume changes to airway caliber. The force oscillates with the inspiratory cycle, and increases during inspiration, increasing airway caliber. The cross-sectional area of the airway decreases with decline in lung volume and airways may close if the lung volume is driven to critically low ranges of FRC (as may occur through the processes described above). Tethering of airways was shown to be absent or less effective in young experimental animals [11] and most likely in infants in whom alveolization and the associated parenchymal elastic network are still in early stages of development. The effect of reduced tethering is decreased airway stability, increased tendency to closure, increased airway resistance, and, ultimately, a tendency to collapse alveolar units in the lung periphery.

2.2.5 Lessons for the Pediatric Radiologist

With the above observations, the radiologist needs to keep in mind that the predictable deficiencies in lung volume in infants, and in particular when interference occurs with the mechanisms that protect lung volume (e.g., sedation), have an immediate effect on the quality of imaging. Chest radiographs and in particular chest CT scans obtained at low lung volumes have artifactual infiltrates in the lung fields that result from closure of airways and atelectases. This occurs in particular in the periphery of the lung and in dependent areas of the lung that are subjected to gravitational effects. To overcome these effects inflation of the lungs during the acquisition of the imaging is desirable. Most attractive for this purpose is the methodology developed by Long and Castile [12].

Some further physiological concepts related to pediatric respiratory physiology may be of use to the pediatric radiologist. Lung emptying in expiration is under normal circumstances a passive maneuver. Expiratory flow rate is determined by the interplay between a force that expels the air from the lung and the properties of the airways through which this exhaled air traverses. This flow rate is termed the expiratory time constant (τ) and is indeed a product of the compliance of the respiratory system (C) and the resistance of the airways (R) (thus, $\tau = C \times R$). To clarify, the force driving the air out upon relaxation at end inspiration is the elastance of the respiratory system (combined elastic properties of the lung and chest wall); this term is the reciprocal of the previously discussed compliance. In other words, compliant structures such as are the chest wall and the lung in the very young, as discussed above, offer little driving force in exhalation. Small airways, the patency of which is impaired because of relatively small lung volumes and insufficient tethering, offer relatively high resistance to flow. This may be complicated in conditions of uneven structures of airways and parenchyma, because of damage related to trauma to the lung, e.g., by mechanical ventilation, or infection, creating regions that offer uneven emptying profiles, or uneven expiratory time constants, bringing about inhomogeneity in lung emptying.

The need to protect lung volumes through the mechanisms described above results in a rapid breathing rate, short expiratory time, and absent expiratory pauses (rapid transition from expiration to inspiration). In such circumstances, when the breathing rate increases (for reasons such as hypoxia, fever, or infection) there may be insufficient time for full lung emptying, in particular when emptying inhomogeneity is present. This may result in air trapping and a radiological interpretation of *hyperinflation*. While no systematic studies exist on the duration of this phenomenon, it is likely to resolve within the second year of life when the maturational processes bring about a shift to the *adult* pattern of breathing.

References

1. Bryan AC, Wohl ME. Respiratory mechanics in children. In: Macklem P, Mead J, editors. Handbook of physiology, Sect. 3, Vol. 111: Part 1: Mechanics of Breathing, Chap. 12. American Physiological Society, Bethesda; 1986.
2. West JB. Respiratory physiology: the essentials. 8th ed. Philadelphia: Lippincott Williams & Wilkins; 2008.
3. Langston C, Kida K, Reed M, et al. Human lung growth in late gestation and in the neonate. Am Rev Respir Dis. 1984;129(4):607–13.
4. Gerhardt T, Bancalari E. Chestwall compliance in full-term and premature infants. Acta Paediatr Scand. 1980;69(3): 359–64.
5. Papastamelos C, Panitch HB, England SE, et al. Developmental changes in chest wall compliance in infancy and early childhood. J Appl Physiol. 1995;78(1): 179–84.
6. Kosch PC, Davenport PW, Wozniak JA, et al. Reflex control of expiratory duration in newborn infants. J Appl Physiol. 1985;58(2):575–81.
7. Kosch PC, Hutchinson AA, Wozniak JA, et al. Posterior cricoarytenoid and diaphragm activities during tidal breathing in neonates. J Appl Physiol. 1988;64(5):1968–78.
8. Mortola JP, Milic-Emili J, Noworaj A, et al. Muscle pressure and flow during expiration in infants. Am Rev Respir Dis. 1984;129(1):49–53.
9. Colin AA, Wohl ME, Mead J, et al. Transition from dynamically maintained to relaxed end-expiratory volume in human infants. J Appl Physiol. 1989;67(5):2107–11.
10. Henderson-Smart DJ, Read DJ. Reduced lung volume during behavioral active sleep in the newborn. J Appl Physiol. 1979;46(6):1081–5.
11. Gomes RF, Shardonofsky F, Eidelman DH, et al. Respiratory mechanics and lung development in the rat from early age to adulthood. J Appl Physiol. 2001;90(5):1631–8.
12. Long FR, Castile RG. Technique and clinical applications of full-inflation and end-exhalation controlled-ventilation chest CT in infants and young children. Pediatr Radiol. 2001;31(6):413–22.

The Normal Pediatric Chest

JEANNE S. CHOW AND ROBERT H. CLEVELAND

CONTENTS

can distinguish primary lung disease and congenital heart disease.

The purpose of this chapter is to understand the appearance of a normal chest radiograph and which abnormalities point to cardiovascular disease. This chapter provides a simple approach in the use of a chest radiograph to distinguish patients with cardiovascular disease as the cause of their respiratory symptoms so that further appropriate testing can be performed.

We recommend a standard approach in evaluating a chest radiograph:

- Technical adequacy
- Chamber enlargement
- Pulmonary vascularity
- Situs and side of aortic arch
- Lung parenchyma
- Extracardiovascular structures

If the heart is enlarged or abnormally shaped, if there is abnormal pulmonary vascularity, edema, or effusions, or if there is an abnormal position of the aortic arch, then the patient may have congenital or acquired cardiovascular disease. Unfortunately, a normal chest radiograph does not exclude congenital heart disease. Parenchymal abnormalities due to primary pulmonary disease are discussed in other chapters.

3.1 The Normal Chest Radiograph and Clues to Cardiovascular Disease

JEANNE S. CHOW

Clinical symptoms for patients with respiratory disease and cardiovascular disease often overlap. One of the first tests for patients with respiratory distress is a chest radiograph. A chest film frequently

3.1.1 Technical Adequacy

In an optimal chest radiograph, the intervertebral disc spaces should be seen through the cardiomediastinal silhouette. An underexposed film (one that is too light) may suggest pulmonary edema or pneumonia where it does not exist. An overexposed film (one that is too dark) may cause the interpreter to miss findings. Digital radiography allows for postprocessing so

JEANNE S. CHOW, MD (✉)
Department of Radiology, Harvard Medical School and Children's Hospital Boston, Boston, MA, USA
e-mail: jeanne.chow@childrens.harvard.edu

ROBERT H. CLEVELAND, MD
Department of Radiology, Harvard Medical School, Boston, MA, USA

Departments of Radiology and Medicine, Division of Respiratory Diseases, Children's Hospital Boston, Boston, MA, USA

R.H. Cleveland (ed.), *Imaging in Pediatric Pulmonology*,
DOI 10.1007/978-1-4419-5872-3_3, © Springer Science+Business Media, LLC 2012

images, which originally were improperly exposed, may be remedied without reexposing the child [1]. In infants, the frontal radiograph is frequently taken recumbent and in the AP (anterior–posterior) projection and in older children the film is obtained upright and in the PA (posterior–anterior) projection.

Patient motion, rotation, and angulation may also distort an otherwise normal appearing chest. In a well-centered film, the distance of the medial ends of the clavicles should be equidistant from the adjacent posterior spinous process. The anterior ribs should be equidistant from the lateral margins of the spine and posterior spinous processes of the vertebra. A slight rotation to the left may cause the appearance of enlargement of the left superior mediastium and left cardiac structures. Right mediastinal and cardiac structures appear larger when the patient rotates to the right. A lordotic image can exaggerate the size of the cardiac apex. On the lateral view, there should be a very small distance between the posterior right and left rib margins.

The degree of inspiration should be assessed on every radiograph. Although the degree of inspiration can be measured indirectly, the amount of inspiration is best judged by experience. Films obtained with very high lung volumes may produce an appearance of abnormal uplifting of the cardiac apex, and be confused for right ventricular enlargement. Films obtained in expiration may suggest edema, atelectasis, or pneumonia where it does not exist. These films may also obscure important findings (Fig. 3.1a).

The cardiac silhouette may also be obscured or appear enlarged with poor inspiration. A good inspiratory image is one in which the anterior sixth or posterior eighth rib is visualized above the apex of the left hemidiaphragm. In general, radiographs taken during expiration may show the dome of the left hemidiaphragm above this level. The lateral view and the appearance of flattened hemidiaphragms are also useful in determining the degree of inspiration. Many experienced radiologists rely on the degree of flattening of the diaphragm as the primary criterion of determining lung inflation.

3.1.2 Normal Heart Size, Shape, and Position

In order to be able to determine the size and position of cardiomediastinal structures, the appearance of the normal thymus must be understood. This is especially important in infants and toddlers where the normal thymus fills the anterior mediastinum and can obscure the superior cardiac border and mediastinum, the side and size of the great vessels, and the normal borders of the heart. Normally, the thymus involutes with increasing age and should be relatively inconspicuous by the end of the first decade.

The classic appearance of a newborn thymus is anterior superior mediastinal soft tissue that blends imperceptibly with the cardiac silhouette. A large thymus can

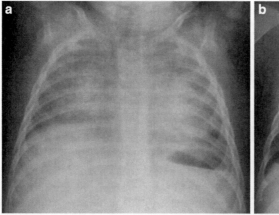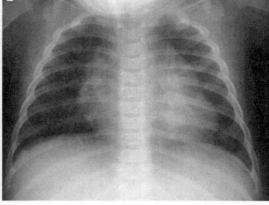

Fig. 3.1. (a, b) Expiratory and inspiratory radiographs with posterior rib fractures. These two frontal radiographs on the same patient emphasize the importance of lung volumes when interpreting a chest radiograph. The first frontal radiograph is performed in expiration, as evidenced by low lung volumes, bilateral atelectasis, and tracheal deviation toward the right. The second radiograph performed moments later in inspiration shows clear lungs and left posterior rib fractures in a patient with non-accidental trauma

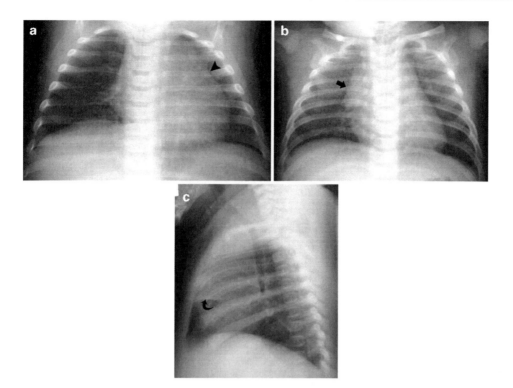

Fig. 3.2. Normal thymus. These three images demonstrate the normal appearance of the thymus in infancy. (**a**) The first image demonstrates a thymus nearly completely filling the left upper chest with a smooth wavy contour (*arrowhead*) due to compression of the adjacent ribs. The thymus blends imperceptibly with the superior and lateral margin of the heart and superior mediastinum. (**b**) The second image demonstrates the *sail sign* of the thymus. The thymus (*arrow*) blends in with the right superior cardiac and mediastinal borders and forms a sharp lateral border mimicking a sail. (**c**) On the lateral view of the chest, the thymus fills the retrosternal clear space and has a sharply defined inferior margin (*curved arrow*)

simulate upper lobe atelectasis [2]. The other classic appearance is of the *sail sign* which is more commonly seen on the right. The lateral edge of the thymus is often undulating, due to adjacent rib compression (the thymic wave sign) [3]. On the lateral view, the thymus fills the anterior superior mediastinum and has a well-defined inferior border. Some of the different appearances of the thymus are pictured in Fig. 3.2.

There is a great variation in the normal size of the thymus [4]. The size varies with inspiration (causing a small appearing thymus) and expiration (causing a larger appearing thymus), may become smaller with infection or medications such as steroids or chemotherapeutic agents (stress atrophy), and rebound in size after recovery (rebound hyptertrophy) [5–8]. A thymus may be pathologically enlarged if the enlargement persists into the second decade, if the borders are unusually lobular in contour, or if adjacent structures are displaced [9].

Both frontal and lateral views are necessary to adequately assess the position, shape, and size of the heart. On a well-centered frontal view of the chest, the heart is centered slightly to the left of the spine,

with the cardiac apex on the left. From superior to inferior, the right cardiac margin is formed by the superior vena cava (upper one third) and right atrium (lower two thirds). The right atrium borders the right middle lobe. The ascending aorta is not normally seen in children. The soft tissue border of the superior vena cava often extends more laterally from the spine in young children than in adults.

The border of the left cardiomediastinal silhouette from superior to inferior is formed by the aortic arch (arrow head), main pulmonary artery (arrow), left atrial appendage (wavy arrow), and left ventricle (curved gray arrow). The left atrial appendage may not be seen in a normal heart (Fig. 3.3a). Normally, the borders of the left atrium and right ventricle do not contribute to the borders of the cardiac silhouette on the frontal view. The borders of the left atrium can be normally seen though the silhouette of the heart in 30% of children [10] (Fig. 3.4).

On the lateral view of the chest, the anterior cardiomediastinal border is formed (from superior to inferior) by the ascending aorta (arrow head), main pulmonary artery (arrow), and right ventricle (curved

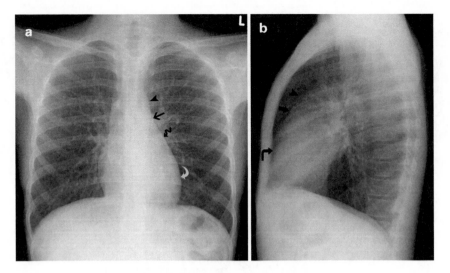

Fig. 3.3. (a, b) Normal PA and lateral radiographs of the chest in a 10 year old

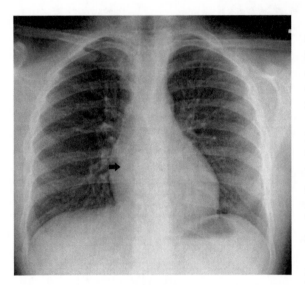

Fig. 3.4. Normal PA radiograph in a 10 year old showing the normal left atrial shadow (*arrow*)

arrow). The retrosternal clear space, or relatively lucent area cephalad to the right ventricle and posterior to the sternum, typically occupies one third to one half of the anterior chest (Fig. 3.3b). In infants, the thymus occupies the anterior mediastinum, and may fill the retrosternal clear space obscuring the anterior superior border of the heart and great vessels.

The posterior cardiomediastinal margin from superior to inferior is composed of the left atrium, left ventricle, and inferior vena cava on the lateral view. Normally, the posterior margin of the left atrium is anterior to the left mainstem bronchus and should not displace the bronchus or extend posterior to the inferior vena cava.

The normal heart size can be judged subjectively and quantitatively. One index, the cardiothoracic ratio, is the ratio between the widest transverse cardiac diameter and the widest internal thoracic diameter. Normal values are less than 60% for newborns and less than 50% for all greater than 1 month of age during quiet respiration [11, 12]. However, neither the left atrium nor the right ventricle is represented in the transverse dimension of the heart, making this measurement unreliable. Thus, a subjective evaluation of the heart size, based on the frontal and lateral views, with attention to each chamber of the heart and the overall cardiac size is preferred. Comparison to prior films is also valuable.

Judging heart size or specific chamber enlargement on an AP view of the chest in an infant with a large thymus is very challenging (Fig. 3.5a, b). The lateral view is particularly helpful. If the posterior aspect of the cardiac silhouette extends over the vertebral bodies, then the heart is enlarged. If the posterior margin of the heart extends posterior to the anterior line of the trachea, the heart may be enlarged. Another way of judging cardiomegaly is if the posterior border of the heart is closer to the anterior edge of the spine than the AP width of the adjacent vertebra, then the heart is too big.

Cardiac silhouette enlargement may be due to global chamber enlargement or due to specific chamber enlargement. Determining which chambers are enlarged provides clues to the type of cardiac abnormality. For example, global cardiac enlargement may be due to a cardiomyopathy or peripheral arterial to venous shunting due to tumors

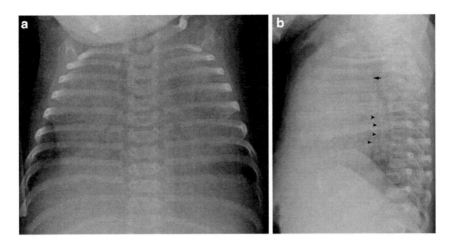

Fig. 3.5. (a, b) AP and lateral radiographs in an infant with a large central soft tissue which nearly opacifies both hemithoracies. The lateral radiograph demonstrates that the posterior margin of the heart (*arrowheads*) does not extend posterior to the anterior margin of the trachea (*arrow*). Ultrasound showed that this mass is a normal large thymus, and the heart was normal

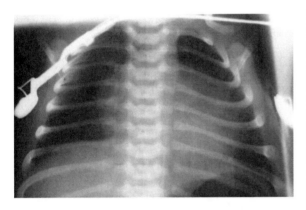

Fig. 3.6. Ebstein anomaly. This frontal view of the chest in an infant with Ebstein's anomaly demonstrates an enlarged box-shaped cardiac silhouette due to a massively enlarged right atrium. The lungs appear hyperlucent because of decreased pulmonary blood flow

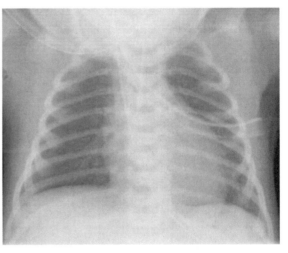

Fig. 3.7. Valvar pulmonary stenosis. This radiograph in a cyanotic infant demonstrates right ventricular enlargement as evidenced by an enlarged left cardiac margin in a patient with pulmonary valve stenosis. This image also demonstrates pulmonary vascular oligemia

(hemangioendothelioma) or vascular malformations (e.g., Vein of Galen aneurysm).

The size and shape of the normal right atrium are variable; thus mild to moderate enlargement of this chamber can be missed. Two signs of right atrial enlargement on the frontal projection are that the border is laterally displaced more than a few centimeters from the spine. When the right atrium is enlarged, the right heart border becomes squared, and the entire heart assumes a box-like appearance. The most common causes of right atrial enlargement in newborns are pulmonary atresia with an intact septum or Ebstein's anomaly (Fig. 3.6).

When the right ventricle is enlarged, the retrosternal clear space becomes smaller. When the right ventricle enlarges, there is a clockwise rotation of the heart and the cardiac apex can point upward (Fig. 3.7). In infants and young children evaluation of the right ventricle on the lateral view may be impossible due to the thymus.

Left atrial enlargement is best seen on the lateral view. An enlarged left atrium extends posterior to the inferior vena cava and pushes the left mainstem bronchus posteriorly. In children, left atrial enlargement may be due to ventriculoseptal defect (Fig. 3.8a, b), patent ductus arteriosus, mitral stenosis, or mitral insufficiency.

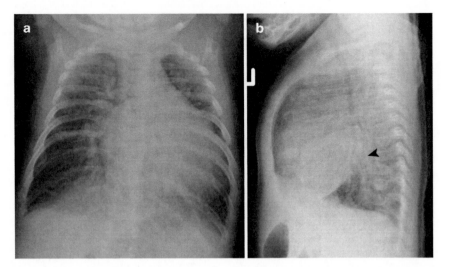

Fig. 3.8. (a, b) AV canal. Frontal and lateral views of the chest in a patient with Trisomy 21 and an unrepaired AV canal defect demonstrate hyperinflation, cardiomegaly, and increased pulmonary vascularity. The lateral view shows left atrial enlargement as evidenced by the posterior margin of the left atrium (*arrowhead*) extending posterior to the inferior vena cava and pushing the left mainstem bronchus posteriorly. Notice that the angle between the left mainstem bronchus and axis of the trachea/right mainstem bronchus increases with left atrial enlargement

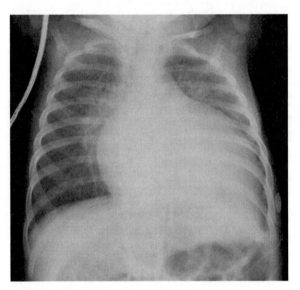

Fig. 3.9. Aberrant coronary artery. This infant presented to the ER with respiratory distress. The frontal radiograph demonstrates cardiomegaly, mainly due to left ventricular dilatation. The patient was found to have an aberrant left coronary artery arising from the left pulmonary artery on echocardiography

Left ventricular enlargement is best seen on the frontal view and is demonstrated by enlargement of the left side of the heart. Left ventricular dilatation may produce a downward pointing cardiac apex. In this patient with an anomalous coronary artery (Fig. 3.9), both the left atrium and left ventricle were enlarged by echocardiography.

3.1.3   Vascular Pattern

Determining normal and abnormal pulmonary vascularity may be the most difficult aspect of evaluating a chest radiograph but is very important to generating the appropriate diagnosis of congenital heart disease. Pulmonary vascularity can be normal, demonstrate increased pulmonary arterial flow, increased pulmonary venous distention, or decreased pulmonary flow. Normally, the right interlobar pulmonary artery is the same size as the trachea at the level of the aortic arch (Fig. 3.10).

The peripheral arteries normally taper gradually from the hilum to the periphery of the lung (see image normal PA of the chest). If the patient is upright, the width of the vessels in the upper lobes is smaller than that of the lower lobes at comparable branch level. If the patient is recumbent, pulmonary vascular markings are more evenly distributed in size. Normally, the margins of the peripheral arteries (seen on end) are approximately the same size as the adjacent bronchi (Fig. 3.11). The borders of the peripheral arteries are normally sharp.

When pulmonary arterial flow is increased, the right interlobar artery will be larger than the trachea, and the apparent number and size of pulmonary arteries will increase. The pulmonary artery seen on end will be larger than the adjacent bronchus (Fig. 3.12). With increased pulmonary venous flow and edema, the margins of the enlarged vessels will

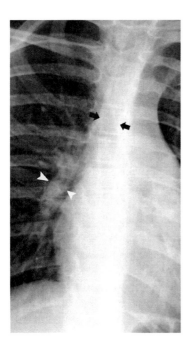

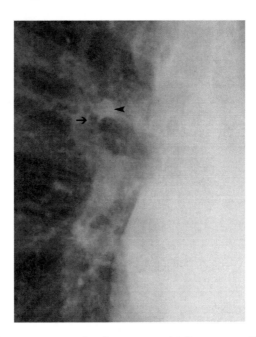

Fig. 3.10. Normal diameter of the right interlobar pulmonary artery relative to the trachea. This magnified view of the chest demonstrates that the width of the normal right interlobar pulmonary artery (*arrowheads*) is the same as the trachea (*arrows*) at the level of the aortic arch. The spinal curvature allows the right hilar structures to be better visualized

Fig. 3.12. Increased pulmonary arterial flow. A magnified view demonstrates that the pulmonary artery (*arrowhead*) is larger than the adjacent bronchiole (*arrow*). Increased pulmonary vascularity is also demonstrated in the previous patient with Trisomy 21 and an AV canal

become poorly defined. Increased pulmonary venous flow is often confused with peribronchial cuffing as seen in viral pneumonia.

Decreased pulmonary vascularity reflects diminished pulmonary blood flow. The main pulmonary artery segment may be decreased in size, the blood vessels appear thin, and the sparseness of the vessels gives an appearance of hyperlucency of the lungs (Fig. 3.6, Ebstein's anomaly).

3.1.4 The Side of the Aortic Arch and Situs

The aorta is normally to the left of the spine, cephalad to the main pulmonary artery. In children, the thymus often obscures direct visualization of the aorta, and the position of the aortic arch is inferred by the deviation of the trachea. The trachea deviates to the opposite side of the aortic arch, especially during expiration [13, 14]. (For an image, refer to the expiratory radiograph in the patient with rib fractures).

A right aortic arch serves as a warning for the presence of congenital heart disease. In the general population, right sided aortic arch is associated with congenital heart disease in 5% of patients, especially truncus arteriosus and tetrology of Fallot (Fig. 3.13),

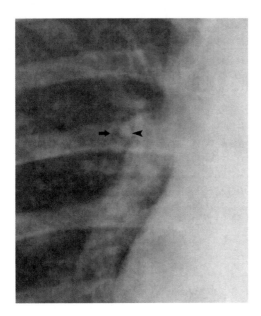

Fig. 3.11. Pulmonary artery on end with bronchus. This magnified view of the chest demonstrates a pulmonary artery (*arrowhead*) and adjacent bronchus (*arrow*) in cross section. Normally the diameter of these two structures is similar

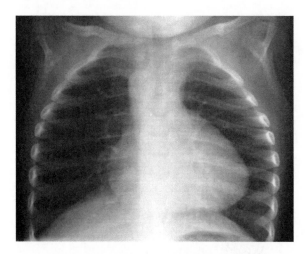

Fig. 3.13. Tetrology of Fallot with right aortic arch. This radiograph in a patient with tetrology of Fallot demonstrates a right aortic arch, and enlarged upturned cardiac apex. The appearance of the heart is due to an enlarged right ventricle which causes clockwise rotation of the heart. There is decreased pulmonary vascularity, due to subpulmonic stenosis with a ventricular septal defect allowing a right to left shunt

and pulmonary atresia with ventricular septal defect [15]. Right sided aortic arches may also indicate the presence of a vascular ring, most commonly due to an aberrant left subclavian or double aortic arch [15, 16].

The situs refers to the position of the chambers of the heart and tracheobronchial tree relative to the stomach, liver, and spleen. Levocardia means that the heart is in the left chest and is normal. Dextrocardia means that the heart is in the right chest. Situs solitus with levocardia is normal. Situs solitus refers to a right sided right atrium, hyparterial left upper lobe bronchus, epiarterial right upper lobe bronchus, right sided liver, left sided stomach, and left sided spleen. A hyparterial bronchus is one below the adjacent pulmonary artery where as an eparterial bronchus is above the adjacent pulmonary artery. Situs inversus is the mirror image of normal.

The importance of situs and the position of the heart is that there is an increased incidence of congenital heart disease in patients with situs abnormalities. The frequency of congenital heart disease in patients with normal anatomy is 1%. In patients with situs solitus and dextrocardia or situs inversus and levocardia, the incidence of congenital heart disease is high approaching 100%.

Practically speaking, the cardiac apex, stomach, and spleen should be on the left and the liver should be centered in the right upper abdomen. If there is discordance between the location of the cardiac apex

and the gastric bubble, there is a very high incidence of congenital heart disease.

3.1.5 Extracardiovascular Structures

Pleural

Cardiovascular disease is one of the many causes of pleural effusions. On the standard PA and lateral chest radiographs, the costophrenic angles should be well visualized and sharp. The lateral view is the most sensitive view of detecting effusions and is represented by blunting of the costophrenic sulci. A lateral decubitus view may be sensitive for showing effusions and if large effusions are free flowing or loculated. Fluid may also track along the fissures so that the fissures appear thickened.

Bony

Certain bony findings on a chest radiograph may also point to the presence of congenital heart disease. Scoliosis, particularly thoracic scoliosis, can be associated with congenital heart disease [17]. Patients with vertebral anomalies may also have the VATER association of anomalies, which include vertebral, anorectal, esophageal atresia, renal, or radial ray anomalies and congenital heart disease [18]. Inferior rib notching may be a very subtle sign of coarctation of the aorta, and is mainly seen in older children. Eleven pairs of ribs or multiple manubrial ossification centers are seen in patients with Down Syndrome. Patients with Down Syndrome have an increased incidence of congenital heart disease [19]. Thoractomy changes or median sternotomy wires may also give clues to prior cardiothoracic surgery. Lack of calcification of the inferior segments of the sternum, the mesosternum, may be also associated with congenital heart disease (Fig. 3.14).

3.1.6 Conclusion

Using a standard approach to interpreting chest radiographs and understanding the normal and abnormal appearances in children can help distinguish primary pulmonary disease from cardiovascular disease.

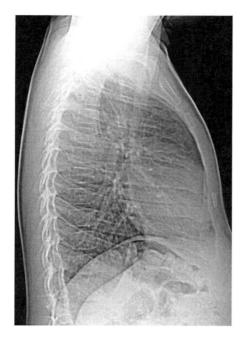

Fig. 3.14. There is absence of the mesosternum

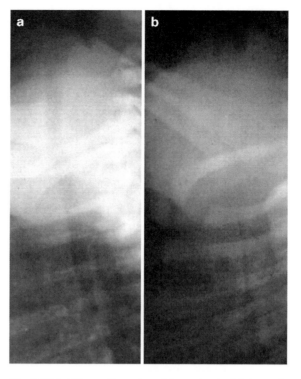

Fig. 3.15. (a) The configuration of the trachea in this 5-month old on inspiration is as seen with a normal adult airway. The trachea assumes a straight, linear course from the infraglottic region to the carina. (b) Moments later on expiration, there is an angular posterior buckling just above the thoracic inlet and then an inferior buckling. The entire intrathoracic trachea is significantly narrowed. (Although image quality is diminished, using *the last image hold* option on fluoroscopy reduces patient radiation exposure and facilitates capturing transient images) (from Cleveland [20], with permission of Contemporary Diagnostic Radiology and from Cleveland [22], with permission of Lippincott Williams & Wilkins)

3.2 Normal Upper Airway in Infants

Robert H. Cleveland

There are two major differences in the infant's upper airway that differ from older children and adults. They are an exaggerated change in diameter of the intrathoracic trachea from inspiration to expiration and a change in course and configuration of the extrathoracic trachea from inspiration to expiration [20–22].

The neonate's tracheal cartilages are less rigid and contribute to less of the circumference of the trachea than in older individuals. This results in significant narrowing of the AP diameter of the intrathoracic trachea on expiration. It is normal as a baby approaches end expiratory volume with crying for the AP diameter of the entire intrathoracic trachea to nearly complete collapse (Fig. 3.15). However if only a portion of the intrathoracic trachea narrows, it is

abnormal and focal tracheomalacia or compression from an extrinsic cause such as a vessel or mass should be suspected.

The normal extrathoracic trachea in infants assumes a very angular buckling on expiration. In frontal projection, this is usually seen as an angular rightward deviation and then inferior deviation just above the thoracic inlet (Fig. 3.16). The buckling is characteristically away from the side of the aortic arch, and hence to the right. On lateral projection, the buckling is posterior and then inferior just above the thoracic inlet (Fig. 3.15b). This will be accompanied by an increased AP diameter of the retropharyngeal soft tissues as the buckling becomes more pronounced with increasing expiration.

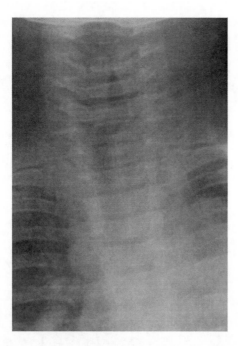

Fig. 3.16. AP image in expiration shows the normal angular buckling away from the side of the aortic arch and then inferiorly just above the thoracic inlet

References

1. Franken Jr EA, Smith WL, Berbaum KS, et al. Comparison of a PACS workstation with conventional film for interpretation of neonatal examinations: a paired comparison study. Pediatr Radiol. 1991;21(5):336–40.
2. Lanning P, Heikkinen E. Thymus simulating left upper lobe atelectasis. Pediatr Radiol. 1980;9(3):177–8.
3. Mulvey RB. The thymic "wave" sign. Radiology. 1963;81: 834–6.
4. Francis IR, Glazer GM, Bookstein FL, et al. The thymus: reexamination of age-related changes in size and shape. AJR Am J Roentgenol. 1985;145(2):249–54.
5. Chen CM, Yu KY, Lin HC, et al. Thymus size and its relationship to perinatal events. Acta Paediatr. 2000;89(8): 975–8.
6. De Felice C, Latini G, Del Vecchio A, et al. Small thymus at birth: a predictive radiographic sign of bronchopulmonary dysplasia. Pediatrics. 2002;110(2 Pt 1):386–8.
7. Hendrickx P, Dohring W. Thymic atrophy and rebound enlargement following chemotherapy for testicular cancer. Acta Radiol. 1989;30(3):263–7.
8. Meyers A, Shah A, Cleveland RH, et al. Thymic size on chest radiograph and rapid disease progression in human immunodeficiency virus 1-infected children. Pediatr Infect Dis J. 2001;20(12):1112–8.
9. Shackelford GD, McAlister WH. The aberrantly positioned thymus: a cause of mediastinal or neck masses in children. Am J Roentgenol Radium Ther Nucl Med. 1974;120(2):291–6.
10. Rosario-Medina W, Strife JL, Dunbar JS. Normal left atrium: appearance in children on frontal chest radiographs. Radiology. 1986;161(2):345–6.
11. Walmsley R, Monkhouse WS. The heart of the newborn child: an anatomical study based upon transverse serial sections. J Anat. 1988;159:93–111.
12. Ablow R. Radiologic diagnosis of the newborn chest. Curr Probl Pediatr. 1971;1:1–55.
13. Strife JL, Matsumoto J, Bisset III GS, et al. The position of the trachea in infants and children with right aortic arch. Pediatr Radiol. 1989;19(4):226–9.
14. Chang LW, Lee FA, Gwinn JL. Normal lateral deviation of the trachea in infants and children. Am J Roentgenol Radium Ther Nucl Med. 1970;109(2):247–51.
15. Stewart JR, Kincaid OW, Titus JL. Right aortic arch: plain film diagnosis and significance. Am J Roentgenol Radium Ther Nucl Med. 1966;97(2):377–89.
16. Felson B, Palayew MJ. The two types of right aortic arch. Radiology. 1963;81:745–59.
17. Luke MJ, McDonnell EJ. Congenital heart disease and scoliosis. J Pediatr. 1968;73(5):725–33.
18. Quan L, Smith DW. The VATER association. Vertebral defects, anal atresia, T-E fistula with esophageal atresia, radial and renal dysplasia: a spectrum of associated defects. J Pediatr. 1973;82(1):104–7.
19. Noonan JA. Association of congenital heart disease with syndromes or other defects. Pediatr Clin North Am. 1978;25(4):797–816.
20. Cleveland RH. The pediatric airway. Contemp Diagn Radiol. 1996;19:1–6.
21. Bramson RT, Griscom NT, Cleveland RH. Interpretation of chest radiographs in infants with cough and fever. Radiology. 2005;236:22–9.
22. Cleveland RH. The pediatric airway. In: Taveras JM, Ferrucci JT, editors. Radiology: diagnosis, imaging, intervention. Philadelphia: JB Lippincott; 1997, vol. 1, Chap. 48A, p. 1–13.

Congenital Lung Masses

4

Edward Y. Lee

CONTENTS

Congenital lung masses are common in pediatric patients. While these masses may be incidental findings in some children, they can also result in various symptoms and imaging findings depending on their size, location, and mass effect upon the adjacent thoracic structures. Imaging plays an important role for early and correct diagnosis, which in turn can improve pediatric patient care by guiding the appropriate next step in management. In this chapter, we discuss clinical presentation and imaging findings of common congenital pulmonary masses in pediatric patients. Familiarity with the characteristic clinical and imaging findings of congenital pulmonary masses can avoid delay in diagnosis and optimize pediatric patient care.

Edward Y. Lee, MD, MPH (✉)
Division of Thoracic Imaging, Department of Radiology and
Medicine, Pulmonary Division, Children's Hospital Boston,
Harvard Medical School, Boston, MA, USA
e-mail: Edward.Lee@childrens.harvard.edu

4.1 The Spectrum of Congenital Lung Masses

Although clinical presentation of pediatric patients with various congenital lung masses is typically related to compression or mass effect upon the tracheobronchial tree, imaging appearance of congenital lung masses varies widely similar to other congenital anomalies involving other body parts. For the purpose of evaluation and diagnosis, congenital pulmonary masses can be classified into two major categories: (1) congenital lung masses with normal vasculature; and (2) congenital lung masses with anomalous vasculature [1]. Additionally, congenital lung masses can also present as a combination of more than one entity such as in cases of congenital pulmonary airway malformation (CPAM) and pulmonary sequestration [1, 2].

4.2 Congenital Lung Masses with Normal Vasculature

4.2.1 Congenital Bronchial Atresia

Congenital bronchial atresia is a rare congenital anomaly which can present as a focal pulmonary lesion. It is also known as congenital bronchocele or mucocele, which results from developmental disconnection of a segmental or subsegmental bronchus from the central airway [3, 4]. Such disconnection of the bronchus results in subsequent mucus accumulation in the segments of bronchus distal to the atretic regions. Air trapping adjacent to the bronchial atresia results from the unilateral collateral air-drift through pores of Kohn and Canals of Lambert from the adjacent normal lung [1, 5]. Such collateral channels act as a check-valve mechanism only allowing air to enter and not leave from the distal lung. Bronchial atresia is most commonly located in the apico-posterior segment of left upper lobe followed by right upper lobe, right middle lobe, and right lower lobe. Bronchial atresia is typically an incidental finding in asymptomatic children on chest radiographs obtained for other indications. However, up to 42% of patients may present with symptoms such as cough, wheezing, hemoptysis, shortness of breath, or recurrent pulmonary infection [6].

On chest radiographs, bronchial atresia typically presents as a round, ovoid, or tubular opacity with or without an associated fluid level [1]. Due to its typical radiographic findings, bronchial atresia can be sometimes confused with a pulmonary nodule or other focal lung abnormality in children. Although CT is not usually obtained for further evaluation when typical imaging findings of bronchial atresia are seen on chest radiographs, CT can be helpful for confirming and further characterizing bronchial atresia. On CT, bronchial atresia is a central mass-like opacity near the hilum that usually has a round, ovoid, or tubular shape [1]. It typically exhibits an attenuation value of 10–25 HU due to internal mucoid contents [6]. After administration of intravenous contrast, there is usually no internal contrast enhancement. Multidetector CT (MDCT) with 2D reconstructions can provide a comprehensive evaluation of spatial relationship of the bronchial atresia and adjacent surrounding air trapping. Although magnetic resonance imaging (MRI) is not currently used for evaluation of bronchial atresia, it has been reported that bronchial atresia shows high 2T signal intensity due to underlying mucoid contents [7]. Unlike CT, MRI cannot demonstrate surrounding air trapping often seen adjacent to the bronchial atresia. Although no treatment is necessary for an incidentally detected bronchial atresia in asymptomatic children, surgical resection may be necessary in symptomatic children particularly with recurrent pulmonary infections.

4.2.2 Bronchogenic Cysts

Bronchogenic cysts are developmental anomalies of airways which result from abnormal ventral budding or branching of the embryonic foregut and tracheobronchial tree, which occurs between 26th and 40th days of gestation [8–10]. Other foregut duplication cysts include enteric cysts and neurenteric cysts. Bronchogenic cysts are usually located within the mediastinum (~67%) or lung parenchyma (~33%) [1, 5]. They account for an approximately 40–50% of all congenital mediastinal cystic masses [5]. Histologically, bronchogenic cysts are characterized by mucoid material collection lined by respiratory ciliated columnar or cuboidal epithelium. Children with small bronchogenic cysts are usually asymptomatic [5]. However, large bronchogenic cysts can result in mass effect upon adjacent airways and the esophagus. Affected children in such situations can present with a variety of clinical symptoms such as respiratory distress, dysphagia, and chest pain.

On chest radiographs, bronchogenic cysts usually present as round opacity located in the mediastinum or lung parenchyma. If they are located in the mediastinum, the most common location of the bronchogenic cysts is the subcarinal region, followed by right paratracheal region and hilar region [1, 5]. Intraparenchymal bronchogenic cysts are typically located in the medial third of the lung [5]. On CT, bronchogenic cysts are characteristically well-circumscribed round or ovoid cystic solitary mass with uniform attenuation (Fig. 4.1a). The attenuation value of the bronchogenic cysts is variable due to variable amount of internal proteinaceous materials and calcium. Approximately 50% of bronchogenic cysts show 0–20 HU on CT images [10–12]. High contents of internal proteinaceous materials and calcium within bronchogenic cysts can result in increased HU of the cysts, which may mimic possible solid masses. In this situation, MRI can be a helpful imaging study for confirmation and further characterization. Although signal intensity of bronchogenic cysts on T1-weighted images may be variable due to variable amount of internal proteinaceous materials [13], the bronchogenic cysts are typically high in signal intensity on T2-weighted images (Fig. 4.1b) [11, 14]. With intravenous contrast, no internal contrast enhancement is typically seen, although wall enhancement may be seen when they are infected. For symptomatic pediatric patients, the current treatment of choice is surgical resection.

4.2.3 Congenital Lobar Emphysema

Congenital lobar emphysema is also known as infantile lobar emphysema or congenital lobar hyperinflation [1]. Although the etiology of congenital lobar

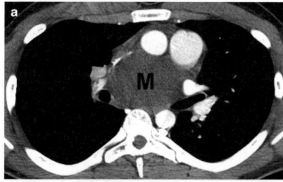

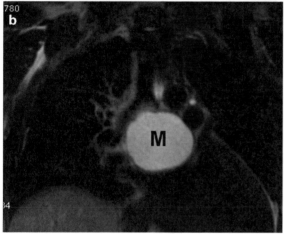

Fig. 4.1. A 18-year-old male with chest pain and respiratory distress. Surgical pathology of the mediastinal cystic mass was consistent with bronchogenic cyst. (**a**) Enhanced axial CT image shows a large round cystic mass (M) located in the subcarinal region. (**b**) Coronal T2-weighted MR image demonstrates a large round cystic mass (M) with high MR signal intensity

emphysema is currently unknown, it has been presumed that underlying airway malacia or stenosis may be the cause of congenital lobar emphysema [5, 9, 12, 15–18]. Such airway malacia or stenosis can cause progressive hyperinflation of the lung by allowing more air to enter the involved lung on inspiration than leaves on expiration as a check-valve mechanism. This results in hyperinflation of an affected lobe without destruction of alveolar walls or septa [1]. The most common location of congenital lobar emphysema is left upper lobe followed by right middle lobe, and lower lobes [5]. Occasionally, more than one lobe can be affected. Most pediatric patients with congenital lobar emphysema present during the neonatal period with respiratory distress due to mass effect upon adjacent airway and lung from the hyperinflated lobe. Congenital lobar emphysema is associated with other congenital anomalies such as cardiovascular anomalies in up to 12–14% of patients [19, 20].

On newborns' chest radiographs, congenital lobar emphysema may present as an opacity due to retention of fetal lung fluid just after birth. However, the affected lobe typically shows hyperlucency as fetal lung fluid is cleared by subsequent lymphatic resorption and replaced by air (Fig. 4.2a). Due to the hyperinflation of affected lobe, adjacent lobes may be compressed or atelectatic. Large and markedly hyperinflated congenital lobar emphysema can result in separation of ipsilateral ribs and hemidiaphragm depression. Due to hyperlucency on chest radiographs, congenital lobar emphysema may be confused with pneumothorax or cystic lung abnormalities. In this situation, CT can be a helpful imaging modality which can show a hyperinflated lobe with attenuating and displaced pulmonary vessels (Fig. 4.2b, c) [1]. Surgical resection is the current management of choice for symptomatic children with congenital lobar emphysema.

4.2.4 Congenital Pulmonary Airway Malformation

CPAM is a congenital lung mass, which results from disorganized adenomatoid and hamartomatous proliferation of bronchioles that are in communication with the adjacent normal bronchial tree [1, 5, 9, 12, 20–25]. The etiology of CPAM is currently unknown. In the past, CPAM has been referred to as congenital cystic malformation of the lung (CCAM) and classified into three different types by Stoker et al. based on its radiological, gross pathological, and histological findings. However, it has been recently reclassified into five types (types 0–4) based on the location or stage of development of the abnormality involving the tracheobronchial airway [26, 27]. Type 0 CPAM is the rarest type which involves an abnormality of the trachea and mainstem bronchi. While type 1 CPAM, which is the most common type (60–70%), involves an abnormality of the bronchial and/or proximal bronchiolar region, type 2 CPAM (15–20%) involves an abnormality of the bronchiolar region. Type 3 CPAM (5–10%) involves an abnormality of the terminal bronchiolar/alveolar duct region. Type 4 CPAM involves an abnormality of the distal acinus or alveolar saccular/alveolus region. Affected children with small CPAM are typically asymptomatic. However, pediatric patients with large CPAM usually present with respiratory distress or superimposed infection.

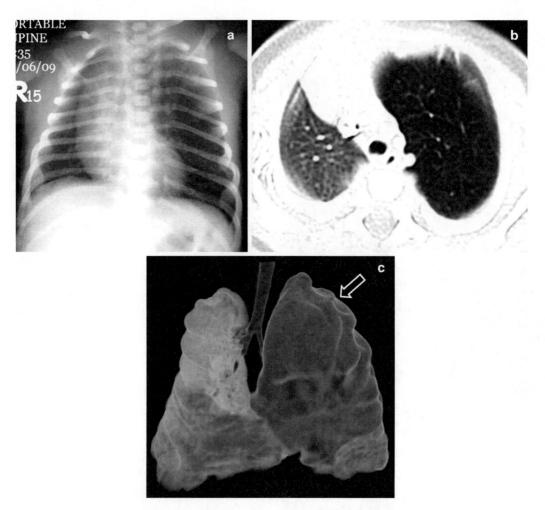

Fig. 4.2. A 3-day-old boy presented with respiratory distress. Surgical pathology was consistent with congenital lobar emphysema. (a) Frontal chest radiograph shows increased lucency and hyperinflation of the left upper lobe. Also noted is mass effect upon mediastinum. (b) Axial lung window CT image demonstrates markedly hyperinflated left upper lobe with attenuating and displaced pulmonary vessels. (c) 3D volume rendered image of the lung shows hyperinflated left upper lobe (*arrow*)

On chest radiographs, CPAMs typically present as solitary or multiple air-filled thin-walled cysts that vary in size [1, 25]. Additionally, they may also present as a focal mass-like opacity. CT is a helpful imaging modality for identifying CPAMs, characterizing CPAMs, evaluating mass effect on adjacent structures, and distinguishing CPAMs from other congenital lung anomalies. On CT, CPAMs are usually solitary or multiple air-filled cystic masses (Fig. 4.3) [1, 25]. However, it may also present as a solid soft tissue mass without associated anomalous vasculature. Surgical resection is the current management of choice particularly due to an increased risk of superimposed infection, if left untreated, or potential development of pulmonary neoplasms such as bronchoalveolar carcinoma or pleuropulmonary blastoma [1].

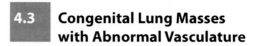

4.3   Congenital Lung Masses with Abnormal Vasculature

4.3.1   Pulmonary Sequestration

Pulmonary sequestration is an aberrant lung mass, which is characterized by dysplastic and nonfunctioning pulmonary tissue without a normal connection with the tracheobronchial tree [1, 25]. Traditionally, pulmonary sequestration is divided into two types: extralobar sequestration (25%) and intralobar sequestration (75%) [1, 25, 28–34] (Table 4.1). Histologically, extralobar sequestration

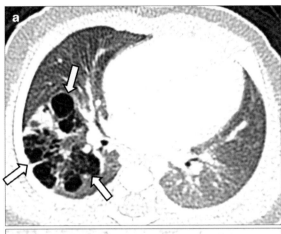

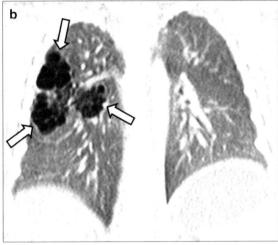

Fig. 4.3. One-month-old girl with prenatal diagnosis of right lung mass is shown. Surgical pathology confirmed congenital pulmonary airway malformation (CPAM). (**a**) Axial lung window image shows type 2 CPAM (*arrows*) manifested as multiple small cystic lesions within the right upper lobe. (**b**) Coronal lung window image again demonstrates type 2 CPAM (*arrows*)

Table 4.1 Characteristics of extralobar and intralobar sequestrations

	Extralobar sequestration	Intralobar sequestration
Cause	Congenital	Acquired (postinfectious) vs. congenital
Patient age	Infants or young children	Older children
Presentation	Focal lung mass	Recurrent infection
Morphology	With its own lung pleura	Without its own lung pleura
Common location	Lower lobes (L > R)	Lower lobes (L > R)
Arterial supply	Abdominal aorta	Thoracic/abdominal aorta/branch arteries
Venous drainage	Systemic veins	Pulmonary veins

has its own lung pleura while intralobar sequestration is located within the lung parenchyma without its own lung pleura. Both extralobar and intralobar sequestrations have anomalous arterial supply generally arising from the descending aorta. However, intralobar sequestration may have an arterial supply from secondary or tertiary branches, possibly relating to prior infection. Anomalous venous drainage associated with extralobar and intralobar sequestrations differs. While anomalous venous drainage of the intralobar sequestration is into a pulmonary vein, extralobar sequestration has an anomalous venous drainage into systemic veins such as the azygous vein, portal vein, or subclavian vein [1, 25]. It has been reported that information regarding anomalous venous drainage associated with pulmonary sequestration can help differentiating the two types of pulmonary sequestration [1, 35]. Such information can be helpful for preoperative evaluation. While most intralobar sequestrations require lobectomy, extralobar sequestration can be surgically removed via segmentectomy without excising adjacent normal lung tissue [1, 36]. Occasionally, extralobar sequestration can coexist with CPAM and appear as a mixed lesion [1, 2]. Clinical presentation of pediatric patients with intralobar and extralobar sequestrations also often differs. While extralobar sequestration typically presents in neonates or young children with a focal lung mass, intralobar sequestration typically presents in older children with recurrent pulmonary infection in the lower lobes [1, 25].

On chest radiographs, a focal lung opacity in the lower lobes, left side more often than right side, is typically seen [1, 25]. When there is superimposed infection, associated lung parenchymal inflammation and/or even abscess formation may be present. CT is helpful imaging modality in diagnosing pulmonary sequestration by demonstrating the abnormally sequestrated portion of the lung and associated anomalous vessels (Fig. 4.4). It has been reported that MDCT with 3D imaging can help radiologists to make a correct detection of anomalous arterial supply and anomalous venous drainage associated with pulmonary sequestration in 100 and 100% of cases, respectively [36, 37]. Surgical resection is the current management of choice for children with pulmonary sequestrations.

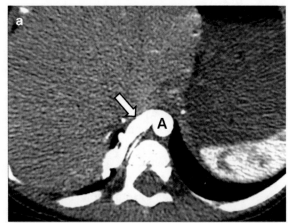

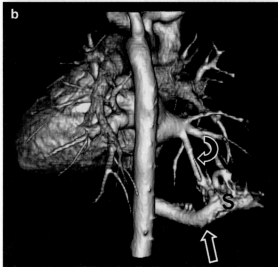

Fig. 4.4. A 5-week-old girl with prenatal diagnosis of focal lung mass located in the right lower hemithorax. Surgical pathology was consistent with pulmonary sequestration. (**a**) Enhanced axial CT image shows an anomalous artery (*arrow*) arising from the descending aorta (letter A). (**b**) 3D volume rendered image demonstrates a pulmonary sequestration (letter S) with associated anomalous artery (*arrow*) and anomalous vein (*curved arrow*)

4.3.2 Pulmonary Arteriovenous Malformation

Pulmonary arteriovenous malformation (AVM) is characterized by a congenital anomalous direct connection between pulmonary veins and arteries due to an underlying defect in the formation of normal pulmonary capillaries [1]. In children, pulmonary AVM is usually congenital in etiology. However, pulmonary AVM can also be acquired typically in children with prior congenital cyanotic heart surgeries (i.e., Glenn and Fontan procedures) or chronic liver disease [28, 38–43]. If there are multiple pulmonary AVMs, hereditary hemorrhagic telangiectasis,

also known as Rendu–Osler–Weber syndrome, should be considered in children. Hereditary hemorrhagic telangiectasis is an autosomal dominant syndrome, which is characterized by a clinical triad of epistaxis, telangiectasis, and a family history of pulmonary AVMs [28, 44, 45]. Although pediatric patients may be asymptomatic if the size of pulmonary AVM is less than 2 cm. However, a large pulmonary AVM (>2 cm) or multiple pulmonary AVMs in children likely result in anatomic right-to-left shunts [1]. Affected children can present with symptoms such as hemoptysis, dyspnea, chest pain, palpitations, and cyanosis [1]. Rarely, serious complications such as stroke or brain abscess due to paradoxical embolization or pulmonary hemorrhage may also occur [28, 45–47].

On chest radiographs, round or oval shaped opacities often with associated curvilinear opacities representing a feeding artery and a draining vein may be seen. They are often located in the lower lobe in 50–70% of cases [27, 45]. In the past, conventional catheter-based pulmonary angiography has been used for the evaluation of pulmonary AVM. However, in recent years, MDCT has become an imaging modality of choice for assessing pulmonary AVM in children (Fig. 4.5). MDCT with 3D imaging is particularly useful in detecting and characterizing the angioarchitecture of the feeding arteries and draining veins [1]. For pulmonary AVMs larger than 2 cm, the current treatment of choice is endovascular coil embolization or balloon occlusion [45–47].

4.3.3 Pulmonary Varix

Pulmonary varix is a localized enlarged segmental pulmonary vein, which anatomically enters the left atrium normally [1]. It may present as a pulmonary mass-like opacity on chest radiographs. It can be congenital or acquired. Chronic pulmonary hypertension and mitral valvular disease are often associated with acquired pulmonary varix [3, 28]. Pulmonary varix is usually discovered incidentally in asymptomatic patients. However, it may also result in serious complications such as systematic embolus from a clot in the varix and rupture leading to the death [28, 48].

On chest radiographs, pulmonary varix typically presents as a well-defined round mass-like opacity near the heart border [1]. Pulmonary varix is usually not clinically significant and it is important

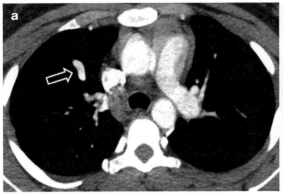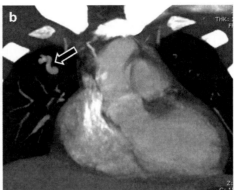

Fig. 4.5. A 17-year-old girl with an abnormal chest radiograph showing possible nodular opacity in the right upper lobe. (**a**) Enhanced axial CT image shows a vascular tubular structure mass (*arrow*) located in the right upper lobe. (**b**) Enhanced coronal CT image demonstrates a tubular structure (*arrow*) with contrast enhancement, consistent with pulmonary arteriovenous malformation

not to confuse it with a true pulmonary mass. CT is currently the best imaging modality for diagnosing pulmonary varix and in differentiating it from other possible diagnostic considerations such as pulmonary AVM or nodule [1]. Confirmation of pulmonary varix can be made when contiguity of pulmonary varix with the adjacent pulmonary vein is visualized on contrast enhanced CT. It is typically located near its point of entry into the left atrium. While asymptomatic children should be closely followed with periodic chest radiographs, symptomatic patients require urgent surgical resection of the pulmonary varix.

4.4   Conclusion

Congenital lung masses, which can be incidental findings or may cause symptoms, are common in pediatric patients. Imaging evaluation can provide the precise information of the congenital lung masses regarding their location, appearance, size, and mass effect upon the adjacent thoracic structures. Such information is crucial for early and correct diagnosis, which in turn can lead to optimal pediatric patient management.

References

1. Lee EY, Boiselle PM, Cleveland RH. Multidetector CT evaluation of congenital lung anomalies. Radiology. 2008;247(3):632–48.

2. McLean SE, Pfeifer JD, Siegel MJ, Jensen ER, Schuler PM, Hirsch R, et al. Congenital cystic adenomatoid malformation connected to an extralobar pulmonary sequestration in the contralateral chest: common origin? J Pediatr Surg. 2004;39(8):e13–7.

3. Fraser R, Colman N, Muller NL, Pare PD. Developmental and metabolic lung disease. In: Fraser R, Colman N, Muller NL, Pare PD, editors. Synopsis of diseases of the chest. 3rd ed. Philadelphia: Elsevier Saunders; 2005. p. 188–221.

4. Webb W, Higgins CB. Congenital bronchopulmonary lesions. In: Webb WR, editor. Thoracic imaging: pulmonary and cardiovascular radiology. Philadelphia: Lippincott Williams & Wilkins; 2005. p. 1–29.

5. Berrocal T, Madrid C, Novo S, Gutierrez J, Arjonilla A, Gomez-Leon N. Congenital anomalies of the tracheobronchial tree, lung, and mediastinum: embryology, radiology, and pathology. Radiographics. 2004;24(1):e17.

6. Rahalkar A, Rahalkar MD, Rahalkar MA. Pictorial essay: all about bronchial atresia. Ind J Radiol Imag. 2005;15(3): 389–93.

7. Matsushima H, Takayagi N, Satoh M, Kurashima K, Kanauchi T, Hoshi T, et al. Congenital bronchial atresia: radiologic findings in nine patients. J Comput Assist Tomogr. 2002;26(5):860–4.

8. Chapman KR, Rebuck AS. Spontaneous disappearance of a chronic mediastinal mass. Chest. 1985;87:235–6.

9. Zylak CJ, Eyler WR, Spizarny DL, Stone CH. Developmental lung anomalies in the adult: radiologic-pathologic correlation. Radiographics. 2002;22(Spec Issue):S25–43.

10. Aktogu S, Yuncu G, Halilcolar H, Ermete S, Buduneli T. Bronchogenic cysts: clinico-pathological presentation and treatment. Eur Respir J. 1996;9:2017–21.

11. McAdams HP, Kirejczyk WM, Rosado-de-Christenson ML, Matsumoto S. Bronchogenic cyst: imaging features with clinical and histopathologic correlation. Radiology. 2000;217:441–6.

12. Williams HJ, Johnson KJ. Imaging of congenital cystic lung lesions. Paediatr Respire Rev. 2002;3:120–7.

13. Ashizawa K, Okimoto T, Shirafuji T, Kusano H, Ayabe H, Hayashi K. Anterior mediastinal bronchogenic cysts: demonstration of complicating malignancy by CT and MRI. Br J Radiol. 2001;74:959–61.

14. Winters WD, Effmann EL. Congenital masses of the lung: prenatal and postnatal imaging evaluation. J Thoracic Imaging. 2001;16:196–206.

15. Karnak I, Senock ME, Ciftci AO, Buyukpamukcu N. Congenital lobar emphysema: diagnostic and therapeutic considerations. J Pediatr Surg. 1999;34:1347–51.

16. Olutoye OO, Coleman GB, Hubbard AM, Adzick NS. Prenatal diagnosis and management of congenital lobar emphysema. J Pediatr Surg. 2000;35:792–5.

17. Mei-Zahav M, Konen O, Manson D, Langer JC. Is congenital lobar emphysema a surgical disease? J Pediatr Surg. 2006;41:1058–61.

18. Ozcelik U, Gocmen A, Kiper N, Dogru D, Dilber E, Yalcin EG. Congenital lobar emphysema: evaluation and long-term follow up of thirty cases at a single center. Pediatr Pulmonol. 2003;35:384–91.

19. Kuga T, Inoue T, Sakano H, Zempo N, Oga A, Esato K. Congenital cystic adenomatoid malformation of the lung with an esophageal cyst: report of a case. J Pediatr Surg. 2001;36(6):E4.

20. Stocker J, Madewell J, Drake R. Congenital cystic adenomatoid malformation of the lung: classification and morphologic spectrum. Hum Pathol. 1977;8:155–71.

21. Wilson RD, Hedrick HL, Liechty KW, et al. Cystic adenomatoid malformation of the lung: review of genetics, prenatal diagnosis, and in utero treatment. Am J Med Genet A. 2006;140:151–5.

22. Sauvat F, Michel JL, Benachi A, Edmond S, Revillon Y. Management of asymptomatic neonatal cystic adenomatoid malformations. J Pediatr Surg. 2003;38:548–52.

23. Usui N, Kamata S, Sawai T, et al. Outcome predictors for infants with cystic lung disease. J Pediatr Surg. 2004;39:603–6.

24. Khosa JK, Leong SL, Borzi PA. Congenital cystic adenomatoid malformation of the lung: indications and timing of surgery. Pediatr Surg Int. 2004;20:505–8.

25. Yikilmaz A, Lee EY. CT imaging of mass-like nonvascular pulmonary lesions in children. Pediatr Radiol. 2007;37(12):1253–63.

26. Stocker J. Congenital pulmonary airway malformation: a new name and expanded classification of congenital cystic adenomatoid malformations of the lung. Histopathology. 2001;41 Suppl 2:424–58.

27. McSweeney F, Papagiannopoulos K, Goldstarw P, et al. An assessment of the expanded classification of congenital cystic adenomatoid malformations and their relationship to malignant transformation. Am J Surg Pathol. 2003;27:1139–46.

28. Remy-Jardin M, Remy J, Mayo JR, Muller NL. Vascular anomalies of the lung. In: Remy-Jardin M, Remy J, Mayo JR, Muller NL, editors. CT angiography of the chest. Philadelphia: Lippincott Williams & Wilkins; 2001. p. 97–114.

29. Corbett HJ, Humphrey GM. Pulmonary sequestration. Paediatr Respir Rev. 2004;5:59–68.

30. Freedom RM, Yoo SJ, Goo HW, Mikailian H, Anderson RH. The bronchopulmonary foregut malformation complex. Cardiol Young. 2006;16:229–51.

31. Frush DP, Donnelly LF. Pulmonary sequestration spectrum: a new spin with helicial CT. AJR Am J Roentgenol. 1997;169:679–82.

32. Bolca N, Topal U, Bayram S. Bronchopulmonary sequestration: radiologic findings. Eur J Radiol. 2004;52:185–91.

33. Ahmed M, Jacobi V, Vogl TJ. Multislice CT and CT angiography for non-invasive evaluation of bronchopulmonary sequestration. Eur Radiol. 2004;14:2141–3.

34. Lee EY, Dillon JE, Callahan MJ, Voss SD. 3D multidetector CT angiographic evaluation of extralobar pulmonary sequestration with anomalous venous drainage into the left internal mammary vein in a paediatric patient. Br J Radiol. 2006;79:e99–102.

35. Lee EY, Siegel MJ, Sierra M, Foglia RP. Evaluation of angio-architecture of pulmonary sequestration in pediatric patients using 3D MDCT angiography. AJR Am J Roentgenol. 2004;183(1):183–8.

36. Lee EY, Boiselle PM, Shamberger RC. Multidetector computed tomography and 3-dimensional imaging: preoperative evaluation of thoracic vascular and tracheo-bronchial anomalies and abnormalities in pediatric patients. J Pediatr Surg. 2010;45(4):811–21.

37. Kang M, Khandelwal N, Ojili V, Rao KL, Rana SS. Multidetector CT angiography in pulmonary sequestration. J Comput Assist Tomogr. 2006;30(6):926–32.

38. Srivastava D, Preminger T, Lock JE, et al. Hepatic venous blood and the development of pulmonary arteriovenous malformations in congenital heart disease. Circulation. 1995;92:1217–22.

39. Shah MJ, Rychik J, Fogel MA, Murphy JD, Jacobs ML. Pulmonary AV malformations after superior cavopulmonary connection: resolution after inclusion of hepatic veins in the pulmonary circulation. Ann Thorac Surg. 1997;63:960–3.

40. Schraufnagel DE, Kay JM. Structural and pathologic changes in the lung vasculature in chronic liver disease. Clin Chest Med. 1996;17:1–15.

41. Lee KN, Lee HJ, Shin WW, Webb WR. Hypoxemia and liver cirrhosis (hepatopulmonary syndrome) in eight patients: comparison of the central and peripheral pulmonary vasculature. Radiology. 1999;211:549–53.

42. Oh YW, Kang EY, Lee NJ, Suh WH, Godwin JD. Thoracic manifestations associated with advanced liver disease. J Comput Assist Tomogr. 2000;24:699–705.

43. McAdams HP, Erasmus J, Crockett R, Mitchell J, Godwin JD, McDermott VG. The hepatopulmonary syndrome: radiologic findings in 10 patients. AJR Am J Roentgenol. 1996;166:1379–85.

44. Shovlin CL, Letarte M. Hereditary haemorrhagic telangiectasia and pulmonary arteriovenous malformations: issues in clinical management and review of pathogenic mechanisms. Thorax. 1999;54:714–29.

45. Donnelly LF. Chest. In: Donnelly LF, editor. Diagnostic imaging pediatrics. Salt Lake City: Amirsys; 2005. p. 118–20.

46. White Jr RI, Lynch-Nyhan A, Terry P, et al. Pulmonary arteriovenous malformations: techniques and long-term outcome of embolotherapy. Radiology. 1988;169:663–9.

47. Lee DW, White Jr RI, Egglin TK, et al. Embolotheraphy of large pulmonary arteriovenous malformations: long-term results. Ann Thorac Surg. 1997;64:930–40.

48. Ferretti GR, Arbib A, Bertrand B, Coulomb M. Haemoptysis associated with pulmonary varices: demonstration using computed tomography angiography. Eur Respir J. 1998;12:989–92.

Congenital and Miscellaneous Abnormalities

5

Jason E. Lang, Robert H. Cleveland, Kara Palm, Neil Mardis,
Edward Y. Lee, and Umakanth Khatwa

Jason E. Lang, MD (✉)
Department of Pulmonology, Allergy and Immunology,
Nemours Children's Clinic/Mayo Clinic College of Medicine,
Jacksonville, FL, USA
e-mail: jelang@nemours.org

Robert H. Cleveland, MD
Department of Radiology, Harvard Medical School,
Boston, MA, USA

Departments of Radiology and Medicine, Division of Respiratory
Diseases, Children's Hospital Boston, Boston, MA, USA

Kara Palm, MD
Division of Respiratory Diseases, Children's Hospital Boston,
Boston, MA, USA

Neil Mardis, DO
Department of Radiology, University of Missouri-Kansas City
School of Medicine, Kansas City, MO, USA

Edward Y. Lee, MD, MPH
Division of Thoracic Imaging, Department of Radiology and
Medicine, Pulmonary Division, Children's Hospital Boston,
Harvard Medical School, Boston, MA, USA

Umakanth Khatwa, MD
Division of Respiratory Diseases, Department of Medicine,
Children's Hospital Boston, Boston, MA, USA

5.1 Bronchobiliary Fistula

Jason E. Lang

Bronchobiliary fistula (BBF) is a rare condition characterized by communication between the tracheobronchial and biliary ductal systems. When BBF occurs, it typically is associated with trauma, cancer or liver infection, although congenital BBF has been described [1–3].

R.H. Cleveland (ed.), *Imaging in Pediatric Pulmonology*,
DOI 10.1007/978-1-4419-5872-3_5, © Springer Science+Business Media, LLC 2012

5.1.1   Congenital Bronchobiliary Fistula

Congenital bronchobiliary fistula (cBBF) was first described in 1952 by Neuhauser. From histologic examination of cases, cBBF appears to result from anomalous liver and bronchial buds connecting and remaining connected after birth [4]. The fistula nearest to the lung often displays respiratory histology such as cartilaginous rings, respiratory epithelium, and airway smooth muscle. Likewise, the fistula closest to the biliary tract displays stratified squamous epithelium of the GI tract. Congenital BBF has been associated with malformations in the biliary tree, diaphragmatic hernia, and esophageal atresia [5–7]. The fistula typically arises from the left hepatic lobe and connects to the distal main trachea or proximal right mainstem bronchus [1] (Figs. 5.1 and 5.2).

Presentation typically occurs within the first year of life with a median age of 4 months, however, adult presentation has also been described [3, 8]. Infants most commonly present with respiratory distress, bilious vomiting or expectoration (biliptysis), and the notable absence of intestinal obstruction [1]. Symptoms in this age group might be mistaken for gastroesophageal reflux, tracheoesophageal fistula, malrotation, or aspiration pneumonia and should be included in the differential diagnosis. Helpful diagnostic testing for BBF includes CT, bronchoscopy, and hepatobiliary scintigraphy. Hepatobiliary scintigraphy (HS) has been recommended to determine adequacy of hepatic drainage and to define associated biliary tract malformations [4, 6]. HS will also allow detection of bilious drainage to the respiratory tract. Reconstruction of CT images may also provide

virtual bronchoscopy that may be more useful and feasible than traditional bronchoscopy. Recommended treatment includes total surgical removal of the BBF. Prognosis related to cBBF is generally good when not associated with more severe congenital anomalies. Typically, if the left hepatic duct can drain normally, total resection of the fistula is performed. Other surgical options may be considered in cases with impaired left hepatic drainage. These can include

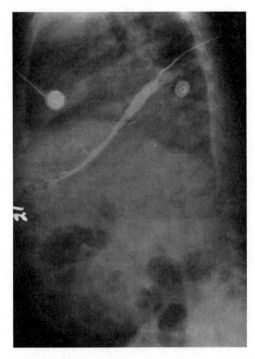

Fig. 5.2. This lateral projection from a percutaneous fistulogram demonstrates the fistula communicating with the intrahepatic branching biliary system

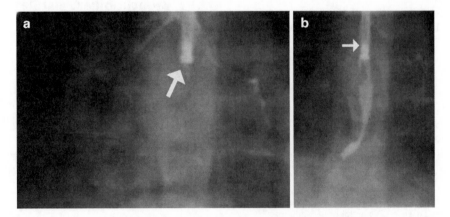

Fig. 5.1. (a) The *arrow* points to the biliary proximal fistula arising from the carina (the two main bronchi are seen partially opacified by contrast material arising from the carina at the uppermost limit of the image). (b) The contrast is seen to fill more of the fistula extending to the level of the liver (*arrow* points to the more superior portion of the fistula)

anastomoses such as a Roux-en-Y or a type of fistula-enteric procedure.

5.1.2   Acquired Bronchobiliary Fistula

Acquired bronchobiliary fistula (aBBF) was first described in 1850 by Peacock complicating hydatid cystic disease of the liver [9]. Most cases of noncongenital BBF occur as a result of acquired hepatic lesions such as hepatobiliary abscess (with or without biliary stones), hydatid disease, hepatic tumors, recurrent pancreatic, blunt or penetrating thoraco-abdominal trauma, or following liver surgery [10–13]. Hepatic infections from tuberculosis [14], echinococcus [15], and ameba have all been described. Overall, aBBF is rare, and can prove difficult to diagnose. A common mechanism of liver disease-associated BBF involves erosion through the diaphragm into the apposing bronchial tree. In cases of trauma with both diaphragmatic and hepatic injury, impaired biliary drainage may act as a nidus for fistula formation.

Acquired BBF should be considered in cases involving liver disease or thoracoabdominal trauma with biliptysis (bilious expectoration). Acquired BBF is associated with significant morbidity and mortality due in part to associated comorbidities and bilious pneumonitis due to the fact that bile is caustic to the respiratory tract. Other common presenting signs and symptoms include respiratory distress, cough, abdominal or chest pain, and fever. When presenting in a subacute manner, symptoms typically include chronic congestion, cough, recurrent pneumonia, and fever. Delayed diagnosis and treatment of BBF can lead to lower lobe bronchiectasis and in some cases the need for lung resection. Several diagnostic imaging studies have been helpful in diagnosis including bronchoscopy [12], hepatobiliary imino-diacetic (HIDA) scan [13], ERCP [16, 17], MR cholangiopancreatography [17], or percutaneous transhepatic cholangiographic fistulogram. Case reports suggest that ERCP with stent- or sphincterotomy-induced bile drainage may be therapeutic by preventing continued intrathoracic bile drainage through the acquired fistula [11, 16, 18]. Additionally, sputum analysis for bilirubin may be helpful. An immediate complication of acquired BBF is bile chemical pneumonitis, which can be severe, leading to respiratory failure. With trauma-induced BBF, both surgical and conservative management approaches are warranted depending on severity

and associated complications. No management guidelines have yet been established; however, resolving biliary obstruction is a well-accepted priority following diagnosis. In cases with severe trauma or pulmonary injury, more definitive surgical resection of BBF may be needed [19].

5.2   Cast Bronchitis

ROBERT H. CLEVELAND AND KARA PALM

Cast or plastic bronchitis is a potentially fatal disorder seen relatively rarely in children. It derives its name from mucoid material which forms within the tracheobronchial tree in the form of a branching tubular cast of the airway (Fig. 5.3). It characteristically has a rubbery consistency. These may be expectorated piecemeal or removed at bronchoscopy as extensive casts of the airway.

5.2.1   Classification of Cast Bronchitis

There are several classifications systems for cast bronchitis [20]. The original system, proposed by Seear [21] described two types. Type I, inflammatory casts, is comprised mainly of fibrin, eosinophils, polymorphonuclear leukocytes, and Charcot-Leyden crystals [20–22]. This form is associated with allergic and inflammatory conditions, most commonly

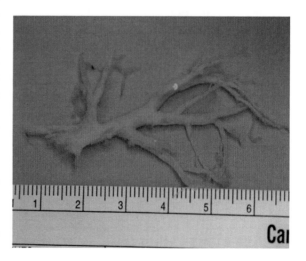

Fig. 5.3. This cast of much of the left bronchial system was retrieved at bronchoscopy

asthma and CF [20, 21]. Type II, noninflammatory casts, is comprised mainly of mucin. This form is associated mainly with cyanotic congenital heart disease, notably with single ventricle physiology, most particularly following the Fontan procedure (right atrium to pulmonary artery conduit). Others have felt this classification to be too restrictive. Brogan [23] has proposed an expanded classification, among other reasons, to include the idiopathic cases. This classification is based on clinical presentation and includes the following three groups: allergic and asthmatic; cardiac; and idiopathic [20, 23]. Although these classifications will include the majority of associated diseases, several other causative or related conditions have been recognized. These include acute chest syndrome of sickle cell disease [20], allergic bronchopulmonary aspergillosis (ABPA) [24], pneumonia [24, 25], lymphangiomatosis [25], bronchiectasis [22, 25], and smoke inhalation [25]. Cases of cast bronchitis have been reported in patients with rheumatoid arthritis, amyloidosis, membranous colitis, and those with large thymuses [22]. In addition to heart disease with single ventricle physiology, isolated cases of associated teratology of Fallot, atrial septal defect with partial anomalous pulmonary venous return, constrictive pericarditis [25], and chronic pericardial effusion [22] have been reported.

The cause of cast formation is unknown. Type I casts are generally acute and occur in association with an acute inflammatory process [24]. Type II casts are generally recurrent or chronic [24]. It has been theorized that Type II casts are caused by disturbances in lymphatic drainage [24] with endobronchial lymph leakage [25] and elevated pulmonary venous pressure [22]. Whereas Type I casts may resolve with airway clearance and treatment of the underlying disorder, Type II casts have a worse prognosis [24].

5.2.2 Treatments

Treatment has had mixed results, frequently with limited poor response and continued high mortality rate (as high as 50% for type I casts), with asphyxiation secondary to airway obstruction as the primary cause of death [24, 25]. Mechanical removal by simple expectoration may be effective; however, bronchoscopic removal may be required and remains the most effective current intervention [20]. Bronchial lavage, hydration, and physical therapy may aid in expectoration of casts [22]. Treatment aimed at cast destruction or disruption has been used with limited success including endobronchial administration of tissue plasminogen activator [24, 25], acetylcysteine [25], urokinase, oral and endobronchial steroids, mucolytic agents, anticoagulants [20, 24], bronchodilators, and azithromycin [24]. Although Type I casts may respond to these therapeutic maneuvers, Type II casts, which may be caused by disturbances in lymphatic drainage, may respond to thoracic duct ligation or diet [24, 25]. Pericardectomy may be effective [25].

5.2.3 Clinical Presentation

Clinical presentation is nonspecific and varied. Signs include dyspnea, wheezing, fever, and cough [20, 22, 24]. As such, presentation may mimic status asthmaticus or foreign body aspiration [20]. A classic adult finding of a *bruit de drapeau* (the sound produced by a flapping flag) has not been reported in children [20, 22].

Imaging findings, likewise, are nonspecific. Findings include atelectasis (sometimes of an entire lung) or airspace consolidation, obstructive emphysema, or compensatory hyperinflation (Figs. 5.4 and 5.5) [20, 22]. An elongated endobronchial opacity with undulating borders may be apparent [20]. Air leakage may rarely occur, including, rarely, pneumomediastinum (Fig. 5.4) [20, 22].

As presenting signs and symptoms and imaging findings are nonspecific, a high index of suspicion is necessary to make the correct diagnosis, particularly in the absence of an expectorated cast which may be mistaken for aspirated food [22, 25]. Acute respiratory failure, with wheezing which is refractory to asthmatic therapy should raise concern for the diagnosis of cast bronchitis, particularly if an aspirated foreign body is not suspected [20]. A low threshold for bronchoscopy is warranted under these circumstances [24]. With the presence of an air leak, emergency bronchoscopy should be performed [20].

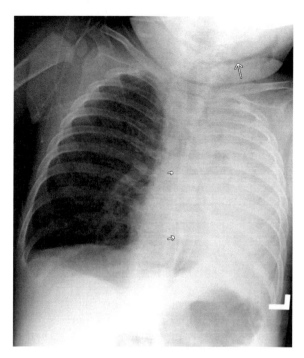

Fig. 5.4. Initial CXR reveals collapse of the left lung. There is subcutaneous air in the left aspect of the neck (*large arrow*) consistent with a pneumomediastinum (*small arrows*). There is compensatory overinflation of the right lung, the mediastinum is shifted to the left

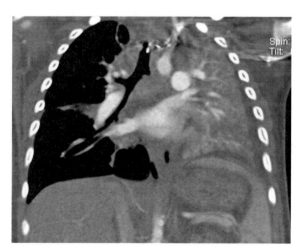

Fig. 5.5. CT confirmed a complete obstruction of the proximal left main bronchus, but did not determine the exact nature of the obstructing process

5.3 Congenital Diaphragmatic Hernia

Neil Mardis

CDH describes an inborn defect in the diaphragm which allows protrusion of abdominal fat and/or viscera through the opening into the thoracic cavity. The cause of this defect is not fully understood and likely is multifactorial. Patients with diaphragmatic hernias suffer from severe, often lethal, pulmonary hypoplasia. The prevalence of CDH has been reported from 1:2,500 to 1:4,000 live births [26, 27]. Mortality rates are upwards of 60% and have arguably remained relatively unaffected by the adoption of new therapies [28]. In addition to the startlingly high mortality despite medical advances, short- and long-term morbidity is significant. Although a majority of cases are sporadic, some cases of CDH are associated with other anomalies or syndromes. Association with another malformation portends a worse prognosis [29].

5.3.1 Embryology and Pathophysiology

Lung formation begins during the third gestational week and continues throughout fetal life. Lung development is often divided into five overlapping stages: embryonic, pseudoglandular, canalicular, saccular, and alveolar. The reader is directed to Chap. 2, for a more detailed examination of pulmonary embryogenesis.

The diaphragm forms between the 4th and 12th gestational weeks. Until recently, the accepted hypothesis of diaphragmatic formation was based upon a developmental scheme in which four separate substratums contributed to the overall structure. The widely taught theory held that the central portion of the diaphragm was formed by the septum transversum, the dorsal esophageal mesentery contributed to the posterior aspect of the structure, the posterolateral portions arose from the pleuroperitoneal folds, and the periphery was formed by contributions from the adjacent body wall [30, 31]. Recent research in a rodent model, however, has questioned the contributions of all elements but the pleuroperitoneal folds [32]. Myogenic cells and axons appear to coalesce within the pleuroperitoneal folds and expand to form the diaphragm. There is compelling evidence to suggest that abnormal formation of the nonmuscular mesenchyme of the pleuroperitoneal folds leads to CDH in rodents and humans [33].

The exact etiology of CDH and the associated pulmonary hypoplasia is not yet fully understood. Interference with the retinoid-signaling pathway has been implicated as a possible causative factor. Retinoids are known to play an important part in all stages of lung development ranging from formation of the lung buds to proliferation of type II pneumocytes, stimulation of phospholipids synthesis, and alveologenesis [34]. When evaluating the retinoid pathway's potential link to CDH, it is helpful to consider the nitrofen rat model. Fetal rodents exposed to nitrofen between the 8th and 11th days post conception experience a high rate of CDH and pulmonary hypoplasia [35]. Although the similarity of this model to human CDH has been questioned [36], nitrofen has recently been shown to decrease retinoic acid levels [37]. Furthermore, retinol and retinol-binding protein have been shown to be decreased in the cord blood of newborns with CDH and increased in their mothers, suggesting a failure of placental transport [38].

The final pathophysiologic theory worthy of consideration is the "dual-hit hypothesis." This concept holds that the pulmonary hypoplasia present in patients with CDH stems not only from compression of the lung by herniated abdominal viscera, but also from a direct insult to the developing lung. This is supported by the nitrofen model in which pulmonary hypoplasia is evident prior to normal diaphragm closure [39]. The importance of retinol in the formation of not only the diaphragm but also the lung helps to explain the severity of pulmonary disease experienced in this population.

5.3.2 Types of Hernias

Diaphragmatic hernias can be subcategorized according to location. The most common form of hernia occurs posterolaterally (Fig. 5.6). Though reported by McCauley in 1754, the Czech anatomist Bochdalek's 1848 description yields the eponymous title of a posterolateral defect. It is postulated that this type of hernia results when the pleuroperitoneal folds fail to fuse to the adjacent body wall. Bochdalek hernias are the most common form of congenital diaphragmatic defect accounting for greater than 80% in most series [40, 41]. Of these, a majority are left-sided. True hernia sacs are found in only a minority (~15%) of Bochdalek hernias.

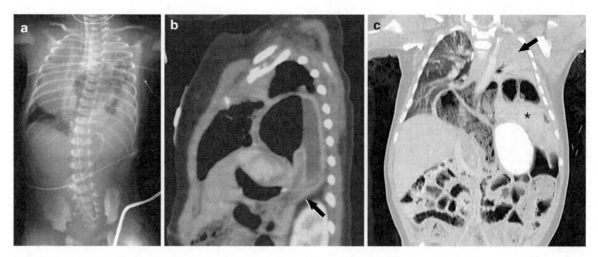

Fig. 5.6. Bochdalek hernia. (a) Frontal view of the chest and abdomen showing numerous loops of air-filled bowel in the left hemithorax. There is significant mediastinal shift to the right. (b) Sagittal CT of the chest and abdomen reveals the posterior diaphragmatic defect (*arrow*) with herniation of bowel through the opening. (c) Coronal lung window image from the same CT shows herniation of bowel and spleen (*asterisk*) into the left thorax. The left lung is hypoplastic and collapsed (*arrow*)

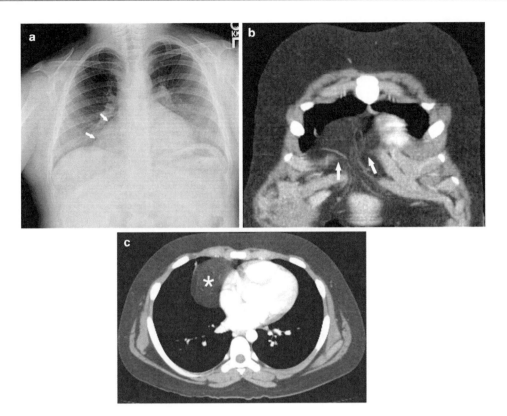

Fig. 5.7. Morgagni hernia. (a) Note the enlarged mediastinal silhouette with abnormal right atrial contour (*arrows*). (b) Coronal CT reveals defect in the anterior diaphragm (*arrows*) with herniation of fat through the defect. (c) Axial CT image shows the fatty mass (*asterisk*) in the anterior mediastinum to the right of the heart

Named for the sixteenth century Italian anatomist and pathologist, Morgagni hernias occur anteriorly between the sternum and 8th rib where the internal mammary artery normally traverses the diaphragm (Fig. 5.7). This type of defect is seen in less than 5% of cases of CDH in many series [26, 41]. Morgagni hernias, though, likely account for a greater percent of CDH in some geographic regions and in patient populations presenting outside the neonatal period [42]. The defect is more often right-sided and typically is contained within a true hernia sac. A less common form of retrosternal hernia is seen in patients with pentalogy of Cantrell. Originally described by J Cantrell in 1958, the condition is typified by an inferior sternal cleft, adjacent anterior diaphragmatic defect, pericardial defect, and omphalocele [43]. The result is an anterior midline defect which permits extrusion of the heart (ectopia cordis). These patients also tend to suffer from complex congenital heart disease. Hiatal hernias constitute the remainder of congenital diaphragmatic defects. Like acquired hiatal hernias, the congenital defect may manifest as a sliding or paraesophageal hernia.

5.3.3   Prenatal

CDH is often detected on routine prenatal ultrasound exams. CDH is suggested when a complex cystic mass representing herniated bowel is noted in the chest. Similarly, the presence of abdominal viscera such as liver or gallbladder adjacent to the fetal heart is indicative of diaphragmatic hernia. Color Doppler may reveal abnormal course or position of the umbilical or portal vein, particularly in hernias containing fetal liver. Often, there is ipsilateral pulmonary hypoplasia and displacement of the mediastinum into the contralateral thorax. Secondary signs such as decreased abdominal circumference and polyhydramnios may also be observed. One important differential consideration in a patient with apparent CDH is congenital diaphragmatic eventration. Congenital eventration implies cephalic displacement of an intact diaphragm and is associated with lower infant morbidity and mortality. Although the prenatal distinction can be difficult to make, high-resolution ultrasound or MRI may allow discrimination. The presence of a pleural and/or pericardial effusion has been suggested as a secondary sign favoring eventration [44].

The lung heart ratio (LHR) has been used to prognosticate cases of diaphragmatic hernia [45–47]. The lung contralateral to the defect is measured in its axial dimensions at the atrial level and this area is divided by the head circumference. A ratio less than 1 is associated with a poor prognosis, with 100% mortality in some series [46, 48]. Conversely, in the same studies a ratio greater than 1.4 was associated with a routinely good prognosis (100% survival). Prognosis appears less predictable for fetuses with ratios between 1.0 and 1.4 [45, 46, 48]. Other studies have questioned the prognostic value of the LHR for survival prediction and the need for extracorporal membrane oxygenation (ECMO) [49–51]. Recently, 3D ultrasonography [52, 53] and fetal MRI have been utilized to obtain fetal lung volumes [54, 55]. Percent predicted lung volumes derived from subtracting mediastinal volume from total thoracic volume on fetal MR have been shown to correlate with ECMO requirement, length of hospital stay, and overall survival [56]. MR fetal lung volume measurements appear to be particularly useful in estimating survival and ECMO requirements beyond 30 weeks gestation [57].

Fetal MRI is also useful in the overall morphologic evaluation of fetuses suspected of having CDH. Presence of liver herniation has been shown to correlate with the need for prosthetic repair and prenatal recognition of this may aid in counseling and surgical planning [58]. Not only can MRI provide information about herniated viscera, coexistent anomalies can be assessed. Fast spin-echo T2-weighted sequences are the mainstay of fetal MRI and provide a detailed anatomic survey in standard imaging planes regardless of fetal position.

Fetal surgery, including CDH repair and tracheal occlusion, are technically possible but have not yet been shown to improve survival [59, 60]. Likewise, pharmacologic therapies such as late prenatal steroids have not demonstrated a benefit [61]. Recent data in an animal model has shown that prenatal treatment with retinoic acid stimulates alveogenesis in hypoplastic lung, leading to increased lung volumes in CDH [62].

5.3.4 Postnatal

The first postnatal imaging study in CDH is typically a frontal chest radiograph. Often, air-filled loops of bowel can be visualized in the chest with mass effect

from the hernia resulting in contralateral mediastinal shift (Fig. 5.8). If the radiograph is acquired early after delivery, the herniated bowel may not yet be air-filled, presenting as opacification of the affected hemithorax. Secondary signs of CDH include abnormal positions or deviations of enteric tubes and umbilical catheters (Fig. 5.9). Severe respiratory

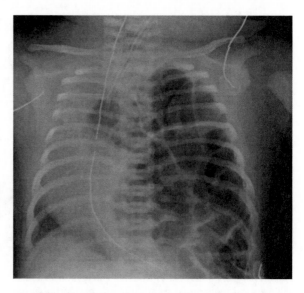

Fig. 5.8. Diaphragmatic hernia with mediastinal shift. Multiple loops of air-filled bowel are herniated into the left hemithorax resulting in marked contralateral mediastinal shift. Note the deviation of the endotracheal and enteric tubes to the right

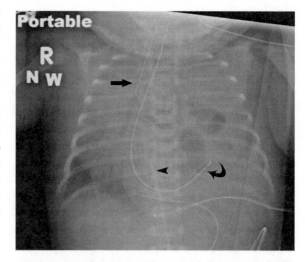

Fig. 5.9. Diaphragmatic hernia with abnormal tube positions. Typical appearance of a left-sided Bochdalek hernia. The endotracheal tube (*arrow*) and umbilical arterial catheter (*arrowhead*) are deviated to the right due to mass effect from the left-sided hernia. Also note the abnormal position of the enteric tube (*curved arrow*) which ends in the lower left hemithorax indicating herniation of the stomach through the defect

failure at birth is common and many patients require rapid ventilatory support. The inherent pulmonary hypoplasia coupled with aggressive ventilation may result in a pneumothorax (Fig. 5.10). The differential for cystic lucent masses within the chest in a newborn includes congenital cystic adenomatoid malformation (CCAM) and pulmonary sequestration. Often, continuity of bowel loops in the upper abdomen and chest makes the diagnosis of CDH obvious. Also, aberrant enteric tube and catheter positions help solidify the diagnosis. Chest and abdominal radiography is often the only preoperative imaging obtained. If question remains as to the etiology of the thoracic mass, computed tomography may be employed for more detailed anatomic depiction.

The inherent pulmonary and vascular hypoplasia results in low volume, poorly compliant lungs in the perioperative period [63]. Due to the potential of iatrogenic lung injury, many institutions employ permissive hypercapnia and "gentle ventilation" techniques. High-frequency oscillatory ventilation and inhaled nitrous oxide are other practices commonly utilized. Despite these methods, approximately half of patients still require ECMO therapy. Preterm infants with CDH who receive ECMO have been shown to have decreased survival, more complications while on ECMO, and longer ECMO courses and hospital stays than similar late-term infants [64]. ECMO may be venovenous or arteriovenous. Venovenous systems are less commonly seen in CDH patients. The radiodense portion of the efferent catheter should be positioned within the SVC with a radiolucent portion extending into the right atrium. The blood is returned via a large diameter venous catheter which may be placed within the femoral vein often extending into the IVC. With a venoarterial system, the venous cannula should extend into the SVC. A radiolucent portion of the catheter then extends into the atrium with a small radiopaque marker at its tip in the right atrium. The radiopaque portion of the arterial side cannula should follow the expected path of the brachiocephalic artery and terminate at the aortic arch (Fig. 5.11).

5.3.5 Long-Term Pulmonary Function

While the early effects of severe pulmonary hypoplasia and pulmonary hypertension are well documented, the long-term pulmonary function of neonates

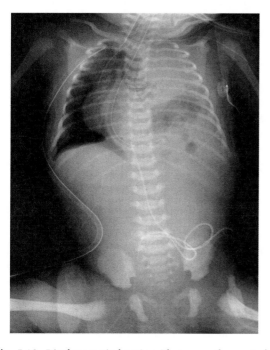

Fig. 5.10. Diaphragmatic hernia with pneumothorax. Left-sided diaphragmatic hernia with typical contralateral mediastinal shift. Note the increased lucency in the right mid and lower thorax with sharply marginated right atrial margin and right diaphragm consistent with an anterior pneumothorax

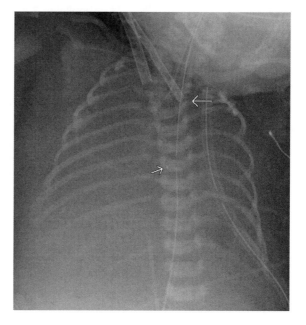

Fig. 5.11. Diaphragmatic hernia on ECMO. Patient with a left-sided hernia on ECMO. The arterial catheter (*large arrow*) courses through the brachiocephalic artery ending in the expected location of the distal aortic arch. The marker at tip of the venous cannula (*small arrow*) projects in the distribution of the right atrium. As expected, on ECMO, the lungs are almost completely airless

surviving CDH repair is less well documented. Recent studies have shown that lung function does improve over time with the most dramatic improvements occurring in the first 6 months of life [65]. Despite normal results on pulmonary function tests, though, there does appear to be residual effects on ventilation distribution and airway patency at the end of the first year of life [66]. While varying degrees of chronic lung disease are encountered, long-term oxygen requirement after the second year is uncommon [67]. A recent study found that adult survivors of CHD repair suffered only mild pulmonary function impairment consistent with residual small airways disease [68]. Other studies, however, have shown that ventilatory impairment and thoracic deformities are common in adult survivors of CDH [69].

5.3.6   Associated Anomalies and Related Morbidity

Congenital Heart Disease

The most common anomaly associated with CDH is congenital heart disease, occurring in 10–35% of patients [70–75]. While the most frequent heart defect reported in association with CDH is a ventricular septal defect (42%), aortic arch obstruction and hypoplastic left heart are also commonly seen [75, 76]. Other reported heart diseases include tetralogy of Fallot, double outlet right ventricle, total anomalous pulmonary venous connection, transposition of the great arteries, pulmonic stenosis, and tricuspid atresia. Overall, there appears to be approximately a 20-fold increase in heart disease in patients with CDH compared to the normal population with the incidence of hypoplastic left heart and obstructive arch lesions disproportionately inflated (100 and 75 times the general population, respectively) [76]. The coexistence of CDH in patients with heart disease yields a worse prognosis than experienced in isolated diaphragmatic hernia. The pulmonary vascular changes inherent in CDH aggravate, and are themselves exacerbated by, congenital heart disease. The effects of increased pulmonary resistance secondary to CDH are greatest in types of heart disease themselves governed by elevated pulmonary pressures. Therefore, patients with arch obstruction, transposition, or monoventricular morphology tend to have a worse prognosis than patients with VSD.

Gastrointestinal Morbidity

Gastrointestinal morbidity is ubiquitous in CDH. As with other malformations resulting in disruption of the normal contour and shape of the peritoneal cavity, intestinal malrotation is inherent in patients with diaphragmatic hernia resulting in intestinal displacement. Obstruction has been reported in up to 20% of patients with CDH [77]. Although the mechanisms are incompletely understood, gastroesophgeal reflux disease (GERD) is commonly encountered in association with CDH. Whether due to abnormal formation of the gatroesophageal junction, esophageal ectasia, or altered thoracic-abdominal pressure gradients post repair, GERD is frequently encountered in patients surviving surgery. The published incidence of GERD varies, but most studies report a prevalence exceeding 50% [78–80]. Reflux and oral aversion are thought to play a significant role in the poor growth and failure to thrive noted in CDH survivors. Other gastrointestinal abnormalities reported in association with CDH include small bowel atresia, colonic agenesis, and Meckel diverticula [81, 82].

Musculoskeletal Deformities

Musculoskeletal deformities are observed in a significant percentage of patients with CDH. Scoliosis has been described in up to 27% of CDH survivors [83]. Chest wall deformities ranging from asymmetry to pectus excavatum have also been reported [83–85]. The pulmonary hypoplasia and increased negative intrathoracic pressure intrinsic to CDH are felt to contribute to the chest wall deformities. The thoracic and spinal abnormalities in turn lead to long-term impairment of pulmonary function.

Neurologic Abnormalities

While morphologic abnormalities of the central nervous system may be seen, acquired neurologic disease secondary to hypoxia, ischemia, and/or hemorrhage is more frequently encountered. The immediate issues of anticoagulation are encountered in patients who require ECMO. These patients undergo regular cranial ultrasound to survey for germinal matrix and parenchymal bleeds. It has been shown that while CDH is not an independent risk factor for ECMO, patients with CDH are more likely to have complications while on ECMO [86]. CDH requiring ECMO is associated with worse long-term cognitive outcome than seen in ECMO patients without

CDH [86]. Also, patients with CDH who require ECMO have a poor neurologic outcome compared to CDH patients who are not treated with ECMO.

5.3.7 Associated Syndromes

Diaphragmatic defects are noted in association with a chromosomal anomaly or syndrome approximately 40% of the time in most series [29, 72], although occurred in over 60% of patients in one large review [87]. The most common chromosomal aberrations seen with CDH are the trisomies 13, 18, and 21 [88]. Turner syndrome (45,X) has also been reported in association with diaphragmatic defects [89]. A vast array of translocations, deletions, duplications, and inversions has been reported with CDH [30]. CDH has been identified as a defining feature of Fryns and Donnai-Barrow syndrome. Fryns syndrome (MIM 229850) is an autosomal recessive condition which consists of CDH, coarse facies, distal limb deformities, cleft lip or palate, congenital heart disease, and cerebral anomalies. Congenital diaphragmatic defect in association with omphalocele, agenesis of the corpus callosum, hypertelorism, and hearing loss constitute Donnai-Barrow syndrome (MIM 222448), an autosomal recessive disorder linked to a mutation in the LRP2 gene (2q23-q31). Other syndromes which do not require, but may have, an associated diaphragmatic hernia include: Beckwith-Wiedemann, Brachmann-de Lange, CHARGE association,

craniofrontonasal, Denys-Drash, Goldenhar, Fraser, Smith-Lemli-Opitz, Noonan, Pallister-Killian, Pierre Robin, Simpson-Golabi-Behmel, thoracoabdominal (including pentalogy of Cantrell), multiple pterygium syndrome, spondylocostal dysostosis, and Wolf-Hirschhorn [26, 27, 30, 87].

5.3.8 Treatment and Outcome Prediction

As previously stated, although fetal repair is technically possible in some cases of CDH, there is no discernable improvement in morbidity or mortality compared to standard postnatal repair. Previously considered a surgical emergency, many institutions now employ a delayed surgical repair. The standard postnatal surgical repair of CDH is via subcostal incision, although thoracotomy may also be performed [90]. The herniated viscera are reduced to the abdominal cavity and the defect is examined. If a hernia sac is present, it is excised to decrease the chance of recurrence. Depending on the extent of the defect, a primary closure or patch repair is then performed. The size of the diaphragmatic defect appears to be an important factor in the outcome of these patients. Infants with small defects which can be closed without a patch have improved survival when compared to patients having moderate sized defects requiring patch closure or those with near complete absence of the diaphragm necessitating a more extensive patch reconstruction [40] (Fig. 5.12).

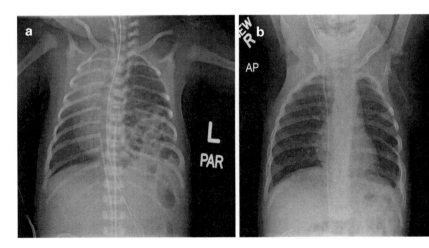

Fig. 5.12. Large diaphragmatic defect requiring patch graft. (a) Preoperative image showing left diaphragmatic hernia. (b) Postoperative image revealing a tight, flattened left hemidiaphragm with ipsilateral small lung. This combination is highly suggestive of prior diaphragmatic hernia repair

EDWARD Y. LEE

5.4   Hepatopulmonary Fusion

Primary hepatopulmonary fusion is an extremely rare condition in patients with a right-sided CDH, in which there is a fusion between the right lung and the herniated liver parenchyma through a defect in the diaphragm [91, 92]. There may be varying degrees of pulmonary hypoplasia associated with this condition [93]. Although the etiology for the development of hepatopulmonary fusion is currently not clearly known, it is speculated that incomplete fusion of the diaphragm may contribute to the fusion between the liver and lung.

5.4.1   Fusion of Four Embryonic Components

Development of an intact diaphragm requires a complete fusion between the four embryonic components: septum transversum, pleuro-peritoneal membrane, muscular component, and dorsal mesentery [94]. Among these four embryonic components of diaphragm, the septum transversum may be hypoplastic which leads to incomplete formation of the diaphragm preventing separation between the liver and lung during embryogenesis [94]. On the other hand, others suspect that hepatopulmonary fusion may be due to the intrauterine inflammatory or ischemic events during organogenesis [95]. Secondary hepatopulmonary fusion which occurs after primary right-sided CDH repair, is also a rare condition. In this condition, the liver herniates through the recurrent diaphragmatic defect resulting in a fusion of the herniated liver and lung parenchyma. Postoperative inflammatory changes and scar formation may be a nidus for a fusion of the herniated liver and lung parenchyma.

5.4.2   Clinical Presentation

There are very few reports consisting of a small patient size or case reports of hepatopulmonary fusion in the literature, limiting the clear understanding of how these patients present clinically [92, 94, 96, 97].

However, the clinical presentations of patients in the reported literature with hepatopulmonary fusion present with similar symptoms as patients with CDH without hepatopulmonary fusion. Typical symptoms include severe respiratory distress, cyanosis, and retraction with scaphoid abdomen immediately following birth [92, 95]. However, patients with small CDH defect and hepatopulmonary fusion may be asymptomatic at birth [97, 98]. They may later present with recurrent respiratory distress.

Radiological Finding

The most reported common radiological finding of hepatopulmonary fusion is the opacification of the right hemithorax without (more common) or with mediastinal shift to the contralateral hemithorax or toward the lesion [93]. Bowel loops, sometimes seen within the right hemithorax in patients with right congenital diaphragm, are not usually seen. Hepatic and pulmonary tissue fused by a fibrous band [95] and broncho-fistula formation [2] are other reported findings associated with hepatopulmonary fusion. Anomalous venous drainage from the right lung to the intrahepatic inferior vena cava was also reported in one patient who was evaluated with MRI [93].

Early Diagnosis

An early and correct diagnosis of hepatopulmonary fusion is difficult due to its rarity; however, high clinical suspicion coupled with the familiarity of this condition is important for correct diagnosis and for proper patient management [99]. It has been reported that reducing the herniated liver into the peritoneal cavity in patients with hepatopulmonary fusion can be particularly challenging during surgical repair, requiring more operation time than the repair of a typical right-sided CDH [91, 92]. Furthermore, intra-operative complication such as kinking of the inferior vena cava and associated intractable hypotension has been reported during hepatopulmonary fusion repair [91].

Once possible hepatopulmonary fusion is suspected in a neonate with a right-sided CDH, a complete preoperative evaluation of the precise anatomy is paramount in order to plan for surgical repair and to minimize possible intraoperative complications. Although plain radiographs are typically an initial postnatal diagnostic imaging study, findings are often nonspecific in patients with hepatopulmonary fusion. MRI has been reported to be useful for evaluation of the fused portion of lung parenchyma and its associated abnormal venous drainage into the intrahepatic inferior vena cava [93]. However, with the advent of multidetector CT (MDCT), MDCT with multiplanar and 3D imaging can be helpful for the preoperative evaluation of hepatopulmonary fusion. Although there is an associated ionizing radiation exposure associated with MDCT, CT has several advantages over the MRI due to its fast scan time and decreased sedation rate. Furthermore, a precise evaluation of lung parenchyma and central airway with axial, multiplanar, and 3D imaging can be achieved with MDCT, unlike MRI, which provides a limited evaluation of the lung parenchyma and central airway. Furthermore, in patients with hepatopulmonary fusion, an evaluation of possible anomalous arterial and venous vessels is crucial for preoperative evaluation. MDCT with multiplanar and 3D imaging has proven to be useful and diagnostic in the evaluation of small anomalous vascular structures in children [100–102].

5.4.3   Conclusion

Treatment of CDH with hepatopulmonary fusion is surgical repair, which may require partial hepatectomy and/or pneumonectomy [91]. Due to the complexity of abnormal anatomy, some patients may need several staged surgical procedures. Unfortunately, the prognosis of patients with hepatopulmonary fusion is poor. Most patients usually die during the perioperative period due to various complications including respiratory distress, right heart failure, persistent pulmonary hypertension, and thrombosis of inferior vena cava [91, 92, 95].

5.5   Horseshoe Lung Malformation

UMAKANTH KHATWA AND EDWARD Y. LEE

Horseshoe lung is a rare congenital lung anomaly first described in 1962 by Spencer, who reported a lung malformation characterized by the fusion of two lungs via a posterior midline isthmus associated with unilateral lung hypoplasia (Fig. 5.13) [103]. In this condition, the posteroinferior bases of the right and left lungs are fused by a narrow band of normal

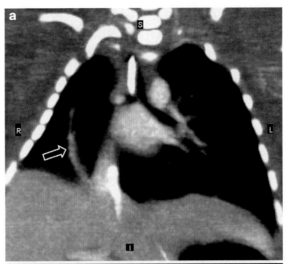

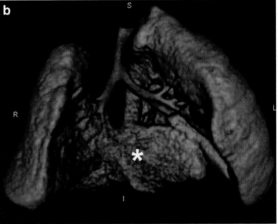

Fig. 5.13. Hypogenetic lung syndrome (Scimitar syndrome) with horseshoe lung in a young child. (**a**) Enhanced coronal CT image shows a scimitar vein (*arrow*) and hypoplastic right lung. (**b**) Anterior view of 3D volume rendered image of the central airway and lungs demonstrates a horseshoe lung. Inferior medial portions (*asterisk*) of both lungs are fused. Case courtesy of David Stringer, M.D. (From Lee et al. [112])

lung tissue referred to as an *isthmus* without an intervening pleural fissure. The isthmic portion of the horseshoe lung originates from the hypoplastic sides of lung; it is located posterior to the heart, but anterior to the aorta and to the esophagus. The blood supply for the isthmus usually originates from the right pulmonary artery and is aerated by a bronchial extension from the right bronchus [103, 104].

5.5.1   Classification

Some investigators believe that horseshoe lung represents one variation on the spectrum of a single lung malformation complex; specifically, an example of *pair organ* maldevelopment associated with various other anomalies of tracheobronchial tree and pulmonary vasculature including scimitar syndrome and *crossover lung segment* [104]. In particular, horseshoe lung malformation association with scimitar syndrome (80%) is well reported [103, 105–107]. The horseshoe lung and scimitar syndrome share several features including hypoplasia of the right lung, anomalous systemic arterial supply to the right lung, and absence or hypoplasia of the bronchus and artery to the right lung. The horseshoe lung is also morphologically similar to crossover lung segment [104]. In the case of *crossover lung*, part of one lung extends into the contralateral side thorax without connection; this displaced pulmonary segment is referred to as the *crossover segment*. Similar to horseshoe lung, the blood supply for the crossover isthmus usually originates from an ipsilateral pulmonary artery and is aerated by a bronchial extension from an ipsilateral bronchus. In addition to scimitar syndrome and crossover lung segment, bilateral pulmonary sequestrations with a bridging isthmus also may mimic horseshoe lung [104, 108, 109].

Horseshoe lung malformation is associated with various tracheobronchial anomalies as listed in Table 5.1 [104]. Horseshoe lung is also associated with various cardiac anomalies; the most common among these is dextraposition of heart (Table 5.2). Other reported anomalies include hypoplastic right thorax, diaphragmatic eventration, diaphragmatic hernia, horseshoe kidney hemivertebrae, and absent radius [104].

5.5.2 Presentation

The age of presentation in patients with horseshoe lung varies greatly (from neonates to adults) and depends on the extent of other associated malformations such as congenital heart disease [103, 104, 107]. Patients with horseshoe lung malformation are commonly symptomatic in the neonatal period (50%) and the diagnosis is usually made by year one (75%). There is greater prevalence among females [104]. In symptomatic patients, the most common presenting symptom is respiratory distress manifested by tachypnea, tachycardia, chest retraction, dyspnea, coughing, wheezing, hypoxia, and cyanosis. Less common symptoms include heart murmur, failure to thrive, chest wall asymmetry, and pulmonary hypertension. Following the neonatal period, recurrent respiratory tract infections (i.e., pneumonia, bronchitis, and empyema) are most frequently reported [104]. In asymptomatic children, diagnosis is often made incidentally when routine chest radiographs show abnormalities associated with horseshoe lung such as unilateral lung haziness and dextraposition of heart [110].

5.5.3 Radiographic Findings

No plain radiographic findings are pathognomonic of horseshoe lung malformation. The most common radiographic findings in patients with horseshoe lung include rightward shift of the heart (dextraposition), mediastinal structures (75%), lung hypoplasia (50%), and Scimitar shadow (40%) [103, 104]. As unilateral pulmonary hypoplasia is a constant finding, horseshoe lung should be looked for in every case of hypoplasia. Other less common plain radiographic findings include eventration of the right diaphragm, hypoplastic right thorax, fusion of ribs, and varying degrees of lung density suggestive of pulmonary sequestration [103, 104, 110]. In the past, bronchography has been used to detect abnormal bronchial branching patterns with an oblique bronchus coursing from right main stem bronchus to the isthmus of the horseshoe lung. Conventional pulmonary

Table 5.1. Tracheobronchial anomalies associated with horseshoe lung malformation

1. Disorganized bronchial branching
2. Abnormal bronchial bifurcation
3. Bridging bronchus
4. Bronchial stenosis
5. Tracheal stenosis
6. Tracheal dilatation
7. Tracheo-esophageal fistula
8. Persistent foregut (common esophaotrachea)

Table 5.2. Cardiac anomalies associated with horseshoe lung malformation

1. Dextraposition
2. ASD
3. VSD
4. Patent foramina ovale
5. Persistent left superior vena cava
6. Pulmonary valvular stenosis
7. Hypoplastic left heart syndrome

angiography (in frontal projection) has also been utilized in evaluating the vascular supply to the isthmus of the horseshoe lung since it accurately depicts the variable degree of hypoplasia, the decreased number of hypoplastic cells, and the abnormal distribution of the segmental branches. Scintigraphy lung perfusion imaging can also show perfusion defects throughout the right lung if these areas are supplied by the systemic arteries [104, 106].

However, in recent years, especially with development of MDCT which clearly depicts lung parenchymal and associated vascular anomalies in congenital lung disease; the diagnosis of horseshoe lung malformation is most often made by CT, thus obviating the need for invasive bronchography and angiography (Fig. 5.13) [104, 111]. Although abnormal lung parenchyma and associated vascular anomalies can be evaluated with axial CT images alone; multiplanar reformations and 3D imaging has proven particularly helpful in confirming the diagnosis well as in further characterizing the anomalous locations and courses of vessels and airways associated with horseshoe lung. 2D and 3D CT imaging have also been established as effective tools in generating useful preoperative evaluations that ultimately improve surgical outcomes and enhance physician--patient/parent communication.

5.5.4 Conclusion

The management of patients with horseshoe lung malformation depends on their clinical symptoms. While asymptomatic patients are managed conservatively, surgery is generally recommended for cases of horseshoe lung malformation (with or without scimitar syndrome) in presence of functional impairment and chronic infection, left to right shunt (Qp: Qs > 2), congenital heart disease, recurrent pneumonias, and progressive pulmonary hypertension [103, 104].

References

1. Tommasoni N, Gamba PG, Midrio P, Guglielmi M. Congenital tracheobiliary fistula. Pediatr Pulmonol. 2000;30(2):149–52.
2. Neuhauser E, Elkin M, Landing B. Congenital direct communication between biliary system and respiratory tract. AMA Am J Dis Child. 1952;83(5):654–9.
3. de Carvalho CR, Barbas CS, Guarnieri RM, et al. Congenital bronchobiliary fistula: first case in an adult. Thorax. 1988;43(10):792–3.
4. Gunlemez A, Tugay M, Elemen L, et al. Surgical experience in a baby with congenital broncho-biliary fistula. Ann Thorac Surg. 2009;87(1):318–20.
5. Tekant GA, Joseph VT, Cheah SL. Congenital tracheobiliary fistula. J Pediatr Surg. 1994;29(5):594–5.
6. Egrari S, Krishnamoorthy M, Yee CA, et al. Congenital bronchobiliary fistula: diagnosis and postoperative surveillance with HIDA scan. J Pediatr Surg. 1996;31(6):785–6.
7. Kalayoglu M, Olcay I. Congenital bronchobiliary fistula associated with esophageal atresia and tracheo-esophageal fistula. J Pediatr Surg. 1976;11(3):463–4.
8. Bringas Bollada M, Cabezas Martin MH, Martinez Sagasti F, et al. Congenital bronchobiliary fistula diagnosed in adult age. Med Intensiva. 2006;30(9):475–6.
9. Peacock TB. Case in which hydatids were expectorated and one of suppuration of a hydatid cyst of the liver communicating with the lungs. Edinburgh Med Surg J. 1850;74:33–46.
10. Eryigit H, Urek S, Olgac G, et al. Management of acquired bronchobiliary fistula: 3 case reports and a literature review. J Cardiothorac Surg. 2007;2:52.
11. Gandhi N, Kent T, Kaban JM, et al. Bronchobiliary fistula after penetrating thoracoabdominal trauma: case report and literature review. J Trauma. 2009;67(5):E143–5.
12. Mitra S, Bhatia N, Dey N, Dalal U. Bronchobiliary fistula: an anesthetic challenge! J Clin Anesth. 2009;21(5):360–2.
13. Annovazzi A, Vicecomte G, Romano L, et al. Detection of a suspected bronchobiliary fistula by hepatobiliary scintigraphy. Ann Nucl Med. 2008;22(7):641–3.
14. Flemma RJ, Anlyan WG. Tuberculous bronchobiliary fistula. Report of an unusual case with demonstration of the fistulous tract by percutaneous transhepatic cholangiography. J Thorac Cardiovasc Surg. 1965;49:198–201.
15. Borrie J, Shaw JH. Hepatobronchial fistula caused by hydatid disease. The Dunedin experience 1952–79. Thorax. 1981;36(1):25–8.
16. Singh B, Moodley J, Sheik-Gafoor MH, et al. Conservative management of thoracobiliary fistula. Ann Thorac Surg. 2002;73(4):1088–91.
17. Oettl C, Schima W, Metz-Schimmerl S, et al. Bronchobiliary fistula after hemihepatectomy: cholangiopancreaticography, computed tomography and magnetic resonance cholangiography findings. Eur J Radiol. 1999;32(3):211–5.
18. Sheik-Gafoor MH, Singh B, Moodley J. Traumatic thoracobiliary fistula: report of a case successfully managed conservatively, with an overview of current diagnostic and therapeutic options. J Trauma. 1998;45(4):819–21.
19. Chua HK, Allen MS, Deschamps C, et al. Bronchobiliary fistula: principles of management. Ann Thorac Surg. 2000;70(4):1392–4.
20. Kruger J, Shpringer C, Picard E, Kerem E. Thoracic air leakage in the presentation of cast bronchitis. Chest. 2009;136:615–7.
21. Seear M, Hui H, Magee F, Bohn D, Cutz E. Bronchial cast in children: a proposed classification based on nine cases and a review of the literature. Am J Respir Crit Care Med. 1997;155:364–70.
22. Bowen A'D, Oudjhane K, Odagiri K, Liston SL, Cumming WA, Oh KS. Plastic bronchitis: large, branching, mucoid bronchial casts in children. Am J Roentgenol. 1985;144:371–5.

23. Brogan TV, Finn LS, Pyskaty DJ, Reddding GJ, Ricker D, Inglis A, et al. Plastic bronchitis in children: a case series and review of the medical literature. Pediatr Pulmonol. 2002;34:482–7.

24. Schultz KD, Oermann CM. Treatment of cast bronchitis with low-dose oral azithromycin. Pediatr Pulmonol. 2003;35:139–43.

25. Costello JM, Steinhorn D, McColley S, Gerber ME, Kumar SP. Treatment of plastic bronchitis in a Fontan patient with tissue plasminogen activator: a case report and review of the literature. Pediatrics. 2002;109:e67.

26. Wenstrom KD, Weiner CP, Hanson JW. A five-year state-wide experience with congenital diaphragmatic hernia. Am J Obstet Gynecol. 1991;165:838–42.

27. Langham Jr MR, Kays DW, Ledbetter DJ, Frentzen B, Sanford LL, Richards DS. Congenital diaphragmatic hernia: epidemiology and outcome. Clin Perinatol. 1996;23:671–88.

28. Stege G, Fenton A, Jaffray B. Nihilism in the 1990s: the true mortality of congenital diaphragmatic hernia. Pediatrics. 2003;112:532–35.

29. Sweed Y, Puri P. Congenital diaphragmatic hernia: influence of associated malformations on survival. Arch Dis Child. 1993;69:68–70.

30. Holder AM, Klaassens M, Tibboel D, de Klein A, Lee B, Scott DA. Genetic factors in congenital diaphragmatic hernia. Am J Hum Genet. 2007;80:825–45.

31. Moore KL, Persaud TVN. The developing human: clinically oriented anatomy. 8th ed. Philadelphia: Saunders; 2008.

32. Babiuk RP, Zhang W, Clugston R, Allan DW, Greer JJ. Embryological origins and development of the rat diaphragm. J Comp Neurol. 2003;455:477–87.

33. Clugston RD, Klattig J, Englert C, Clagett-Dame M, Martinovic J, Benachi A, et al. Teratogen-induced, dietary and genetic models of congenital diaphragmatic hernia share a common mechanism of pathogenesis. Am J Pathol. 2006;169:1541–49.

34. Montedonico S, Nakazawa N, Puri P. Congenital diaphragmatic hernia and retinoids: searching for an etiology. Pediatr Surg Int. 2008;24:755–61.

35. Mortell A, Montedonico S, Puri P. Animal models in pediatric surgery. Pediatr Surg Int. 2006;22:111–28.

36. Baglaj SM, Czernik J. Nitrofen-induced congenital diaphragmatic hernia in rat embryo: what model? J Pediatr Surg. 2004;39:24–30.

37. Noble BR, Babiuk RP, Clugston RD, Underhill TM, Sun H, Kawaguchi R. Mechanisms of action of the congenital diaphragmatic hernia-inducing teratogen nitrofen. Am J Physiol Lung Cell Mol Physiol. 2007;293:L1079–87.

38. Major D, Cadenas M, Fournier L, Leclerc S, Lefebvre M, Cloutier R. Retinol status of newborn infants with congenital diaphragmatic hernia. Pediatr Surg Int. 1998;13:547–49.

39. Keijer R, Liu J, Deimling J, Tibboel D, Post M. Dual-hit hypothesis explains pulmonary hypoplasia in the nitrofen model of congenital diaphragmatic hernia. Am J Pathol. 2000;156:1299–306.

40. The Congenital Diaphragmatic Hernia Study Group. Defect size determines survival in infants with congenital diaphragmatic hernia. Pediatrics. 2007;120:e651–57.

41. Torfs CP, Curry CJ, Bateson TF, Honore LH. A population-based study of congenital diaphragmatic hernia. Teratology. 1992;46:555–65.

42. Al-Salem AH, Nawaz A, Matta H, Jacobsz A. Herniation through the foramen of Morgagni: early diagnosis and treatment. Pediatr Surg Int. 2002;18:93–7.

43. Cantrell JR, Haller JA, Ravitch MM. A syndrome of congenital defects involving the abdominal wall, sternum, diaphragm, pericardium, and heart. Surg Gynecol Obstet. 1958;107:602–14.

44. Jeanty C, Nien JK, Espinoza J, Kusanovic JP, Goncalves LF, Qureshi F, et al. Pleural and pericardial effusion: a potential ultrasonographic marker for the prenatal differential diagnosis between congenital diaphragmatic eventration and congenital diaphragmatic hernia. Ultrasound Obstet Gynecol. 2007;29:378–87.

45. Metkus AP, Filly RA, Stringer MD, Harrison MR, Adzick NS. Sonographic predictors of survival in fetal diaphragmatic hernia. J Pediatr Surg. 1996;31:148–51.

46. Lipshutz GS, Albanese CT, Feldstein VA, Jennings RW, Housley HT, Beech R, et al. Prospective analysis of lung-to-head ratio predicts survival for patients with prenatally diagnosed congenital diaphragmatic hernia. J Pediatr Surg. 1997;32:1634–36.

47. Jani J, Keller RL, Benachi A, Nicolaides KH, Favre R, Gratacos E. Prenatal prediction of survival in isolated left-sided diaphragmatic hernia. Ultrasound Obstet Gynecol. 2006;27:18–22.

48. Laudy JA, Van Gucht M, Van Dooren MF, Wladimiroff JW, Tibboel D. Congenital diaphragmatic hernia: an evaluation of the prognostic value of the lung-to-head ratio and other prenatal parameters. Prenatal Diagn. 2003;23:634–39.

49. Sbragia L, Paek BW, Filly RA, Harrison MR, Farrell JA, Farmer DL, et al. Congenital diaphragmatic hernia without herniation of the liver: does the lung-to-head ratio predict survival? J Ultrasound Med. 2000;19:845–48.

50. Heling KS, Wauer RR, Hammer H, Bollman R, Chaoui R. Reliability of the lung-to-head ratio in predicting outcome and neonatal ventilation parameters in fetuses with congenital diaphragmatic hernia. Ultrasound Obstet Gynecol. 2005;25:112–18.

51. Arkovitz MS, Russo M, Devine P, Budhorick N, Stolar CJ. Fetal lung-head ratio is not related to outcome for antenatal diagnosed congenital diaphragmatic hernia. J Pediatr Surg. 2007;42:107–10.

52. Bahmaie A, Hughes SW, Clark T, Milner A, Saunders J, Tilling K, et al. Serial fetal lung volume measurements using three-dimensional ultrasound. Ultrasound Obstet Gynecol. 2000;16:154–58.

53. Ruano R, Joubin L, Sonigo P, Benachi A, Aubry MC, Thalabard JC, et al. Fetal lung volume estimated by 3-dimensional ultrasonography and magnetic resonance imaging in cases with isolated congenital diaphragmatic hernia. J Ultrasound Med. 2004;23:353–58.

54. Jani JC, Cannie M, Peralta CF, Deprest JA, Nicolaides KH, Dymarkowski S. Lung volumes in fetuses with congenital diaphragmatic hernia: comparison of 3D US and MR imaging assessments. Radiology. 2007;244:575–82.

55. Büsing KA, Kilian AK, Schaible T, Endler C, Schaffelder R, Neff KW. MR relative fetal lung volume in congenital diaphragmatic hernia: survival and need for extracorporeal membrane oxygenation. Radiology. 2008;248:240–46.

56. Barnewolt CE, Kunisaki SM, Fauza DO, Nemes LP, Estroff JA, Jennings RW. Percent predicted lung volumes as measured on fetal magnetic resonance imaging: a useful biometric parameter for risk stratification in congenital diaphragmatic hernia. J Pediatr Surg. 2007;42:193–7.

57. Büsing KA, Kilian AK, Schaible T, Dinter DJ, Neff KW. MR lung volume in fetal congenital diaphragmatic hernia: logistic regression analysis – mortality and extracorporeal membrane oxygenation. Radiology. 2008;248:233–39.

58. Kunisaki SM, Barnewolt CE, Estroff JA, Nemes LP, Jennings RW, Wilson JM, et al. Liver position is a prenatal factor of prosthetic repair in congenital diaphragmatic hernia. Fetal Diagn Ther. 2008;23:258–62.

59. Harrison MR, Adzick NS, Bullard KM, Farrell JA, Howell LJ, Rosen MA, et al. Correction of congenital diaphragmatic hernia in utero VII: a prospective trial. J Pediatr Surg. 1997;32:1637–42.

60. Harrison MR, Keller RL, Hawgood SB, Kitterman JA, Sandberg PL, Farmer DL, et al. A Randomized trial of fetal endoscopic tracheal occlusion for severe fetal congenital diaphragmatic hernia. N Engl J Med. 2003;349: 1916–24.

61. Lally KP, Bagolan P, Hosie S, Lally PA, Stewart M, Cotton CM, et al. Corticosteroids for fetuses with congenital diaphragmatic hernia: can we show benefit? J Pediatr Surg. 2006;41:668–74.

62. Montedonico S, Sugimoto K, Felle P, Bannigan J, Puri P. Prenatal treatment with retinoic acid promotes pulmonary alveologenesis in the nitrofen model of congenital diaphragmatic hernia. J Pediatr Surg. 2008;43:500–7.

63. Nakayama DK, Motoyama EK, Mutich RL, Koumbourlis AC. Pulmonary function in newborns after repair of congenital diaphragmatic hernia. Pediatr Pulmonol. 1991;11:49–55.

64. Stevens TP, Chess PR, McConnochie KM, Sinkin RA, Guillet R, Maniscalco WM, et al. Survival in early- and late-term infants with congenital diaphragmatic hernia treated with extracorporeal membrane oxygenation. Pediatrics. 2002;110:590–96.

65. Koumbourlis AC, Wung JT, Stolar CJ. Lung function in infants after repair of congenital diaphragmatic hernia. J Pediatr Surg. 2006;41:1716–21.

66. Dotta A, Palamides S, Braguglia A, Crescenzi F, Ronchetti MP, Calzolari F, et al. Lung volumes and distribution of ventilation in survivors to congenital diaphragmatic hernia (CDH) during infancy. Pediatr Pulmonol. 2007;42: 600–4.

67. Jaillard SM, Pierrat V, Dubois A, Truffert P, Lequien P, Wurtz AJ, et al. Outcome at 2 years of infants with congenital diaphragmatic hernia: a population-based study. Ann Thorac Surg. 2003;75:250–56.

68. Peetsold MG, Vonk-Noordegraaf A, Heij HH, Gemke R. Pulmonary function and exercise testing in adult survivors of congenital diaphragmatic hernia. Pediatr Pulmonol. 2007;42:325–31.

69. Vanamo K, Rintala R, Sovijärvi A, Jääskeläinen J, Turpeinen M, Lindahl H, et al. Long-term pulmonary sequelae in survivors of congenital diaphragmatic defects. J Pediatr Surg. 1996;31:1096–100.

70. Greenwood RD, Rosenthal A, Nadas AS. Cardiovascular abnormalities associated with congenital diaphragmatic hernia. Pediatrics. 1976;57:92–7.

71. Cuniff C, Jones KL, Jones MC. Patterns of malformation in children with congenital diaphragmatic defects. J Pediatr. 1990;116:258–61.

72. Fauza DO, Wilson JM. Congenital diaphragmatic hernia and associated anomalies: their incidence, identification, and impact on prognosis. J Pediatr Surg. 1994;29:1113–7.

73. Martínez-Frías ML, Prieto L, Urioste M, Bermejo E. Clinical/epidemiological analysis of congenital anomalies associated with diaphragmatic hernia. Am J Med Genet. 1996;62:71–6.

74. Migliazza L, Otten C, Xia H, Rodriguez JI, Diez-Pardo JA, Tovar JA. Cardiovascular malformations in congenital diaphragmatic hernia: human and experimental studies. J Pediatr Surg. 1999;34:1352–8.

75. Cohen MS, Rychik J, Bush DM, Tian ZY, Howell LJ, Adzick NS, et al. Influence of congenital heart disease on survival in children with congenital diaphragmatic hernia. J Pediatr. 2002;141:25–30.

76. Graziano JN. Cardiac anomalies in patients with congenital diaphragmatic heria and their prognosis: a report from the congenital diaphragmatic hernia study group. J Pediatr Surg. 2005;40:1045–50.

77. Vanamo K, Rintala RJ, Lindahl H, Louhimo I. Long-term gastrointestinal morbidity in patients with congenital diaphragmatic defects. J Pediatr Surg. 1996;31:551–54.

78. Koot VC, Bergmeijer JH, Bos AP, Molenaar JC. Incidence and management of gastroesophageal reflux after repair of congenital diaphragmatic hernia. J Pediatr Surg. 1993;28:48–52.

79. Kieffer J, Sapin E, Berg A, Beaudoin S, Bargy F, Helardot PG. Gastroesophageal reflux after repair of congenital diaphragmatic hernia. J Pediatr Surg. 1995;30:1330–3.

80. Su W, Berry M, Puligandla PS, Aspirot A, Flageole H, Laberge JM. Predictors of gastroesophageal reflux in neonates with congenital diaphragmatic hernia. J Pediatr Surg. 2007;42:1639–43.

81. van Dooren MF, Goemaere N, de Klein A, Tibboel D, de Krijger RR. Postmortem findings and clinicopathological correlation in congenital diaphragmatic hernia. Pediatr Dev Pathol. 2004;7:459–67.

82. Benjamin DR, Juul S, Siebert JR. Congenital posterolateral diaphragmatic hernia: associated malformations. J Pediatr Surg. 1988;23:899–903.

83. Vanamo K, Peltonen J, Rintala R, Lindahl H, Jääskeläinen J, Louhimo I. Chest wall and spinal deformities in adults with congenital diaphragmatic defects. J Pediatr Surg. 1996;31:851–54.

84. Lund DP, Mitchell J, Kharasch V, Quigley S, Kuehn M, Wilson JM. Congenital diaphragmatic hernia: the hidden morbidity. J Pediatr Surg. 1994;29:258–62.

85. Arena F, Romeo C, Calabrò MP, Antonuccio P, Arena S, Romeo G. Long-term functional evaluation of diaphragmatic motility after repair of congenital diaphragmatic hernia. J Pediatr Surg. 2005;40:1078–81.

86. Stolar C, Crisafi MA, Driscoll YT. Neurocognitive outcome for neonates treated with extracorporeal membrane oxygenation: are infants with congenital diaphragmatic hernia different? J Pediatr Surg. 1995;30: 366–71.

87. Stoll C, Alembik Y, Dott B, Roth MP. Associated malformations in cases with congenital diaphragmatic hernia. Genet Couns. 2008;19:331–9.

88. Tibboel D, Gaag A. Etiologic and genetic factors in congenital diaphragmatic hernia. Clin Perinatol. 1996;23: 689–99.

89. Cigdem MK, Onen A, Okur H, Otcu S. Associated malformations in Morgagni hernia. Pediatr Surg Int. 2007;23: 1101–3.

90. Stolar CJ, Dillon PW. Pediatric surgery. 6th ed. Philadelphia: Mosby; 2006.

91. Tanaka S, Kubota M, Yagi M, et al. Treatment of a case with right-sided diaphragmatic hernia associated with an abnormal vessel communication between a herniated liver and the right lung. J Pediatr Surg. 2006;41(3):E25–8.

92. Robertson DJ, Harmon CM, Goldberg S. Right congenital diaphragmatic hernia associated with fusion of the liver and the lung. J Pediatr Surg. 2006;41(6):E9–10.

93. Slovis TL, Farmer DL, Berdon WE, et al. Hepatic pulmonary fusion in neonates. Am J Radiol. 2000;174:229–33.
94. Kluth D, Tenbrinck R, Ekesparre M, et al. The natural history of congenital diaphragmatic hernia and pulmonary hypoplasia in embryo. J Pediatr Surg. 1993;28:456–63.
95. Katz S, Kidron D, Litmanovitz I, et al. Fibrous fusion between the liver and the lung: an unusual complication of right congenital diaphragmatic hernia. J Pediatr Surg. 1998;33(5):766–7.
96. Van MK, Lou SB. Congenital diaphragmatic hernia: the neonatologist's perspective. Pediatr Rev. 1999;20:e79–87.
97. Keller RL, Aaroz PA, Hawgoog S, et al. MR imaging of hepato pulmonary fusion in neonates. Am J Radiol. 2003;180:438–40.
98. Nadroo AM, Levshina R, Tugertimur A, et al. Congenital diaphragmatic hernia: atypical presentation. J Perinat Med. 1999;27(4):276–8.
99. Bohn D. Congenital diaphragmatic hernia. Am J Respir Crit Care Med. 2002;166:911–5.
100. Lee EY, Siegel MJ, Hildebolt CF, Gutierrez FR, Fallah JH, Bhalla S. Evaluation of thoracic aortic anomalies in pediatric patients and young adults: comparison of axial, multiplanar, and 3D images. AJR. 2004;183:777–84.
101. Lee EY, Siegel MJ, Sierra LM, Foglia RP. Evaluation of angio architecture of pulmonary sequestration in pediatric patients using 3D MDCT angiography. AJR. 2004;183:183–8.
102. Lee EY, Dillon JE, Callahan MJ, Voss SD. 3D MDCT angiographic evaluation of extralobar sequestration with anomalous venous drainage into left internal mammary vein in a pediatric patient. Br J Radiol. 2006;79(945): e99–e102.
103. Frank JL, Poole CA, Rosas G. Horseshoe lung: clinical, pathologic, and radiologic features and a new plain film finding. Am J Roentgenol. 1986;146:217–26.
104. Kelly D, Mroczek EC, Galliani CA, et al. Horseshoe lung and cross over segment: a unifying concept. Perspect Pediatr Pathol. 1995;18:183–213.
105. Paterson A. Imaging evaluation of congenital lung anomalies in infants and children. Radiol Clin N Am. 2005;43:303–23.
106. Freedom RM, Burrows PE, Moes CA. Horseshoe lung: report of five cases. Am J Roentgenol. 1986;146:211–5.
107. Dupuis C, Remy J, Remy-Jardin M, et al. The "horseshoe" lung: six new cases. Pediatr Pulmonol. 1994;17(2):124–30.
108. Hawass ND, Badwai AM, Al-Muzrakehi M, et al. Horseshoe lung: differential diagnosis. Pediatr Radiol. 1990;20: 580–4.
109. Chen SJ, Li YW, Wu MH, et al. Crossed ectopic left lung with fusion to the right lung: a variant of horseshoe lung? Am J Roentgenol. 1997;168:1347–8.
110. Takeda K, Kato N, Nakagawa T, et al. Horseshoe lung without respiratory distress. Pediatr Radiol. 1990;20(8):604.
111. Takahashi M, Murata K, Yamori M, et al. Horseshoe lung: demonstration by electron-beam CT. Br J Radiol. 1997; 70:964–6.
112. Lee EY, Dorkin H, Vargas SO. Congenital pulmonary malformations in pediatric patients: review and update on etiology, classification, and imaging findings. Radiol Clin North Am. 2011;49:921–48.

Further Reading

Figa FH, Yoo SJ, Burrows PE, et al. Horseshoe lung-A case report with unusual bronchial and pleural anomalies and a proposed new classification. Pediatr Radiol. 1993;23:44–7.

Hawass ND, Badawi MG, Fatani JAETAL. Horseshoe lung with multiple congenital anomalies. Case report and review of the literature. Acta Radiol. 1987;28(6):751–4.

Manner J, Jakob C, Steding G, et al. Horseshoe lung: report on a new variant-"inverted" horseshoe lung – with embryological reflections on the formal pathogenesis of horseshoe lungs. Ann Anat. 2001;183(3):261–5.

Takeda K, Kato N, Nakagawa T, et al. Horseshoe lung without respiratory distress. Pediatr Radiol. 1990;20:604.

Tilea B, Garel C, Delezoide A, et al. Prenatal diagnosis of horseshoe lung: contribution of MRI. Pediatr Radiol. 2005;35:1010–3.

The Pediatric Airway

6

Robert H. Cleveland, Edward Y. Lee, Mary Shannon Fracchia, and Dennis Rosen

In addition to the various developmental and normal physiologic factors that influence the airway [1–4] (see Chap. 3), certain diseases and congenital defects may cause structural abnormalities. Many of these

Portions of the text and illustrations from Cleveland RH. The pediatric airway. Contemp Diagn Radiol. 1996;19:1–6 [1]; Bramson RT, Griscom NT, Cleveland RH. Interpretation of chest radiographs in infants with cough and fever. Radiology. 2005;236:22–29 [2]; and Cleveland RH. The pediatric airway. In: Taveras JM, Ferrucci JT, editors. Radiology: diagnosis, imaging, intervention. Philadelphia: JB Lippincott; 1997, Vol. 1, Chap. 48A, p. 1–13 [3], with permission.

Robert H. Cleveland, MD (✉)
Department of Radiology, Harvard Medical School,
Boston, MA, USA

Departments of Radiology and Medicine, Division
of Respiratory Diseases, Children's Hospital Boston,
Boston, MA, USA
e-mail: Robert.Cleveland@childrens.harvard.edu

Edward Y. Lee, MD, MPH
Division of Thoracic Imaging, Departments of Radiology and
Medicine, Pulmonary Division, Children's Hospital Boston,
Harvard Medical School, Boston, MA, USA

Mary Shannon Fracchia, MD
Pediatric Pulmonary Department, Massachusetts General
Hospital, Harvard Medical School, Boston, MA, USA

Dennis Rosen, MD
Division of Respiratory Diseases, Harvard Medical School,
Children's Hospital Boston, Boston, MA, USA

may present with upper airway obstruction. The differential diagnosis for extra-thoracic airway obstruction is extensive and includes obstructions of the nasal passages, oropharynx, larynx and the glottis. Anatomic abnormalities of the chin and tongue, such as micrognathia and macroglossia, can cause obstruction. In the naso-pharynx, obstruction is caused by nasal polyps and a persistence of the bucconasal membrane, as seen in choanal atresia (Fig. 6.1a) [5] or nasal piriform aperture stenosis (Fig. 6.1b). Within the oropharynx, adenoid-tonsillar enlargement (Fig. 6.2), as well as peri-tonsillar and retropharyngeal abscesses, can obstruct the airway.

Obstructive sleep apnea (OSA) is a condition wherein the upper airway undergoes partial or total collapse during inspiration, resulting in a significant (greater than 50%) decrease in airflow [6]. The decrease in airflow during the obstructive event(s) leads to decrease in the hemoglobin oxygen saturation (SaO_2) and increase in end tidal carbon dioxide ($ETCO_2$) levels, prompting autonomic, physical and electroencephalographic (EEG) arousals. OSA has been associated with a large array of short and long term behavioral and metabolic deficits and disorders.

There are many causes of OSA, often acting in combination and include adenotonsillar hypertrophy, gastroesophageal reflux disease (GERD), or environmental tobacco smoke exposure with resultant inflammation of the soft tissues of the upper airway, low muscle tone, attenuated upper airway reflexes to PCO_2 and negative pressure stimuli, craniofacial dysplasia and mandibular hypoplasia. OSA is present in approximately 2% [7] of the pediatric population and is more prevalent in obese children [8] and children with central hypotonia, craniofacial and chromosomal abnormalities [9].

The diagnosis of OSA is made by a sleep study, also termed polysomnography, which entails parallel determination of multiple physiological parameters

R.H. Cleveland (ed.), *Imaging in Pediatric Pulmonology*,
DOI 10.1007/978-1-4419-5872-3_6, © Springer Science+Business Media, LLC 2012

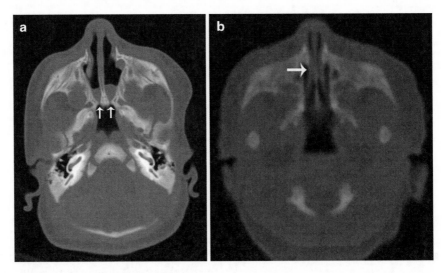

Fig. 6.1. (a) Choanal atresia is caused by bony or soft tissue obstruction of the posterior (*arrows*) nasopharynx. (b) Nasal piriform aperture stenosis causes relatively anterior (*arrow*) obstruction of the nasal passages

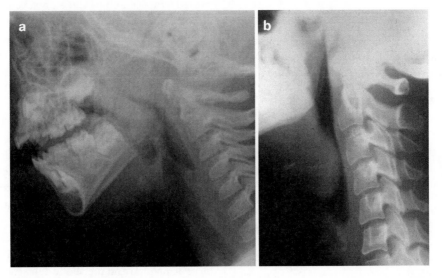

Fig. 6.2. (a) Large hypertrophied tonsils and adenoids are often the cause of obstruction in otherwise normal children. (b) There are enlarged pharyngeal tonsils in this child with infectious mononucleosis (similarly enlarged tonsils may be seen with lymphoma)

(EEG, EKG, EMG), eye movements, pulse oximetry, $ETCO_2$ levels, air flow and respiratory effort while the subject sleeps [10]. A lateral neck film (Fig. 6.2) is sometimes used to assess for evidence of adenoidal or tonsillar hypertrophy, but this is not considered a sensitive modality for diagnosing OSA [11], since it does not account for sleep related dynamic changes in airway patency.

In children, the first line of therapy for OSA is removal of the adenoids and tonsils. This is curative in as many as 85–90% of children with OSA [12].

However, in certain segments of the pediatric population, including older children, children who are obese [13], those with craniofacial abnormalities [14], chromosomal disorders, central hypotonia, as well as some otherwise healthy children, this surgery is not sufficient, and further treatment is necessary. In these cases, continuous positive airway pressure (CPAP) while sleeping is usually prescribed.

Common causes of extra-thoracic obstruction at the larynx include laryngomalacia and laryngostenosis. Laryngomalacia is the most common cause

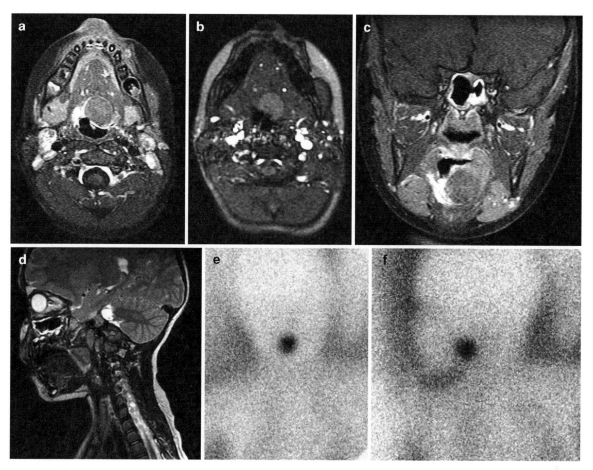

Fig. 6.3. A lingual thyroid is demonstrated posteriorly, slightly to the left of midline. (**a**) Cross section MRI, T1 post gadolinium with fat suppression. (**b**) Cross-section MRI, SPGR. (**c**) Coronal MRI T1 post gadolinium with fat suppression. (**d**) Sagittal MRI T2 FSE with fat suppression. (**e**) 1^{123} radionuclide study in frontal projection. (**f**) 1^{123} radionuclide study in lateral projection

of stridor in children under two, and results from delayed maturation of the supporting structures of the larynx [15]. A flaccid epiglottis, arytenoids, and aryepiglottic folds prolapse into the airway during inspiration. The malacia is pronounced when supine or agitated. Although this is a relatively common abnormality, it is difficult to accurately document with radiologic imaging. Therefore the diagnosis is usually made by laryngoscopy. Laryngostenosis is a congenital or acquired narrowing of the airway, often termed subglottic stenosis. Although it may be congenital, it most commonly occurs after endotracheal intubation.

A lingual thyroid, due to failure of thyroid descent, may cause obstruction in the midline (Fig. 6.3). Remnants of the thyroglossal duct may form a cyst, which presents as a smooth mass in the midline of the neck, and typically moves upward when the

tongue is protruded [15]. Laryngoceles, webs, and cysts, are rarer causes of midline obstruction. A web results from failure of the embryonic airway to reacanalize, while a cyst occurs in the aryepiglottic fold and contains mucus from salivary glands. A laryngocele arises as a dilatation of the saccule of the laryngeal ventricle [15].

Vallecular cysts are rare causes of upper airway obstruction. They usually present at birth or within the first week of life. Presenting symptoms range from hoarse cry, inspiratory stridor, apnea, and cyanosis to chest retractions, feeding difficulties, reflux, and failure to thrive [16]. Laryngomalacia is a common association [17]. Vallecular cysts are usually assessed by laryngoscopy and are seen on the lingual surface of the epiglottis obstructing the upper airway [18, 19]. They may be detected by ultrasound (Fig. 6.4) or cross-sectional imaging. Careful visualization of the base of the tongue is imperative to visualize the cyst. The differential includes thyro-glossal cysts, as well as dermoid cysts, hemangiomas, and lymphatic malformations (cystic hygromas) [20]. Lymphatic malformations are collections of lymphatic sacs that contain clear, colorless lymph, while a hemangioma is the collection of blood vessels located submucosally in the subglottic region.

When there is incomplete development of the elastic and connective tracheal tissue (tracheomalacia), only a *portion* of the intrathoracic trachea may collapse with expiration; while the remainder of

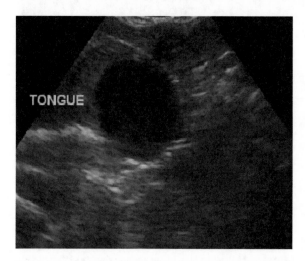

Fig. 6.4. This sagittal ultrasound image reveals a vallecular cystic mass at the base of the tongue

airway maintains normal in caliber during inspiration and expiration. In diagnosing tracheomalacia in infants and children, conventional fluoroscopy guided airway studies are typically recommended. Computed tomography (CT) may be more effective, however, in depicting the location, extent, and degree of tracheomalacia by utilizing a paired inspiratory-expiratory airway protocol that images the central airway at the end of inspiration and expiration. Further, multi-detector CT (MDCT) with 3D central airway reconstruction produces exquisitely detailed images of the entire central airway [21]. Cervical tracheal size is affected by the pressure within its lumen. An excellent illustration of this is when the extrathoracic airway is obstructed or partially obstructed (as in croup). Under these circumstances, the entire cervical trachea may collapse with vigorous inspiration. Moreover, the cervical trachea may become significantly enlarged as the vocal cords close and there is a corresponding increase in positive pressure within the chest [22].

Disease processes such as prevertebral abscess, adenopathy or tumor can also impact airway configuration. These pathologies are frequently characterized by prominent soft tissues (Fig. 6.5a), but without the angled configuration that takes place during normal expiration [1–4] (Chap. 3). Rhabdosarcoma, lymphoma, primitive neuroectodermal tumors (PNET), and mesenchymal cell sarcomas (including germ cell and yolk sac tumors), most commonly

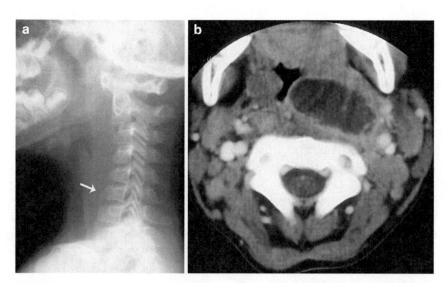

Fig. 6.5. (a) A focal soft tissue prominence, which is out of proportion to the soft tissues inferior to it, is suggestive of a localized abnormality. Lending further evidence of a pathological process is obliteration of the normal fat planes (*arrow points to the normal fat plane*) in the region of the soft tissue prominence. (b) CT of the neck of the child imaged in Fig. 6.5a reveals a large left-sided retropharyngeal abscess (from Cleveland [3], with permission of Lippincott Williams & Wilkins)

develop in this location. These lesions generally obscure the normal prevertebral soft tissue plains (Fig. 6.5a). Further, if the retropharyngeal soft tissue fullness is more pronounced superiorly than inferiorly, it likely reflects pathology (Fig. 6.5a). Once retropharyngeal pathology is suspected on conventional imaging, CT should be performed to establish the extent of disease and the presence of a drainable abscess (Fig. 6.5b).

6.1 Laryngeal and Subglottic Airway

The junction of the underside of the true vocal cords and infraglottic larynx is less acute in infants and small children than it is in older children and adults; this results in a less prominent normal subglottic "shoulder" effect (Fig. 6.6a, b). However, subglottic narrowing can and should be distinguished from the normal sloping of the infraglottic larynx. In addition, during active breathing, the vocal cords are abducted producing a normal loss of the infraglottic "shoulders" (Fig. 6.6c), which is recognized by the lack of vocal cord apposition.

The edema that causes subglottic narrowing, associated with "croup," is characterized by labored breathing and a hoarse, brassy cough. It is usually associated with infection by a parainfluenza virus. But the term *croup* is also used to refer to the expanded complex of laryngotracheobronchitis. This disease primarily affects children of 6 months to 3 years of age, during the winter months. Whereas epiglottitis presents with high probability of life-threatening airway obstruction, croup is generally more benign (Fig. 6.7). In severe circumstances, intubation may be necessary. In the most severe cases, intrathoracic pressure may exceed oncotic pressure on inspiration resulting in pulmonary edema (Fig. 6.8).

Inflammation of the epiglottis (epiglottitis) is classically associated with infection by hemophilus influenza type b (HIB) infection. Fortunately, relatively few cases of this disease are now reported since HIB vaccinations are widely available and strongly encouraged. Infections by non-type b hemophilus influenza, however, occasionally occur. Other types of bacteria may also give rise to epigottitis. The edema that is caused by the ingestion of hot foods or liquids may also resemble epiglottitis. Edema that results from hypersensitivity (e.g., an allergic reaction) may also appear anatomically similar to infection. Epiglottitis generally occurs in winter months and primarily affects children aged 3–6 years. The most clinically apparent symptom is epiglottic swelling, although the aryepiglottic folds and subglottic larynx may show evidence of inflammation as well.

Imaging by plain film or fluoroscopy may be used to definitively diagnose a suspected case of epiglottitis, but extreme caution must be exercised, and should be avoided if possible, because the child's airway may become completely obstructed during imaging. If the head and neck are moved or

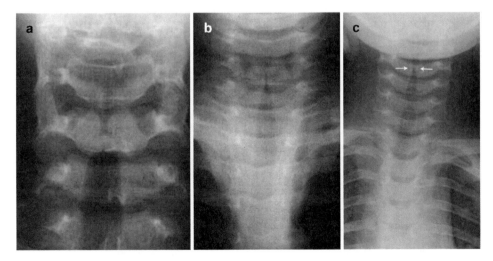

Fig. 6.6. (a) The normal adult subglottic airway ("shoulder") is typically angularly squared off. (b) The normal subglottic "shoulder" in infants and small children is much less angular and squared off than in older children and adults (from Cleveland [3], with permission of Lippincott Williams & Wilkins). (c) With abduction of the vocal cords (*arrows*), there is normally a loss of the subglottic "shoulders." This should not be confused with croup where the vocal cords will be apposed with a loss of the "shoulders"

straightened, the airway may become completely occluded. At times, the aryepiglottic folds or subglottic airway are involved, further complicat-

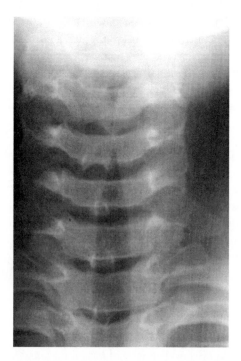

Fig. 6.7. Croup causes subglottic edema and narrowing which is much better seen on frontal projection. Note that there is apposition of the vocal cords in conjunction with loss of the subglottic "shoulders" producing the typical "church steeple" or "pencil point" configuration (from Cleveland [3],with permission of Lippincott Williams & Wilkins)

ing an imaging study (Fig. 6.9). In certain cases, the epiglottis may be relatively spared, but the aryepiglottic folds and/or subglottic airway are affected (Fig. 6.10).

Bacterial organisms, frequently staphylococcal, may give rise to tracheal bacterial infections known as bacterial croup or pseudomembraneous tracheitis (Fig.6.11).This process may present with pseudomembrane formation and croup-like symptoms.

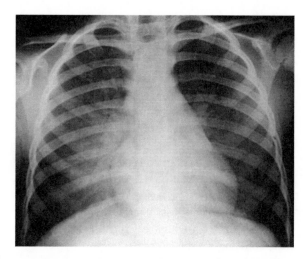

Fig. 6.8. The subglottic obstruction of croup may be so severe that attempts to inflate the lungs will produce such negative intrathoracic pressure that oncotic pressure will be exceeded producing pulmonary edema (from Cleveland [3], with permission of Lippincott Williams & Wilkins)

a

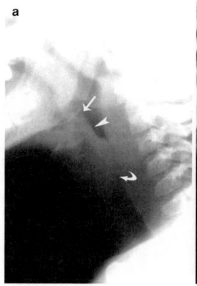

b

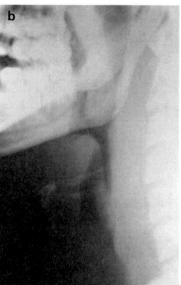

Fig. 6.9. (a) This child with H. flu disease exhibits swelling of the epiglottis (*arrow*), the aryepiglottic folds (*arrow head*), and the subglottic airway (*curved arrow*). This is an example of panglottitis. (b) More often the swelling will be limited mainly

to the epiglottis. In this child with H. flu disease, there is also mild swelling of the aryepiglottic folds (from Cleveland [3], with permission of Lippincott Williams & Wilkins)

In infants and children, focal masses may appear in the subglottic airway. Focal granulation tissue may develop secondary to previous intubation or tracheotomy (Fig. 6.12). Lesions may also be secondary to a subglottic hemangioma, which often arise concomitantly with cutaneous hemangiomata, often of the head or neck. Most often located posterolaterally, usually within 1–1.5 cm below the vocal cords, subglottic hemangiomas frequently involute spontaneously by age 5 or 6 years (Fig. 6.13). Although the detection of subglottic hemangioma can be accomplished by plain radiographs or conventional fluoroscopy guided airway study, CT, especially MDCT with its multiplanar

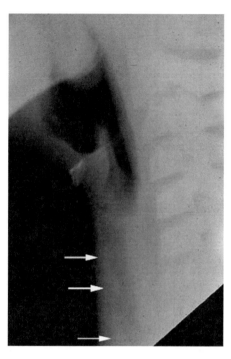

Fig. 6.11. Multifocal and irregular filling defects (*arrows*) may be seen in the infraglottic airway and upper trachea with pseudomembraneous tracheitis. This is caused by the presence of an apple peel configured pseudomembrane. The filling defect is usually more apparent on lateral projection than on the frontal projection

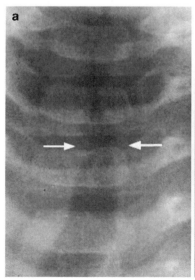

Fig. 6.10. Occasionally, the swelling will be primarily of the aryepiglottic folds, with a normal appearing epiglottis

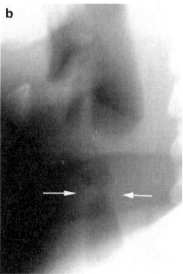

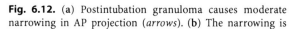

Fig. 6.12. (a) Postintubation granuloma causes moderate narrowing in AP projection (*arrows*). (b) The narrowing is more pronounced in AP direction as seen in comparison with this lateral projection (*arrows*)

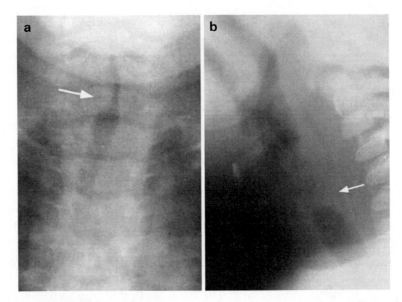

Fig. 6.13. Subglottic hemangiomas (*arrow*) typically arise 1–1.5 cm below the vocal cords. Symptoms of partially obstructing upper airway lesions may be confused with asthma. (**a**) AP projection (from Cleveland [1], with permission of Contemporary Diagnostic Radiology and from Cleveland [3], with permission of Lippincott Williams & Wilkins) (**b**) lateral projection

and 3D imaging capabilities, can be helpful. Virtual tracheobronchoscopy is particularly useful for evaluating the degree of airway obstruction, which is proven to correlate well with the conventional tracheobronchoscopy (Fig. 6.14). After 5 years of age, it is more likely that an isolated subglottic mass is a papilloma (Fig. 6.15) than it is a hemangioma. The papillomata are caused by innoculation with the human papaloma virus, acquired during vaginal delivery. In up to 20% of patients, the viral infection may propagate down the airway and into the lung parenchyma producing nodular, cavitary lung lesions (Fig. 6.16) [23]. Other tumors of the subglottic airway and trachea are seen only rarely in children [24].

6.2   Trachea and Mainstem Bronchi

The most commonly found intraluminal airway abnormalities in children are aspirated foreign bodies. Among very young children, single aspirated foreign bodies are distributed nearly equally between the two lungs. By age 15, the bronchial angles subtended from the trachea acquire a more adult configuration; at this stage, twice as many foreign bodies occur in the right lung [25]. Even when a foreign body is suspected, an initial inspiratory chest film may not show this conclusively. In cases where the diagnosis is uncertain, different imaging strategies can be adopted. For example, an obstructed lung or segment of lung is usually clearly depicted with fluoroscopy. When the lung is obstructed, the abnormal side or lobe does not respond to respiration. In other words, a lung that is filled with trapped air will remain filled (Fig. 6.17a, b). Likewise, a partially collapsed lung will remain similarly collapsed throughout respiration. The failure of a lung, or segment of lung, to exhibit a change in volume through the respiratory cycle is the critical observation. Under these circumstances, diaphragmatic excursion is unequal. On inspiration, when there is air trapped in the obstructed lung, the mediastinum moves toward the abnormal side; on expiration, away from the side of obstruction. An alternative is to use bilateral decubitus chest images (Fig. 6.17c, d). However, this approach often provides less convincing information since the decubitus images are often inadvertently obtained in an oblique position which compromises the ability to accurately assess comparative lung volumes. When viewing right lateral or left lateral decubitus films, the normal dependent lung should appear deflated when compared to the normal non-dependent lung. In older, more cooperative children, these altered dynamics are clearly demonstrated with comparative inspiration and expiration X-rays.

Relatively radiolucent foreign bodies within the airway are sometimes visible in only one projection. Esophageal foreign bodies lodged for extended periods may result in significant edema

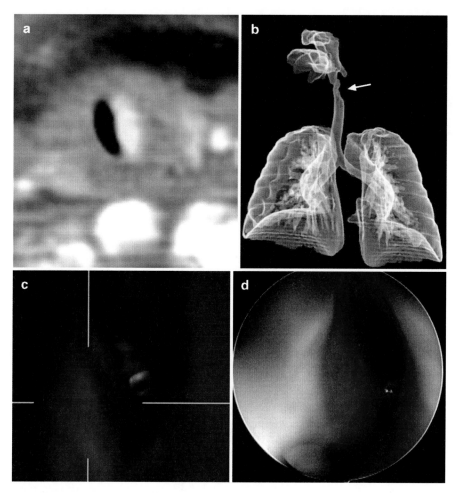

Fig. 6.14. (a) Contrast enhanced CT shows enhancing intraluminal lesion located on the left lateral subglottic region. CT study was performed since the patient had cutaneous hemangiomas and respiratory distress. (b) 3D CT image better demonstrates location, extent, as well as degree of airway obstruction resulted from subglottic hemangioma (*arrow*) (**a** from Lee and Siegel [30], with permission). (c) 3D virtual tracheobronchoscopy shows the degree of subglottic narrowing in a patient with suglottic hemangioma. (d) Subglottic hemangioma seen on conventional tracheobronchoscopy correlates well with that of 3D virtual tracheobronchoscopy image (c)

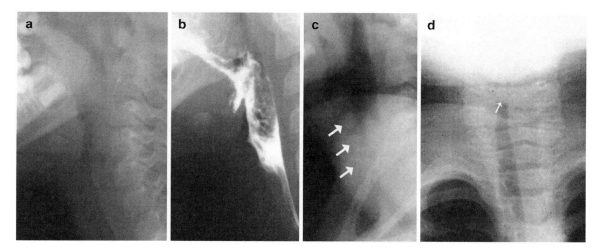

Fig. 6.15. (a) The verrucose lesions of laryngotracheal papillomatosis may present as a laryngeal mass, as seen in this lateral projection of the pharynx. (b) With oral contrast, the extent of the pharyngeal mass is better appreciated. (c) More commonly the lesions will be encountered in the trachea as in this girl, with multiple lesions (*arrows*) (from Cleveland [3], with permission of Lippincott Williams & Wilkins). (d) As with other focal lesions of the upper airway, papillomata may be more difficult to image in frontal projection (*arrow*), than the lateral (c) (from Cleveland [3], with permission of Lippincott Williams & Wilkins)

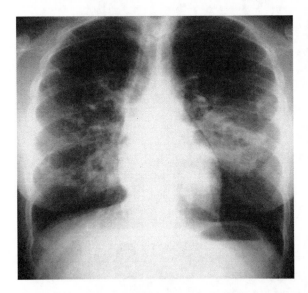

Fig. 6.16. In a few children, the papillomata may eventually spread to the lower airway presenting as multiple solid and eventually cavitating nodules. These predominate in the perihilar and posterior portions of the lungs, especially in the bases (from Cleveland [3], with permission of Lippincott Williams & Wilkins)

and inflammation, creating, at times, obstruction of the adjacent airway (Fig. 6.18) [26]. Extrinsic compression on the airway may result from mediastinal masses such as bronchopulmonary foregut malformations (i.e., bronchogenic cysts, GI duplications, neurenteric cysts) as well as abnormal mediastinal vessels (i.e., double aortic arch, aberrant subclavian artery, pulmonary sling, anomalous innominate artery) [27]. Central airway compression resulting from the abnormal mediastinal vessels may be identified [28, 29] based on plain radiographs (Fig. 6.19); cross-sectional imaging by CT and MRI confirms this finding and provides useful preoperative data. The advantage of MRI is its ability to depict lung structure and function *without exposing* the patient to ionizing radiation. CT, on the other hand, offers more precise detail of the central airway and lung parenchyma. With the introduction of MDCT and its multiplanar and 3D imaging capabilities, the diagnosis and preoperative assessment of mediastinal vascular anomalies resulting in central airway

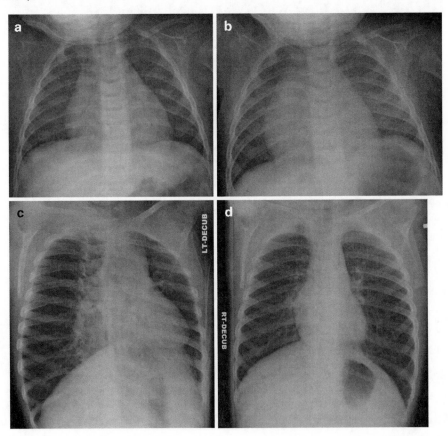

Fig. 6.17. (a) In this moderately inspiratory image, there is essentially equal lung inflation. (b) With expiration, it becomes clear that the right lung is trapping air, confirming the suspected foreign body in the right main bronchus. (c) In a separate child, this left lateral decubitus image shows deflation of the dependent left lung. (d) The right lateral decubitus image of the same child as (c) shows little change in the volume of the dependent right lung, confirming air trapping on the right

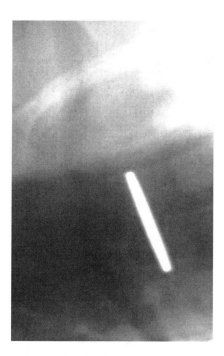

Fig. 6.18. This coin has been in the esophagus long enough to produce a degree of inflammatory response adequate to deviate the trachea anteriorly and to narrow it

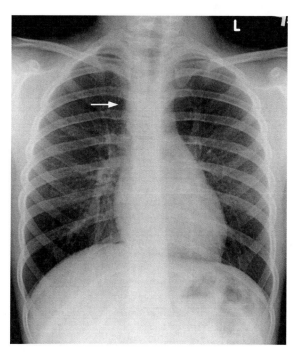

Fig. 6.19. Frontal radiograph of chest demonstrating tracheal narrowing due to right aortic arch (*arrow*)

compression has been significantly enhanced [21]. Mediastinal vascular anomalies, central airway compression, and lung parenchyma can be separately evaluated with the same CT data by applying different CT reconstruction algorithms. The efficient use of imaging data thus minimizes exposure to the potentially harmful effects of radiation, which is of particular concern in evaluating children (Fig. 6.20).

When in utero extrinsic compression of the airway occurs, airway cartilage development is impaired, which, in turn, may cause bronchomalacic or tracheomalacic segments to develop. With esophageal atresia, the dilated upper pouch compresses the trachea compromising tracheal cartilage development in the segment adjacent to the dilated upper esophageal pouch. This structural aberration often produces significant tracheal narrowing and tracheomalacia (Fig. 6.21). The narrowed, malacic segment of the trachea may persist even after the esophageal atresia is surgically corrected. Less commonly the entire esophagus may be distended by obstruction at the esphagogastric junction. This may relate to chalasia, ectopic tracheal cartilages, Chaga's disease, or any lesion causing relative obstruction at the gastroesophageal junction (Fig. 6.22). Significant tracheal narrowing is less common with these lesions than

with esophageal atresia. Congenital tracheal or bronchial stenosis caused by a complete ring or "o" configuration of the cartilages is often associated with pulmonary sling, which passes between the esophagus and trachea (Figs. 6.23 and 6.24).

Peribronchial adenopathy that causes obstruction or endobronchial extension leading to obstruction is often associated with inflammatory processes, particularly tuberculosis (Fig. 6.25). CT is especially useful in evaluating the location, extent, and associated airway compression or obstruction that arises from tuberculosis (Fig. 6.25) [30]. It is also important to evaluate airways that are distal to the obstruction. CT has an advantage over conventional tracheobronchoscopy for evaluation of high-grade airway obstruction resulting from the peribronchial or mediastinal adenopathy. Although the airway distal to the obstruction can be evaluated with CT, conventional tracheobronchoscopy cannot be utilized if the obstruction is high-grade and the bronchoscope cannot be passed beyond the obstruction. Lymphoma, primary mediastinal tumors, or metastatic disease occurring in the mediastinum may cause similar extrinsic obstructions (Fig. 6.26).

Several congenital variations are viewed as failures of tracheoesophageal differentiation from the

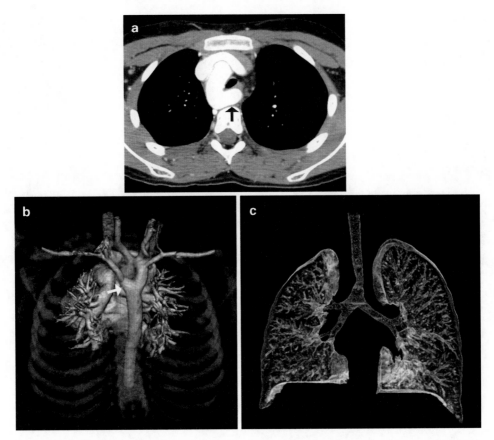

Fig. 6.20. (a) Contrast enhanced CT study showing right aortic arch with aberrant left subclavian artery resulting in trachea compression in an infant girl who presented with respiratory distress. As is often the case, there is a diverticulum of Kommerell (*arrow*) at the origin of the aberrant left subclavian. This diverticulum may produce the dominant obstruction to the airway. (b) 3D volume rendered image of the mediastinal vessels from the posterior view shows right aortic arch with an aberrant left subclavian artery. The *arrow* indicates the diverticulum of Kommerell. (c) 3D volume rendered lumenogram of the central airway and lung demonstrates trachea compression due to the right aortic arch and an aberrant left subclavian artery (from Lee and Siegel [30], with permission)

primitive foregut. There may be complete absence of differentiation with absence of the trachea where the mainstem bronchi arise directly from the distal esophagus (Fig. 6.27). There may be laryngeotracheal clefts extending from the larynx to the carina (sometimes referred to as a common tracheoesophagus) or the cleft may be limited to the larynx, a laryngeal cleft. The least severe is an H-type tracheoesophageal fistula (Fig. 6.28). Duplication of the trachea occurs rarely [31]. Bronchial hypoplasia (or atresia), typically associated with pulmonary artery hypoplasia/atresia and congenitally hypoplastic/absent lung, are occasionally seen (predominantly on the right). In addition, "scimitar syndrome," a rare congenital disorder (1–3 in 100,000 live births), may also give rise to hypoplasia. This condition presents with an anomalous draining, usually right, upper lobe pulmonary vein emptying into the inferior vena cava. Although

the crescent-shaped "scimitar" vein (Fig. 6.29) may be isolated and asymptomatic (scimitar sign), it may be associated with ipsilateral pulmonary, bronchial, and pulmonary artery hypoplasia (scimitar syndrome). There may also be associated congenital heart disease, especially atrial septal defect (ASD); and less commonly, ventricular septal defect (VSD) [32]. Scimitar syndrome is also associated with pulmonary sequestration [33].

Yet another unusual condition known as "pig bronchus" occurs when the right upper lobe bronchus, multiple bronchi or a bronchial segment arises directly from the trachea. Although this configuration is normal in pigs (and sheep), it can be problematic for human beings. While adults with this defect are generally asymptomatic, it may be the source of recurrent right upper lobe atelectasis or pneumonia in children (Fig. 6.30). This anatomic variant should

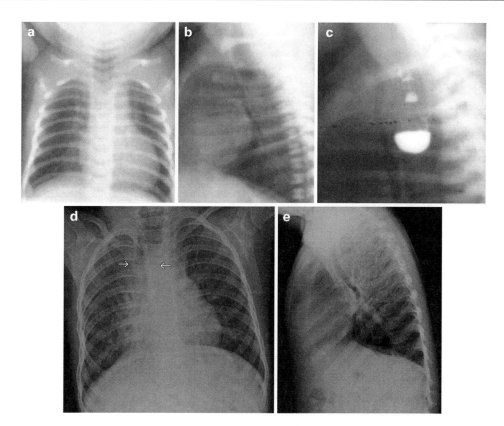

Fig. 6.21. The air distended upper pouch of an esophageal atresia pushes upon the adjacent trachea from posteriorly. The trachea is deviated anteriorly and narrowed. (**a**) AP projection. (**b**) Lateral projection. (**c**) Lateral projection with barium in the blind ending upper pouch. (**d**) When the obstruction is severe, there may be a demonstrable air fluid level above the obstruction (*arrows*). This child had repaired esophageal atresia; however, air fluid levels may result from esophageal obstruction at any level. (**e**) Lateral view in the same child as (**d**) also reveals an air fluid level in the dilated esophagus. The trachea is anteriorly displaced

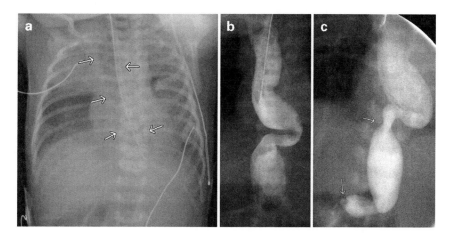

Fig. 6.22. (**a**) Portable AP CXR reveals gaseous distention of the entire esophagus (*arrows*). (**b**) Contrast injection via esophageal tube demonstrates a distended esophagus almost identical to that seen on CXR (**a**). (**c**) There is microgastria causing the esophageal dilatation. The *upper arrow* marks the gastroesophageal junction, the *lower arrow* points to the pylorus

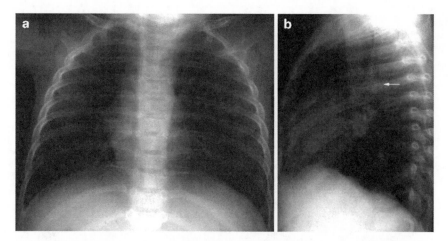

Fig. 6.23. (a) PA projection revealing findings of an aberrant left pulmonary artery including a slightly inferiorly positioned right main bronchus, a leftward deviation of the distal, supracarinal portion of the trachea, partial obscuration of the distal, supracarinal portion of the trachea ("tracheal cut-off sign") and a slightly hyperlucent, slightly enlarged left lung. (b) Lateral projection reveals a soft tissue process (the aberrant left pulmonary artery) (*arrow*) posterior to the distal trachea deviating the trachea anteriorly and narrowing it

be particularly suspected if a child is noted to develop right upper lobe atelectasis associated with placement of an ET tube deep within the trachea but not with less advanced ET tubes. A small accessory cardiac bronchus rarely arises from the medial wall of the bronchus intermedius (Fig. 6.31). It may be associated with recurrent infection or hemoptysis and may trap debris [34].

There are a few rare congenital abnormalities of the trachea and main bronchi which may lead to atelectasis, pneumonia and bronchiectasis. William-Campbell Syndrome (deficient branchial cartiledges) may cause reduced airway clearance leading to recurrent atelectasis, infection and bronchiectasis [35]. Congenital tracheobronchomegaly, Mounier-Kuhn syndrome, and acquired tracheomegaly/tracheobronchomegaly can also lead to recurrent atelectasis, pneumonia and bronchiectasis. This may be associated with pulmonary fibrosis, Ehlers-Danlos syndrome, ankylosing spondyliltis, rheumatoid arthritis or cystic fibrosis [36].

6.3   Peripheral Bronchi

Among the most common acute inflammatory processes that occur in infants and very young children is bronchiolitis, which is characterized by coughing, wheezing, and fever [2]. It is typically viral (most often respiratory syncytial virus), and primarily affects the peripheral bronchi. From a radiographic standpoint, bronchiolitis is depicted by "air trapping,"

often with little or no other radiographic abnormalities (Fig. 6.32). Diffuse bronchial wall thickening (peribronchial thickening), however, is frequently apparent. Atelectasis appears less often; and on sequential imaging typically shows a shift in its distribution. Unfortunately, the radiographic course of bronchiolitis can create some confusion. Although hyperinflation is the most prevalent initial finding, as the process resolves the lungs generally show less air trapping but more atelectasis. Paradoxically, this apparent deterioration of multifocal lung disease is a sign that the inflammation is improving.

Bronchiolitis is the most common cause of acute bronchial wall thickening. Chronic bronchial wall thickening is most commonly seen in children with reactive airways disease or asthma. Radiographs of children with asthma or reactive airway disease generally show diffuse air trapping when acutely symptomatic. Diffuse bronchial wall thickening is present even when asymptomatic. The recognition of bronchial wall thickening is complicated since the prominence of the bronchial walls increases with age. As a guide, infants have only a minimal number of visible bronchial walls in the lung periphery, but many may be normally detected in the perihilar regions (Fig. 6.33). With pathologic bronchial wall thickening, more evidence of the process can be detected in the lung periphery, seen as "o rings" and "tram tracking" (Figs. 6.34 and 6.35). Since the process effects the bronchi, which converge on the hilar regions, the process may be most noticeably abnormal centrally, which may be recognized as large poorly marginated hilae, especially on the lateral image (Fig. 6.35a).

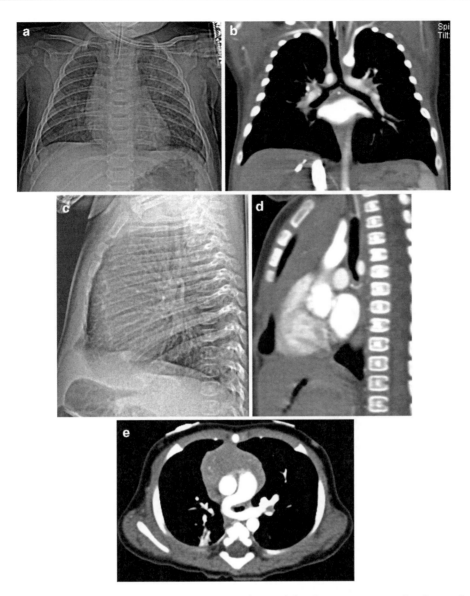

Fig. 6.24. Pulmonary sling. (**a**) PA CXR reveals a slight leftward deviation of the trachea just above the carina. (**b**) Coronal reconstruction from CT shows the aberrant left pulmonary artery adjacent to the inferior trachea causing the leftward deviation. (**c**) Lateral CXR reveals a slight anterior deviation of the inferior trachea. (**d**) Sagittal CT reconstruction reveals the aberrant left pulmonary artery causing the anterior bowing of the trachea. (**e**) Cross-sectional image shows the left pulmonary artery arising from the main pulmonary artery then coursing to the right of the trachea and then to the left between the trachea and esophagus

Diffuse bronchial wall thickening is also the most common initial radiographic indicator of cystic fibrosis in infants and young children [37, 38]. In older children and adults, this often progresses to coarse bronchiectatic changes frequently perceived as nodules when fluid-filled, or as cysts when air-filled (Fig. 6.36) [37, 38]. Less commonly, chronic recurrent pneumonia may result in bronchial wall thickening. This is most commonly a consequence of one of two processes: (1) it may be secondary to recurrent aspiration associated with a swallowing abnormality or a tracheoesophageal fistula; or (2) it

may relate to an immune deficiency. In these instances the process may be uneven in distribution, as opposed to the more evenly distributed process seen with early CF and asthma/reactive airway disease. Other rarer causes include those entities discussed in the chapter on interstitial lung disease.

In congenital lobar emphysema (CLE), an estimated 50% of cases show some evidence of focal bronchial obstruction that manifests itself as an over inflated, hyperlucent lobe (Fig. 6.37) [39]. However, in the first few days of life this may present with preferential trapping of fetal lung liquid in the abnormal

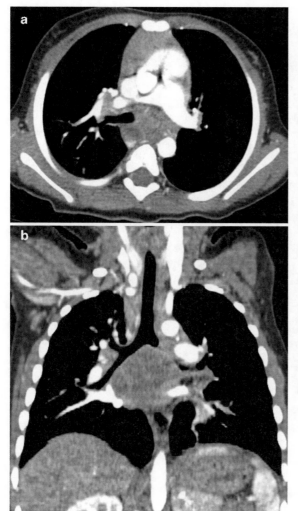

Fig. 6.25. (a) Contrast enhanced CT demonstrates a heterogeneous posterior mediastinal mass obstructing the left main stem bronchus. (b) The location, extent, and left main stem bronchial obstruction resulted from the tuberculous mediastinal lymphadenopathy are better evaluated with coronal multiplanar CT image

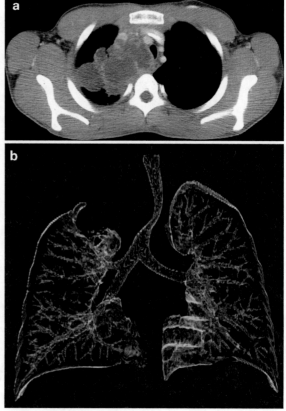

Fig. 6.26. (a) Contrast enhanced CT shows heterogenous metastatic lymphadenopathy resulting in tracheal compression in a child with metastatic prostate rhabdomyosarcoma. (b) 3D volume rendered image shows a compressed trachea, which shifts to the contralateral side of the mass. Also noted is a metastatic mass compressing the right upper lung (from Lee and Siegel [30], with permission)

lobe. This, in turn, produces an overinflated, opaque lobe (Fig. 6.38), which slowly drains the fluid over ensuing days, subsequently becoming hyperlucent. The distribution of CLE is roughly 43% in the left upper lobe, 32% in the right middle lobe, 20% in the right upper lobe and 5% in two lobes [40]. With an overinflated hyperlucent lobe and associated mediastinal shift to the contralateral side, CLE may be mistaken as tension pneumothorax. When this occurs, CT is useful in visualizing the underlying, overinflated, and hyperlucent lung parenchyma (Fig. 6.39).

Further complicating a definitive diagnosis is a condition known as "polyalveolar lobe," which is clinically and radiographically indistinguishable from CLE. Although polyalveolar lobe shares a similar distribution and demographics with CLE; it has a normal tracheobronchial tree but a greater number of alveoli [40]. It has been suggested that cases of suspected CLE that preferentially retain fetal lung liquid are actually polyalveolar lobe [40].

Chronic lung disease of prematurity (bronchopulmonary dysplasia) develops over a period of several days as supplemental oxygen is delivered to the neonatal patient via an ET tube. It typically presents in premature infants with hyaline membrane disease, in which ciliated epithelial cells of the trachea and bronchi are destroyed and replaced with non-ciliated cells. The replacement of ciliated cells with

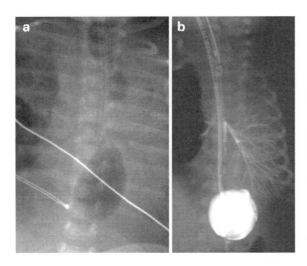

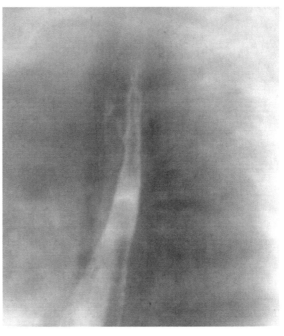

Fig. 6.27. (a) Attempts at intubation of this newborn consistently resulted in the tube being placed in the esophagus. This image shows the main bronchi abutting the esophageal tube at right angles. This scenario suggests an absent trachea (from Cleveland [3], with permission of Lippincott Williams & Wilkins). (b) Postmortem injection of an esophageal tube confirms the origin of the bronchi from the distal esophagus

Fig. 6.28. "H" type tracheoesophageal fistula. The fistula courses upward from the esophagus to the trachea. This is a consistent finding suggesting that the abnormality possibly should be referred to as an "N" type fistula. Barium is the best contrast agent to use in assessing for this lesion with the patient positioned with the right side down on a horizontal fluoroscopy table

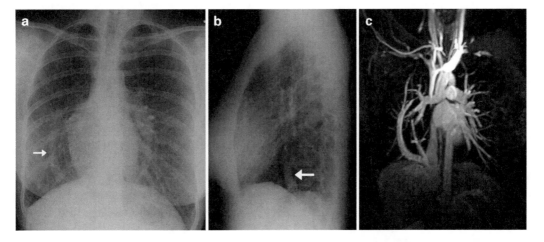

Fig. 6.29. An aberrant right upper lobe pulmonary vein, a scimitar vein, is easily recognized (*arrow*). (**a**) PA projection. (**b**) Lateral projection. (**c**) Coronal MRI

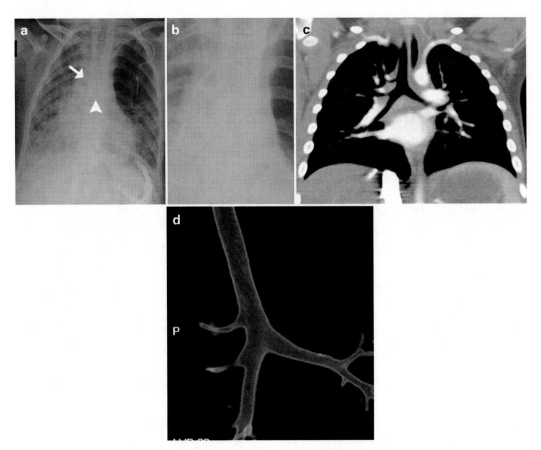

Fig. 6.30. (a) This frontal chest X-ray reveals a "pig" bronchus (*arrow*). The trachea distal to the anomalous bronchus is proportionately diminished in caliber (*arrow head* indicates the carina). (b) Coned image of the main intrathoracic airway from (a). (c) This coronal reconstruction from a CT of a different child shows a "pig" bronchus but without the associated narrowing of the distal trachea. (d) 3D rendering of the airway illustrated in (c)

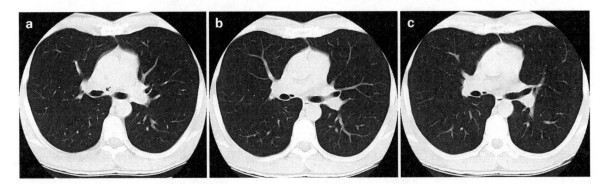

Fig. 6.31. Accessory cardiac bronchus. (a) CT image approximately 5 mm below the carina shows the orifice of an accessory cardiac bronchus (*arrow*) arising from the medial wall of the bronchus intermedius. (b) Five millimeters below the orifice of the accessory bronchus, the accessory bronchus is separated from the bronchus intermedius. (c) The accessory bronchus approximately 1 cm from its origin. It was no longer present on the next contiguous image

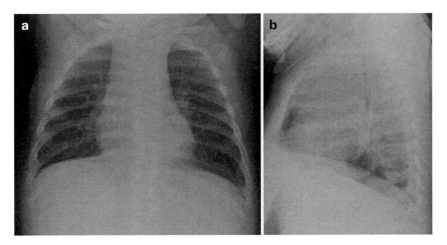

Fig. 6.32. (a, b) The chest radiograph on this infant with RSV positive bronchiolitis reveals diffuse air trapping. The flattening of the diaphragm is the most reliable indicator of overinflation. There is also multifocal subsegmental atelectasis and diffuse bronchial wall thickening

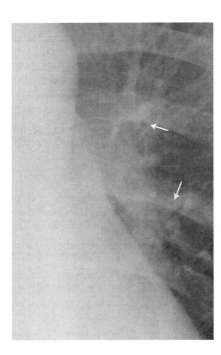

Fig. 6.33. Normal bronchial walls (*arrows*) in the perihilar regions are prominent enough to be easily recognized

non-ciliated cells leads to recurrent atelectasis and infections. There are also multifocal areas of atelectasis and fibrosis alternating with areas of focal overexpansion [39]. In premature infants with bronchopulmonary dysplasia who survive for several months or years, the radiographic and clinical depiction of the disease may closely resemble that of children with acute bronchiolitis or asthma. In addition, older children diagnosed with pulmonary disorders at birth including hyaline membrane disease, meconium aspiration, neonatal pneumonia, and diaphragmatic hernia frequently develop reactive airway disease that is clinically recognizable or confirmed by pulmonary function studies [41].

Bronchiolitis obliterans (Swyer-James syndrome or McLeod syndrome) generally develops secondary to viral infection, although it can also arise from a bacterial or parasitic infection (i.e., mycoplasma). In adults, bronchiolitis obliterans is characterized by hyperlucent small volume lung; but in children, by an overexpanded hyperlucent lung, a discrepancy explained by diminished lung growth following onset of the disease. While air trapping is initially evident on imaging, proportionately less growth results in reduced lung volume compared to the more normal lung. In addition, it has been established that many cases of bronchiolitis obliterans feature diffuse and irregularly affected lungs. Specifically, on CT both lungs may show abnormalities, including bronchiectasis [42], but one lung typically dominates (Fig. 6.40).

Other inflammatory diseases may add to the diagnostic confusion. The early stages of follicular

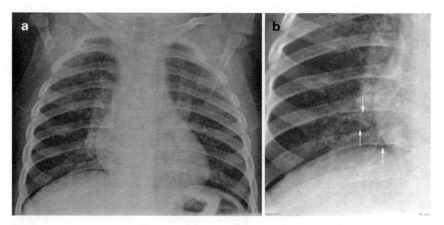

Fig. 6.34. (a) Peribronchial thickening (bronchial wall thickening) is seen diffusely on this PA chest X-ray in a child with bronchiolitis. (b) Coned image of the right lung base from (a) more clearly shows the "ring shadows" of thickened bronchial walls seen in cross-section (*arrows*)

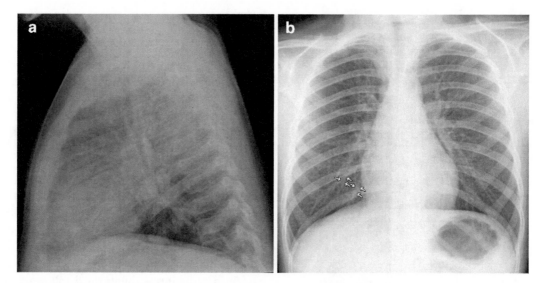

Fig. 6.35. (a) Lateral projection of the chest seen as Fig. 6.34 again reveals diffuse bronchial wall thickening. The convergence of the prominent bronchi has produced abnormally prominent hilar configuration which is ill-defined ("shaggy"). (b) Tram tracking of thickened bronchial walls is seen in the right lung base in a different patient (*arrows*)

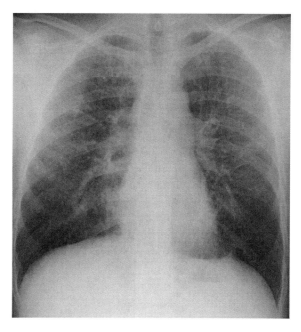

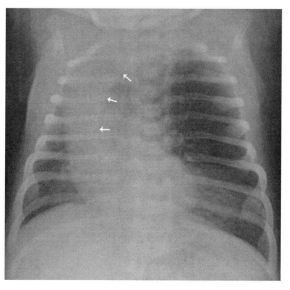

Fig. 6.36. This teenager with cystic fibrosis has the typical radiographic changes of her disease. There is diffuse bronchial wall thickening, with areas of bronchiectasis, prominent hilae, areas of atelectasis or fibrosis and high lung volumes. In approximately 50% of patients with bronchiectasis, it will be most accentuated in the upper lobes

Fig. 6.37. There is congenital lobar emphysema of the left upper lobe with overinflation and increased lucency of the left upper lobe. This has resulted in mediastinal shift to the right and bilateral lower lobe atelectasis (left greater than the right). The *arrows* point the anterior junction line, where the pleural margins of the two lungs meet anteriorly. It is shifted to the right secondary to "herniation" of the overinflated left upper lobe

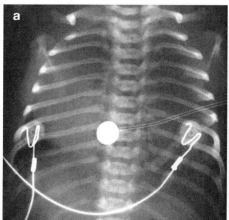
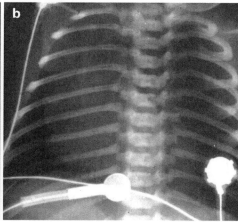

Fig. 6.38. (a) Polyalveolar left upper lobe with retained fetal lung liquid producing and over-distended and opaque left upper lobe in this 2 h old girl. (b) By 4 days of life most of the fetal lung liquid has drained from the left upper lobe (from Cleveland [3], with permission of Lippincott Williams & Wilkins)

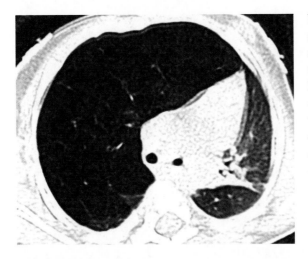

Fig. 6.39. Lung window CT image in an infant with right upper lobe congenital lobar emphysema demonstrates markedly hyperinflated right upper lobe resulting in mediastinal shift to the left side. Underlying lung parenchyma of the right upper lobe despite hyperinflation was well seen on lung window CT image

bronchitis [43] may radiographically and clinically resemble bronchiolitis. This disease which some equate with "neuroendocrine cell hyperplasia" (NeHi), usually presents within the first 6–8 weeks of life. However, contrary to the typically short-lived clinical course of bronchiolitis, the tachypnea and wheezing characteristic of follicular bronchitis persist for 2–3 years. Radiographic findings initially suggest bronchiolitis because of air trapping, bronchial wall thickening, and occasional instances of atelectasis. By approximately 5 or 6 months of age, a diffuse, essentially interstitial process has evolved; and by 8 years of age, symptoms and radiographic indicators have generally reverted to normal. Recent work has identified a CT configuration specific for NeHi (Fig. 6.41) with anteriorly dominate interstitial disease [44].

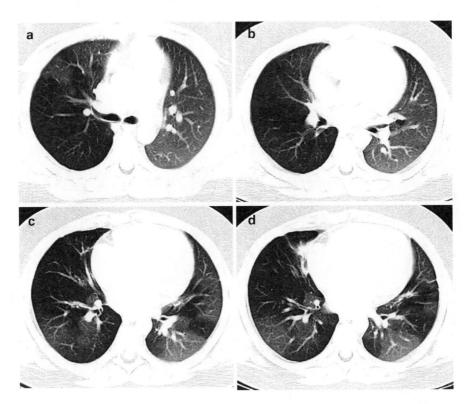

Fig. 6.40. CT of bonchiolitis obliterans presents with accentuated hyperlucent oligemic segments of lung, usually worse in one lung with associated mild to moderate bronchiectasis. (**a–d**) Images at discontiguous levels from cranial to caudal

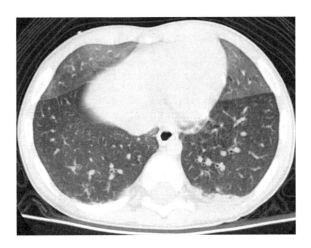

Fig. 6.41. CT study with lung window settings demonstrates ground-glass opacity in the right middle lobe and lingula in a 23-month-old infant with biopsy proven NeHi

References

1. Cleveland RH. The pediatric airway. Contemp Diagn Radiol. 1996;19:1–6.
2. Bramson RT, Griscom NT, Cleveland RH. Interpretation of chest radiographs in infants with cough and fever. Radiology. 2005;236:22–9.
3. Cleveland RH. The pediatric airway. In: Taveras JM, Ferrucci JT, editors. Radiology: diagnosis, imaging, intervention. Philadelphia: JB Lippincott; 1997, vol. 1, Chap. 48A, p. 1–13.
4. Cleveland R. The pediatric airway. Syllabus IDKD: diseases of the heart, chest & breast. Milan: Springer-Verlag Italia; 2007. p. 204–8.
5. Leung KC, Cho H. Diagnosis of Stridor in children. Am Fam Physician. 1999;60:2289–96.
6. AASM Manual for the Scoring of Sleep and Associated Events. Rules, terminology and technical specifications. Westchester: American Academy of Sleep Medicine; 2007.
7. Lumeng JC, Chervin RD. Epidemiology of pediatric obstructive sleep apnea. Proc Am Thorac Soc. 2008;5(2):242–52.
8. Redline S, Tishler PV, Schluchte M, Aylor J, Clark K, Graham G. Risk factors for sleep-disordered breathing in children. Associations with obesity, race, and respiratory problems. Am J Respir Crit Care Med. 1999;159:1527–32.
9. Dyken ME, Lin-Dyken DC, Poulton S, et al. Prospective polysomnographic analysis of obstructive sleep apnea in Down syndrome. Arch Pediatr Adolesc Med. 2003;157:655–60.
10. Chesson Jr AL, Ferber RA, Fry JM, Grigg-Damberger M, Hartse KM, Hurwitz TD, et al. The indications for polysomnography and related procedures. Sleep. 1997;20(6):423–87.
11. Brooks LJ, Stevens BM, Bacevice AM. Adenoid size is related to severity but not the number of episodes of obstructive apnea in children. J Pediatr. 1998;132(4):682–6.
12. Mitchell RB. Adenotonsillectomy for obstructive sleep apnea in children: outcome evaluated by pre- and postoperative polysomnography. Laryngoscope. 2007;117(10):1844–54.
13. Mitchell RB, Kelly J. Outcome of adenotonsillectomy for obstructive sleep apnea in obese and normal weight children. Otolaryngol Head Neck Surg. 2007;137(1):43–8.
14. Muntz H, Wilson M, Park A, et al. Sleep disordered breathing and obstructive sleep apnea in the cleft population. Laryngoscope. 2008;118(2):348–53.
15. Leung KC, Cho H. Diagnosis of Stridor in children. Am Fam Physician. 1999;60:2289–96.
16. Gutierrez JP, Berkowitz RG, Robertson C. Vallecular cysts in newborns and young infants. Pediatr Pulmonol. 1999;27:282–5.
17. Chow PY, Nag DK, Poon G, Hui Y. Vallecular cyst in a neonate. Hong Kong Med J. 2002;8:464.
18. Myer CH. Vallecular cyst in the newborn. Ear Nose Throat J. 1988;67:122–4.
19. Gluckman PG, Chu TW, Van-Hasselt CA. Neonatal vallecular cyst and failure to thrive. J Laryngol Otol. 1992;106:448–9.
20. Santiago W, Rybak LP, Bass RM. Thyroglossal duct cyst of the tongue. J Otolaryngol. 1985;14:261–4.
21. Lee EY, Siegel MJ, Hildebolt CF, Gutierrez FR, Fallah JH. MDCT evaluation of thoracic aortic anomalies in pediatric patients and young adults: comparison of axial, multiplanar, and 3D images. AJR Am J Roentgenol. 2004;182:777–84.
22. Wittenborg MH, Gyepes MT, Crocker D. Tracheal dynamics in infants with respiratory distress, stridor, and collapsing trachea. Radiology. 1967;88:653–62.
23. Gruden JF, Webb WR, Sides DM. Adult onset disseminated tracheobronchial papillomatosis: CT features. J Comp Assist Tomogr. 1994;18:640–2.
24. Mahboubi S, Behhah RD. CT evaluation of tracheobronchial tumors in children. Int J Pediatr Otorhinolaryngol. 1992;24:135–43.
25. Cleveland RH. Symmetry of bronchial angles in children. Radiology. 1979;133:89–93.
26. Jaramillo D, Cleveland RH, Blickman JG. Radiologic management of esophageal foreign bodies. Semin Intervent Radiol. 1991;8:198–203.
27. Berdon WE, Baker DH. Vascular anomalies and the infant lung: rings, slings, and other things. Semin Roentgenol. 1972;7:39–64.
28. van Son JA, Konstantinov IE, Burckhard F. Kommerell and Kommerell's diverticulum. Tex Heart Inst J. 2002;29:109–12.
29. Mossad E, Ibraim F, Youssef G, et al. Diverticulum of Kommerell: a review of a series and a report of a case with tracheal deviation compromising single lung ventilation. Anesth Analg. 2002;94:1462–4.
30. Lee EY, Siegel MJ. MDCT of tracheobronchial narrowing in pediatric patients. J Thorac Imaging. 2007;22:300–9.
31. Karcaaltincaba M, Haliloglu M, Ekinci S. Partial tracheal duplication: MDCT bronchoscopic diagnosis. AJR Am J Roentgenol. 2004;183:290–2.
32. Dupuis C, Charaf LA, Breviere GM, Abou P. "Infantile" form of the scimitar syndrome with pulmonary hypertension. Am J Cardiol. 1993;71:1326–30.
33. Horcher E, Helmer F. Scimitar syndrome and associated pulmonary sequestration: report of a successfully corrected case. Prog Pediatr Surg. 1987;21:107–11.
34. McGuinness G, Naidich DP, Garay SM, Davis AL, Boyd AD, Mizrachi HH. Accessory cardiac bronchus: CT features and clinical significance. Radiology. 1993;189:563–6.
35. Cleveland RH, Mark EJ. Case records of the Massachusetts General Hospital: Case #31-1998. New Eng J Med 1998;339:1144–1152.

36. Woodring JH, Barrett PA, Rehm SR, Nurenberg P. Acauired tracheomegaly in adults as a complication of diffuse pulmonary fibrosis. AJR 1989;152:743–747.

37. Cleveland RH, Neish AS, Nichols DP, Zurakowski D, Wohl MEB, Colin AA. Cystic fibrosis: a system for assessing and predicting progression. AJR Am J Roentgenol. 1998;170:1067–72.

38. Cleveland RH, Neish AS, Nichols DP, Zurakowski D, Wohl MEB, Colin AA. Cystic fibrosis: predictors of accelerated decline and distribution of disease in 230 patients. AJR Am J Roentgenol. 1998; 171:1311–5.

39. Cleveland R. Congenital lobar emphysema: case 4. In: Siegel MJ, Bisset GS, Cleveland RH, Donaldson JS, Fellows KE, Patriquin HB, editors. ACR pediatric disease (fourth series) test and syllabus. Reston: American College of Radiology; 1993. p. 96–130.

40. Cleveland RH, Weber B. Retained fetal lung liquid in congenital lobar emphysema: a possible predictor of polyalveolar lobe. Pediatr Radiol. 1993;23:291–5.

41. Cleveland RH. A radiologic update on medical diseases of the newborn chest. Pediatr Radiol. 1995;25:631–7.

42. Padley SP, Adler BD, Hansell DM, Muller NL. Bronchiolitis obliterans: high resolution CT findings and correlation with pulmonary function tests. Clin Radiol. 1993;47:236–40.

43. Bramson RT, Cleveland RH, Blickman JG, Kinane TB. The radiographic appearance of follicular bronchitis in children. AJR Am J Roentgenol. 1996;166:1447–50.

44. Brody AS, Crotty EJ. Neuroendocrine cell hyperplasia of infancy (NEHI). Pediatr Radiol. 2006;36:1328.

Newborn Chest*

7

ROBERT H. CLEVELAND AND LAWRENCE RHEIN

CONTENTS

*Portions of this chapter are reprinted from Cleveland RH. A radiologic update on medical diseases of the newborn chest. Pediatr Radiol. 1995;25:631–7; and Cleveland R, Donoghue V. Imaging of the newborn chest. Syllabus IDKD: diseases of the heart, chest & breast. Milan: Springer-Verlag Italia; 2007. p. 55–62, with permission.

ROBERT H. CLEVELAND, MD (✉)
Department of Radiology, Harvard Medical School,
Boston, MA, USA
e-mail: Robert.Cleveland@childrens.harvard.edu

Departments of Radiology and Medicine, Division
of Respiratory Diseases, Children's Hospital Boston,
Boston, MA, USA

LAWRENCE RHEIN, MD
Center for Healthy Infant Lung Development,
Divisions of Newborn Medicine and Respiratory Diseases,
Children's Hospital Boston, Boston, MA, USA

This chapter reviews the common spectrum of disorders of the neonatal chest. Emphasis is on radiographic changes that have been produced by the introduction of new therapeutic maneuvers, particularly the use of artificial surfactant in treating hyaline membrane disease (HMD) and the survival of profoundly premature newborns (less than 650 g). A discussion of meconium aspiration syndrome (MAS), neonatal pneumonia, transient tachypnea of the newborn (TTN), congenital lymphangiectasia, and congenital heart disease is also included. The effect on the neonatal chest radiograph of extracorporeal membrane oxygenation (ECMO) and high-frequency ventilation are also mentioned [1, 2]. Some have paid particular attention to lung volume as a differentiating criterion of these lesions. Generally, HMD and neonatal pneumonia have been associated with low lung volumes, while congenital lymphangiectasia, MAS and transient tachypnea have been associated with normal or increased lung volumes. However, many initial images are obtained only after the baby has been intubated and the lungs have been artificially inflated. There is also a considerable occurrence of concomitant diseases, i.e., HMD with pneumonia or transient tachypnea. Hence, there is no discussion of differentiating diseases based on lung volume. A review of *surgical* lesions is provided elsewhere (see Sects. 11.2, 11.3, and 11.5).

Although cross-sectional and ultrasound imaging have specific but limited roles in assessing the newborn chest, the standard chest radiograph remains the most common imaging tool. The spectrum of diseases that affect the neonate's chest have significant overlap in their radiographic and clinical appearances. Therefore, an open exchange of information between the neonatologist and the radiologist is critical to the intelligent interpretation of these images.

The main disease entities of concern are HMD, bronchopulmonary dysplasia (BPD), MAS, neonatal pneumonia, and TTN. Congenital lymphangiectasia may mimic the findings of TTN, MAS or neonatal pneumonia. Congenital heart disease may be present in a fashion that is easily confused with a pulmonary parenchymal process. This is most common when the heart remains normal in size, but there is pulmonary venous hypertension. Specific infective organisms such as *Chlamydia trachomatis* or viruses, which are acquired during or following birth, may be present within the neonatal period with clinical and radiographic findings. These findings may be easily confused with one or several of the above-mentioned entities.

7.1 Hyaline Membrane Disease

HMD is the nonspecific histological name, used interchangeably with the term respiratory distress syndrome (RDS), which reflects the clinical manifestation of pulmonary immaturity, seen predominantly in children less than 36–38 weeks of gestational age weighing less than 2.5 kg. Rates of HMD are inversely proportional to gestational age. However, while HMD is most common in the extremely premature infant, HMD due to relative surfactant deficiency in the late preterm or even term infant are commonly observed. Term infants of mothers with poorly controlled diabetes may present with RDS because fetal hyperinsulinism interferes with the glucocorticoid axis that governs surfactant biosynthesis. HMD remains the leading cause of death in live born infants. The death rate is highest in the most premature with few deaths occurring in infants weighing more than 1.5 kg. Males are affected almost twice as often as females, and HMD is more common in whites than blacks.

The disease results from deficiency of surfactant in the lungs, which leads to the inability to maintain acinar distention. Exposure to air can then rapidly lead to the development of hyaline membranes containing fibrin and cellular debris. There frequently is epithelial necrosis beneath the hyaline membranes. By the second day of life, repair has begun with proliferation of type 2 pneumocytes (which produce surfactant) and increased secretions [3]. In the current era of available surfactant replacement and/or early use of continuous positive airway pressure (CPAP) most cases of HMD improve. In severe cases, the lungs can become almost impossible to inflate and on gross inspection, may appear similar to liver.

Infants that survive HMD but go on to require continued ventilatory support, including positive pressure ventilation and supplemental oxygen, develop a significant chance of developing bronchopulmonary dysplasia (BPD), which is discussed in further detail in a later section.

Clinically, infants with HMD are usually symptomatic within minutes of birth, with grunting, nasal flaring, retractions, tachypnea and cyanosis. It may be a few hours before symptoms are recognized, however. Although the initial radiographic findings may be noted minutes after birth, occasionally the maximum radiographic findings are not present until 12–24 h of life. For most premature infants with HMD, the radiographic finding is an evenly distributed, finely granular opacification seen throughout both lungs (Fig. 7.1). This is so characteristic, that if the opacification is uneven it suggests a different, or multiple etiologies, such as TTN, or neonatal pneumonia. The exception is seen occasionally in near term boys where there may be mild accentuation of opacification in the lung bases (Fig. 7.2). Bile acid pneumonia [4] may produce a pattern identical to HMD. This diagnosis may be suspected in newborns of mothers with severe intrahepatic cholestasis of pregnancy. This is especially true if indices of lung maturity are good and the baby has high serum bile acid levels.

The rigid, noncompliant lungs and the associated hypoxia and acidosis of HMD often result in persistent pulmonary hypertension. As pulmonary resistance decreases, there may be the onset of left to right shunting across a patent ductus arteriosus (Fig. 7.3). This may be recognized radiographically before clinical symptoms of a murmur develop. It is heralded by the development of pulmonary edema and, on occasion, a suddenly enlarging heart size. The ductus arteriosus can only respond to stimuli to close if it is term or near term in development. These stimuli include a normal oxygen level, a normal pH, and normal levels of prostaglandin E1 and E2. In the premature newborn with HMD, the ductus is open, but the pulmonary and systemic pressures may be equal or the pulmonary pressure may exceed systemic, precluding left to right shunting. These babies are usually hypoxic and acidotic with high levels of prostaglandin E1 and E2 [5]. By several days of life, as the pulmonary resistance drops, if the ductus is not responsive or the stimuli are not present, the ductus arteriosus will remain open allowing left to right shunting and the development of congestive heart failure. Treatment with cyclooxygenase inhibitors such as ibuprofen or indomethacin (by inhibiting production of prostaglandin) may produce ductal closure but also increase the risk of inducing gastrointestinal perforation and/or osteoarthropathy.

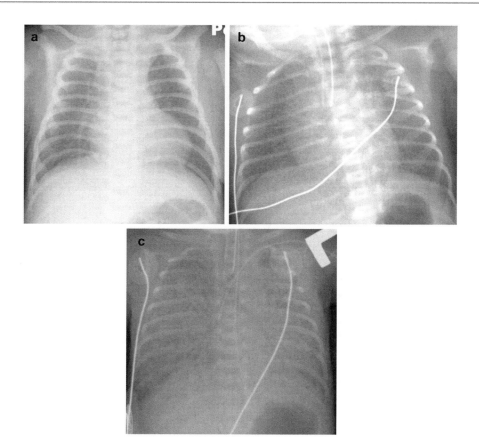

Fig. 7.1. Uncomplicated HMD is an evenly distributed, fine granular opacification. It may vary from patient to patient in its clinical and imaging severity. (**a**) Mild HMD. (**b**) Moderate HMD. (**c**) Severe HMD

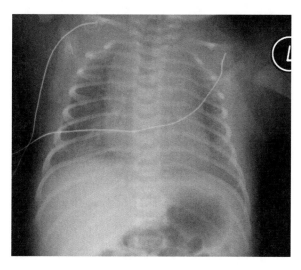

Fig. 7.2. HMD in near term boys may be irregular in its distribution, usually accentuated in the lung bases as in this 36-week gestational age newborn boy

Surgery may be required to close a persistent patent ductus arteriosus.

Sudden diffuse opacification of the lungs in HMD may be seen with other conditions in addition to pulmonary edema from a PDA or fluid overload (Fig. 7.4).

A frequent cause is atelectesis due to decreasing ventilatory support. Less commonly, diffuse pulmonary hemorrhage may be a cause. Rarely, sudden catastrophic intracranial hemorrhage may produce pulmonary edema that is central nervous system-mediated.

Since Northway's original description of bronchopulmonary dysplasia (BPD) in 1967 [6], many changes have occurred in the management and outcome of children with HMD, as well as in the definition of BPD itself. Much has been learned about the specific toxic effects of oxygen and assisted ventilation. Babies of much lower gestational age and birth weight are surviving with HMD, particularly since the advent of high-frequency ventilation and the use of artificial surfactant. The likelihood of developing BPD or retinopathy of prematurity and their severity has diminished with successful attempts at keeping inspired oxygen at or below 60% (FiO_2 less than 0.6), keeping ventilatory pressures and rate as low as possible, and extubating as soon as possible. Infants at greatest risk for developing BPD (also referred to as chronic lung disease of prematurity or CLD) are the profoundly premature who require longer courses of assisted ventilation at greater pressures and rate and

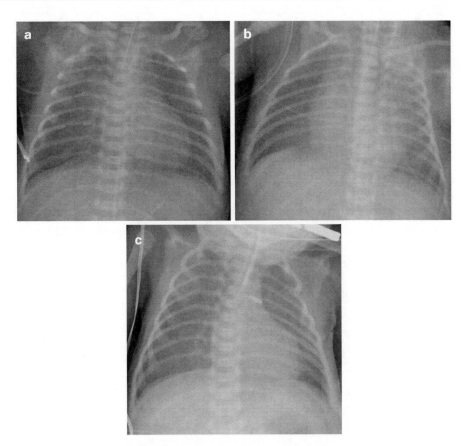

Fig. 7.3. Pulmonary edema, usually the result of left to right shunting across a patient ductus arteriosus, is a relatively common complication in premature infants. (**a**) Moderately severe HMD in a 1 day old. (**b**) Increased hazy opacification, accentuated centrally, on the third day of life consistent with the interval development of pulmonary edema. (**c**) The edema has diminished following surgical closure of the PDA (a ductus clip overlies the left hilus)

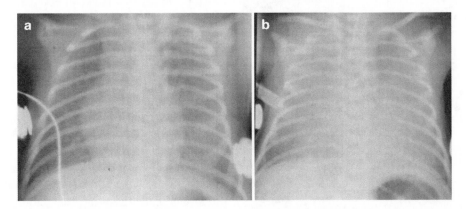

Fig. 7.4. Sudden onset of a *white out* has several possible explanations. (**a**) Moderately severe HMD on day 2 of life. (**b**) This image was obtained 2 days later, approximately 15 min after a moderate decrease in peek end expiratory pressure
(PEEP). There is a dramatic increase in diffuse pulmonary opacification. The baby was stable at this time with a subsequent image no longer showing the *white out*

higher inspired oxygen concentration (FiO$_2$ of 0.6–1.0). Infants with barotrauma and resultant air leak phenomenon (pulmonary interstitial emphysema [PIE], pneumothorax, pneumomediastinum, or pneumopericardium) (Fig. 7.5) also usually require prolonged

treatment with higher oxygen concentration. With improvements in neonatal intensive care, it is now rare to see the development of the classic four stages of BPD as described by Northway et al. [6] (Fig. 7.6). However, in cases of severe classic BPD, the

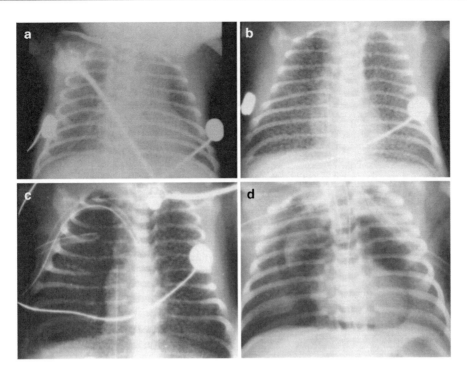

Fig. 7.5. The incidence of air leak phenomenon has decreased with the use of high-frequency ventilation. (**a**) Moderate HMD on day 1 of life. (**b**) Diffuse PIE has developed by day 3. (**c**) Right pneumothorax developed shortly afterward. (**d**) Air surrounding the heart, lifting the right lobe of the thymus off the heart indicates the presence of a pneumomediastinum or pneumopericardium. Air outlining the inferior heart is more commonly seen in pneumopericardium, but may be seen with a pneumomediastinum as is the case in this baby with air in the subcutaneous tissues of the right shoulder/neck

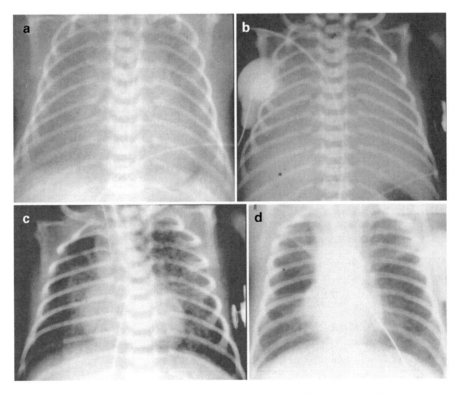

Fig. 7.6. With modern management of HMD, the four stages of BPD as originally described by Northway [6] is rarely encountered. (**a**) Stage 1: HMD on day 1. (**b**) Stage 2: *white out* on day 3. (**c**) Stage 3: BPD on day 21. (**d**) Stage 4: BPD at 6 weeks

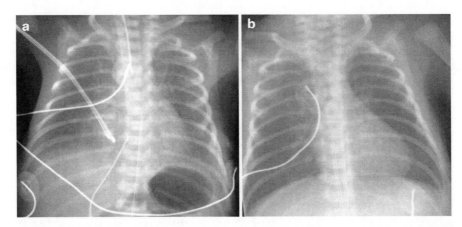

Fig. 7.7. Most cases of mild to moderate HMD resolve without developing BPD. (a) Moderate HMD on day 1. (b) By day 6, the crisp, finely granular appearance of HMD seen on day 1 has become less distinctly defined and is now irregular in its distribution. The baby's HMD resolved without pulmonary sequelae

histopathology reveals alternating areas of overinflation with fibrosis and atelectasis, associated with severe airway injury. In children successfully managed with short courses of assisted ventilation and FiO_2 below 0.4–0.6, the usual radiographic course is to evolve from HMD to a hazy diffuse opacification of the lungs to normal over a period of several days to 2 or 3 weeks (Fig. 7.7).

A different form of BPD was described in 1999 [7] referred to as *new BPD* which occurs in immature infants with minimal lung disease after birth. Symptoms often develop after the first week of life. The disease is attributed to aberrant lung development with inhibition of alveolar and vascular development. Some suspect that this *new BPD* is in fact what has been previously referred to as Wilson–Mikity syndrome [8]. Radiographically, BPD and *new BPD* or Wilson–Mikity syndrome are indistinguishable.

Several emerging technologies have greatly altered the clinical and radiographic evolution of children with HMD. Randomized controlled trials have shown that antenatal corticosteroid administration reduces the incidence of RDS, based on the rationale that glucocorticoids accelerate lung maturation. Current National Institutes of Health consensus guidelines on antenatal corticosteroid use recommend that all pregnant women should be considered eligible for a single course of corticosteroids during 24–34 weeks gestation.

Two different strategies in the early perinatal period also have helped decrease sequelae of HMD: (1) prophylactic use of CPAP to maintain acinar distension and (2) prophylactic administration of exogenous surfactant. Although the number of institutions that have successfully managed most of their prema-ture infants with prophylactic nasal CPAP in the delivery room has been limited, more recent studies suggest that this strategy will be more commonly utilized.

The efficacy and safety of surfactant replacement therapy to improve oxygenation, decrease the need for mechanical ventilation, and reduce mortality in neonates with respiratory failure from RDS have been established in multiple randomized controlled clinical trials. However, the long-term consequences of HMD, such as BPD, have not been clearly altered [9–11]. The use of artificial surfactant has produced several significant changes in radiographic configurations. The surfactant is given as liquid boluses via an ET tube. Frequently the surfactant is not evenly distributed throughout the lungs. Therefore, it is common to see areas of lung which may rapidly improve in aeration alternating with areas of unchanged HMD. The uneven distribution produces a radiograph that may simulate other entities such as neonatal pneumonia or MAS. In addition, the surfactant may reach the level of the acinae causing sudden and effective distention of multiple acinar units producing a radiographic configuration quite suggestive of PIE [12]. In these situations, close communication with the neonatologist to ascertain clinical status is mandatory to the intelligent interpretation of the radiograph. Babies with positive response to surfactant generally improve at this point, while those with PIE deteriorate. Those babies with PIE usually resolve the interstitial air over a period of a few days. However, rarely, the interstitial air may persist and enlarge. This may be severe enough to expand the involved segment of lung causing mass effect and further respiratory distress. Occasionally the PIE may coalesce into a giant interstitial bleb. Many of these eventually resolve spontaneously, but some will require

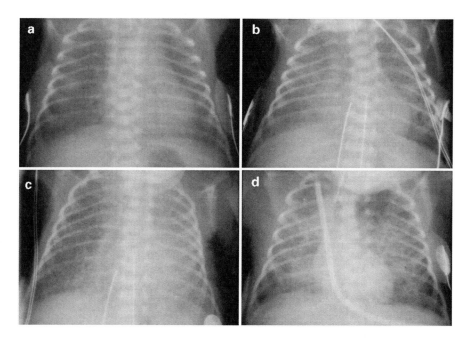

Fig. 7.8. BPD developing within the first few days is now being encountered with the survival of babies of very low birth weight. (**a**) 550 g premature with HMD at 2 h of age with mild HMD. (**b**) By 36 h of age a configuration similar to Northway's Stage 3 BPD is noted. (**c**) By day 4 there is continued evolution of BPD, or as it has become known, chronic lung disease of prematurity. (**d**) By the ninth day of life, the BPD is well established

surgical resection. Although not usually necessary to establish the diagnosis, CT may show a characteristic *line and dot* pattern [13].

High-frequency ventilation (HiFi) (10–15 Hz, 600–900 cycles/min) has also been employed to reduce the incidence of barotrauma [14]. The peaks and valleys of conventional ventilation with abruptly alternating peak inspiratory pressure and end expiratory pressure produce a *water hammer* effect. HiFi with its more consistently even pressure reduces the degree of barotrauma. For both of these modalities the overall improvement in long-term prognosis is yet to be determined. The radiographs of babies receiving HiFi are not significantly altered from that noted with conventional ventilator therapy. However, the degree of pulmonary inflation is used to adjust mean airway pressure (MAP). Ideally, the dome of the diaphragm should project over the 8–10 posterior rib if MAP is appropriately adjusted.

With advances in medical management, more profoundly premature babies are being maintained and salvaged. It is not uncommon today for babies weighing as little as 650 g to be successfully treated and survive their prematurity. The radiographic presentation of these babies may differ from that of the more gestationally mature. In this profoundly premature age group, it is common that initial radiographs performed within the first few hours to 2 days

of life may be normal or nearly normal with only minimal evidence of HMD. Then, suddenly, over a period of 2–3 days the radiographic pattern (Fig. 7.8) may evolve into a much coarser and somewhat irregularly distributed lung disease similar to that seen in Northway's stage three BPD (a situation originally described as occurring at several weeks of age) [6].

In spite of the advances in management of these babies, many of the survivors develop the chronic pulmonary manifestations of Northway's stage 4 BPD [6]. This consists of alternating areas of fibrosis/atelectasis and focal overexpansion of lung. These findings have been documented by CT in older children and adults and expectedly are represented by areas of linear opacities and areas of ground glass opacification alternating with areas of decreased attenuation and perfusion (focal overinflation). There is diffuse bronchial wall thickening and decreased bronchus to pulmonary artery diameter ratios [15].

7.2 Meconium Aspiration Syndrome

MAS is the result of intrapartum or intrauterine aspiration of meconium. It most commonly occurs in babies who are post mature; the mean gestational age for MAS has been reported as 290 days or 10 days past the expected date of delivery. MAS may also occur in infants who are small for gestational age, or in infants that have been exposed to intrauterine stress causing hypoxemia. Although there is meconium staining of the amniotic fluid in approximately 10–15% of live births, MAS, which is diagnosed by the presence of meconium in the airway below the vocal cords, is seen in 1–5% of newborns.

The radiographic findings in MAS vary, in part secondary to the severity of the aspiration. The tenacious meconium often will cause both medium and small airway obstruction, even after vigorous endobronchial suctioning. This typically will cause areas of atelectasis alternating with areas of overinflation (Fig. 7.9). The meconium is an irritant to bronchial mucosa and may cause a chemical pneumonia. This increases the risk for subsequent gram-negative bacterial infection. Hypoxia usually results, with all factors combining to produce pulmonary hypertension, referred to as persistent fetal circulation (PFC). As vigorous suctioning and aggressive therapy with endotracheal intubation and ventilatory support are often required, it is not surprising that air leak phenomenon is encountered, with pneumothorax present in 25–40% of cases. Occasionally, however, babies with MAS requiring ventilatory support will have a normal chest X-ray or possibly only a pneumothorax. Small pleural effusions are also seen in approximately 10% of cases. The chest X-rays of infants with MAS may be indistinguishable from children with neonatal pneumonia. Because of the difficulty in excluding neonatal pneumonia and the possibility of

developing a superimposed pneumonia in MAS, most of these infants are treated with antibiotics. On rare occasions, an early follow-up radiograph shortly after initiation of aggressive suctioning will show dramatic improvement in pulmonary opacifications (possibly mimicking the clearing of TTN). However, in these cases of MAS, the clinical condition does not improve in parallel with the radiograph and subsequent images fail to show similar continued rapid clearing of the abnormality (as would be expected with TTN).

In spite of optimal care, there is a persistent mortality rate of up to 25% in babies with MAS. This has been partly mitigated by the use of inhaled nitric oxide (iNO) to treat severe pulmonary hypertension, and ECMO. Since ECMO has potentially life-threatening side effects including hemorrhage, frequently into the brain, its use is limited to babies who have failed conventional therapy. Survival rates with ECMO have been excellent. The most critical factor in weaning from ECMO is not simply improved pulmonary mechanics, but reduction of pulmonary vascular pressure to below systemic. Some have postulated a primary abnormality of pulmonary microcirculation in MAS. However, others feel that the increased pressures within the airways, produced by assisted ventilation, are the cause of PFC in these babies. ECMO, which bypasses the lungs, allows pulmonary inflation to be at a minimum while maintaining physiologic levels of oxygen tension and saturation [16–18]. In addition, there is significant third space fluid deposition while on ECMO. Therefore, on ECMO the lungs are usually nearly or

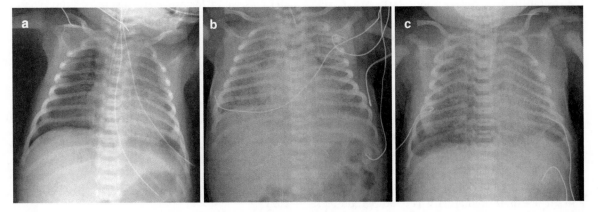

Fig. 7.9. MAS may present radiographically in several manners. (**a**) It may present as ill defined focal opacifications as in this baby's left lower lobe and to a lesser degree the right lower lobe. There is a right pneumothorax seen as a lucent line paralleling the superior mediastinum (medial pneumothorax) and inferolaterally. (**b**) More typically, MAS may present as course irregular opacification. (**c**) There may be a combination of coarse, irregular opacifications and focal consolidations (left lower lobe in this baby). There is a right pneumothorax

completely airless (Fig. 7.10). There are two types of ECMO. One technique is to place a venous catheter into a jugular vein, usually the right, with the tip in the superior vena cava (SVC)/right atrium distribution. This catheter withdraws unoxygenated blood for passage through the membrane oxygenator. An arterial catheter is placed into a carotid artery, usually the right, with its tip in the distal aortic arch to provide oxygenated blood to the patient's systemic circulation. This is referred to as VA ECMO. This almost inevitably leads to occlusion of the carotid artery after the catheter is removed. To avoid sacrificing the carotid artery, an alternative technique was developed referred to as VV ECMO. This employs a single double lumen venous catheter, also placed in the jugular vein. The tip is situated at the level of the

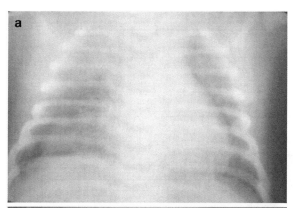

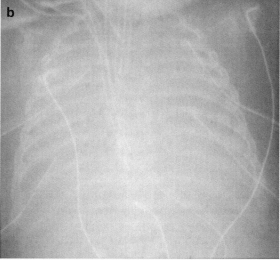

Fig. 7.10. The survival of infants with MAS may require the use of ECMO. (**a**) Eight hour old with severe MAS. (**b**) Once this baby was placed on ECMO, the lungs became airless. The ECMO cannulae are appropriately placed with the venous line tip in the right atrium and the arterial line tip in the distal aortic arch

tricuspid valve. A venous port withdraws unoxygenated blood; an arterial port perfuses oxygenated blood directed at the tricuspid valve for access to the patient's circulation.

7.3 Neonatal Pneumonia

Neonatal pneumonia is seen in less than 1% of live born infants. Premature infants are at increased risk. It may be acquired in utero, during labor, at delivery or shortly after birth. The major risk factor for intra-uterine development of pneumonia is prolonged rupture of the membranes, particularly if labor is active during this period. Some organisms, particularly viruses, may cross the placenta. Group B streptococcus infections are currently the most common cause of pneumonia in the newborn with an incidence of 3/1,000 live births and are acquired in utero or during labor and delivery [19]. Both clinically and radiographically, it may be difficult to distinguish this infection from HMD. Chest radiographs may reveal lung disease identical to HMD; however, pleural effusions are more commonly associated with pneumonia (in up to 67%) and essentially never with uncomplicated HMD [19]. In neonatal pneumonia, the lungs may reveal irregular patchy infiltrates (Fig. 7.11) or occasionally be normal. There may be mild cardiac enlargement with pneumonia but it is unusual with uncomplicated HMD (Fig. 7.12) [20]. Infections with other bacterial organisms may produce radiographic findings identical to those described above in group B streptococcal infections [21, 22]. Although initially the specific infecting organism may not be discernable except by culture, an unusual clinical and imaging course has been described with *Ureaplasma urealyticum*. This has been characterized as having a milder acute course but early onset of chronic lung disease [22]. HMD and neonatal pneumonia frequently coexist.

Both neonatal pneumonia and MAS most commonly present with irregularly distributed, somewhat coarse airspace opacifications. Generally the coarseness of the opacifications is more accentuated in MAS, but not consistently enough to allow precise differentiation. These imaging findings may also be seen with TTN. However, with TTN the radiographic and clinical courses improve rapidly in parallel over the first 1–3 days of life.

There have been several infants reported [23] with late onset (at several days of life) right-sided

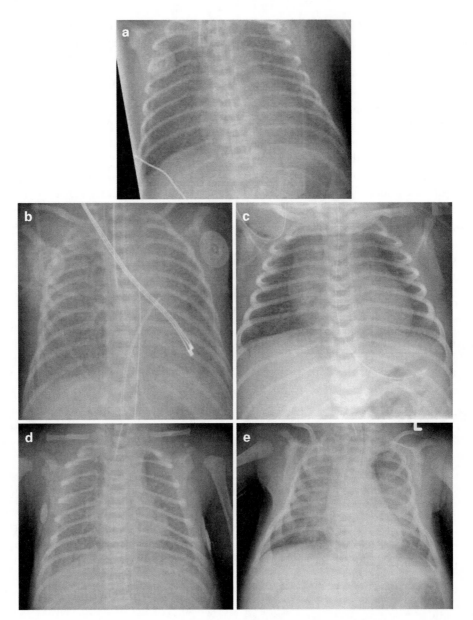

Fig. 7.11. Neonatal pneumonia has variable radiographic characteristics. (**a**) It may simulate mild HMD, except in this patient it is somewhat accentuated in the left lower lobe. (**b**) It may simulate severe HMD, except in this baby there are slightly accentuated focal opacities in the left upper lobe and left lower lobe. (**c**) It may present as a focal infiltrate as in this baby's left lower lobe. (**d**) The opacification may be coarse and irregularly distributed. There are bilateral effusions as well. (**e**) The opacifications may be classically alveolar

diaphragmatic hernia in association with neonatal pneumonia. At surgery, there are no distinguishing characteristics of the hernia to suggest a specific effect of the pneumonia or of sepsis. These cases presumably represent late onset of herniation of liver and intestine through a preexisting, congenital diaphragmatic defect.

The presence of pleural effusions or pneumothorax differ based on the underlying pathology and may be an aid to determining the correct diagnosis (Fig. 7.13). The location of a pneumothorax in a newborn, as is true for all individuals imaged in supine position, may best be seen medially, along the mediastinal border [24]. The anteriormedial chest in a supine patient is the most superior portion of the thorax. Without pleural adhesions to restrict free flow of air in the pleural space, the air will accumulate anteriorly and first be apparent as an air/pleural interface medially adjacent to the heart border. As the pneumothorax enlarges, it will become apparent inferiorly, subpulmonic. As it further increases, it will be seen laterally and inferiorly and finally over the pulmonary apex. The opposite is true for free flowing pleural effusions. Small effusions are most apparent over the pulmonary apex and in the medial, inferior costophrenic sulcus.

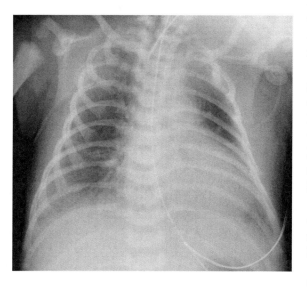

Fig. 7.12. The presence of moderate cardiac enlargement in a baby with coarse, irregularly distributed disease (left lower and right lower lobes) suggests neonatal pneumonia

7.4 Transient Tachypnea of the Newborn

TTN is also referred to as retained fetal lung liquid. Fetal lung liquid is an ultrafiltrate of fetal serum. Under normal circumstances it is cleared from the lungs at or shortly after birth via the tracheobronchial system (30%), the interstitial lymphatics (30%) and the capillaries (40%). TTN is most commonly seen in infants born by cesarean section but may also be identified in children who are quite small or who have experienced a precipitous delivery. The lungs usually are diffusely affected with a variable characterization, which may range from an appearance similar or identical to HMD, a coarse interstitial pattern similar to pulmonary edema (Fig. 7.14) or an irregular opacification as may be seen with meconium aspiration or neonatal pneumonia (Fig. 7.15). A pleural effusion is a common accompaniment. A transient slight cardiac enlargement may occur. The hallmark of this process is a relatively benign clinical course (i.e., tachypnea) as compared to the overall severity of disease suggested by chest X-ray, i.e., if there is no endotracheal tube (ETT) or other ventilatory support in a child with significant lung abnormalities on chest X-ray.

Clearing of the process should occur rapidly (1–2 days). In particularly severe cases, where clearing may require up to 3 days, there should be a rapid improvement on each successive image.

Focal retention of fetal lung liquid within congenital lobar emphysema has been recognized for several years. One publication suggests that the focal retention of fetal lung liquid occurs only, or mainly,

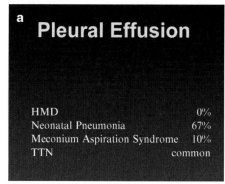
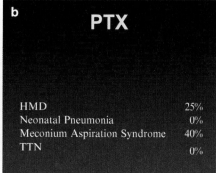

a Pleural Effusion		b PTX	
HMD	0%	HMD	25%
Neonatal Pneumonia	67%	Neonatal Pneumonia	0%
Meconium Aspiration Syndrome	10%	Meconium Aspiration Syndrome	40%
TTN	common	TTN	0%

Fig. 7.13. The presence of a pneumothorax or pleural effusion is an aid in making the correct diagnosis. (**a**) Causes of pleural effusion. (**b**) Causes of pneumothorax. With the advent of the use of artificial surfactant and HiFi, the incidence of pneumothorax in HMD has dramatically diminished below 25%

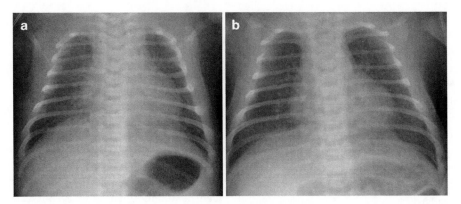

Fig. 7.14. TTN may mimic the image of HMD or neonatal pneumonia. (**a**) At 1.5 h of age there is a diffuse granular opacification with bibasilar alveolar accentuation, but no ET tube. (**b**) By 10 h, the opacifications have almost resolved

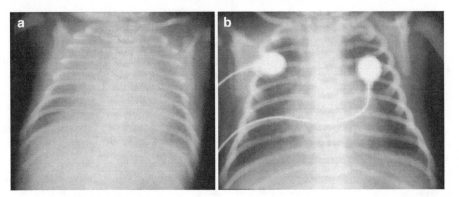

Fig. 7.15. Severe TTN may mimic MAS or alveolar infiltrates of neonatal pneumonia. (**a**) At 3 h of age there are dense multifocal alveolar opacifications, bilateral effusions, and possible heart enlargement, but no ET tube. (**b**) By the third day of life, the focal opacifications have markedly improved, the effusions have resolved and the heart is at the upper limits of normal

within polyalveolar lobes rather than classic congenital lobar emphysema [25].

7.5   Congenital Lymphangiectasia

Babies with congenital lymphangiectasia may present with symptoms similar to HMD. The lungs may be normal or reveal a course interstitial infiltrate secondary to the distended and abnormally draining lymphatics. There may be generalized overinflation. Pleural effusions may be present [26]. A particularly large pleural effusion should suggest this diagnosis or may be related to a traumatic chylous or hemorrhagic effusion (Fig. 7.16). The presence of a chylous effusion without a history of trauma is suggestive of congenital lymphangiectasia although isolated chylous effusions do occur. This diagnosis is best made by sampling of the pleural effusion following the administration of fatty foods. Although prominent interlobular septae, ground glass opacifications and subpleural fluid/pleural fluid demonstrated on CT are suggestive of this

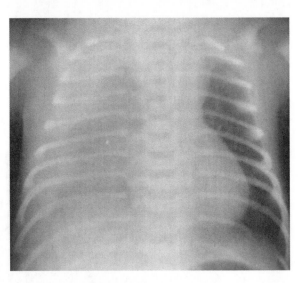

Fig. 7.16. The presence of the large right effusion suggests hemothorax or chylothorax

diagnosis [27], the findings are very nonspecific. Although historical descriptions of neonatal congenital pulmonary lymphangiectasia suggested that it was uniformly fatal, more recent experience suggests that a milder form exists. Conservative nutritional management with parenteral nutrition, high-MCT formula feeding, and gradual transition to normal feeds may be successful in such cases.

7.6 Congenital Heart Disease

Cases of congenital heart disease may closely mimic several of the entities mentioned previously. The presence of pulmonary interstitial edema may be difficult to distinguish from HMD, neonatal pneumonia or TTN.

A particularly confusing constellation of chest findings may occur in congenital heart lesions producing obstruction to pulmonary venous return but without significant cardiac enlargement. This includes congenital obstructing lesions which occur at the level of the mitral valve or between the mitral valve and the pulmonary venous system. Specifically, these lesions include mitral valve stenosis, supravalvular mitral stenosis, cor triatriatum, stenosis of a common pulmonary vein or total anomalous pulmonary venous connection (TAPVC) with obstruction. TAPVC physiologically may present with or without obstruction. If obstruction is sufficient, children will present in the first week of life with cyanosis (in severe cases) or with signs of pulmonary edema, dyspnea, and feeding difficulties (in less severe cases). A chest radiograph will show evidence of pulmonary venous hypertension but without an enlarged heart (Fig. 7.17). If there is little or no obstruction to venous return, the children usually present with high output failure at 6–12 months of age with a radiograph suggestive of congestive heart failure. Several reviews have revealed an overall incidence of obstruction in TAPVC of 50–65%. With supradiaphragmatic draining veins, obstruction has been noted in up to 53% of cases. Essentially, all subdiaphragmatic draining veins are obstructed [19].

If the heart is significantly enlarged, the likelihood that the baby has true congestive heart failure is suggested. Within the first week of life, before the pulmonary vascular resistance drops sufficiently to allow left to right shunting, congestive heart failure is usually secondary to pressure overload, obligatory volume overload or myocardial dysfunction. The lesions most commonly producing this phenomenon include critical aortic stenosis, hypoplastic left heart syndrome, coarctation of the aorta (interruption of the aortic arch), myocarditis,

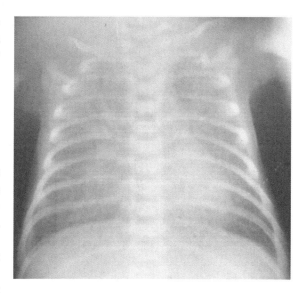

Fig. 7.17. The presence of pulmonary edema with a normal sized heart suggests mechanical obstruction of pulmonary venous return. In this child with cor triatriatum, there is also a small right effusion. In the correct clinical setting, this image could have represented TTN, neonatal pneumonia or MAS

dysrhythmias, myocardial ischemia, and arterial venous fistula. Significant arterial shunting outside the heart, such as vein of Galen aneurysm, hepatic hemangioma or hemangioendothelioma may also produce congestive failure in this time period. By the second week of life, after pulmonary resistance has dropped sufficiently, volume overload lesions are the predominant cause for congestive failure. This includes ventricular septal defect, endocardial cushion defect, patent ductus arteriosus, aortopulmonic window, as well as milder forms of those lesions potentially presenting within the first week of life. Children with untreated hypoplastic left heart syndrome may live beyond the first week and are therefore a potential category of children having congestive heart failure in the older age group [28].

7.7 Chlamydia Pneumonia

Chlamydia pneumonia is caused by a bacterial-like intracellular parasite, C. trachomatis [29–31], which is acquired from the mother by direct contact during vaginal delivery. This organism is widely distributed, having been identified in the vagina of up to 13% of women tested. Up to 50% of babies infected become symptomatic with conjunctivitis. This most common manifestation usually appears around 5–14 days of life. Pneumonia develops in 10–20% of infected

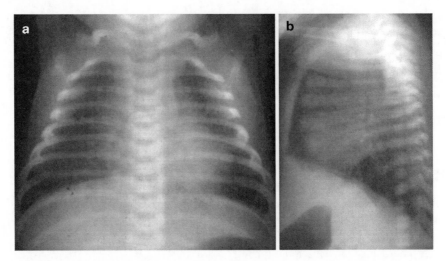

Fig. 7.18. This 26-day-old girl presented at the time of a well baby checkup with no symptoms but faint crackles heard in both lungs. There is a diffuse interstitial infiltrate, bibasilar ill defined alveolar opacifications and hyperinflation. The imaging findings are worse than anticipated based on the clinical findings. (**a**) PA image. (**b**) Lateral image

babies, appearing between 2 weeks and 3 months of age. However, the average age of onset is 6 weeks; therefore, Chlamydia pneumonia is somewhat unusual in the neonatal age group. Cough, sometimes paroxysmal and associated with tachypnea, is the most common symptom of this disease. It may be preceded by nasal obstruction or discharge. Up to 50% of infants with Chlamydia pneumonia will have conjunctivitis and up to 50% will have peripheral eosinophilia with absolute blood eosinophil levels in excess of 300/mm^3. Not uncommonly, the findings on chest radiograph are far worse than would be predicted by physical examination (Fig. 7.18). The findings may range from a purely interstitial process to a focal alveolar infiltrate. Hyperinflation is generalized, and pleural effusions are uncommon. Occasionally there will be a diffuse linear opacification closely mimicking congenital lymphangiectasia, obstructed pulmonary venous return, or possibly bacterial pneumonia or meconium aspiration.

7.8   Lines and Tubes

What is considered to be the *correct* position of various lines and tubes used for support purposes varies from institution to institution. The following discussions reflect the current practice in our institution. Since opinion concerning *safe and appropriate* positioning changes frequently and varies from institution to institution and physician to physician, the following should not be taken as recommendations

but merely a reporting of current practice at the author's institution.

7.8.1   Endotracheal Tubes

ETTs in neonates commonly do not have inflatable cuffs. Therefore many neonatalogists attempt to maintain the ETT tip within the intrathoracic trachea, i.e., between the thoracic inlet and the carina. The thoracic inlet is anatomically defined as a plane extending from the first thoracic vertebral body (T1) to the medial end of the clavicles. At the level of the thoracic inlet, the trachea is midway between the T1 vertebral body and the medial end of the clavicles. Therefore, for purposes of chest X-ray assessment, the level of the thoracic inlet in reference to the trachea is the midpoint between the body of T1 and the medial end of the clavicles.

It has been demonstrated that the tip of the ETT in neonates may move a distance equal to the length of the intrathoracic trachea when the head is moved from complete flexion to complete extension. Therefore, the *correct* position of an ETT must relate to head position and the level of the ETT tip. The ETT tip moves inferiorly with flexion of the head and superiorly with extension of the head [32]. Therefore, if the chin is flexed upon the chest wall, the ETT tube tip should be very slightly above the carina. If the head is quite extended and rotated laterally, the ETT tip should be slightly below a point midway between the TI vertebral body and the clavicles. Some institutions will reference the ETT tip to a vertebral body.

Since differences in X-ray beam angle, i.e., straight anterior–posterior vs. lordotic, will alter the way the ETT tip projects over the spine, using only the vertebral level is a less accurate means of assessment.

7.8.2 Enteric Tubes

Nasogastric and orogastric tubes should be positioned so that the tip projects in the expected region of the stomach. Because of the relative sizes of premature and full term neonates and commercially available tubes, an appropriately positioned tube often unavoidably will have the side port in the esophagus.

Enteric tubes are often placed into the small bowel for feeding purposes. Ideally these tubes should follow a course that corresponds to the normal positioning of the stomach, pylorus, duodenum and proximal jejunum, with the duodenal–jejunal junction (DJJ) (also referred to as the Ligament of Treitz) in the left upper quadrant of the abdomen, roughly at the craniocaudal level of the pylorus. However, enteric tubes, particularly if in place for several days, will often cause a straightening of their course, mimicking the positioning of midgut malrotation. In these situations, it may be prudent to slightly withdraw the tube to proximal to the DJJ and perform a bedside injection of opaque contrast material to document the placement of the DJJ.

7.8.3 Central Venous Lines

The *correct* position of central venous lines (CVLs), including peripherally inserted central catheters (PICC) is highly controversial. Some authorities insist that these lines should never be within the right atrium (RA), while others insist that they must be within the RA. Potential concerns include erosion of the endothelium with subsequent development of cardiac tamponade. Arrhythmias have also been attributed to incorrect CVL placement. The best policy is to know the manufacturers' recommendation, the planned use of the catheter, and any existing institutional or governmental policies concerning the *correct* position of the CVL in use.

For most PICC placed through an upper extremity, many neonatologists prefer to have the tip situated within the SVC. Based on the course of the PICC, the level of the confluence of the innominate veins can usually be estimated. This represents the superior extent of

the SVC. The junction of the SVC and right atrium (SVC/RA junction) has been estimated by projecting the lateral margin of the right atrium to its junction with the SVC. However, the most precise localization, based on CT evidence, places the SVC/RA junction two vertebral bodies (±0.4 vertebral body) below the carina on frontal CXR imaging [33]. PICCs placed via the lower extremity optimally will have the tip situated at the inferior vena cava/right atrium (IVC/RA) junction. As discussed in the section concerning ETT, some institutions use the thoracic spine level as the point of reference; however, because of reasons discussed in connection with ETT position, this is felt by many to be a less accurate method of determining intravascular position. The position of a PICC tip will move up to several centimeters with changes in position of the extremity into which the line is placed (Fig. 7.19).

7.8.4 Umbilical Arterial Catheters

There are two commonly used practices for umbilical arterial catheter (UAC) placement. Both are meant to minimize the potential for development of thromboembolic propagation into the main braches of the aorta. These are the *high line* position and *low line* position. Occasionally there may be the need or preference for placement of peripheral arterial lines.

Since the aorta lies adjacent to the spine, UAC tip position can be reliably referenced to the vertebral level. The branching of the aorta in newborns is slightly different from that of older children and adults. The ductus arteriosus is frequently initially open in both full term and premature newborns. It joins with the aorta at the level of the fourth thoracic vertebra (T4). The expected level of abdominal aortic branching in newborns is two vertebral bodies higher than in adults. In newborns, the best assumptions are that the celiac axis arises at T10–11, the superior mesenteric artery at T11, the renal arteries at T12–L1, the inferior mesenteric artery at L1 and the iliac bifurcation at L3.

The goal of UAC placement following a *high line* positioning is to have the tip between the ductus arteriosus and the celiac axis, i.e., between T4 and T10. Most neonatologists, therefore, attempt to have the tip between T6 and T9.

For *low line* placement, the tip should be at or below L3. However, the iliac bifurcation lies roughly at L3. Lines with their tips in the iliac artery risk being displaced. As a result most institutions follow a *high line* policy.

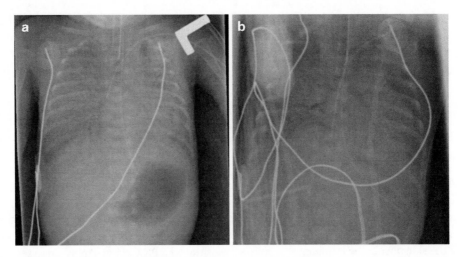

Fig. 7.19 Vascular catheter tip positions change with changing position of the body part into which the catheter is inserted. (**a**) With the left arm slightly abducted, the left arm PICC tip is per-fectly positioned at the SVC–RA junction. (**b**) Five hours later, without the PICC having been manipulated, but with the left arm now elevated above the baby's head, the PICC tip in deep within the RA

7.8.5 Umbilical Venous Catheters

Unlike for UAC, umbilical venous catheter (UVC) tip position is not reliably referenced to the vertebral level. The explanation is as explained for ETT and CVL. Since the venous anatomy is not adjacent to the spine, variability in patient positioning and X-ray beam angle will significantly alter the projected UVC tip position in relation to the spine. Therefore, reference should be to the venous anatomy. This may be stated as below the liver, within the liver, or above the liver. Rarely the UVC will descend in the inferior vena cava. Most consider the preferred UVC tip position to be at the inferior vena cava and right atrial junction (IVC/RA junction). When the catheter extends more superiorly, a statement should be made as to where the tip resides, i.e., in the right atrium, the right ventricle, the pulmonary artery, across the foramen ovale into the left atrium or pulmonary veins, up the SVC, into the neck, etc.

References

1. Cleveland RH. A radiologic update on medical diseases of the newborn chest. Pediatr Radiol. 1995;25:631–7.
2. Cleveland R, Donoghue V. Imaging of the newborn chest. Syllabus IDKD: diseases of the heart, chest & breast. Milan: Springer-Verlag Italia; 2007. p. 55–62.
3. Welty S, Hansen TN, Corbet A. Respiratory distress in the preterm infant. In: Taeusch HW, Ballard RA, Gleason CA, editors. Avery's diseases of the newborn. Philadelphia: Elsevier Saunders; 2005. p. 687–703.
4. Zecca E, Costa S, Lauriola V, et al. Bile acid pneumonia: a "new" form of neonatal respiratory distress syndrome? Pediatrics. 2004;114:269–72.
5. Clyman RI. Patent ductus arteriosus in the premature infant. In: Taeusch HW, Ballard RA, Gleason CA, editors. Avery's diseases of the newborn. Philadelphia: Elsevier Saunders; 2005. p. 816–26.
6. Northway WH, Rosan RC, Porter DY. Pulmonary disease following respirator therapy of hyaline-membrane disease: bronchopulmonary dysplasia. N Engl J Med. 1967;276:357–68.
7. Jobe AH. The new BPD: an arrest of lung development. Pediatr Res. 1999;66:641–3.
8. Hodgman JE. Relationship between Wilson-Mikity syndrome and the new BPD. Pediatrics. 2003;112:1414–5.
9. Couser RJ, Ferrara TB, Ebert J, Hoekstra RE, Fangman JJ. Effects of exogenous surfactant therapy on dynamic compliance during mechanical breathing in preterm infants with hyaline membrane disease. J Pediatr. 1990;116:119–24.
10. Leichty EA, Donovan E, Purohit D, et al. Reduction of neonatal mortality after multiple doses of bovine surfactant in low birth weight neonates with respiratory distress syndrome. Pediatrics. 1991;88:19–28.
11. American Academy of Pediatrics committee on Fetus and Newborn: Surfactant replacement therapy for respiratory distress syndrome. Pediatrics 1991;87:946–7.
12. Jackson JC, Troug WE, Standaert TA, et al. Effect of high-frequency ventilation on the development of alveolar edema in premature monkeys at risk for hyaline membrane disease. Am Rev Respir Dis. 1991;143:865–71.
13. Donnelly LF, Lucaya J, Ozelame V, et al. CT findings and temporal course of persistent pulmonary interstitial emphysema in neonates: a multiinstitutional study. AJR Am J Roentgenol. 2003;180:1129–33.
14. Swischuk LE. Bubbles in hyaline membrane disease. Differentiation of three types. Radiology. 1977;122:417–26.
15. Howling SJ, Northway WH, Hansell DM, et al. Pulmonary sequelae of bronchopulmonary dysplasia survivors: high-resolution CT findings. AJR Am J Roentgenol. 2000;174:1323–6.

16. Brudno DS, Boedy RF, Kanto WP. Compliance, alveolar-arterial oxygen difference, and oxygenation index changes in patients managed with extracorporeal membrane oxygenation. Pediatr Pulmonol. 1990;9:19–23.

17. Gregory GA, Gooding CA, Phibbs RH, Tooley WH. Meconium aspiration in infants – a prospective study. J Pediatr. 1974;85:848–52.

18. Lancet (editorial). Lung function in children after neonatal meconium aspiration. Lancet. 1988;2:317–8.

19. Cleveland R. Total anomalous pulmonary venous connection: Case 10. In: Siegel MJ, Bisset GS, Cleveland RH, Donaldson JS, Fellows KE, Patriquin HB, editors. ACR pediatric disease (fourth series) test and syllabus. Reston: American College of Radiology; 1993. p. 272–302.

20. Leonidas JC, Hall RT, Beatty EC, et al. Radiographic findings in early onset neonatal group B *Streptococcal septicemia*. Pediatrics. 1977;59(Suppl):1006–11.

21. Ursi D, Ursi J-P, Ieven M, et al. Congenital pneumonia due to *Mycoplasma pneumoniae*. Arch Dis Child. 1995;72: F118–20.

22. Theilen U, Lyon AJ, Fitzgerald T, et al. Infection with *Ureaplasma urealyticum*: is there a specific clinical and radiological course in the preterm infant? Arch Dis Child Fetal Neonatal Ed. 2004;89:F163–7.

23. McCarten KM, Rosenberg HK, Borden S, Mandell GA. Delayed appearance of right diaphragmatic hernia associated with group B streptococcal infection in newborns. Radiology. 1981;139:385–9.

24. Moskowitz PS, Griscom NT. The medial pneumothorax. Radiology. 1976;120:143–7.

25. Cleveland RH, Weber B. Retained fetal lung liquid in congenital lobar emphysema: a possible predictor of polyalveolar lobe. Pediatr Radiol. 1993;23:291–5.

26. Hagmann C, Berger TM. Congenital pulmonary lymphangiectasia. N Engl J Med. 2003;349:e21.

27. Chung CJ, Fordham LA, Barker P, et al. Children with congenital pulmonary Lymphangiectasia: after infancy. AJR Am J Roentgenol. 1999;173:1583–8.

28. Freed MD. Congenital cardiac malformations. In: Avery ME, Taeusch HW, editors. Schaffer's diseases of the newborn. 5th ed. Philadelphia: WB Saunders; 1984. p. 243–90.

29. Schachter J. Chlamydial infections (first of three parts). New Engl J Med. 1978;298:428–35.

30. Schachter J. Chlamydial infections (second of three parts). New Engl J Med. 1978;298:490–5.

31. Schachter J. Chlamydial infections (third of three parts). New Engl J Med. 1978;298:540–9.

32. Todres ID, deBros F, Kramer SS. Endotracheal tube displacement in the newborn infant. J Pediatr. 1976;89:126–7.

33. Baskin KM, Jimenez RM, Cahill AM, et al. Cavoatrial junction and central venous anatomy: implications for central venous access tip position. J Vasc Interv Radiol. 2008;19: 359–65.

Interstitial Lung Disease in Infants and Children: New Classification System with Emphasis on Clinical, Imaging, and Pathological Correlation

8

Edward Y. Lee, Robert H. Cleveland, and Claire Langston

CONTENTS

Edward Y. Lee, MD, MPH (✉)
Division of Thoracic Imaging, Department of Radiology and Medicine, Pulmonary Division, Children's Hospital Boston, Harvard Medical School, Boston, MA, USA
e-mail:edward.lee@childrens.harvard.edu

Robert H. Cleveland, MD
Department of Radiology, Harvard Medical School, Boston, MA, USA

Departments of Radiology and Medicine, Division of Respiratory Diseases, Children's Hospital Boston, Boston, MA, USA

Claire Langston, MD
Department of Pathology, Texas Children's Hospital, Baylor College of Medicine, Houston, TX, USA

R.H. Cleveland (ed.), *Imaging in Pediatric Pulmonology*,
DOI 10.1007/978-1-4419-5872-3_8, © Springer Science+Business Media, LLC 2012

Interstitial lung diseases in infants and children comprise a rare heterogeneous group of parenchymal lung disorders, with clinical syndromes characterized by dyspnea, tachypnea, crackles, and hypoxemia. They arise from a wide spectrum of developmental, genetic, inflammatory, infectious, and reactive disorders. In the past, there has been a paucity of information and limited understanding regarding their pathogenesis, natural history, imaging findings, and histopathologic features, which often resulted in enormous diagnostic challenges and confusion.

In recent years, there has been a substantial improvement in the understanding of interstitial lung disease in the pediatric patient, due to the development of a structured classification system [1, 2] based on etiology of the lung disease, established pathologic criteria for consistent diagnosis, and improvement of thoracoscopic techniques for lung biopsy [3, 4]. Imaging plays an important role in evaluating interstitial lung diseases in infants and children by confirming and characterizing the disorder, generating differential diagnoses, and providing localization for lung biopsy for pathological diagnosis.

In this chapter, the authors present epidemiology, challenges, and uncertainties of diagnosis and amplify a recently developed classification system for interstitial lung disease in infants and children with clinical, imaging, and pathological correlation. It is not possible to review all of the conditions that are considered to be interstitial lung disorders in infants and children; individually, they are rare and collectively uncommon, but important conditions and particularly challenging ones are considered. The major aim of this chapter is to increase the understanding of interstitial lung disease among pediatric pulmonologists, neonatologists, radiologists, and pathologists who take care of affected infants and children. Increasing understanding of these challenging disorders should result in early and correct diagnosis, which in turn, will improve patient care.

8.1 Epidemiology of Pediatric Interstitial Lung Disease

Although the true prevalence of interstitial lung disease in infants and children is not clearly known, an estimated prevalence of chronic interstitial lung disease in the pediatric population of 3.6 cases per million in immunocompetent children younger than 17 years has been reported, based on a national survey performed in the United Kingdom and Ireland from 1995 to 1998 [5]. This reported prevalence is likely to be substantially underestimated, particularly given the increased recognition of interstitial lung diseases in the pediatric population in recent years, due to: (1) a recently developed classification system for categorizing pediatric interstitial lung disease; (2) increased recognition particularly of the unique interstitial lung diseases which occur in infants; and (3) increased use of thoracoscopic lung biopsy in pediatric patients for definitive diagnosis. Additionally, although the prevalence of any single specific interstitial lung disease is low, the combination of the varied types of interstitial lung diseases in the pediatric population may be sizable as a collective group. A national registry or large prospective multicenter studies focusing on evaluation of the true prevalence of interstitial lung disease in infants and children is currently needed.

Challenges and Uncertainties Regarding Diagnosis of Interstitial Lung Disease in Infants and Children

There are many challenges and uncertainties for the early and correct diagnosis of interstitial lung disease in the pediatric patient. Three major challenges include, first, interstitial lung disease is less common in infants and children compared with adults. Therefore, most clinicians and radiologists are less familiar with considering and recognizing interstitial lung disease in this patient population. Second, the clinical manifestations of interstitial lung disease particularly in infants and the young child are often subtle, highly variable, and typically nonspecific, such as dyspnea, tachypnea, crackles, and hypoxemia. Lastly, there are currently no pathognomonic clinical or laboratory criteria for the diagnosis of interstitial lung disease in pediatric patients. Some of the major uncertainties involving interstitial lung disease in this population include: (1) the paucity of information regarding the natural history of interstitial lung disease in childhood; (2) the lack of understanding of the role of specific host factors in the pathogenesis of interstitial lung disease; and (3) the absence of information on prognostic indicators in interstitial lung disease in childhood, and more particularly in infants. Due to the above stated challenges and uncertainties, evaluation and diagnosis of interstitial lung disease in childhood and particularly in infants has been markedly limited in the past.

New Pediatric Interstitial Lung Disease Classification

8.3.1 Rationale and History Behind the Development of the New Childhood Interstitial Lung Disease Classification

Rationale

Two main factors led to the development of a new classification for new childhood interstitial lung disease (ChILD). First, there has been substantial confusion and difficulty associated with the description and classification of specific interstitial lung diseases in infants and young children with multiple terms used for similar abnormalities and sometimes the same term used for differing conditions; and there has been a tendency to attempt to fit these pediatric disorders into the diagnostic schema used for adults. As the adult ILD classification became more refined and as more knowledge was gained about certain forms of infant ILD, it became clear that using the adult classification was both suboptimal and limiting as conditions common in adults are rare or nonexistent in infants and children and recently recognized infant conditions have no place in the adult classification. Second, the adult ILD classification system did not acknowledge the important role of heritable and genetic disorders that have become widely recognized as an important component of ChILD. The recognition of the role of genetic disorders of the surfactant system was pivotal in changing this understanding. And, now genetic underpinnings are being sought for a wider group of ChILD. Classifying ILD in the pediatric patient based on the adult ILD classification system is no longer a viable approach.

History

Recognition of the substantial differences between pediatric and adult ILD led to the evolution of the current and evolving classification system for ChILD. A European Respiratory Society (ERS) Task Force addressed this issue in a retrospective review of 185 pediatric cases of chronic interstitial lung disease in immunocompetent patients; most, but not all, had lung biopsy and histologic material which was not reviewed as part of this project; the diagnoses made at initial examination were accepted. The ERS review divided the diagnoses made clinically into four categories based on a proposal by Fan and Langston [6]: (1) Diffuse lung parenchymal disease of unknown association (drug reaction, aspiration, connective tissue disorders, infection, environmental disorders); (2) idiopathic interstitial pneumonias (nonspecific interstitial pneumonia [NSIP]), cellular/fibrotic, desquamative interstitial pneumonitis (DIP), lymphoid interstitial pneumonia (LIP), diffuse alveolar damage/acute interstitial pneumonia (DAD/AIP), organizing pneumonia (OP), usual interstitial pneumonitis (UIP) to include familial cryptogenic fibrosing alveolitis, and chronic pneumonitis of infancy (CPI); (3) other forms of interstitial pneumonia to include lymphangioleiomyomatosis, Langerhans cell granulomatosis, pulmonary alveolar proteinosis (PAP), sarcoidosis, eosinophilic pneumonia, idiopathic/infantile pulmonary hemosiderosis; and (4) congenital disorders (DIP, LIP, lipoid pneumonia, NSIP/UIP, and surfactant deficiencies). Although this concept was an important step toward improved understanding and diagnosis of ChILD, there was clearly a need for further refinement, particularly as diagnostic criteria were not provided for these entities, disorders of immunocompromised children were not addressed, and the requirement for chronicity excluded severe and rapidly progressive conditions. Additionally, adult terminology continued to be used in large part for quite different entities including idiopathic pulmonary fibrosis (IPF) and usual interstitial pneumonia (UIP), conditions that are common in adults, but vanishingly rare in childhood. This study was a major advance in redirecting thinking about ChILD, and it is important for this reason, but does not truly present a new classification system, nor did it resolve many of the issues leading to diagnostic confusion.

A truly new classification system for pediatric interstitial lung disease [7] evolved out of the recognition that clinical setting is an important consideration in the diagnosis of pediatric ILD and that combined clinical, imaging, and pathological correlation is a more powerful diagnostic tool, than any one single component. This new pediatric interstitial lung disease classification system was validated for infants and very young children in a retrospective review of 186 lung biopsies done between 1999 and 2004 [2] with accompanying clinical histories and images from children under age 2 contributed by 11 pediatric institutions in North America. The importance of this new classification system lies in its acknowledgment of the unique nature of ILD in infants and the overlap of other lung disorders seen in infants and young children with the varied spectrum of conditions seen in older children and adults. Based on this new classification system, ChILD is classified into three main groups: (1) disorders of infancy; (2) other categories (not specific to infancy); and (3) unclassifiable. This expandable and flexible system for categorization has gained wide clinical recognition. This chapter uses this classification scheme (Table 8.1) as its organizing principal focusing initially on those disorders seen almost exclusively during infancy and not in older children or adults.

Table 8.1. Clinicopathologic classification of diffuse lung disease in childhood

I. Disorders of infancy
  A. Diffuse developmental disorders
    1. Acinar dysplasia
    2. Congenital alveolar dysplasia
    3. Alveolar capillary dysplasia with misalignment of pulmonary veins
  B. Growth abnormalities
    1. Prenatal conditions – secondary pulmonary hypoplasia of varying degree
    2. Postnatal conditions – chronic neonatal lung disease
      a. Prematurity-related chronic lung disease (also known as bronchopulmonary dysplasia [BPD])
      b. Term infants with chronic lung disease
    3. Associated with chromosomal abnormalities
      a. Trisomy 21
      b. Others
    4. Associated with congenital heart disease in chromosomally normal children
  C. Surfactant dysfunction disorders and related abnormalities
    1. Surfactant dysfunction disorders
      a. SpB genetic mutations (pulmonary alveolar proteinosis and variant histologies)
      b. SpC genetic mutations (chronic pneumonitis of infancy is the dominant histologic pattern, others include PAP, DIP, NSIP)
      c. ABCA3 genetic mutations (PAP-dominant histologic pattern, others include CPI, DIP, NSIP)
      d. Congenital GMCSF receptor deficiency (PAP histologic pattern)
      e. TTF1 genetic mutations
      f. Others with histology consistent with surfactant dysfunction disorder without an as yet recognized genetic disorder
    2. Lysinuric protein intolerance (PAP histologic pattern)
  D. Specific conditions of unknown/poorly understood etiology
    1. Neuroendocrine cell hyperplasia of infancy (NEHI)
    2. Pulmonary interstitial glycogenosis
      a. Primary
      b. Associated with other pulmonary conditions
II. Disorders of the normal host
  A. Infectious and postinfectious processes
    1. Postinfectious airway injury ranging from mild airway fibrosis to constrictive/obliterative bronchiolitis with and without preceding history of viral respiratory infection
    2. Specific infections identified
      a. Bacterial
      b. Fungal
      c. Mycobacterial
      d. Viral
  B. Disorders related to environmental agents
    1. Hypersensitivity pneumonia
    2. Toxic inhalation

(continued)

Table 8.1. (continued)

C. Aspiration syndromes
D. Eosinophilic pneumonias
E. Acute interstitial pneumonia/Hamman–Rich syndrome/idiopathic diffuse alveolar damage
F. Nonspecific interstitial pneumonia
G. Idiopathic pulmonary hemosiderosis
H. Others
III. Disorders related to systemic disease processes
A. Immune-mediated disorders
1. Specific pulmonary manifestations
a. Goodpasture's syndrome
b. Acquired pulmonary alveolar proteinosis/autoantibody to GMCSF
c. Pulmonary vasculitis syndromes
2. Nonspecific pulmonary manifestations
a. Nonspecific interstitial pneumonia
b. Pulmonary hemorrhage syndromes
c. Lymphoproliferative disease
d. Organizing pneumonia
e. Nonspecific airway changes including lymphocytic bronchiolitis, lymphoid hyperplasia, and mild constrictive changes
3. Other manifestations of collagen-vascular disease
B. Nonimmune-mediated systemic disorders
1. Storage disease
2. Sarcoidosis
3. Langerhans cell histiocytosis
4. Malignant infiltrates
5. Others
IV. Disorders of the immunocompromised host
A. Opportunistic infections
1. PCP
2. Fungal/yeast
3. Bacterial
4. Mycobacterial
5. Viral
6. Suspected
B. Disorders related to therapeutic intervention – chemotherapeutic drug and radiation injury
1. Chemotherapeutic drug injury
2. Radiation injury
3. Combined
4. Drug hypersensitivity
C. Disorders related to solid organ, lung and bone marrow transplantation, and rejection syndromes
1. Rejection
2. GVHD
3. PTLD
D. DAD of undetermined etiology
E. Lymphoid infiltrates related to immune compromise (for nontransplanted patients)
1. Nonspecific lymphoproliferation
2. With lymphoid hyperplasia
3. With poorly formed granulomas
4. Malignant
V. Disorders masquerading as interstitial disease
A. Arterial hypertensive vasculopathy

(continued)

Table 8.1. (continued)

B. Congestive vasculopathy including veno-occlusive disease
C. Lymphatic disorders
1. Lymphangiectasis
2. Lymphangiomatosis
D. Pulmonary edema
E. Thromboembolic
VI. Unclassified
End-stage disease
Nondiagnostic
Inadequate tissue
Insufficient information

Modified from Deutsch et al. [2]. Reprinted with permission of the American Thoracic Society. Copyright American Thoracic Society. Official Journal of the American Thoracic Society

8.4 Interstitial Lung Disorders in Infants

In the multicenter study, disorders of infancy comprised the largest portion of the 186 reviewed cases. These infant disorders are divided into four important subgroups: (1) diffuse developmental disorders; (2) growth abnormalities; (3) surfactant dysfunction mutations and related disorders; and (4) specific conditions of undefined etiology, currently including pulmonary interstitial glycogenosis (PIG) and neuroendocrine cell hyperplasia of infancy (NEHI). The clinical, imaging, and pathologic features of these different categories of infant ILD [8–16] are summarized in Table 8.2.

8.4.1 Diffuse Developmental Disorders

This category includes acinar dysplasia, congenital alveolar dysplasia (CAD) [17, 18], and alveolar capillary dysplasia with misalignment of pulmonary veins (ACDMPV) [19, 20].

Key Clinical Aspects

Infants with ILD in this category are typically term infants who present with rapidly and progressively worsening hypoxemia often associated with severe pulmonary hypertension (PHT) immediately following birth, or early in the neonatal period.

Table 8.2. Summary of clinical, imaging, and pathologic features of interstitial lung disease in infancy

Types of ILD	Clinical features	Imaging features	Pathologic features
Diffuse developmental disorders			
Acinar Dysplasia	Term infants, mostly female, present at birth, severe hypoxemia, high morality (100%)	Diffuse opacity, hypoinflation	Small lung size, airway without acinar development, growth arrest late pseudoglandular phase
CAD	Term infants, present at birth, severe hypoxemia, high mortality (100%)	Diffuse opacity, hypoinflation, increased size of MPA/pulmonary blood flow if + PHT	Normal or increased lung size if chronic ventilatory support, growth arrest canalicular phase
ACDMPV	Term infants, present soon after birth, severe hypoxemia, associated with other congenital anomalies, high mortality (100%)	Diffuse opacity, hypoinflation, increased size of MPA/pulmonary blood flow if + PHT	Normal or increased lung size if chronic ventilatory support, reduced capillary density, malpositioned veins, arterial hypertensive changes
Growth abnormalities	Most common ILD, both preterm and term infants, variable clinical presentation, associated with underlying causes for growth abnormalities, moderate mortality (~30%)	Variable imaging findings, small cysts often located peripherally in the lungs with chromosomal abnormalities (e.g., Trisomy 21)	Alveolar enlargement related to prenatal or postnatal defective alveolarization
Surfactant dysfunction mutations and related disorders			
SpB defect	Term infants, present at birth, severe hypoxemia, autosomal recessive, high mortality without transplant (100%)	Diffuse hazy or granular opacity on CXR, GGO with variable interlobular septal thickening on HRCT	Prominent diffuse alveolar epithelial hyperplasia, variable proteinosis material, foamy macrophages, lamellar body abnormalities on EM PAP or variant pattern
SpC defect	Term infants, present at birth, severe hypoxemia, autosomal-dominant, moderate early mortality	Diffuse hazy or granular opacity on CXR, GGO with variable interlobular septal thickening on HRCT	Prominent diffuse alveolar epithelial hyperplasia, variable proteinosis, foamy macrophages, no specific EM change CPI or DIP pattern
ABCA3 defect	Term infants, during postnatal period, persistent tachypnea and hypoxemia, autosomal recessive, moderate early mortality (~30%)	Diffuse hazy or granular opacity on CXR, GGO with variable interlobular septal thickening on HRCT	Prominent diffuse alveolar epithelial hyperplasia, variable proteinosis material, foamy macrophages, tiny lamellar bodies with dense inclusion on EM CPI or DIP pattern
Specific conditions of undefined etiology			
NEHI	Term infants, initially well, present by 3 months with persistent tachypnea, retractions, hypoxemia, and crackles without cough or wheeze, no steroid response no morality	Hyperinflation with variable increased perihilar opacity on CXR, Geographic GGO with central predominance especially in the lingula and RML on HRCT, air trapping in both the areas on HRCT	Essentially normal lung histology occasionally mild peri-airway lymphocytic inflammation, increased numbers bombesin for immunopositive cells in airways and prominent neuroepithelial bodies
PIG	Both preterm and term infants, presents at birth, severe tachypnea and hypoxemia, often associated with other conditions that affect lung growth, pulse steroids mortality related to associated disorders	Hyperinflation and diffuse increased interstitial markings on CXR, diffuse segmental or subsegmental GGO, interlobular septal thickening and reticular change predominantly subpleural with few centrilobular nodules on HRCT	Large clear rounded, glycogen-laden, vimentin immunopositive mesenchymal cells expand the lobular interstitium. Monoparticulate glycogen on EM

ILD interstitial lung disease; *CAD* congenital alveolar dysplasia; *MPA* main pulmonary artery; *PHT* pulmonary hypertension; *ACDMPV* alveolar capillary dysplasia with misalignment of pulmonary veins; *SpB* surfactant protein B; *CXR* chest radiographs; *GGO* ground glass opacity; *HRCT* high-resolution CT; *SpC* surfactant protein C; *ABCA3* ATP-binding cassette transport proteins (ABC); *NEHI* neuroendocrine cell hyperplasia of infancy; *RML* right middle lobe; *TX* treatment; *PAP* - pulmonary alveolar proteinosis; *EM* - electron microscopy; *CPI* - chronic pneumonitis of infancy; *DIP* - desquamative interstitial pneumonia.

Due to their rapid clinical course of respiratory failure, most infants with this type of interstitial lung disease die during the first 2 months of life despite supportive management including advanced ventilation support strategies, extracorporeal membrane oxygenation, and therapeutic interventions for PHT. Infants with acinar dysplasia, the rarest of these conditions, present at birth and their survival is shortest. While most reported cases are female infants, male infants may be affected as well. Those with CAD typically present within hours of birth and require continuous and often maximal supportive measures for survival with such support they may survive weeks, but cannot be weaned from these measures. Infants with ACD/MPV typically present within the first few days of birth, but a few have a delayed presentation at weeks or sometimes a few months of age. Once they present, their course with respiratory failure and PHT rarely ameliorates and death by 1 month following presentation is the usual outcome.

Familial cases have been reported in all and account for about 10% of ACD/MPV cases; they have been identified rarely in each of the other disorders. This feature has suggested a genetic basis for all these disorders. In addition, the majority of infants with ACD/MPV have other congenital anomalies most commonly involving the cardiovascular, gastrointestinal (including absence of the gallbladder), and/or genitourinary system. A search for the genetic basis of ACD/MPV has resulted in the recent recognition of mutation/microdeletion of the FOXF1 gene in a proportion of ACD/MPV cases and the recognition of familial cases highlights the need for genetic testing and counseling in cases with suspected ACD/MPV. As genetic abnormalities have not been found for acinar dysplasia or CAD, and as all ACD/MPV cases have not yet had a genetic mechanism identified, the definitive diagnosis of these developmental disorders currently rests on pathological analysis of lung tissue from biopsy and/or postmortem specimens.

Imaging Features

Due to the rarity of these diffuse developmental disorders and the often precarious clinical status of these patients, detailed imaging findings for this category of ChILD are currently not available. Plain chest radiographs of affected infants with diffuse developmental abnormalities typically show normal to decreased lung volume associated with diffuse opacities related to hypoinflation resembling hyaline membrane disease (Fig. 8.1); however, with long-term ventilation support as often occurs with CAD (Fig. 8.2) and ACD/MPV (Fig. 8.3), lung volume may be increased, and the increased size of the main pulmonary artery and increased pulmonary blood flow may also be seen on plain chest radiographs in affected infants who have concurrent PHT.

Pathological Features

The diffuse developmental disorders are thought to originate early in lung development. On gross examination, the lungs in acinar dysplasia are small (Fig. 8.1); histologically, they suggest growth arrest in the pseudoglandular stage with only airway structures, bronchi, and larger bronchioles, embedded within loose mesenchyme; although occasionally there is minimal early acinar formation. For CAD (Fig. 8.2) and ACD/MPV (Fig. 8.3), lung size is typically normal or even large particularly when there has been long-term ventilatory support. Histologically, CAD (Fig. 8.2) suggests growth arrest in the canalicular stage of lung development showing acinar formation with simplified lung structure and sometimes, but not always, reduced capillary density. Histologic changes in ACD/MPV (Fig. 8.3) are less clearly reminiscent of a specific stage in lung development, but there is lobular underdevelopment with variable and sometimes marked alveolar enlargement and reduced capillary density. In addition to the structural changes in the lobule, there are vascular changes including prominent medial hyperplasia of small pulmonary arteries and malposition of pulmonary veins adjacent to arteries and small airways, as well as sometimes prominent regional or diffuse lymphangiectasis.

8.4.2 Growth Disorders

The commonest form of infant ILD is that related to alveolar growth disorders. These differ from the diffuse developmental disorders in that the lung is not programed to be abnormal, rather some superimposed condition or event alters normal programed development. Conditions in this category include (1) pulmonary hypoplasia associated with prenatal conditions such as oligohydramnios, space-occupying lesions, or neuromuscular disease; (2) postnatal conditions such as prematurity-related chronic lung disease (i.e., bronchopulmonary dysplasia) and term infants with chronic lung disease; (3) the structural pulmonary changes seen with

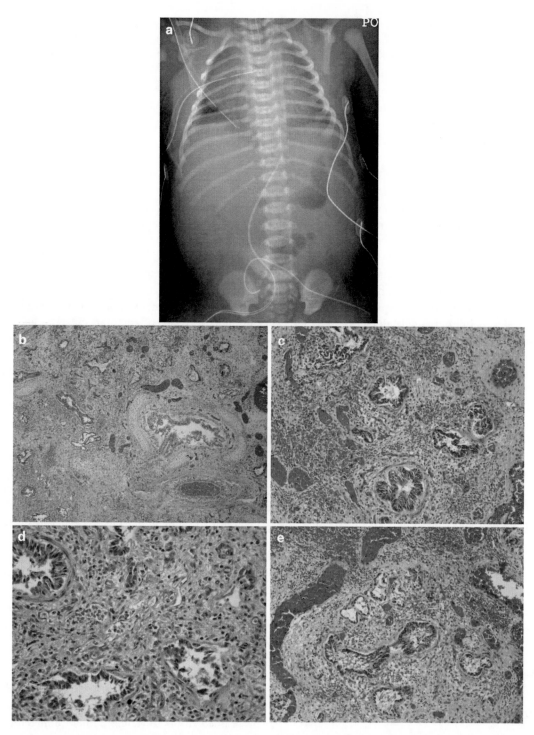

Fig. 8.1. (**a**) Acinar dysplasia: As is expected with the diffuse developmental disorders, the CXR on this baby with acinar dysplasia revealed nonspecific diffuse lung opacification resembling that seen with hyaline membrane disease. (Image courtesy of Dr. Paul Guillerman, Baylor College of Medicine, Texas Children's Hospital, Department of Radiology.) (**b–e**) Acinar dysplasia: The lung is from the autopsy of a near-term male infant who survived with continuous maximal support for only 14 h. The findings are typical for acinar dysplasia with arrest of development in the pseudoglandular stage. It shows multiple airways, both bronchi (**b**) and bronchioles (**b–e**), but very little acinar development (**e**) with only a very few airspaces among the prominent airways. The few airspaces seen are at the periphery of only a few lobular regions in the lower lobes. Bronchioles are surrounded by small amounts of smooth muscle (**c**, **e**) and are dispersed in loose mesenchyme. There is often prominent vascular dilatation and hemorrhage (**b**, **c**, **e**) related to hypoxia

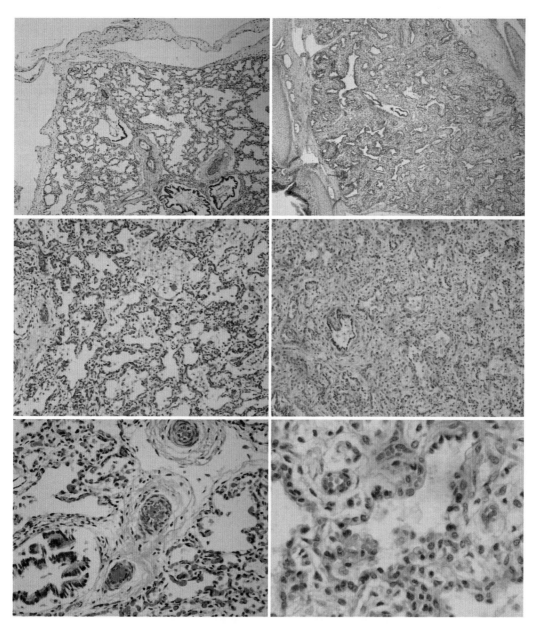

Fig. 8.2. Congenital alveolar dysplasia (CAD): The *left* and *right panels* are from two different examples of CAD and show the range of developmental delay that can be seen in this condition. CAD shows developmental arrest that ranges from the canalicular to the early saccular stage. The *left column* shows images from the lung of a near-term male infant who developed respiratory distress at a few hours of age and was supported with supplemental oxygen and mechanical ventilation for 2 weeks. An echocardiogram showed pulmonary hypertension. The *upper left panel* is an overview of the lung histology and also shows dilated lymphatic channels in the pleura and an interlobular septum, but not adjacent to airways and arteries. The lobules are formed of simple saccular structures that in the *left middle panel* are seen to have the somewhat irregular internal configuration seen with secondary crest formation and the wider airspace walls consistent with the early saccular stage of development. In the *lower left panel,* a well-developed pattern of capillaries is evident oriented to the airspace epithelium in a normal fashion. There is no deficiency of capillary development in this case, although it may be seen occasionally in association with CAD. Small pulmonary arteries in the *lower left panel* have mildly increased medial smooth muscle. A single small bronchiole is also evident in the *lower left panel.* The *right hand panels* show images from the lung of a near-term female infant who developed hypoxia and respiratory failure shortly after birth. She survived 3 days. This lung shows an earlier developmental stage with far less advanced acinar development. Development is consistent with the canalicular stage. The *upper right panel* is an overview of lung with only small numbers of simple elongated airspaces disposed in loose mesenchyme. This is better seen in the *middle right panel* where somewhat irregular airspaces lined by cuboidal epithelium are separated by abundant mesenchyme. In the *lower right panel,* the airspace epithelium and capillary development are better seen with capillaries becoming apposed to the epithelium with the formation of small regions with thin air-blood barriers

chromosomal abnormalities particularly Trisomy 21 are grouped here, as the genesis of their alveolar growth abnormalities is postnatal in origin, but this is a programed abnormality; and (4) changes seen in some chromosomally normal infants with congenital heart disease.

Key Clinical Aspects

In the multicenter review, this was the most common of the infant interstitial lung disorders, accounting for 43% of diffuse lung disease in infants. Because of the varied underlying conditions and associations, clinical presentations of these infants vary substantially. If the clinical setting includes any of the various conditions associated with alveolar growth abnormality, including prematurity, oligohydramnios, chromosomal abnormality, or congenital heart disease, the possibility of a lung growth abnormality should be considered and further investigations might include lung biopsy for diagnosis and prognosis as the mortality rate in this patient population is often substantial, being as high as 34% in the multicenter study.

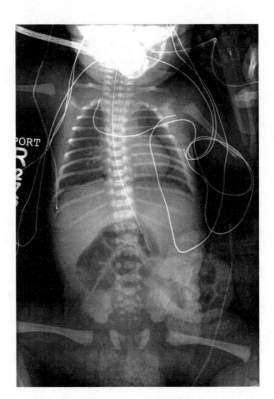

Fig. 8.3. (a) Alveolar capillary dysplasia: Newborn with alveolar capillary dysplasia with misalignment of pulmonary veins. Even with the lung volumes increased with positive pressure ventilation, there is still evidence of a nonspecific diffuse granular interstitial opacification similar to that seen with hyaline membrane disease. There is a left pneumothorax and an omphalocele. (Image courtesy of Dr. Paul Guillerman, Baylor College of Medicine, Texas Children's Hospital, Houston, TX.) (b) Alveolar capillary dysplasia with misalignment of pulmonary veins: All cases of alveolar capillary dysplasia with misalignment of pulmonary veins have a constellation of histologic features that include: (1) Medial thickening of small pulmonary arteries (*upper right* and *left* and *lower right* panels) with extension of arterial smooth muscle into small intralobular vessels (*middle right and left panels*); (2) abnormal position of pulmonary veins adjacent to small pulmonary arteries in their normal parabronchiolar location (*upper right* and *left* and *lower right*) and within the lobular parenchyma adjacent to small abnormally muscularized intralobar vessels (*middle left panel*); (3) lobular maldevelopment with enlarged, simple, and often thick-walled airspaces (*all panels*); (4) deficient numbers of normally positioned alveolar capillaries (*middle left* and *bottom right* panels); and (5) in some cases, there is also lymphangiectasis (*lower left panel*). Photographs are from two different cases of ACD/MPV, one in the *left panels* and another in the *right panels* and illustrate the variability in lobular maldevelopment, airspace size, and other associated changes

b   ACD

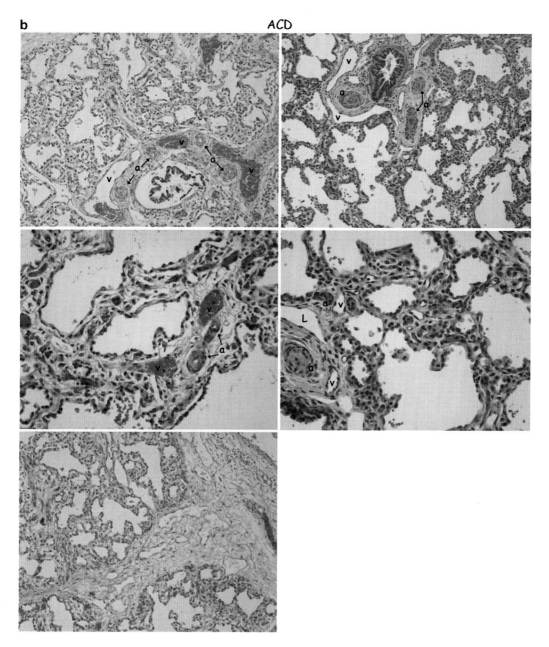

Fig. 8.3. (continued)

Imaging Features

Variable imaging findings in infants with alveolar growth abnormalities are seen in both plain radiographs and high-resolution computed tomography (HRCT). However, small cysts, often located peripherally in the lungs, may suggest this diagnosis and are particularly common in infants with chromosomal abnormalities such as Trisomy 21 (Fig. 8.4) or Turner syndrome.

Pathological Features

Histologically, the alveolar growth abnormalities share the common feature of alveolar enlargement and simplification, often marked and often more prominent at the lobular periphery and in subpleural regions (Fig. 8.5). This alveolar enlargement may be subtle or severe and is sometimes accompanied by vascular changes of pulmonary hypertensive arteriopathy with muscularization of alveolar wall ves-

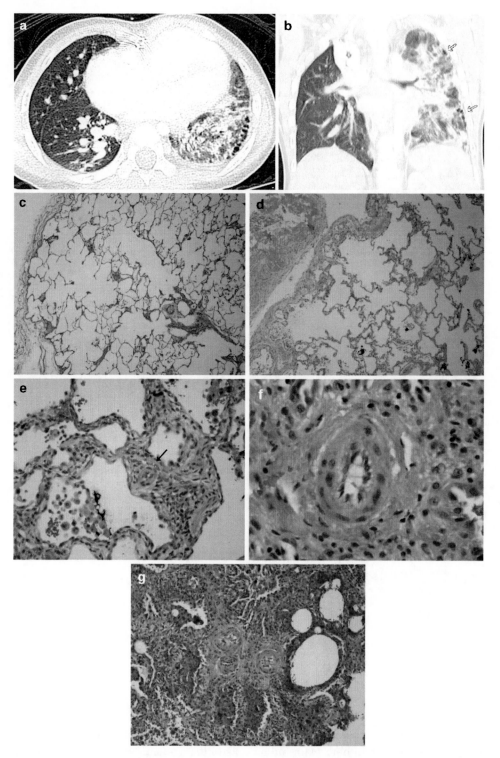

Fig. 8.4. (a) Trisomy 21: CT of a teenager with Trisomy 21 shows multiple peripheral cysts along the left posterolateral hemithorax. (b) Coronal reconstruction again shows multiple peripheral cysts along the left lateral hemithorax (*arrows*). The lung in Down syndrome (c–g) shows a distinctive form of pulmonary hypoplasia that is postnatally acquired and can be quite subtle (c) with mild-to-moderate alveolar enlargement, widening of alveolar ducts, and more prominent patchy enlargement of subpleural alveoli. This process may progress over early childhood and the subpleural alveolar enlargement may become more prominent (d). This particular growth abnormality is generally accompanied, even in its early manifestations by arterial changes with increased arterial smooth muscle, beginning with muscularization of alveolar wall vessels (e) and proceeding to more prominent arterial changes with increased medial smooth muscle (f) and evidence of tortuosity (g) with clustered profiles of a tortuous small artery

sels and medial thickening of small pulmonary arteries.

8.4.3 Surfactant Dysfunction Disorders

Interstitial lung diseases of infancy in this category include surfactant dysfunction disorders due to genetic abnormalities [21] in the surfactant proteins B (SpB) [22] and C (SpC) [23,24], and in the ATP-binding cassette transporter protein A3 (ABCA3) [25, 26].

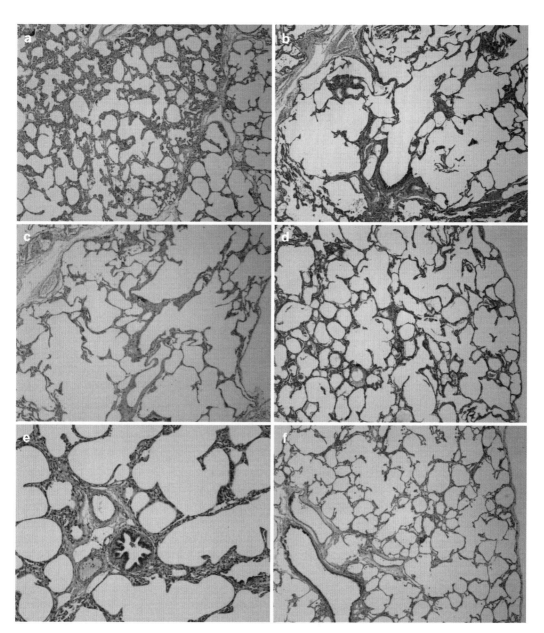

Fig. 8.5. (a–j) Alveolar growth abnormalities. All cases of alveolar growth abnormality show enlargement of alveolar spaces, which may vary in degree from mild (**a**) to extreme (**b, c**) and may be uniform (**a–f**) or variable (**b, c, g**). They may show a variety of associated changes, although none need be present, including typically mild pulmonary hypertensive arteriopathy (**h**) with muscularized alveolar wall vessels and/or the presence of PIG, typically in a patchy fashion (**a**) which shows the patchy nature best, (**i**) with quite mild PIG. The appearance is similar regardless of the underlying condition which may include various forms of pulmonary hypoplasia (**b, c, g**), chronic lung disease of prematurity (bronchopulmonary dysplasia) (**d, h–j**), or a combination of prenatal and postnatal insults (**a, e, f**). Comparison of alveolar size with that of small membranous bronchioles (**e**) can be useful in estimating alveolar size, as alveoli should be much smaller than these distal airways

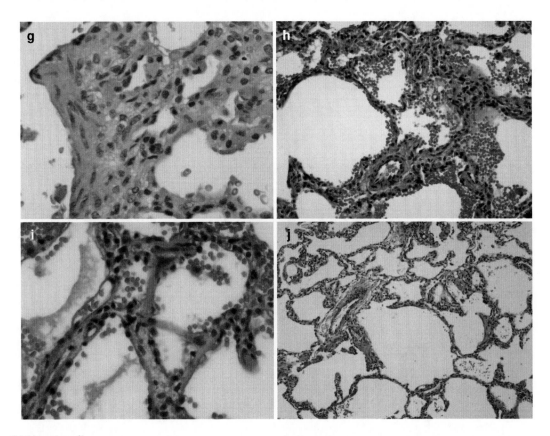

Fig. 8.5. (continued)

While inherited genetic mutations in SpB and ABCA3 are autosomal recessive, SpC mutations are autosomal-dominant loss of function mutations. Other rare genetic disorders also impact surfactant function and belong in this category, including abnormalities of TTF1 and lysinuric protein intolerance. There also may be other, as yet unrecognized, disorders in this category and interstitial lung disease in infants with histology consistent with surfactant dysfunction disorder without a yet recognized genetic disorder is also included here.

Key Clinical Aspects

Infants with surfactant dysfunction disorders typically present either immediately at birth with respiratory failure (SpB and ABCA3) or later postnatally with persistent tachypnea and hypoxemia (SpC and ABCA3). A family history of lung disease may be present in such infants and is common in those with SpC mutations. On laboratory examination, PAS-positive material identified in bronchoalveolar lavage (BAL) fluid and elevation of serum lactate dehydrogenase (LDH) can be potential clues in the diagnosis of surfactant dysfunction disorders. Genetic analysis is considered the definitive diagnostic test, although lung biopsy is often done for categorization and for prognosis and treatment considerations while awaiting the results of genetic testing. Lung biopsy is also definitive for those without as yet recognized genetic mutation and often guides the workup of those with rare genetic disorders in this category. The current treatment for infants with surfactant dysfunction disorders presenting with interstitial lung disease varies based on the degree of clinical symptoms and the underlying genetic defect. Aggressive chronic ventilation for infants with respiratory failure is currently most often performed for infants with a SpC mutation and lung transplant is the only effective therapeutic option for infants with SpB mutation. Those with ABCA3 mutations have a more varied presentation and course, at least in part depending on the specific mutation involved. In older children with ABCA3, there is a high incidence of pectus excavatum [27]. There are a few cases of SpB and ABCA3 mutations that have been noted anecdotally to respond to hydroxychloroquine therapy.

Imaging Features

The characteristic imaging findings of infants with surfactant dysfunction disorders are the early appearance of diffuse hazy or granular parenchymal opacities (ground glass opacities) on plain chest radiographs (Fig. 8.6). On HRCT, the most characteristic imaging findings of surfactant dysfunction disorders include ground glass opacity (GGO) with variable interlobular septal thickening. These imaging findings, however, can change over time.

Pathological Features

Surfactant dysfunction mutations in infants are histopathologically characterized (Fig. 8.6) by: (1) prominent diffuse uniform alveolar epithelial hyperplasia; (2) variable amounts of proteinosis material; and (3) increased and often foamy macrophages with occasional cholesterol clefts, variable interstitial widening, and sometimes mild interstitial inflammation that may increase with age. These changes typically are described as one of several possible histologic patterns seen in these disorders, including PAP pattern, desquamative interstitial pneumonia (DIP) pattern, CPI pattern, and NSIP pattern, all of which in this setting suggest an underlying surfactant dysfunction mutation. While each of these patterns may be seen with any one of the specific surfactant dysfunction mutations, PAP is uncommon and when seen suggests an SpB abnormality, DIP is more often seen with SpC or ABCA3 abnormalities, and CPI is more characteristic of SpC but may also be seen with ABCA3 mutations. An NSIP pattern is more often seen in older infants and children with SpC or ABCA3 abnormalities. Histologic variants outside these typical definable patterns also occur, but all are marked by the key features of alveolar epithelial hyperplasia, an element of proteinosis, and an element of lipid accumulation most often as a few scattered cholesterol clefts. Electron microscopic examination of lung tissue can be helpful as well, as ABCA3 and SpB have specific ultrastructural abnormalities of lamellar bodies in type 2 alveolar epithelial cells. ABCA3 has tiny lamellar bodies with a prominent dense inclusion and SpB shows reduced numbers of lamellar bodies with reduced lamellations and sometimes fusion of lamellar and multivesicular bodies.

Other Conditions in the Spectrum of the Surfactant Dysfunction Disorder

There are several rare conditions that should be considered in the differential of surfactant disfunction disorders. These include mutations in TTF-1 (Fig. 8.7) [28–31] which may present with proteinosis in the neonate and in older infants and young children histology resembling that of surfactant disfunction disorders often in combination with congenital hypothyroidism and benign chorea as part of the brain-thyroid-lung syndrome [32]. Lysinuric protein intolerance, another rare genetic disorder with mutation in the amino acid transporter gene *SLC7A7*, may also present with alveolar proteinosis in early infancy. Congenital deficiency of the GMCSF alpha receptor also results in alveolar proteinosis, although with presentation in early childhood, rather than in infancy. It is also important to remember that in a proportion of infants with typical histologic and imaging findings for surfactant dysfunction disorders, no genetic abnormality may be identified and that other genetic disorders impacting surfactant function may yet be discovered.

8.4.4 Specific Conditions of Undefined Etiology

There are two important and relatively common interstitial lung disorders in this category of ILD in infancy, NEHI and PIG.

Key Clinical Aspects

Neuroendocrine cell hyperplasia of infancy (NEHI) [33–37] has also been known as persistent tachypnea of infancy, or chronic idiopathic bronchiolitis of infancy and sometimes as follicular bronchitis [38]. This recently described entity accounts for a substantial portion of ILD in infants. Affected infants are usually term and typically present with clinical symptoms of persistent tachypnea, retractions, hypoxemia, and crackles without substantial cough or wheezing by 3 months of age often beginning after an initial period of well-being and sometimes following an uncomplicated viral respiratory infection. Infant pulmonary function test may show evidence of substantial hyper-

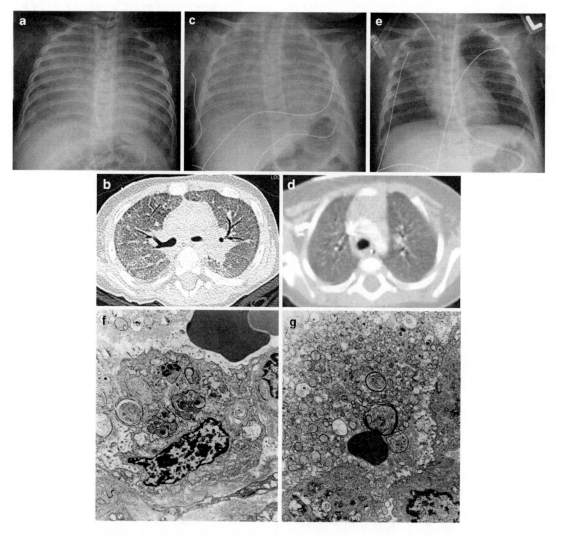

Fig. 8.6. (a) ABCA3 deficiency: Newborn with ABCA3 deficiency. As is typical for the surfactant protein deficiencies, there is a hazy severe diffuse opacification. (b) Typical of the CT findings of the surfactant protein deficiencies, this image from the infant shown in Fig. 8.4a has diffuse ground glass opacity with intralobular septal thickening. (c) Another infant with ABCA3 shows similar findings by CXR. (Image courtesy of Dr. Mike Tsifansky, Advocate Lutheran General Children's Hospital, Pediatric Pulmonology and Critical Care Medicine, Park Ridge, IL.) (d) CT on the infant shown in (c) has a ground glass opacity similar to that in Fig. 8.4b, but less pronounced intralobular septal thickening. (Image courtesy of Dr. Mike Tsifansky, Advocate Lutheran General Children's Hospital, Pediatric Pulmonology and Critical Care Medicine, Park Ridge, IL.) (e) The baby shown in (c, d) was treated with aerosolized hydroxychloroquine with significant, but transient, improvement in respiratory and imaging conditions. (Image courtesy of Dr. Mike Tsifansky, Advocate Lutheran General Children's Hospital, Pediatric Pulmonology and Critical Care Medicine, Park Ridge, IL.) Surfactant dysfunction disorders and related abnormalities (f–i) are all surfactant B deficiency images, (j–n) are all surfactant C deficiency images, and (o–t) are all ABCA3 images. Surfactant dysfunction mutations: Histologic changes in the infant lung in the surfactant dysfunction mutations are stereotypical with lobular remodeling (surfactant B (**h**)), surfactant C (**j**), ABCA3 (**q**) uniform diffuse alveolar epithelial hyperplasia (surfactant B (**i**)), surfactant C (**j**, **k**), ABCA3 (**o**), at least some element of proteinosis (surfactant B (**i**)), surfactant C (**j–m**), ABCA3 (**r**, **s**), and often at least

a few cholesterol clefts (ABCA3 (**o**, **s**)). These changes are present in all cases regardless of the underlying abnormality or the histologic pattern. While a variety of histologic patterns have been described in surfactant dysfunction mutations, including pulmonary alveolar proteinosis (PAP), desquamative interstitial pneumonia, and chronic pneumonitis of infancy (surfactant C (**j**)), most cases do not present a single clearly defined pattern. An atypical proteinosis pattern is more frequent with surfactant B mutations (surfactant B (**h**, **i**)), a chronic pneumonitis of infancy pattern is more frequent with surfactant C mutations (surfactant C (**j**)), and ABCA3 shows proteinosis in a chunky fashion (**r**, **s**); however, no pattern is specific to a particular abnormality. While mutation analysis is the definitive diagnostic modality, ultrastructural changes in the lamellar bodies of type 2 pneumocytes can be quite helpful for more rapid categorization for prognosis and treatment decisions. These changes are quite specific for ABCA3 where there is a paucity of lamellar bodies (ABCA3 (**p**)) and those present are tiny, poorly lamellated, and contain a dense central inclusion (ABCA3 (**t**)). SpB mutations also show characteristic ultrastructural changes with fusion of lamellar and multivesicular bodies (surfactant B (**f**)) and absence of tubular myelin (surfactant B (**g**)); there are also reduced numbers of lamellar bodies, which are typically poorly lamellated (not shown). There are no characteristic lamellar body ultrastructural findings with SpC mutations, the type 2 pneumocytes may appear normal (surfactant C (**m**)), or there may be mild changes in the size and distribution of lamellar bodies (surfactant C (**n**))

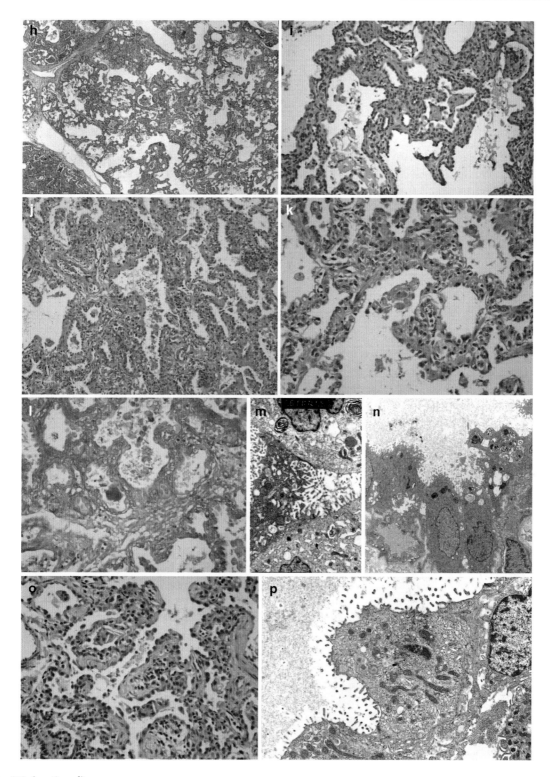

Fig. 8.6. (continued)

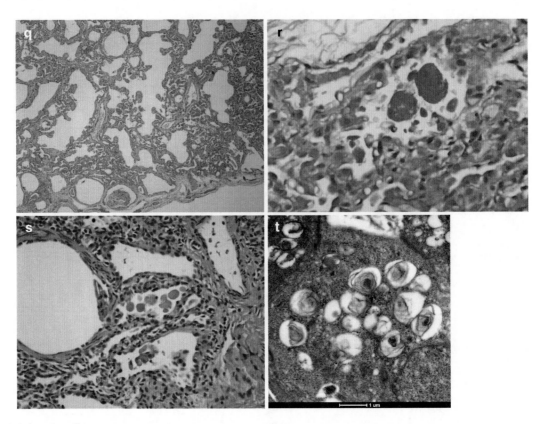

Fig. 8.6. (continued)

inflation and bronchoscopy and BAL are usually normal. The treatment for NEHI is currently supportive and aimed at preventing hypoxemia and infection while maintaining nutritional support. Many affected infants develop failure to thrive with time. Corticosteroids are not helpful for improving symptoms in infants with NEHI as underlying inflammation is not a component of the disorder, evidenced by the lack of inflammatory cells on BAL or in lung tissue at biopsy. Despite persistent symptoms and a prolonged need for oxygen therapy, infants with NEHI usually have a favorable long-term outcome with no reported deaths directly related to NEHI, no respiratory failure, and no progression to end-stage lung disease or lung transplantation. However, some patients with NEHI have long-term morbidity with persistent symptoms due to hyperinflation and reactive airway disease and may relapse with hypoxemia during intercurrent respiratory infection.

Pulmonary interstitial glycogenosis (PIG) [39, 40] has been previously known as infantile cellular interstitial pneumonitis and histiocytoid pneumonia, and as such, has been recognized for many years. PIG may occur in both preterm and full-term infants who usually present with tachypnea and hypoxemia either immediately or soon after birth. It is very unusual for PIG to occur or persist beyond 6 months of age. Although PIG has been described as an isolated finding, it is more often associated with the variety of conditions that affect lung growth, the alveolar growth abnormalities. Most affected infants do not require specific treatment; however, in those more severely affected clinically, pulse steroids have been recommended. Clinical outcomes of infants with PIG are varied and are thought to be related to the underlying condition rather than to PIG itself. There has been no reported death in infants with pure diffuse PIG; however, death has been reported in infants with patchy PIG who also had underlying growth abnormalities and PHT.

Imaging Features

Neuroendocrine cell hyperplasia of infancy (NEHI). The typical imaging findings of NEHI are hyperinflation with variable increased perihilar opacity on

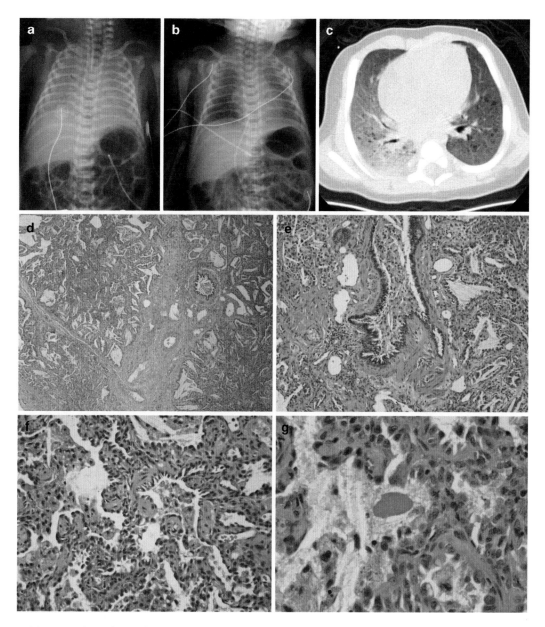

Fig. 8.7. (**a**) TTF-1: This infant with TTF-1 on the first day of life 1 has a severe nonspecific diffuse granular interstitial opacification similar to that seen with hyaline membrane disease. (**b**) TTF-1: With positive pressure ventilation, there is increased lung volume but persistent granular interstitial lung opacification. (**c**) TTF-1: CT at 11 weeks reveals diffuse ground glass opacification with multiple posterior cysts. (**a–c**, from Galambos et al. [31]. Reprinted with permission of the American Thoracic Society. Copyright American Thoracic Society. Official Journal of the American Thoracic Society.) TTF-1 Histologic changes in the lung with TTF-1 mutations (**d–k**) clearly vary, but there is limited information on the variety of changes seen. These images are from one case with quite severe lung disease that shows histologic abnormalities within the spectrum of the surfactant dysfunction mutations with diffuse involvement with lobular remodeling (**d**), intralveolar and distal airway debris with prominent numbers of cholesterol clefts (**e**), diffuse alveolar epithelial hyperplasia (**f**), proteinosis seen here as globular eosinophilic material (**g**), and mild patchy interstitial lymphoplasmacytic infiltrates (**h**). In addition to these changes that clearly link this disorder histologically with the surfactant dysfunction mutations, there may be other changes with metaplastic bronchiolar epithelium with lepidic spread i, somewhat atypical features (**j**), and mucin content (Movat stain (**k**)) that suggest the possibility of bronchioloalveolar carcinoma

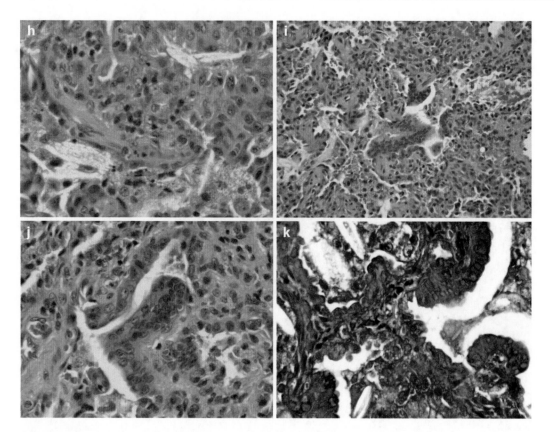

Fig. 8.7. (continued)

plain chest radiographs (Fig. 8.8). HRCT findings are quite characteristic with geographic GGO with central predominance especially in the lingula and right middle lobe without other interstitial abnormalities. Additionally, marked air trapping often affecting both the areas of GGO and the remaining lung can be seen. It has been reported that the sensitivity and specificity of HRCT for the diagnosis of NEHI are 78 and 100%, respectively, based on a recent study of 29 CT examinations from 23 patients with biopsy-proven NEHI and 6 patients with other forms of pediatric interstitial lung disease.

Pulmonary interstitial glycogenosis (PIG). Similar to the imaging findings of NEHI, infants with PIG typically show changes of bilateral hyperinflation and diffuse interstitial markings on plain chest radiograph. On HRCT, diffuse, segmental, or subsegmental ground-glass opacities, interlobular septal thickening and reticular change predominantly in a subpleural distribution with few centrilobular nodules have been reported. Recently, multiple small variably sized scattered air-filled cystic changes in conjunction with diffuse ground-glass opacities, interlobular septal

thickening, and reticular change have been reported in an infant boy with PIG in the setting of alveolar growth abnormality (Fig. 8.9) [41]; the contribution of PIG and of the growth abnormality to these changes cannot be apportioned with any certainty. The concomitant appearance of PIG with alveolar growth abnormalities suggests that imaging findings in these conditions typically share this uncertainty.

Pathological Features

Neuroendocrine cell hyperplasia of infancy (NEHI). On routine histopathological evaluation, NEHI (Fig. 8.8) typically shows only minor and nonspecific changes including mildly increased airway smooth muscle, mildly increased numbers of alveolar macrophages, and occasional mild peri-airway lymphocytic inflammation, although some biopsies also show mild and focal airway changes likely related to intercurrent infection. Histologic diagnosis rests on the identification of increased numbers of bombesin immunopositive neuroendocrine cells in bronchioles and prominent neuroepithelial bodies in the lobular parenchyma in the absence of other significant pathologic changes. A recent study documents the absence of neuroendocrine cell hyperplasia in the focally injured airways sometimes seen within these biopsies, suggesting that NEHI is not an abnormal reaction to viral infection; and another documents familial association suggesting a genetic propensity for the development of NEHI. The pathophysiology of the disorder remains unknown, although the role of the neuroendocrine system in regulating bronchial and vasomotor tone in the lung may be central to disease manifestation.

Pulmonary interstitial glycogenosis (PIG). The diagnosis of PIG requires examination of lung tissue. It is characterized by the expansion of the lobular interstitium by rounded, glycogen-laden undifferentiated mesenchymal cells without fibrosis, airway disease, or underlying inflammation on pathological analysis (Fig. 8.9). The interstitial cells in patients with PIG are immunoreactive for vimentin and are negative for muscle, epithelial, macrophage, and leukocyte markers suggesting that they are poorly differentiated mesenchymal cells. The most reliable means of diagnosis is the ultrastructural identification of characteristic deposits of monoparticulate glycogen within these mesenchymal cells. These interstitial cells may rarely contain small amounts of lipid by ultrastructural examination. PIG has been classified as: diffuse or patchy; the patchy form is more common and is

typically seen in association with alveolar growth abnormalities of varied etiology.

8.5 Conclusions: Disorders More Prevalent in Infancy

The early and correct diagnosis of ILD in infants has been a major challenge for clinicians, radiologists, and pathologists mainly due to the rarity of these disorders coupled with nonspecific clinical symptoms and the absence of a coherent classification system. With the advent of the new ChILD classification system, our understanding of ILD in infants has markedly improved. Knowledge of clinical, imaging, and pathological features of ILD in infants will enhance accurate diagnosis and improve timeliness, both are crucial as prognosis and treatment vary considerably among the different infant interstitial lung disorders. Although the etiology is currently unknown, several of these abnormalities of lung parenchyma have been shown to have multiple cysts. This includes infants with TTF-1, alveolar growth disturbance, and PIG, as well as children with Trisomy 21 and Turner syndrome and in some chromosomally normal infants with congenital heart disease.

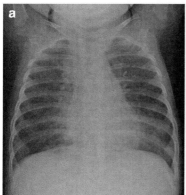
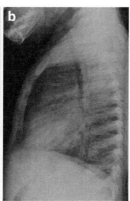
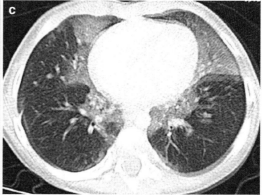

Fig. 8.8. (a) NEHI: PA CXR of this baby with NEHI shows a centrally accentuated hazy interstitial opacification bilaterally with hyperinflation. (b) NEHI: Lateral CXR confirms that the central opacifications are accentuated anteriorly. Hyperinflation is again evident. (c) CT reveals the classic centrally, anteriorly accentuated ground glass opacities of NEHI. (d) Neuroendocrine cell hyperplasia of infancy (NEHI): Cases of NEHI generally have a near normal histologic appearance, illustrated in the *left upper two panels* with hematoxylin and eosin stain where there are mild nonspecific changes including mild prominence of airway smooth muscle and a mild increase in alveolar macrophages; however, occasional cases may show prominence of airway-associated lymphoid tissue and mild peri-airway lymphocytic infiltrates, illustrated in the *right upper two panels* with hematoxylin and eosin stain, which overshadow the similar mild airway smooth muscle and macrophage increase. With this quite bland background, the histologic hallmark of NEHI is an increase in the proportion of neuroendocrine cells in small airways (*lower four panels* with immunostain for bombesin), where they often appear clustered in small groups and sheets, rather than as isolated cells; neuroepithelial bodies (*bottom right*) may be enlarged and/or numerous

d

NEHI

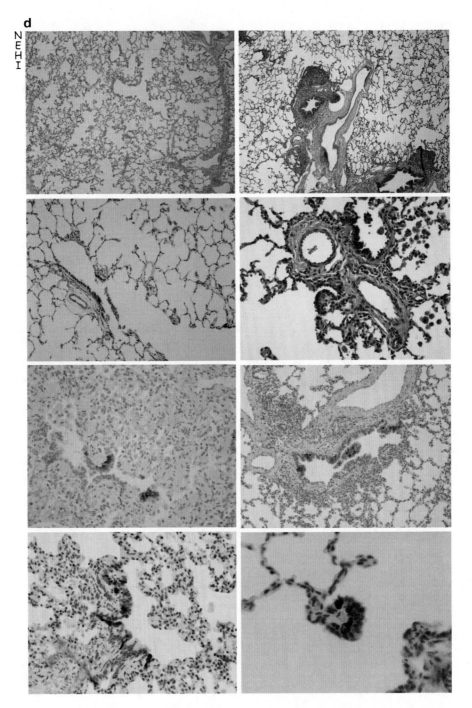

Fig. 8.8. (continued)

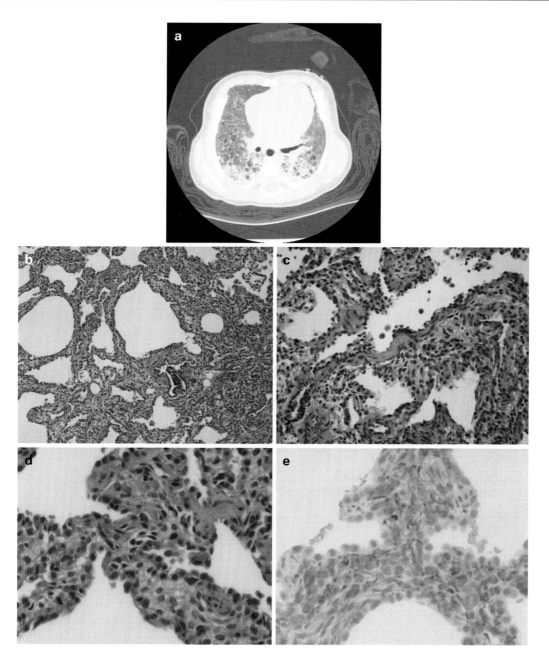

Fig. 8.9. (**a**) PIG: CT of an infant with alveolar growth abnormality and PIG shows ground glass opacities, intralobular septal thickening, reticular changes, and multiple posterior cysts. (Image courtesy of Dr. Paul Guillerman, Baylor College of Medicine, Texas Children's Hospital, Houston, TX.) Cases of PIG typically show at least some element of alveolar growth abnormality in the background as seen in (**b**) with enlarged airspaces. In PIG, the lobular interstitium is widened by an accumulation of bland appearing cells with abundant pale to bubbly cytoplasm (**b–d**). Other features vary depending on the underlying conditions affecting the infant. There may be mild and patchy alveolar epithelial hyperplasia (**b–d**); it is not a necessary feature and is almost never prominent and diffuse; there also may be pulmonary arterial changes of hypertensive vasculopathy (not illustrated). The large pale interstitial cells are immunopositive for vimentin (**e**), but not for macrophage or epithelial markers, suggesting that they are mesenchymal in type. Definitive diagnosis requires the identification of these large bland interstitial cells by electron microscopy. These cells widen the alveolar interstitium (**f**); they have bland nuclei and a paucity of cytoplasmic organelles (**g**), and their cytoplasm contains abundant monoparticulate glycogen (**e**). The cells stain similarly to the glycan-rich matrix of early fibrosis with Movat pentachrome stain (**h**) and as fibrous tissue with trichrome stain(not shown), although there is no actual collagen deposition by electron microscopy. While in occasional cases the intracellular glycogen may be demonstrated by PAS staining with PAS-positive, diastase-sensitive interstitial staining (not illustrated), in most the glycogen is washed out during processing and the PAS stain is not positive

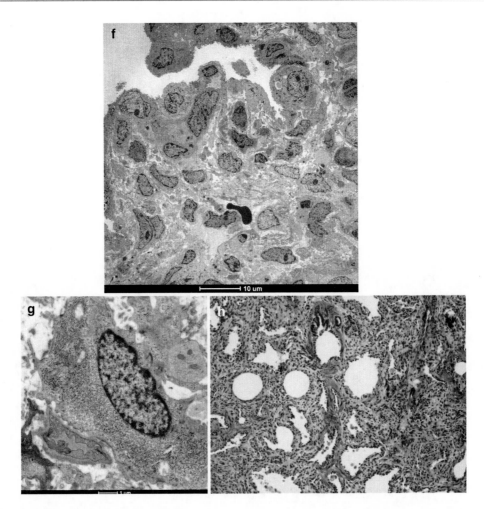

Fig. 8.9. (continued)

8.6 Other Childhood Interstitial Lung Disorders

Infant lung disorders are only rarely seen in older children. Occasionally, children with alveolar growth disorders or NEHI may not come to biopsy until the third year, and some children with surfactant dysfunction mutations present later in childhood, or as adolescents or young adults. While the lung disorders more specific to infancy predominate in infants and young children, almost 40% of the lung biopsies in the multicenter institutional study revealed diagnoses in other categories of ChILD (Table 8.1). This narrow predominance of lung disorders more specific to infancy was also documented in a single institutional study of diffuse lung disease in infancy [42]. The other categories for infants and also for older children are detailed below according to the ChILD classification system beginning with disorders of the normal host and are supported by both the under two multicenter study [2] and by a multicenter review of almost 200 lung biopsies from children 2–18 years of age, similar to that done in infants and young children. In this older group, nearly equal numbers of biopsies were from immunocompetent as from immunocompromised children. Those from immunocompromised patients, the largest single group, account for nearly half the classifiable biopsies, followed by those from children with underlying systemic disorders, accounting for another quarter of the biopsies.

8.7 Disorders of the Normal Host

Previously normal children are less likely to come to lung biopsy for the diagnosis of ILD than are those with immune compromise of underlying systemic disease. In these normal children, infectious and postinfectious disorders predominate with noninfectious disorders including hypersensitivity pneumonia, aspiration syndromes, eosinophilic pneumonia, DAD, and idiopathic pulmonary hemosiderosis being individually uncommon.

8.7.1 Infectious Etiology

Acute Infectious Disease

Acute lower respiratory infections are common causes of pulmonary infections in children and continue to result in substantial morbidity and mortality globally. In immunocompetent pediatric patients, various pathogens, both viral and bacterial, can cause primary pulmonary infections. In fact, viruses are the cause of approximately 50% of all pneumonias in children less than 5 years old. Table 8.3 lists common pathogens that can cause pulmonary infection in the pediatric population, categorized by age group. It is important to recognize that more than one pathogen can concomitantly cause pulmonary infection in children. For example, a recent review showed that approximately 23% of children with pneumonia have a viral infection together with a bacterial infection.

Imaging features. Although a characteristic imaging finding of pulmonary infection such as consolidation in pediatric patients with bacterial pneumonia can be easily recognized, various other imaging findings of pulmonary infections sometimes can be mistaken for interstitial lung disease in immunocompetent pediatric patients. Such imaging findings can result from abnormalities caused by an acute infectious process involving airways and interstitium. Airway abnormalities (e.g., bronchial wall thickening, irregular aeration, atelectasis) and interstitial abnormalities (e.g., fine linear markings, interlobular septal thickening, small nodular opacities) can mimic interstitial lung disease in children with normal immune function. In general, viral rather than bacterial pulmonary infection results in imaging findings similar to those of interstitial lung disease in children (see Fig. 14.1, Chap. 14). Clinical history, laboratory findings, prior imaging studies, and follow-up imaging studies can provide helpful information to differentiate abnormal pulmonary imaging findings due to acute pulmonary infection from those of underlying interstitial lung disease.

Pathologic findings. Infection is a relatively common finding in diffuse lung disease in the normal host and is usually readily diagnosed by consideration of clinical history, imaging findings, and laboratory, particularly culture results. Sometimes diagnosis is elusive, and in such circumstances, BAL for culture and even lung biopsy may be done. In children who come to lung biopsy in such circumstances, viral and mycobacterial disease, sometimes atypical, as well as fungal infection, are more common findings than bacterial infection. The pathologic changes vary with the responsible organism from diffuse to patchy interstitial inflammation with associated airway

Table 8.3. Common pathogens for pulmonary infections in pediatric patients by age group

Age group	Pathogen	
	Virus	Bacteria and mycoplasma
Neonates	Cytomegalovirus (CMV) Herpes simplex virus Respiratory syncytial virus (RSV)	Group B streptococcus Gram-negative bacilli *Escherichia coli* *Klebsiella pneumoniae* *Proteus*
1–3 months	RSV CMV	*Chlamydia* *Streptococcus pneumoniae* *Haemophilus influenzae* type B *Staphylococcus aureus*
4 months to 5 year	RSV Parainfluenza Adenovirus Influenza Rhinovirus	*S. pneumoniae* *H. influenzae* *S. aureus*
>5 year	–	*Myocoplasma* *S. pneumoniae*

epithelial changes for respiratory viral infections, to granulomatous pneumonitis for mycobacterial and most fungal disorders.

8.7.2 Postinfectious Airway Injury

Postinfectious airway disease includes a spectrum of changes. This may be mild airway wall and peri-airway fibrosis with or without organization of intraluminal contents as tufts of proliferated fibroblasts or granulation tissue within distal airways and streaming fibroblasts within distal airways and alveolar ducts. At the other end of the spectrum, there may be severe airway fibrosis with significant luminal narrowing to complete airway obliteration (constrictive/obliterative bronchiolitis). For many, the term *constrictive/obliterative bronchiolitis* has replaced the terms bronchiolitis obliterans (BO) and bronchiolitis obliterans organizing pneumonia (BOOP), although none of these diagnostic terms convey the full spectrum of changes that may be seen. Within this context, what was previously called BO and BOOP are now considered points within a spectrum encompassed by the diagnosis of constrictive/obliterative bronchiolitis. Also, the radiology, pathology, and clinical use of the terms BO and BOOP differ from and are frequently at odds with each other. Consequently, these terms will not be used in this chapter.

Since historically within the pediatric imaging literature, the terms BO [44] and BOOP [45] have been widely used, a brief discussion of them is warranted for clarity's sake.

Historically, within the radiology community, BO and BOOP were described as secondary to a common set of predisposing conditions. These included pulmonary infection, Stevens–Johnson syndrome, connective tissue disease, toxic inhalation, hypersensitivity pneumonitis, drug-induced lung disease, rejection in lung or heart-lung transplantation, and graft-versus-host disease in bone marrow transplantation, among others. In the radiology literature, in children, most commonly BO was described as following previous lung infection and BOOP was often seen following organ transplantation. When BOOP was encountered as an idiopathic condition, many came to refer to it as cryptogenic organizing pneumonia. BO was considered irreversible, but BOOP often resolved, especially following successful treatment of the underlying condition (such as acute rejection). The imaging findings described with BO were irregular hyperinflation and mosaic attenuation, usually with one lung dominantly affected, and bronchiectasis (also referred to as Swyer–James or McLeod syndrome) (Fig. 8.10). BOOP was described as irregular hyperaeration, patchy interstitial lung disease, and scattered pulmonary nodules (often peripheral) (Fig. 8.11).

Nonetheless, postinfectious airway injury is the most common cause of irreversible chronic small airway disease in children. While there may be non-infectious etiologies for this pathologic process, in children it is most commonly a sequela of prior viral or bacterial infection. Rare cases follow inhalation of toxic gases, collagen-vascular disease, or are seen in special settings complicating bone marrow and lung transplants. Among the many pulmonary infections known to have an association with the development of postinfectious airway injury, adenovirus pulmonary infection during early life (<5 years), especially with types 21 and 7 has been considered the most important cause of this condition.

Imaging Findings

Imaging plays an important role in the diagnosis of postinfectious airway injury with constrictive/obliterative bronchiolitis because the clinical findings are often nonspecific; however, a prior history of prolonged recovery from a pulmonary infection with subsequent development of wheezing and shortness of breath as well as abnormal pulmonary function test characterized by fixed airway obstruction should raise suspicion for postinfectious airway injury with constrictive/obliterative bronchiolitis. The imaging appearance, particularly by CT, in affected children can be characteristic and may avoid subsequent invasive procedures such as lung biopsy. On plain chest radiographs, the affected lung is hyperlucent and relatively underperfused while maintaining normal or decreased lung volume, although it can be normal in appearance. CT findings of constrictive/obliterative bronchiolitis are characterized by: (1) air trapping, accentuated on expiration; (2) mosaic attenuation pattern; (3) bronchial wall thickening; (4) bronchiectasis; and (5) diminished small vessels. Although these CT findings should suggest a diagnosis of constrictive/obliterative bronchiolitis in children, other more common entities, such as acute viral bronchiolitis, should be considered unless air trapping and bronchiectasis are both present. Follow-up imaging study can be helpful in differentiating the changes of chronic postinfectious airway injury from acute viral bronchiolitis. In cases of acute

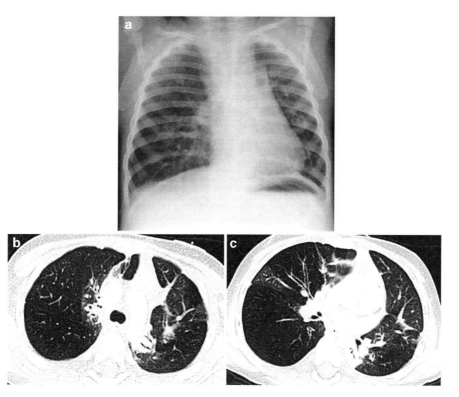

Fig. 8.10. (a) Bronchiolitis obliterans: This 2.5-year-old boy had a normal CXR prior to an adenovirus type 3 infection several months previously. The current CXR shows asymmetric lung inflation with multifocal coarse parenchymal opacifications. CT images at the level of the carina (b) and inferior hilus (c) both show a mosaic pattern of hyperlucent and over-inflated lung segments with oligemia and segments of ground glass interstitial lung disease. The right lung is again shown to be relatively more inflated than the left. There is diffuse bronchiectasis. The findings are those of BO

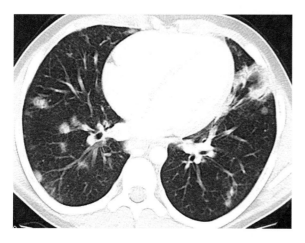

Fig. 8.11. BOOP: CT shows diffuse nodules with mild intral-obular septal thickening and mild patchy ground glass opacifications consistent with BOOP

viral bronchiolitis, follow-up imaging studies will show normalization of the previously abnormal imaging findings after resolution of symptoms (although imaging abnormalities may persist for up to a few months),

while persistent or worsening abnormalities will be present in cases of irreversible constrictive/oblitera-tive bronchiolitis.

Pathologic Findings

Histologically, postinfectious airway injury is a patchy condition in which some, but not all, airways show signs of previous injury and repair with airway nar-rowing by subepithelial and peri-airway fibrosis. Typically, smaller membranous bronchioles and termi-nal bronchioles are affected, rarely larger airways. Such fibrosis may eventuate in marked luminal narrowing and complete airway obliteration may occur. This can be difficult to identify histologically. Clues to its presence include the identification of small pulmonary arteries without associated airways and residual air-way smooth muscle fibers embedded in fibrotic tissue. This latter finding may be subtle and may require spe-cial stains to highlight smooth muscle. There is often variable hyperexpansion of pulmonary lobules in affected regions. Inflammation may highlight affected airways, but late in the process or following steroid treatment this may not be a prominent feature.

8.7.3   Noninfectious Disorders

Hypersensitive Pneumonia

Hypersensitive pneumonia, also known as extrinsic allergic alveolitis, is characterized by the development of alveolar inflammation due to hypersensitivity to inhaled organic dusts. While it has been thought to be uncommon in childhood, it is more likely that it is rarely suspected and therefore poorly investigated. When children are affected, it is usually through an environmental exposure and only occasionally through close contact with family members who are exposed to an organic dust through their occupation or hobbies. Hypersensitivity pneumonia is traditionally classified into three forms based on the duration of illness: acute, subacute, and chronic.

The acute form of hypersensitivity pneumonia usually develops within 4–6 h after exposure to the causative dust antigen. Affected children typically present with nonspecific symptoms such as fever, chills, malaise, cough, dyspnea, and headache. These symptoms usually resolve within 12 h to several days after initial exposure. In children with the subacute form of hypersensitivity pneumonia, symptoms are similar to the acute form of hypersensitivity pneumonia, but usually less severe and more prolonged. The clinical presentation of children with the chronic form of hypersensitivity pneumonia is characterized by insidious onset of cough, progressive dyspnea, fatigue, and weight loss.

Imaging findings. On plain chest radiographs, the common imaging findings of the acute form of hypersensitivity pneumonia are diffuse micronodular interstitial prominence often with ground-glass opacities predominately in the middle and lower lung zones (Fig. 8.12). High-resolution CT (HRCT) can further characterize the chest radiographic findings of acute hypersensitivity pneumonia; these include small (1–3 mm), poorly defined centrilobular nodules representing bronchiolitis and ground-glass opacity representing alveolitis. Both chest radiographic and CT imaging findings of the subacute

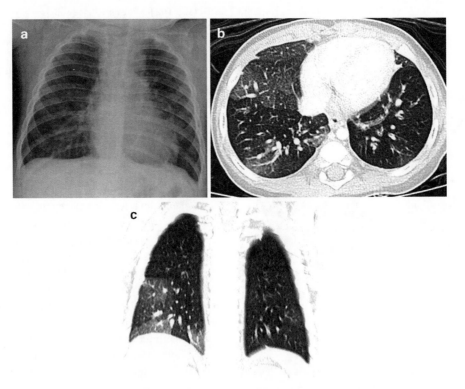

Fig. 8.12. (a) Acute hypersensitivity: CXR reveals a coarse interstitial process accentuated in the bases. (b) Acute hypersensitivity: CT shows that there are scattered ground glass nodular-like opacities in both lung bases. (c) Acute hypersensitivity: Coronal CT shows that the process is accentuated in the bases

form of hypersensitivity pneumonia are similar to those of the acute form. In chronic hypersensitivity pneumonia, imaging findings on plain chest radiographs and CT include progressive fibrotic changes with volume loss without substantial nodular or ground-glass opacity predominately affecting the mid lung zone (Fig. 8.13). The location of fibrotic lung changes can be helpful in differentiating this entity from IPF which is predominately located in the lung bases.

Pathologic findings. Lung biopsy is rarely done during acute disease and there is limited information regarding pathologic findings at this stage. Histologic changes are similar in the subacute and chronic forms of hypersensitivity pneumonia with fibrosis supervening in chronic forms. The changes are characteristic and include lymphoplasmacytic inflammation centered around small airways and extending into alveolar walls with occasional multinucleate giant cells and small poorly formed granulomas in

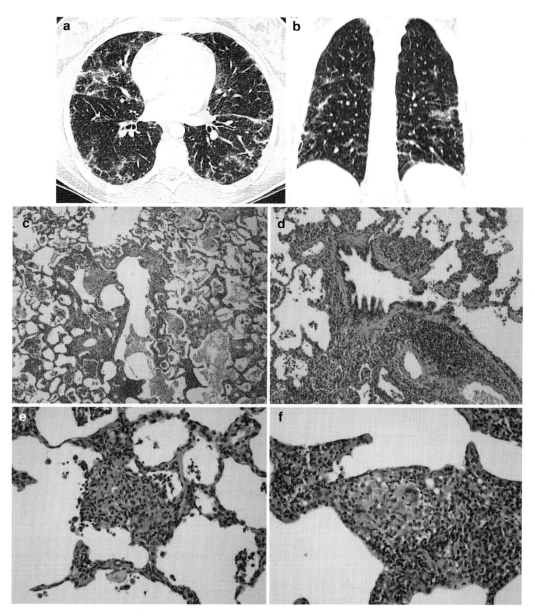

Fig. 8.13. (a) Chronic hypersensitivity: CT shows coarse diffuse fibrosis. (b) Chronic hypersensitivity: Coronal CT reveals the fibrosis is somewhat accentuated in the mid-lungs. Hypersensitivity pneumonia: Hypersensitivity pneumonia or extrinsic allergic alveolitis is seen histologically in its subacute or chronic phase. It shows a picture of chronic interstitial pneumonia with bronchiolocentric lymphoplasmacytic infiltration (c) and lymphocytic bronchiolitis (d) with poorly formed granulomas (e) and giant cells (f) in airspaces and interstitial tissues, typically most prominent adjacent to small airways or at the lobular margins

the walls of distal bronchioles and in alveoli and small airway lumens (Fig. 8.13).

For the diagnosis of hypersensitivity pneumonia, lung biopsy alone may be suggestive, but is rarely diagnostic. A careful investigation of clinical history and imaging findings can provide important clues to the correct diagnosis, and serologic investigations for specific antigens, guided by the clinical history, may be diagnostic in cases of hypersensitivity pneumonia in children.

8.7.4   Aspiration Syndromes

Aspiration syndromes in children can result in acute and chronic lung changes. There are a wide variety of causes for aspiration in children including: (1) swallowing disorders (due to neurogenic abnormalities, neuromuscular disorders, immaturity, cleft palate, laryngeal cleft); (2) H-type fistula or bronchobiliary fistula; (3) esophageal stricture or obstruction (e.g., vascular ring, foreign body, achalasia); and (4) gastroesophageal reflux.

Imaging Findings

Imaging findings of aspiration syndromes largely depend on the timing and amount of aspiration. The typical plain radiographic and CT findings of aspiration syndromes are diffuse alveolar consolidations in the dependent portions of lungs such as posterior lower lobes. In children with persistent aspiration syndrome, advanced lung disease such as abscess can also develop. For evaluation of causes of aspiration due to underlying swallowing disorders or anatomic malformation, barium swallow study is a useful imaging study. Chronic aspiration, without acute aspiration, may produce a diffuse, but irregularly distributed interstitial prominence (Fig. 8.14).

Pathologic Findings

Except in its more extreme manifestations, such as prolonged chronic aspiration with H-type fistula, aspiration can be a difficult pathologic diagnosis; however, there should always be some degree of airway injury and repair, typically with reactive epithelial changes (hyperplasia or metaplasia), an element of inflammation (acute, chronic, and/or with foreign body giant cells and granuloma formation), and in severe cases often prominent lobular changes with inflammation and fibrosis.

8.7.5   Eosinophilic Pneumonia

Eosinophilic pneumonia is a component of eosinophilic lung diseases, a diverse group of pulmonary disorders characterized by peripheral or tissue eosinophilia. Eosinophilic lung diseases are traditionally classified into three groups: eosinophilic lung diseases of unknown cause, eosinophilic lung disease of known cause, and eosinophilic vasculitis. Eosinophilic lung diseases of unknown cause include simple pulmonary eosinophilia, acute eosinophilic pneumonia, chronic eosinophilic pneumonia, and idiopathic hypereosinophilic syndrome. Eosinophilic lung diseases of known cause include allergic bronchopulmonary aspergillosis, bronchocentric granulomatosis, parasitic infections, and drug reactions. Eosinophilic vasculitis includes allergic angiitis and granulomatosis (i.e., Churg–Strauss syndrome). Churg–Strauss is now typically a clinical diagnosis made in the presence of a constellation of signs and symptoms in the setting of known asthma; it is not a pathologic diagnosis, although the histologic demonstration of extravascular eosinophils is one diagnostic sign. It may present with multiple pulmonary nodules, but does not always do so (Fig. 8.15a, b). In this section, only acute eosinophilic pneumonia and chronic eosinophilic pneumonia will be reviewed.

Acute eosinophilic pneumonia was first recognized in 1989, but its exact cause remains unknown. It is characterized by: (1) an acute febrile illness of less than 5 days duration; (2) hypoxemia; (3) diffuse alveolar or mixed alveolar-interstitial opacities on chest radiographs; (4) BAL fluid consisting of more than 25% eosinophils; (5) absence of parasitic, fungal, or other infection; (6) prompt and complete response to corticosteroids; and (7) absence of relapse after discontinuation of corticosteroids. It is more often seen in adolescents than in young children.

Imaging Findings

Typical chest radiographic findings of children with acute eosinophilic pneumonia include bilateral reticular opacities with or without patchy consolidation and pleural effusion (Fig. 8.15c). On CT, there is bilateral patchy GGO frequently associated with interlobular septal thickening, consolidation, or poorly defined nodules (Fig. 8.15d). Due to its rarity and the similarity of its imaging findings to those of other more common entities such as hydrostatic pulmonary edema, acute respiratory distress syndrome, AIP, and atypical bacterial or viral pneumonia, correct diagnosis of acute eosinophilic

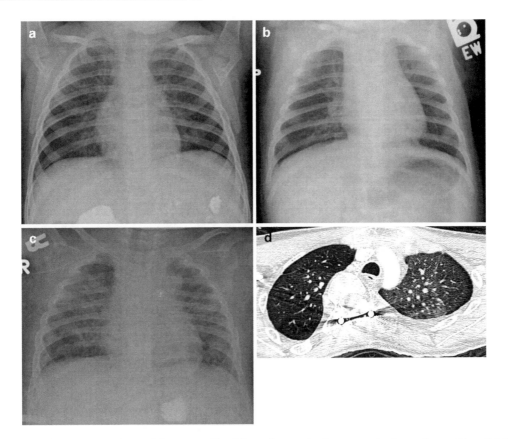

Fig. 8.14. (a) Chronic aspiration mild: 1-year-old with hypotonia and chronic cough and wheeze. There is diffuse peribronchial thickening (PBT), somewhat exaggerated in the right upper and lower lobes and the left perihilar region. The initial chronic manifestations of recurrent aspiration may mimic that seen in early CF or asthma. However, with aspiration, the PBT may be irregularly distributed, particularly in the right upper and lower lobes and left perihilar region, as these are the locations most commonly affected when aspiration occurs in the supine position. (b) Chronic aspiration moderate: 4-month-old with chronic congestion and cough. There is moderately severe PBT accentuated in the same distribution as in (a). (c) Chronic aspiration severe: 2-year-old with seizures and aspiration. There is severe diffuse interstitial lung disease (ILD) with areas of atelectasis and/or fibrosis. (d) CT in an 18-year-old with chronic aspiration shows a mosaic distribution of ground glass ILD

pneumonia may be initially missed or delayed particularly in children. This delay may be critical as failure to rapidly institute treatment may be accompanied by severe clinical deterioration and death. Peripheral blood eosinophilia is not a frequent feature of this disorder, although it may be present.

Pathologic Findings

On histology, acute eosinophilic pneumonia shows changes of DAD associated with interstitial and intra-alveolar eosinophils.

8.7.6 Chronic Eosinophilic Pneumonia

Chronic eosinophilic pneumonia is characterized by chronic and progressive respiratory and systemic symptoms. Although it is more common in middle-aged patients with asthma, chronic eosinophilic pneumonia can be seen in pediatric patients. In patients with chronic eosinophilic pneumonia, elevated peripheral blood eosinophilia, increased serum IgE levels, elevated erythrocyte sedimentation rate, and high percentage of eosinophils in the BAL fluid are typically present. Unlike patients with acute eosinophilic pneumonia, symptoms may relapse after discontinuation of corticosteroid treatment.

Imaging Findings

Plain chest radiographic findings in patients with chronic eosinophilic pneumonia are often characteristic and include nonsegmental peripheral airspace consolidation predominantly affecting upper lobes (Fig. 8.15e). Peripheral infiltrates with a "reversed pulmonary edema pattern" is also considered highly suggestive of chronic

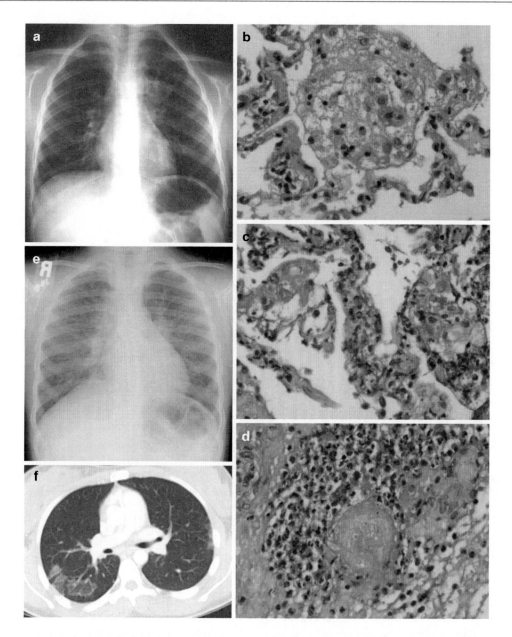

Fig. 8.15. (**a**) Churg–Strauss: This child presented with acute asthmatic symptoms. CXR reveals multiple nodules, most evident in the left perihilar region consistent with the diagnosis of Churg–Strauss syndrome. Churg–Strauss: Histologic findings in Churg–Strauss Syndrome depend on the stage of disease. Early, eosinophilic pneumonia is common (**b, c**) and eosinophils may appear extravascularly at other sites. In the vasculitic phase, there are also eosinophilic granulomas and eosinophilic vasculitis. The granulomas have a necrotic center of eosinophils with palisaded histiocytes. The vasculitis may involve any category of vessel and can include other inflammatory cells in addition to eosinophils (**d**). (**e**) Acute eosinophilic pneumonia: 4-year-old with acute onset of elevated temperature. There is severe reticular ILD accentuated centrally with the suggestion of a small left pleural effusion. (**f**) CT in a different child with acute eosinophilic pneumonia shows multiple ground glass peripheral opacifications. (**g**) CXR shows multiple peripheral nodules typical of chronic eosinophilic pneumonia. (**h**) CT in a different patient with chronic eosinophilic pneumonia shows multiple peripheral airspace consolidations. In chronic eosinophilic pneumonia, there is multifocal consolidation (**i**) with interstitial and intralveolar collections (**j**) of eosinophils with associated macrophages and an often mild interstitial lymphoplasmacytic infiltrate. There may be associated small poorly formed granulomas (**k**) as well as variable interstitial fibrosis (**i, l**) and epithelial hyperplasia (**j, l**)

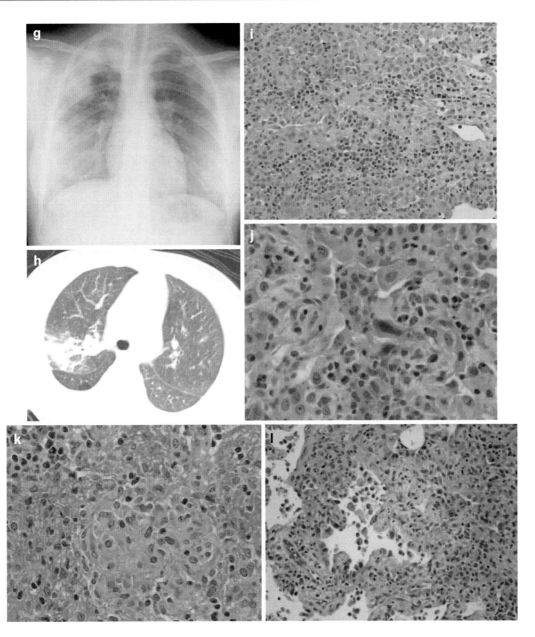

Fig. 8.15. (continued)

eosinophilic pneumonia. On CT, typical nonsegmental areas of airspace consolidation with peripheral predominance are usually seen (Fig. 8.15f). Less common additional CT findings in patients with chronic eosinophilic pneumonia include ground-glass opacities, nodules, and reticulation.

Pathologic Findings

Histologic changes include dense accumulations of eosinophils, often with associated macrophages which may contain eosinophil granules, in alveoli and in the interstitium where the eosinophils are accompanied by lymphocytes and plasma cells (Fig. 8.15g). Eosinophils may be seen in the walls of blood vessels, but a true vasculitis with reactive vascular change or necrosis is never seen. Eosinophil abscesses with central necrosis and palisaded histiocytes with intermixed eosinophils may also be seen. There is usually organizing pneumonia and sometimes poorly formed granulomas; with continued chronicity, interstitial fibrosis may occur. Prebiopsy treatment with corticosteroids may strikingly diminish the numbers of eosinophils hampering accurate diagnosis.

8.7.7   Acute Interstitial Pneumonia/ Hamman–Rich/Idiopathic Diffuse Alveolar Damage

AIP, also known as Hamman–Rich syndrome, was first described in 1935 by Louis Hamman and Arnold Rich. It is a rare lung disease of unknown etiology that typically affects adults older than 40 years old, but it can be seen in childhood and even occasionally in infancy resulting in severe lung disease in otherwise healthy children with intact immune function. Affected patients usually present with nonspecific symptoms such as cough, fever, and difficulty breathing. Unfortunately, these nonspecific symptoms can rapidly progress to severe respiratory failure requiring ventilatory support within days or weeks after symptom onset. Approximately half of the affected children recover, and half of those who recover do so without significant pulmonary sequelae. This improvement in survival is largely due to improved ICU care as there is not yet any clear understanding of the pathogenesis of this condition and treatment remains supportive.

Imaging Findings

Due to its rarity, imaging findings of AIP are not well described; however, those reported are those of acute respiratory distress syndrome with diffuse bilateral alveolar opacities, septal thickening, and often pleural effusion.

Pathologic Findings

Biopsy of the lung in patients with AIP shows DAD usually in an exudative and early organizing stage.

8.7.8   Idiopathic Pulmonary Hemosiderosis

Idiopathic pulmonary hemosiderosis, first described by Virchow in 1864 as *brown lung induration*, is a rare lung disease that affects both children and adults. It is characterized by recurrent episodes of pulmonary hemorrhage with hemoptysis, iron deficiency anemia, and diffuse lung infiltrates on chest radiographs (Fig. 8.16). Due to recurrent concealed blood loss, the anemia of idiopathic pulmonary hemosiderosis is hypochromic, microcytic, and characteristic of iron deficiency. The clinical course of children with idiopathic pulmonary hemosiderosis is characterized by remissions and exacerbations of symptoms despite therapy. The causes of death in such patients include progressive pulmonary insufficiency resulting in chronic respiratory failure and acute pulmonary hemorrhage. With advances in early diagnosis and therapeutic management, 86% of patients now survive beyond 5 years after the diagnosis of idiopathic pulmonary hemosiderosis.

Imaging Findings

Imaging findings in idiopathic pulmonary hemosiderosis depend on the stage of disease progression. At early stages where pulmonary hemorrhage predominates pathologically, ground-glass opacity often associated with consolidation in a central distribution on CT is typically seen (Fig. 8.16).

Pathologic Findings

In early stages on lung biopsy, there are prominent intra-alveolar accumulations of hemosiderin-laden macrophages, usually without prominent associated hemorrhage. At later stages following recurrent clinical episodes, there are prominent reactive lung changes with continuing abundance of hemosiderin-laden macrophages. In later stages, there is progression of these changes including deposition of hemosiderin in interstitial tissue with thickening of interlobular septa and alveolar walls, as well as bronchiolar and arterial walls, sometimes with prominent ferrocalcific deposits, and with eventual progression to irreversible pulmonary fibrosis.

8.8   Disorders Related to Systemic Disease Process

Approximately one fourth of biopsies for ILD in a multicenter study in older children were from children with preexisting systemic disease, and in this study immune-mediated disorders with nonhemorrhagic parenchymal disease were slightly more common than immune-mediated hemorrhage syndromes. Other nonimmune-mediated systemic conditions were distinctly rare.

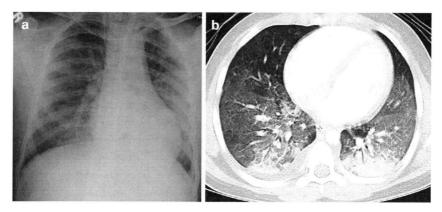

Fig. 8.16. (a) Hemosiderosis: 10-year-old with hemoptysis. There is diffuse moderate ILD increased in the right lower lobe and airspace opacification of the left lower lobe. There is a small left effusion. (b) Hemosiderosis: CT reveals diffuse patchy ground glass ILD with nodular/confluent airspace disease and a right effusion

8.8.1 Immune-Related Disorders

Acquired Pulmonary Alveolar Proteinosis

PAP is a rare lung disease, first described in 1958 by Rosen and his coworkers. It is characterized by abnormal accumulation of surfactant, lipoproteinaceous material, within the alveoli which prevents normal gas exchange. PAP has been traditionally classified into congenital and acquired forms. Congenital PAP is discussed in the infant lung disorder section as it relates to surfactant dysfunction disorders. In older children and adults, PAP is an acquired disorder and is seen in two settings. The first is with macrophage dysfunction typically associated with chemotherapeutic drug use in malignancies. It is then categorized with disorders in the immunocompromised host. The form of PAP that belongs in this section on immune disorders is a manifestation of an autoimmune condition in which an autoantibody to GM-CSF is formed. It is not seen in early childhood, but may affect school-age children or adolescents, as well as adults. Affected children present with slowly progressive dyspnea and nonproductive cough. Diagnosis is by the demonstration of proteinosis material either on BAL or lung biopsy coupled with identification of the autoantibody. Current treatment for this acquired PAP is repeated lung lavage, which has been successful in older children and adults.

Imaging findings. Imaging studies do not differentiate among the various forms of PAP and show bilateral symmetric perihilar opacities that often extend into the peripheral portions of the lungs on plain chest radiographs. These opacifications are frequently not as consolidative and dense as those of a typical bacterial pneumonia (Fig. 8.17). On CT, particularly on HRCT, bilateral ground-glass opacities with smooth intra- and interlobular septal thickening in polygonal shapes, also known as a *crazy-paving* pattern, are commonly seen (Fig. 8.17). After treatment with lung lavage, improvement of these CT findings has been reported in patients with autoimmune PAP.

Pathologic findings. Biopsy findings vary depending on the underlying etiology of the alveolar proteinosis, but all share the common feature of variably abundant PAS-positive granular to globular material with contained small cholesterol clefts filling alveolar spaces. The associated changes in infants with surfactant deficiency disorders are noted above. With PAP due to autoantibodies to GM-CSF, the background lung structure is relatively normal appearing, although there are often scattered interstitial plasma cells, and alveolar macrophages sometimes have atypical appearances.

Pulmonary Hemorrhage Syndromes

Immune-mediated pulmonary hemorrhage, usually with capillaritis [46], can be seen in a variety of disorders including microscopic polyangiitis, collage-vascular disease (systemic lupus erythematosus, rheumatoid arthritis, systemic sclerosis, polymyositis, and mixed connective-tissue disease), Wegener's granulomatosis, and Goodpasture syndrome. Not all pulmonary hemorrhage is immune-

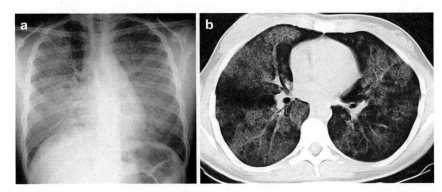

Fig. 8.17. (**a**) PAP: 13-year-old with known pulmonary alveolar proteinosis. There is diffuse severe *ground glass* opacification of both lungs typical of PAP. This CXR pattern is also frequently seen with subacute/chronic hemosiderosis. (**b**) PAP: CT shows diffuse ground glass opacification with septal thickening representing *crazy-paving* appearance

mediated; other conditions leading to pulmonary hemorrhage include drug-induced coagulopathy and hemorrhage-associated malignancy. The clinical and imaging findings are often similar in all such disorders. Affected patients typically present with hemoptysis and dyspnea as well as anemia.

Imaging findings. Bilateral symmetric geographic areas of ground-glass opacities with interlobular septal thickening are typical imaging findings of symptomatic patients with pulmonary hemorrhage syndrome. Focal, sometimes multifocal and nodular-like opacities may also be present representing sites of acute hemorrhage. Chest radiographic findings, particularly in the subacute phase, may be quite similar to that seen in PAP.

Pathologic findings. The definite diagnosis of pulmonary hemorrhage syndrome is based on the identification of blood within BAL fluid or the demonstration of abundant hemosiderin-laden alveolar macrophages. Serologic demonstration of antineutrophil cytoplasmic antibodies (ANCA) may avert lung biopsy to evaluate for the presence of capillaritis (Fig. 8.18), but when these are negative or not obtainable in an appropriate time-frame, lung biopsy is often done. Active immune-mediated hemorrhage is associated with pulmonary capillaritis, often necrotizing.

Nonhemorrhagic Parenchymal Disease

Rheumatologic disorders (collagen-vascular disease). These conditions include systemic lupus erythematosus, rheumatoid arthritis, dermatomyositis, scleroderma, Sjogren's syndrome, and mixed connective tissue disease. The clinical presentation, physical findings, and laboratory findings of these collagen-vascular diseases vary; however, imaging findings of early disease are often those of NSIP.

Imaging findings. For collagen-vascular disease in general, early imaging findings include ground-glass opacity intermixed with septal thickening, while lower lobe-predominant ground-glass opacity, irregular septal thickening, honeycombing, and traction bronchiectasis are the usual imaging findings of later advanced disease or progressive collagen-vascular disease (Fig. 8.19). Characteristic CT findings of NSIP, a common histologic manifestation of many of these conditions, include ground-glass opacity with reticular abnormality, traction bronchiectasis, and lower lobe volume loss predominately located in the peripheral portions of the lower lobes in the absence of nodules, cysts, and areas of low attenuation (Fig. 8.19). The presence of areas of low attenuation interspersed with areas of interstitial abnormality should raise the possibility of hypersensitivity pneumonitis rather than NSIP.

Pathologic findings. Although there are a variety of pathologic manifestation of these disorders in the lung, one of the commoner is of NSIP. Despite its name, this manifestation has a very specific histologic appearance with a mixture of lymphoplasmacytic inflammation and fibrosis and is typically divided into cellular and fibrotic subtypes (Fig. 8.19). It is seen in a variety of settings in childhood. It is one of the histologic patterns of the surfactant dysfunction disorders, particularly in patients with late-onset disease or prolonged survival.

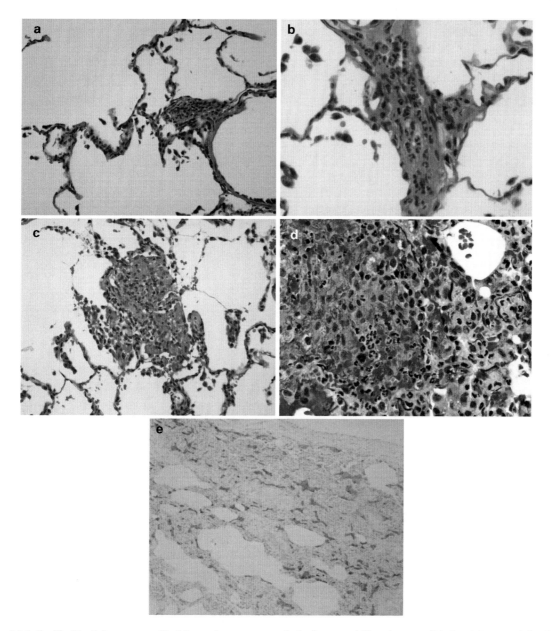

Fig. 8.18. Capillaritis: Pulmonary capillaritis may be seen as a component of immune-mediated hemorrhage in a variety of situations. It may be seen in rheumatologic and autoimmune disorders, usually as a component of multicompartment involvement (see Fig. 8.19e, f) or it may be an isolated feature in microscopic polyangiitis or the only manifestation of Wegener's granulomatosis. In these situations, there may be foci of neutrophilic microvasculitis involving arterioles (**a**), small arteries (**b**), and capillaries often with regions of alveolar wall disruption (**c**) with focal fibrinous and cellular exudate in the region of alveolar wall disruption. Acute hemorrhage, neutrophils, and fibrin may be seen focally (Movat stain) (**d**) and there may be regionally prominent hemosiderin-laden macrophages (Iron stain) (**e**)

It is also a common manifestation of lung involvement by rheumatologic disorders (collagen-vascular disease) in children and adults and has been seen in the setting of systemic sclerosis, polymyositis and dermatomyositis, Sjogren syndrome, lupus, and rheumatoid arthritis.

Wegener's Granulomatosis

Wegener's granulomatosis is a rare systemic disorder primarily affecting the upper and lower respiratory tract and the kidney. It is thought to be immunologically mediated via a T-cell reaction and the frequent ANCA

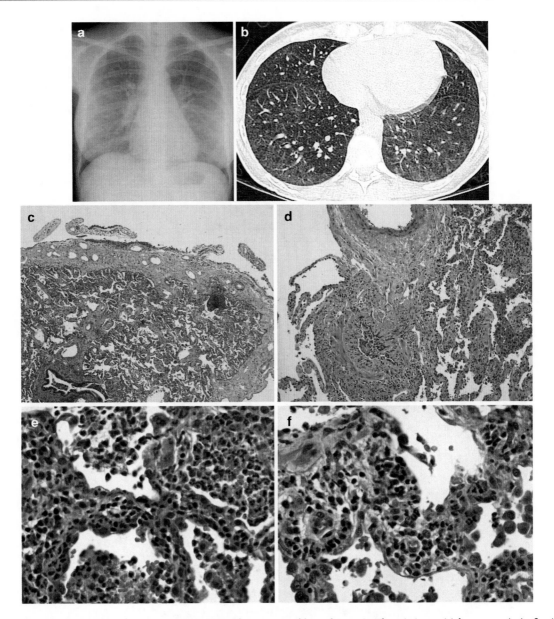

Fig. 8.19. (a) NSIP: 17-year-old with restrictive PFTs. There is moderate ILD worse in the lung bases. (b) NSIP: CT shows ground glass ILD worse in the periphery of the lower lobes with associated mild bronchiectasis. The connective tissue diseases, now called rheumatologic disorders and auto immune disorders, have myriad manifestations in the lung with histologic changes in the interstitium, airways, vasculature, and pleura. It is this multicompartment involvement that characterizes such disorders histologically, sometimes with more specific lesions that implicate a specific disorder. Pleuritis (c) is a common feature of these disorders and may be active with cellular infiltrates or be present as pleural fibrosis with less prominent infiltrates. Airway changes may include lymphocytic or follicular bronchiolitis, constrictive bronchiolitis with subepithelial fibrosis narrowing the bronchiolar lumen (d) and bronchiectasis. Chronic interstitial pneumonia (e, f) with alveolar epithelial hyperplasia and interstitial lymphoplasmacytic infiltrates and exudates is common and may be patchy, but is often widespread; acute alveolitis and capillaritis can be seen in this setting as well. Features of organizing pneumonia are common in this setting as well (g) with streaming fibroblasts in alveolar ducts. In addition to capillaritis, other vascular changes, including thrombosis (h) and evidence of recent (i) and remote hemorrhage (j) (iron stain) with hemosiderin deposition, may also be seen. The pattern of interstitial pneumonia may vary, but in childhood it is most often nonspecific interstitial pneumonia with a variable mixture of cellular and fibrotic components or organizing pneumonia with intralveolar and bronchiolar organization of exudate by proliferated fibroblasts (k)

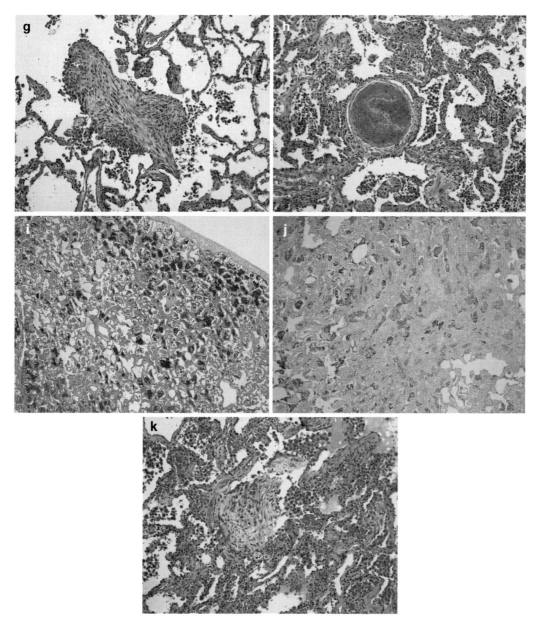

Fig. 8.19. (continued)

positivity suggests an autoimmune-mediated process. It is thought that immunologically mediated endothelial injury leads to activation of inflammatory mediators and cellular inflammation with both vasculitis and parenchymal inflammation of various forms. Although this rare disorder is more common in adults, it is the most common necrotizing systemic vasculitis in the pediatric population. Affected children usually present with nonspecific symptoms such as fever, malaise, weight loss, arthralgias, and chronic rhinitis. Those with lung involvement may be asymptomatic or may present with hemoptysis, dyspnea, or chest pain. On laboratory studies, positive rheumatoid factor, elevated erythrocyte sedimentation rate, and c-ANCA (approximately 85% of patients with active disease) are usually present.

Imaging findings. The pulmonary changes in Wegener's granulomatosis are variable and range from discrete focal opacities to nodular masses (2–4 cm in diameter) with or without cavitation to ill-defined areas of consolidation on plain chest radiographs (Fig. 8.20). On CT, multiple pulmonary nodules typically ranging in size from 2 mm to several centimeters in diameter are often seen in both lungs. Associated cavitation within these nodules has been reported in 50% of nodules larger than 2 cm in diameter. Consolidation often due to pulmonary hemorrhage and/or ischemic necrosis is well evaluated with CT (Fig. 8.20).

Pathologic findings. Pulmonary involvement with Wegner's granulomatosis includes microabscesses, suppurative granulomas, and large geographic areas of necrosis in a background of interstitial inflammation that is typically regional (Fig. 8.20).

8.8.2 Nonimmune-Mediated Systemic Disorders

Sarcoidosis

Sarcoidosis is a systemic disease process of unknown etiology with multisystem involvement. Pulmonary sarcoidosis is traditionally classified into four different stages of disease progression: (1) isolated lymphadenopathy; (2) lymphadenopathy with pulmonary disease; (3) isolated pulmonary disease; and (4) pulmonary fibrosis. Affected patients present with a wide variety of symptoms related to specific end-organ damage. When sarcoid involves lungs, patients usually present with dyspnea, cough, and fever with a minority developing hemoptysis in advanced disease. Sarcoid does occur in childhood, although it is commoner in adults. The clinical presentation, imaging findings, and histologic features in the pediatric patient are not different from those seen in adults.

Imaging findings. Imaging findings of sarcoidosis depend on the stage of disease progression. Small peribronchial nodules (<3 mm in diameter) and interstitial thickening intermixed with the areas of ground-glass opacities and consolidation are typical imaging findings in patients with stage 1 to stage 3 pulmonary sarcoidosis (Fig. 8.21). In contrast, pulmonary fibrosis, architectural distortion, septal thickening, traction bronchiectasis, and honeycombing are predominant imaging findings on CT of patients with advanced stage 4 sarcoidosis. It has been reported that high-resolution CT (HRCT) is superior to conventional CT for detecting parenchymal detail and differentiating alveolitis from fibrosis in patients with sarcoidosis.

Pathologic findings. Sarcoid is characterized histologically by the presence of multiple small and well-circumscribed granulomas without necrosis. These granulomas are often located along lymphatic pathways and thus are seen in interlobular septa and around blood vessels. There is sometimes granulomatous vasculitis. Fibrosis occurs in advanced disease and may replace large regions of the lung parenchyma (Fig. 8.21).

Langerhans Cell Histiocytosis

Langerhans cell histiocytosis (LCH), previously known as eosinophilic granuloma or histiocytosis X, is a multisystem disease characterized by a clonal proliferation of Langerhans cells of bone marrow origin. It usually affects children between 1 and 15 years of age with a yearly incidence of 1 in 200,000. Although it is a sporadic and nonhereditary condition, familial clustering has been reported. In the adult, but not in childhood, pulmonary LCH is known to be strongly associated with smoking. Affected patients typically present with nonspecific respiratory symptoms such as cough and dyspnea.

Imaging findings. On chest radiographs, indistinct nodular opacities intermixed with areas of reticular interstitial opacities predominately located in the upper lung zones are usually seen in patients with early-stage pulmonary involvement from LCH (Fig. 8.22). Pulmonary fibrosis with areas of architectural distortion and honeycombing can be observed on chest radiographs of patients with advanced and long-standing disease. HRCT is the preferred imaging modality for evaluating pulmonary disease caused by Langerhans cell histiocytosis because it can detect characteristic imaging features of small nodules (<5 mm in diameter) in a centrilobular or peribronchiolar distribution intermixed with thin-walled cysts in both lungs with sparing of the lung bases and costophrenic angles (Fig. 8.23).

Pathologic findings. Pulmonary LCH, previously known as pulmonary eosinophilic granuloma, is characterized by infiltration of the lung parenchyma by Langerhans cells. These CD1a and Langerin immunopositive histiocytes are generally seen in an airway-centered distribution that progresses to form symmetrical stellate nodules that also contain eosinophils, lymphocytes, and fibroblasts. In later stages, these nodules may become centrally cystic, but typically central scarring develops with later lesions showing associated honeycombing and surrounding emphysema. Ultrastructural examination shows the characteristic Birbeck granule of the Langerhans cell.

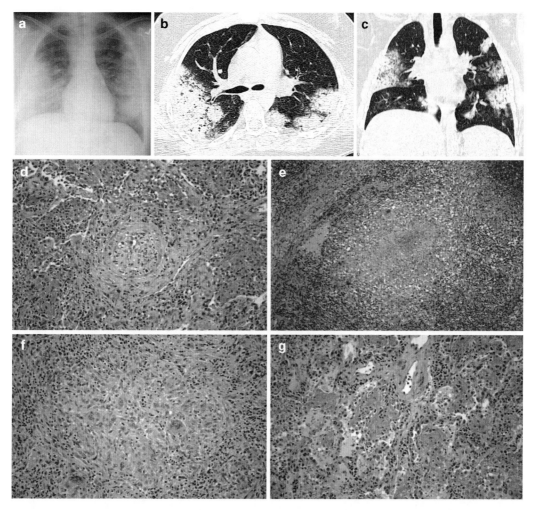

Fig. 8.20. (a) Wegner: There are confluent peripheral nodules. (b) Wegner: CT shows multiple ill-defined nodules some of which are confluent. (c) Wegner: Coronal reconstruction again shows multiple ill-defined nodules some of which are confluent. Wegener's granulomatosis: The histologic picture in Wegener's granulomatosis includes vasculitis, and necrosis with granulomatous inflammation and a widespread inflammatory background. The vasculitis, which is most often chronic, involves medium-sized and small pulmonary vessels (d), here seen involving a small pulmonary artery with lymphocytic infiltration of the perivascular tissue, media, and expanded intima. Large areas of both large geographic and more focal areas of necrosis as here (e) in a dense inflammatory background may be present, with scattered multinucleate giant cells and granulomas (f) within this inflammatory background. Regions of interstitial infiltrate with fibrinous exudate (g) and often hemorrhage are also present

Cystic Fibrosis

Cystic fibrosis (CF), first recognized in 1930s, is the most common genetic disorder resulting in chronic pulmonary disease in children. It is an autosomal recessive disorder with mutations involving the cystic fibrosis transmembrane regulator (CFTR) gene located on the long arm of chromosome 7. Although CF is more common among children of European heritage with an estimated incidence of 1:2,500 white live births, it can also affect children of Asian and African descent. Affected individuals are often dis-covered during infancy when they present with meconium ileus syndrome (18%), failure to thrive, malabsorption syndrome, or chronic recurrent respiratory infections. A definitive diagnosis of CF can be based on abnormal sweat test or via genetic testing, usually employing a panel of more common mutations in specific geographic groups.

Although CF may result in significant gastrointestinal and liver disease, involvement of the respiratory system is the major cause of morbidity and mortality in children and nearly all affected children will eventually develop progressive pulmonary disease.

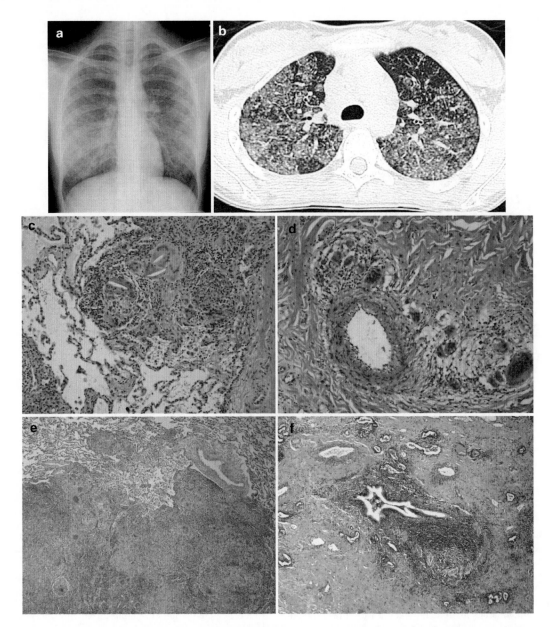

Fig. 8.21. (a) Sarcoid: 17-year-old with hypercalcemia, weight loss, fatigue, and chest pain. There is diffuse coarse micronodular ILD with bilateral paratracheal adenopathy. (b) CT, in another patient with sarcoidosis, shows diffuse nodular and confluent ground glass opacities. Sarcoid: The occurrence of multiple circumscribed nonnecrotizing granulomas (c, d) is the histologic hallmark of sarcoidosis. In the lung these granulomas often are seen in perivascular regions (d) and along lymphatic pathways (e). The granulomas may be confluent (e). With time, granulomas may become hyalinized and there may be dense interstitial fibrosis as in (f) where the remnant of a granuloma is seen in the wall of a narrowed and chronically inflamed small airway in a background of dense lobular fibrosis

Pulmonary disease is the most common cause of death in patients with cystic fibrosis. Imaging findings of CF vary depending on several factors including the age of the patient, the duration and severity of disease, and associated infection.

Imaging. Lungs can be normal or show mild-to-moderate air trapping (hyperinflation) and/or bronchial wall thickening in children with early-stage CF (see Chap. 15). The hyperinflation in CF patients results from the obstruction of the small airways (i.e., terminal and respiratory bronchioles) by abnormally viscid mucus. Imaging findings of later or advanced disease are characterized by the presence of upper lobe predominant bronchiectasis (in 50% of patients with lobe dominate disease) [47], peribronchial wall thickening, centrilobular nodular and tree-in-bud opacities, and mucus plugging with air trapping best detected on expiratory CT images. The reason for

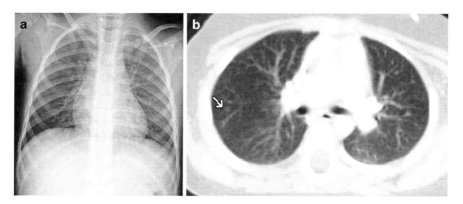

Fig. 8.22. (a) Acute Langerhans cell histiocytosis (LCH): There is mild nonspecific ILD suggesting bronchial wall thickening, which is often the first imaging evidence of LCH. (b) Acute LCH: CT reveals multiple small nodules (*arrow*), dominantly in the upper lobes

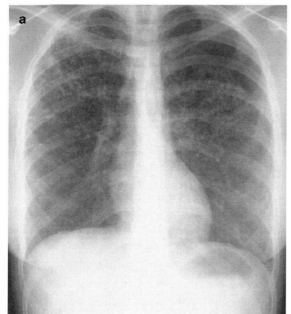

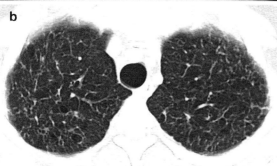

Fig. 8.23. (a) Chronic LCH: There is coarse ILD with multiple cysts, dominantly in the upper lobes. There is a left pneumothorax. (b) Chronic LCH: CT reveals honeycombing with peripheral cysts and intralobular septal thickening

upper lobe predominant lung changes in CF is not known, but it has been postulated that decreased ventilatory excursions in the upper lobe may exacerbate the already impaired drainage of bronchial secretions. Due to chronic and recurrent superimposed infection, concomitant hilar and mediastinal lymphadenopathy is often seen. Several CT scoring systems are available for assessment of the extent and severity of CF disease, although they are not widely used clinically.

Pathologic Findings. The lungs in cystic fibrosis show progressive changes that early may be mistaken for ILD. Initially, there is mucus stasis with impaired clearance and supervening infection. The chronic inflammatory changes progress to alteration of airway walls with epithelial erosion, partial replacement of the mucosa by granulation tissue, progressive airway dilatation resulting in bronchiectasis, and for small airways sometimes fibrotic and obliterative changes. With advanced disease there is progressive loss of lung parenchyma through lobular atrophy and fibrosis, as well as loss of access to the parenchyma due to airway obstruction.

Marfan-Associated Pulmonary Disorders

Marfan syndrome, first described in 1895, is an inherited disorder of connective tissue resulting from an abnormality in the fibrillin gene on chromosome 15. The estimated prevalence of Marfan syndrome is 1 in 5,000 individuals. Although most serious complications of Marfan syndrome result from involvement of the heart valves and aorta, it can also affect other organs, particularly the lungs, eyes, and skeleton. Affected patients are usually tall with long limbs and long thin fingers. Pulmonary involvement in Marfan syndrome is uncommon, occurring in only about 10% of patients. Such involvement may include congenital enlargement of the trachea and bronchi; later findings include pulmonary artery rupture and pneumothorax. A few patients with Marfan have an emphysema-like abnormality with pleural and subpleural bullae and parenchymal cysts.

Imaging. The connective tissues that provide stability and elasticity for the lungs are affected by Marfan syndrome; this may uncommonly result in the development of emphysema, pleural and subpleural bullae, parenchymal cysts, and bronchiectasis. Pneumothorax is the only common respiratory disorder seen in Marfan syndrome and is the commonest imaging finding of pulmonary involvement in Marfan syndrome.

Pathologic findings. Marfan syndrome is a rare cause of spontaneous pneumothorax; the pathologic findings do not differ from those of pneumothorax in unaffected individuals.

Malignant Infiltrates

Malignant infiltrates of the lungs can be seen with a variety of underlying malignancies. In adults this is commonly seen as lymphangitic carcinomatosis, resulting from spread of malignant cells via the lymphatic system in the lung. In children, carcinoma is an uncommon form of malignancy and infiltrative disease in the lung is more commonly related to hematologic malignancy with similar spread via pulmonary lymphatics. Such children usually have known and treated malignancy and present with shortness of breath, cough, or rarely hemoptysis.

Imaging. It has been reported that the sensitivity of chest radiographs for detecting lymphangitic spread of malignancy is only approximately 25%. Therefore, the imaging modality of choice for evaluating lymphangitic tumor spread is CT. Smooth, irregular, or nodular interlobular septal thickening and peribronchial small nodules are the most common CT imaging findings of lymphangitic tumor dissemination. Malignant hilar or mediastinal lymphadenopathy and/or malignant pleural effusion are often concurrently present.

Pathologic findings. With lymphangitic tumor spread, there is typically regional permeation of malignant cells through the lymphatic system in interlobular septa and bronchovascular bundles. This may be coupled with early infiltration of the connective tissue of these regions and sometimes small nodular deposits of malignant cells.

8.9 Disorders of the Immunocompromised Host

In children beyond age 2 years who come to biopsy for the diagnosis of diffuse interstitial lung disease, disorders associated with immune compromise are commoner than any other single group, accounting for nearly half of biopsy diagnoses. In immunocompromised children with diffuse lung disease, opportunistic infection accounts for almost half of diagnoses with interstitial changes resulting from therapeutic intervention in the form of chemotherapeutic drugs and radiation accounting for perhaps another 20% of diagnoses.

8.9.1 Opportunistic Infection

The commonest pulmonary disorder in children with altered immunity on either a congenital or acquired basis is opportunistic infection, and in biopsied cases, fungal disease predominates. Opportunistic infection occurs with organisms that typically do not cause disease in the immunologically normal host. Immune compromise may occur from a variety of underlying conditions, including congenital immunodeficiency, malnutrition, the use of immunosuppressive agents in organ transplant and in chemotherapy for cancer, extensive skin damage, antibiotic treatment, and acquired immunodeficiency syndrome (AIDS). For immune-compromised children with diffuse lung disease leading to biopsy for diagnosis, the commonest underlying conditions are postbone marrow transplantation and in the setting of chemotherapy for malignancy. Common infectious agents in these children include *Pneumocystis jirovecii, Candida albicans, Aspergillus* sp, and viral agents such as *Cytomegalovirus, and Respiratory syncytial virus*; but other organisms including *Toxoplasma gondii, HHV6, Cryptosporidium,* and *Histoplasma capsulatum* may also be implicated.

Imaging

Imaging findings with thoracic infection from these different pathogens widely vary from small pulmonary nodules to masses, ground-glass opacities to consolidations, and increased interstitial markings/thickenings. However, there are sometimes characteristic imaging appearances of opportunistic pulmonary infections in children that can be helpful clues to early and correct diagnosis, which in turn can lead to optimal patient care. Bilateral symmetric hazy ground-glass opacities and cystic lung changes are characteristic imaging findings in *Pneumocystis jirovecii* (Fig. 8.24) infection in children who are immunosuppressed secondary to organ transplantation, hematologic malignancy, or HIV infection (CD4 count <200/mm³), or less commonly with an inflammatory condition requiring steroid therapy. Multiple small diffuse nodules in both lungs are common pulmonary imaging findings in children infected with *Candida albicans* (Fig. 8.25), *Toxoplasma gondii*, and *Cytomegalovirus*. Multiple lung nodules of various sizes often associated with calcification are common in children infected with *Histoplasma capsulatum* (Fig. 8.26). Parenchymal consolidation occasionally surrounded by ground-glass opacity representing alveolar hemorrhage, also known as a halo sign, is characteristic of invasive pulmonary aspergillosis infection (Fig. 8.27).

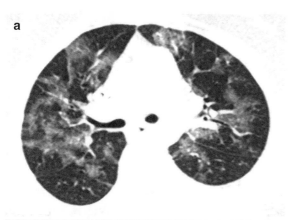

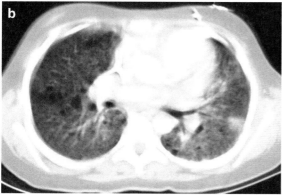

Fig. 8.24. (a) Pneumocystis: CT of this child with *Pneumocystis jirovecli* pneumonia shows bilateral ground glass opacifications although no cysts were evident (which are often present). (b) CT of another child with *Pneumocystis jirovecli* pneumonia shows diffuse coarse interstitial disease with areas of focal consolidation, intralobular septal thickening, and multiple scattered cysts

Pathologic Findings

Appropriate treatment of opportunistic infections depends on identification of the infectious agent, so prompt and accurate diagnosis is paramount. When noninvasive means fail to identify an organism, lung biopsy may be done to provide tissue for both culture and histologic examination.

8.9.2   Congenital Immunodeficiency

In infants the most common congenital immune deficiency leading to lung biopsy for the diagnosis of interstitial lung disease is severe combined immunodeficiency syndrome (SCIDS). In older children, chronic granulomatous disease (CGD) and common variable immune deficiency (CVID), although rare, are the commonest associated inherited conditions. In all these settings, biopsy is most often done for suspected infection that has not been demonstrated by noninvasive methods. For CGD and CVID, there may also be noninfectious complications that should be considered [48].

Chronic Granulomatous Disease

CGD, first described in 1954, is a rare inherited immunodeficiency disorder due to genetic mutations in one of four genes encoding subunits of phagocyte nicotinamide adenine dinucleotide phosphate (NADPH). Most cases (75%) affect boys in an X-linked recessive inheritance pattern, and girls

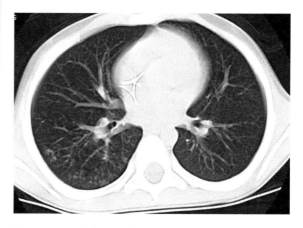

Fig. 8.25. Candida: CT shows multiple small nodules most accentuated in the right lower lobe. The patient had Candidal sepsis

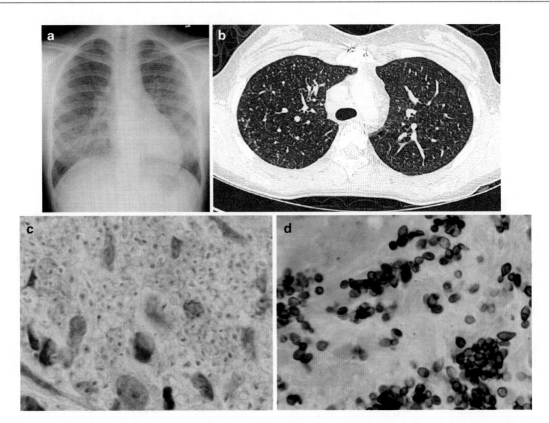

Fig. 8.26. (**a**) Histoplasma: PA CXR shows a diffuse coarse interstitial prominence in this 13-year-old girl with Histoplasmosis 8 weeks following heart transplant with 2 weeks of fever. (**b**) CT reveals diffuse small nodules. (**c**) Lung biopsy (H&E ×1,000). Alveolar macrophages contain numerous yeast often with an artifactual halo as the cytoplasm retracts from the poorly stained cell wall giving the impression of an unstained capsule. This finding is suggestive of *H. capsulatum*. (**d**) Lung biopsy (Gomori methanamine silver ×1,000). Ovoid yeast with occasional narrow-based budding (*upper right*) are most suggestive of *H. capsulatum*. This was confirmed by a urine antigen test and rising serum titres

account for 25% of cases and show both autosomal recessive inheritance and sometimes skewed lyonization of the X-linked gene. The genetic mutations result in impaired phagocyte NADPH oxidase activity leading to reduced superoxide production and impaired oxidative burst. This impaired phagocyte oxidative function results in impaired intracellular killing of catalase-positive bacterial organisms including *Staphylococcus*, *Burkholderia cepacia*, *Klebsiella*, and *Pseudomonas* sp, as well as fungal organisms, particularly *Aspergillus* and *Nocardia* and *Mycobacteria*. CGD affects approximately one in 200,000–250,000 live births in the United States. Affected children typically present within the first 2 years of life with recurrent infections in various locations due to this inability in intracellular killing of catalase-positive organisms. In children with CGD, the lungs are the most common location of infection followed by skin and gastrointestinal tract. Liver or bones may also be affected resulting in hepatic abscess and osteomyelitis, respectively.

Approximately 80% of patients with CGD present with recurrent pneumonia from *Aspergillus*, *Staphylococcus aureus*, and enteric bacteria. The definitive diagnosis of CGD is based on the neutrophile oxidative burst test or previously on the nitroblue-tetrazolium (NBT) test; genetic testing is also available. Early diagnosis of CGD in children is important because they can then be placed on prophylactic antibiotics to prevent infection and appropriate patient education can occur so that prompt and proper treatment can be achieved when infection does occur. With advances in the diagnosis and treatment of CGD in children, their prognosis has improved and affected children now often survive into adulthood.

Imaging. Pulmonary infections in children with CGD typically present as focal consolidation or multiple small pulmonary nodules in a military pattern in cases of hematogenous spread. Development of abscess, pulmonary fibrosis, and honeycomb lung are

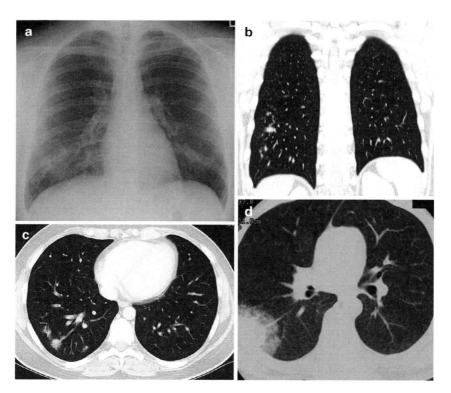

Fig. 8.27. (**a**) Aspergillus: There is an ill-defined right lung base airspace opacification. (**b**) Aspergillus: CT shows multiple right lower lobe nodules some with a questionable "halo" of ground glass opacification. (**c**) Aspergillus: Coronal CT showing the same as (**b**). (**d**) In another patient with diffuse nodular lesions, there is a classic "halo sign" surrounding a large right lower lobe nodule. (Courtesy of Dr. Theresa McLoud, Department of Radiology, Massachusetts General Hospital, Harvard Medical School, Boston, MA)

eventual sequelae of long-standing recurrent pulmonary infections in children with CGD. In these children, additional thoracic involvement may include mediastinal or hilar lymphadenopathy, empyema, and osteomyelitis of adjacent ribs or vertebral bodies. Other common radiological manifestations of CGD in children include osteomyelitis of the small bones of the hands and feet, persistent lymphadenitis, soft tissue calcification from healed infections (Fig. 8.28), and inflammatory obstruction of the gastrointestinal or urinary tract.

Pathologic findings. Histologically, there is granulomatous inflammation, often with necrosis, with surrounding chronic inflammation and fibrosis. It is this prominent granulomatous tissue reaction that has resulted in the name *chronic granulomatous disease.* Even though there is striking granulomatous reaction, the organism burden is typically quite low and biopsy may be done to obtain tissue for culture even in known cases of CGD. Additionally, sometimes even with eradication of the infectious agent, the granulomatous reaction is unchecked and may require immunomodulatory treatment for control.

Common Variable Immune Deficiency

CVID combines a group of varied disorders that result from the defective or deficient immunoglobulin production. The estimated incidence of CVID is approximately 1 in 30,000 live births. Most cases are sporadic, but there are familial cases with varied inheritance pattern. The clinical presentation of CVID widely varies, but all have varying degrees of hypogammaglobulinemia resulting in recurrent pyogenic infections due to common bacteria, virus, and occasionally parasites and protozoa in children. In addition to impaired and immature B-cell function, there may be varied T cell and other abnormalities and autoimmune phenomenon are seen in many patients. About one third of patients are diagnosed in childhood with a bimodal distribution of age of onset with peaks between 1 and 5 years and between 16 and 20. Other causes of humoral immune defects need to be excluded. Because of the difficulty in establishing the diagnosis, which rests on the exclusion of other causes of humoral immune deficiency, there is typically a 5-year delay between symptom onset and diagnosis. While recurrent pulmonary and sinus infections are

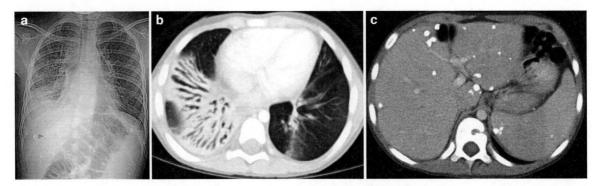

Fig. 8.28. (a) Chronic granulomatous disease (CGD): 8-year-old girl with recurrent infections secondary to CGD. There is diffuse, coarse irregularly distributed ILD with bibasilar airspace opacifications and bronchiectasis. The initial imaging manifestation of recurrent pneumonia is often diffuse ILD. As is also true for recurrent aspiration, the ILD frequently is irregular in its distribution. There are multiple soft tissue calcifications suggesting the diagnosis of CGD of childhood (arrows point to snaps on the patients pajamas). (b) CGD: CT of the lung bases confirms the bronchiectasis. (c) CGD: CT of the upper abdomen shows multiple calcifications

the most common presentations, there may also be lymphoid hyperplasia, autoimmune disease, granulomatous inflammation, and malignancy.

Imaging. Radiological findings of thoracic involvement from CVID are protean but typically include lymph node enlargement, pneumonia, bronchiectasis, and (noncaseating granulomas) in the lungs (Fig. 8.29).

Pathologic findings. Histologically, there are two major manifestations of pulmonary involvement with CVID; one is with infection often leading to chronic pulmonary infection and the development of bronchiectasis; the other is noninfectious diffuse lung disease characterized by lymphoproliferative and often associated granulomatous infiltration. These may progress along the spectrum of lymphoid proliferations to malignancy, typically lymphoma. This latter manifestation is becoming more common as control of infection has been improved by high-dose intravenous gamma globulin administration in CVID patients. The development of granulomatous-lymphocytic lung disease is associated with increased morbidity and shortened survival; however, there are recent reports of response to TNF-alpha antagonists in patients with granulomatous involvement [49–51].

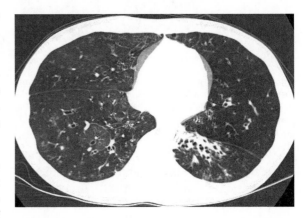

Fig. 8.29. CVID: CT reveals a mosaic attenuation with scattered nodules, bronchiectasis, and volume loss in this patient with CVID

8.9.3   Acquired Immunodeficiency

Disorders Related to Therapeutic Intervention

Chemotherapeutic drug and radiation treatment, typically for the treatment of malignancy and also in other settings, leads to immune compromise and carries a risk of pulmonary complications, both infectious and noninfectious. Opportunistic infection is discussed above, but noninfectious complications of chemotherapeutic drug and radiation treatment may also be seen. Histologic manifestations of chemotherapeutic drug and radiation injury show many commonalities and may be difficult to separate with both showing DAD and varying degrees of organizing pneumonia, and for some chemotherapeutic agents, manifestations of hypersensitivity reactions. With certain drugs, specific histologic features may occur that permit their identification as the mechanism of lung injury and for some hypersensitivity reactions poorly formed granulomas may occasionally occur. Radiation injury in this setting is typically more prominent zonally and is often subpleural; in addition to the common features noted above, there are varying degrees of interstitial and alveolar fibrosis, as well as vascular changes with intimal fibrosis and foamy macrophages within vessel walls; veins are more affected than arteries. In addition, reactive changes affect a wide variety of cell types with nuclear enlargement and hyperchromasia as well as bizarre nuclear forms. In both chemotherapeutic drug injury and radiation injury, changes may resolve spontaneously, or steroid therapy may be used in both to aid in this resolution. Or, they may progress to chronic respiratory compromise with the degree of compromise being related to the degree of fibrosis. Death can occur in this setting and risk depends on the agent and injury pattern.

Imaging Findings

During the early stage of lung injury from chemotherapeutic drugs and radiation, there is nonspecific interstitial prominence and alveolar opacities representing underlying alveolitis. These areas can eventually become fibrotic. Although any portion of the lung may be affected when pulmonary fibrosis resulting from chemotherapeutic drug injury, with radiation injury, changes are in geographic areas in the radiation field and are often zonal in the lung with subpleural accentuation [27] (Fig. 8.30). Additional thoracic manifestations of high-dose radiation treatment include chest wall deformity associated with a loss in the lung volume and decreased functional lung capacity.

8.9.4 Disorders Related to Solid Organ, Lung, and Bone Marrow Transplantation

Rejection

Acute cellular rejection is a cell-mediated process with infiltration of the graft by host-derived lymphocytes targeting endothelial and epithelial cells with immune activation, inflammatory cytokine release, and up-regulation of adhesion molecules. In the lung, it may develop at almost any time in the posttransplant period from as early as 3 days to years later, but is more common in the first year, particularly between 2 and 9 months. Presentation is with fever, cough, and dyspnea, and sometimes with hypoxemia and decrease in pulmonary function. It is thought that infection, and possibly aspiration, may precipitate rejection events, as may lack of compliance with immunosuppressive therapy. Lymphocytic bronchiolitis often accompanies higher grade pulmonary rejection (A2 and above). Acute cellular rejection is assessed by evaluation of lung tissue obtained by transbronchial biopsy.

In the lung, chronic rejection is manifested as constrictive/obliterative bronchiolitis. Its pathogenesis

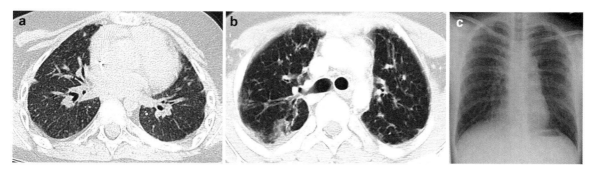

Fig. 8.30. (a) Fibrosis: The patient has had prior chemotherapy and BMT. CT reveals diffuse intralobular septal thickening consistent with pulmonary fibrosis. (b) CT in a different patient also after remote chemotherapy and BMT. There is coarse interstitial thickening with intralobular septal thickening, pleural thickening, and focal airspace/nodular opacifications again consistent with pulmonary fibrosis. (c) CXR in this patient who received mantel radiation therapy for Hodgkin's Disease shows coarse interstitial prominence accentuated centrally in the region of mantel therapy

is incompletely understood, but the airway injury of acute rejection is thought to be an important factor. Clinically there is gradual onset of nonproductive cough and vague generalized symptoms, as well as progressive dyspnea and decline in pulmonary function tests. When this decline exceeds 10% of baseline, a diagnosis of bronchiolitis obliterans syndrome (BOS) can be made and this is graded according to the degree of functional loss. When clinical diagnosis is uncertain, a lung wedge biopsy is done to confirm the clinical suspicion; transbronchial biopsies are considered to be inappropriate in this situation as diagnostic yield is low for airway pathology.

Imaging Findings

Acute rejection. Only approximately 40% of patients with acute lung transplant rejection have signs or symptoms of rejection. In these, noninvasive diagnostic tests including HRCT are notoriously insensitive and nonspecific. Consequently patients are monitored by transbronchial biopsy. At this time, no imaging techniques are accepted as reliable in the diagnosis. There are experimental radionuclide techniques that have been reported [52].

Chronic rejection. Pulmonary imaging findings of BOS can be varied, but typical findings include a subtle pulmonary nodules and GGO with mosaic patterns of lung attenuation. Such mosaic patterns of lung attenuation are due to the presence of areas of increased attenuation (from shunting of blood away from areas with diminished capacity for gas exchange) and decreased attenuation (from hypoxic pulmonary vasoconstriction and peripheral air trapping). CT, particularly high resolution CT technique or thin section (<1 mm) technique with MDCT, is the best currently available imaging modality of choice for diagnosis. It is essential to perform expiratory CT imaging in addition to inspiratory, because air trapping can be more accurately diagnosed with expiratory CT imaging (Fig. 8.11).

Pathologic Findings

Acute cellular rejection. Acute cellular rejection is characterized by lymphocytic infiltration, sometimes with associated eosinophils, neutrophils, and plasma cells, that begins in the perivascular region and extends into adjacent alveolar walls and other tissues. There is a well-defined system for the classification and grading of pulmonary allograft rejection based on the degree of lymphocytic infiltration and associated changes. This is monitored either on a protocol basis and/or in the face of clinical symptoms by transbronchial biopsy, often with associated BAL.

Chronic rejection. In chronic rejection, there is a spectrum of airway changes ranging from lymphocytic bronchiolitis to severe constrictive bronchiolitis and sometimes complete airway obliteration. The important change is subepithelial airway fibrosis which may be patchy or concentric resulting in partial airway obstruction or progressive narrowing, eventuating in complete luminal obliteration. It may be accompanied by lymphocytic infiltration, but inflammatory infiltrates are not always seen. Concomitantly, there is intimal fibrosis and luminal narrowing of small blood vessels. Associated changes include mucus stasis, obstructive lipoid pneumonia, and focal acute bronchiolitis. All changes are patchy in their distribution and may range in severity in any given patient from mild to severe.

Graft-versus-Host Disease

Graft-versus-host disease (GVHD) is seen in the lungs in two settings, in the postlung transplant patient where cells derived from host bone marrow react with the lung allograft, and in the bone marrow transplant patient where cells derived from the allograft marrow react with the host lung. They have quite similar clinical, imaging, and histologic changes and are defined by the setting in which they occur. In the past decade, bone marrow transplant has been increasingly performed to restore hematologic and immunologic competence after chemotherapy or radiation therapy in children with various neoplasms, immune deficiencies, and genetic disorders. In these children, as in children with lung transplantation, GVHD can develop when functional immune cells from the marrow recognize the patient as *foreign* and attack various organ systems in the setting of marrow transplant or only the lung in the setting of lung transplant. Graft-versus-host disease has been classified traditionally into two forms: acute and chronic. The acute form of GVHD usually develops within the first 100 days after bone marrow transplant and is associated with high morbidity and mortality. In contrast, the chronic form of GVHD occurs later, more than 100 days after transplant. The current treatment of choice in children with both acute and chronic forms of GVHD is immune modulation with intravenous administration of corticosteroids.

Imaging. The typical pulmonary imaging findings in children with acute GVHD following bone marrow transplant and lung transplant is diffuse bilateral alveolar opacities which may be related to underlying diffuse alveolar hemorrhage, pulmonary edema, or an ARDS-like process. In chronic GVHD, changes are those of constrictive bronchiolitis described above in the setting of chronic rejection (Fig. 8.31).

Pathologic findings. Acute GVHD in the setting of bone marrow transplantation is rarely biopsied in the lung as more readily accessible sites, including the skin and gastrointestinal tract, are more often affected as well. In chronic GVHD in the setting of lung and bone marrow transplantation, the most prominent lung change is BO with constrictive bronchiolitis and organizing pneumonia (OP) as typical pathologic findings. The airway findings are similar to those seen in chronic rejection in the lung transplant patient with subepithelial airway fibrosis and lymphocytic infiltration.

Posttransplant Lymphoproliferative Disorder

In patients with lung and other solid organ transplants and bone marrow transplants, posttransplant lymphoproliferative disorder (PTLD) is a serious complication. Incidence varies with the organ transplanted, occurring in approximately 0.6% of patients after bone marrow transplantation, 1–5% of those with renal allografts, 2% of those with liver transplants, and in about 5% of heart transplant recipients. It is said to be higher, perhaps up to 10% in lung allograft recipients reflecting the degree of immunosuppression. Lymphoproliferation in the setting of immunosuppression shows a predilection for extranodal sites, and a variety of organs including the lung may be affected. There is a strong association with EBV infection, and infection following transplant is a major risk factor.

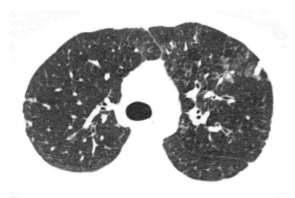

Fig. 8.31. GVHD: This patient with GVHD shows changes of what the radiology literature refers to as BOOP. There are multiple nodules, interlobular septal thickening, and bronchiectasis

Early disease is treated by immune modulation, while more advanced disease is treated as lymphoma.

Imaging. When occurring within the chest, PTLD presents as mediastinal adenopathy, pulmonary nodules, pulmonary parenchymal consolidation or effusion (pleural and pericardial), frequently in combination. The findings are nonspecific and biopsy is required to confirm and stage the process. With lung transplants, pulmonary involvement is approximately four times as common as mediastinal. Whereas, with other transplants, lung and mediastinal involvement is about equal. Nodules tend to be large, frequently in the range of 1–4 cm in diameter. There may be an associated *halo sign* with the nodules as may be encountered with invasive aspergillosis (Fig. 8.27d), but most often the nodules are well defined. The nodules may have evidence of central necrosis with low attenuation on CT. Nodules may be single or multiple [53].

Pathologic findings. This B-cell disorder manifests a range of appearances from benign-appearing lymphoid proliferations that are shown to be polyclonal and polymorphous to monomorphic clonal lymphoid malignancy. It has an infiltrative appearance, but may be focal and nodular or diffuse.

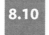

8.10 Disorders Masquerading as Interstitial Lung Disease

As with any set of conditions defined by a common clinical presentation, there are conditions that show similar presentations, but are clearly outside the boundaries of the defined disorder. With pediatric ILD, there are a variety of mimics or disorders that masquerade as ILD. It is important to correctly recognize these; they are individually important and require quite different management from ILD. Almost all such conditions seen in the pediatric patient with suspected ILD are vascular in their origin. In infants, congestive vasculopathy predominates, while in older children arterial hypertensive vasculopathy, lymphatic disorders and pulmonary edema in addition to congestive vasculopathy may also mimic ILD. To identify underlying disorders and to differentiate among the various disorders masquerading as ILD, it is crucial to obtain high-quality high-resolution CT images (either with conventional technique or with thin image reconstruction (<1 mm) from MDCT) often in conjunction with angiographic acquisitions in cases of conditions related to vasculopathy.

8.10.1 Arterial Hypertensive Vasculopathy

PHT is defined as a mean pulmonary artery pressure greater than 25 mmHg at rest or greater than 30 mmHg during exercise in the setting of an increased pulmonary vascular resistance. In children, pulmonary arterial hypertensive vasculopathy can be either idiopathic or in association with various other conditions including parenchymal lung disease, liver disease, thromboembolic disease, and cardiac disease (i.e., left-to-right cardiac shunt lesions).

Imaging Findings

The common pulmonary imaging findings from various causes of pulmonary arterial hypertensive vasculopathy are similar. Enlargement of central pulmonary arteries, abrupt narrowing or tapering of peripheral pulmonary arteries, dilated bronchial arteries, and a mosaic pattern of lung parenchymal attenuation are commonly seen in patients with pulmonary arterial hypertensive vasculopathy. The mosaic pattern of lung parenchymal attenuation in children with arterial hypertensive vasculopathy is due to underlying variable lung perfusion and can sometimes be confused with interstitial lung disease in children. Additional imaging findings such as right ventricular hypertrophy and right ventricular and atrial enlargement in conjunction with information regarding the patient's underlying medical condition can be helpful in differentiating lung changes due to arterial hypertensive vasculopathy from true interstitial lung disease.

Pathologic Findings

Arterial hypertensive vasculopathy is characterized by progressive changes in the pulmonary arteries that begin with extension of arterial smooth muscle into small, normally nonmuscularized, vessels in alveolar walls and progress to involve small pulmonary arteries with medial hypertrophy, followed by intimal cellular proliferation, vascular dilatation, and the development of plexiform lesions.

8.10.2 Congestive Vasculopathy

A variety of conditions related to pulmonary veins and the mitral valve may result in pulmonary venous hypertension and changes of congestive vasculopathy in children. These include pulmonary veno-occlusive disease, extrinsic pulmonary venous compression by mediastinal mass or fibrosis, left-sided cardiac disease, and pulmonary vein stenosis or atresia in pediatric patients.

Imaging

Pulmonary interstitial and alveolar edema are the most common imaging finding of congestive (venous) vasculopathy (see Sect. 9.1).

Pathologic Findings

Congestive vasculopathy is characterized pathologically by thickening of the walls of pulmonary veins with sclerosis and arterialization, lymphatic dilatation, progressive peripheral lobular interstitial edema and fibrosis, and usually small numbers of hemosiderin-laden macrophages reflecting leakage of erythrocytes from the often dilated and congested alveolar capillaries. There are also changes involving the distalmost arteries with mild medial hyperplasia. The pleura and interlobular septa may also be widened by edema and progressive fibrosis. In pulmonary veno-occlusive disease, there will also be prominent cushions of expanded intima in veins that lead to marked luminal compromise or complete obliteration. With severe congestive vasculopathy, there may also be manifestations of pulmonary arterial hypertension due to transmission of venous pressure through the alveolar capillaries into the arterial system.

8.10.3 Lymphatic Disorders

A variety of lymphatic disorders including pulmonary lymphangiectasis and pulmonary lymphangiomatosis [54, 55] may mimic ILD. Pulmonary lymphatics play an essential role by removing extravascular lung fluid and protein. Lymphatics are located adjacent to the blood vessels in the bronchovascular spaces and in the connective tissues of interlobular septa and the pleura. In pulmonary lymphangiectasis, there is enlargement of these lymphatic channels on a congenital or acquired basis, and in some genetic syndromes. In pulmonary lymphangiomatosis, there is proliferation of lymphatic channels expanding the pleura, interlobular septa, and bronchovascular bundles. Both these lymphatic disorders may be isolated to the lung or associated with involvement of other organs sometimes limited to the thorax and sometimes extrathoracic as well.

Congenital pulmonary lymphangiectasis is a rare disorder of poorly understood etiology. It has been suggested that it results from failure of normal regression of lymphatic channels of the fetal lung at 20 weeks of gestation. Affected patients present at birth with severe respiratory distress, tachypnea, and cyanosis, often with pleural effusion that has limited late gestational lung growth. A proportion of affected fetuses are stillborn and in those that are live-born there is early mortality within a few hours of birth likely due to lung hypoplasia. There are, however, less severely affected infants who may survive long-term with variable degrees of respiratory compromise. These infants and young children are typically managed with fluid restriction and diet. Manifestations often improve with age. The diagnosis of congenital pulmonary lymphangiectasis should be strongly considered in term of neonates who present with severe respiratory distress and pleural effusion at birth. In older children with congenital pulmonary lymphangiectasis, the common clinical presentations include recurrent cough, wheeze, increased respiratory effort with inspiratory crackles, and sometimes congestive heart failure.

Imaging

Chest radiographs of affected infants usually show bilateral increased interstitial markings with hyperinflation and often with pleural effusion (Fig. 8.32, also see Sect. 9.2). On CT, diffuse thickening of the peribronchovascular interstitium and interlobular septa is usually seen. On MR, high-signal material within the pulmonary interstitium, often associated with pleural effusion, can be seen on T2-weighted images.

Pathologic Findings

Congenital pulmonary lymphangiectasis is characterized by the presence of dilated and tortuous lymphatic channels in normal numbers in their normal

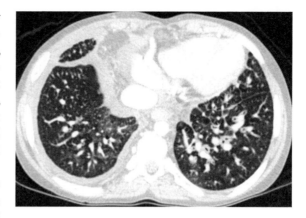

Fig. 8.32. Lymphangiectasis: CT reveals diffuse bronchial wall thickening, intralobular septal thickening, mosaic opacifications, and bilateral pleural effusions in this child with lymphangiectasis. There is incidental fatty infiltration of the mediastinum

locations in the pleura, interlobular septa, and in perivascular and peribronchial connective tissue. The pleural effusion which often accompanies congenital pulmonary lymphangiectasis is not chylous until enteric feeds are instituted, but may contain prominent large lymphocytes of thoracic duct origin. Those who present later will show less prominent lymphatic dilatation, but will have bland fibrosis of the pleura, interlobular septa, and bronchovascular bundles due to the presence of chronic edema in these regions (brawny edema).

8.10.4   Pulmonary Edema

Pulmonary edema results from the excessive accumulation of fluid in lung tissues. It can be due to many causes, but is traditionally categorized into three types: cardiogenic, noncardiogenic (capillary leak), and fluid overload (iatrogenic and renal causes). In children, the majority of cardiogenic pulmonary edema is related to impaired left ventricular function or obstruction of pulmonary venous return. Noncardiogenic pulmonary edema can be due to upper airway obstruction, ARDS, and neurogenic causes (e.g., head trauma and seizures). Fluid overload due to either excessive administration of intravenous fluid or underlying renal dysfunction can result in fluid overload type pulmonary edema in children. Clinical presentation of children with pulmonary edema varies based on the severity of the condition; however, they typically present with difficult breathing, desaturation, and excessive sweating.

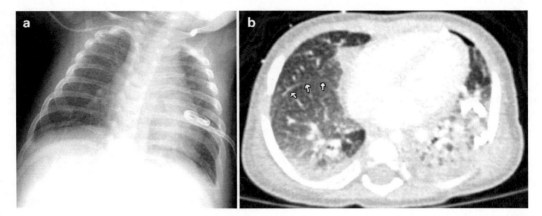

Fig. 8.33. (a) Edema: This infant is recently status post-PDA ligation with mild interstitial pulmonary edema. Note subtle Kerley B lines in the left costophrenic angle. (b) CT reveals bibasilar atelectasis with dependent alveolar pulmonary edema. There is subpleural fluid accentuating the minor fissure (*arrows*). Mild intralobular septal thickening is present. Also noted is a small left pneumothorax

Imaging

The imaging appearance of pulmonary edema usually follows the stages of increasing severity: (1) pulmonary vascular redistribution (on upright but not supine imaging); (2) interstitial edema; and (3) alveolar edema. Characteristic radiographic findings of the early stage of pulmonary edema include vascular redistribution, fuzzy vascular and bronchial walls, Kerley's B lines (i.e., thickening of the interlobular septa presenting as thin, nonbranching lines abutting the pleura), and thickening of the pleural fissures (Fig. 8.33). More advanced degrees of pulmonary edema typically present as increased alveolar opacity and air bronchograms with ill-defined borders. On CT, areas of ground-glass opacity, smooth intralobular septal thickening, fissural thickening, and pleural effusion are often seen (Fig. 8.33). The presence of left atrial and ventricular enlargement on imaging studies can be helpful clues to cardiogenic pulmonary edema.

Pathologic Findings

It is rare for children with isolated pulmonary edema, particularly on an acute basis to come to biopsy, but these would show protein-rich (pink) fluid within alveolar spaces. Occasionally, those with chronic edema mistaken for interstitial disease may have lung biopsy for diagnosis. Such biopsies show, in addition to protein-rich fluid within alveoli, capillary dilatation and congestion, leakage of erythrocytes, hemosiderin-laden macrophages, and widening of alveolar walls and the pulmonary interstitium by edema fluid. Advanced changes are those of congestive vasculopathy.

References

1. Deterding R. Evaluating infants and children with interstitial lung disease. Semin Respir Crit Care Med. 2007;28:333–41.
2. Deutsch GH, Young LR, Deterding RR, et al. Diffuse lung disease in young children: application of a novel classification scheme. Am J Respir Crit Care Med. 2007;176:1120–8.
3. Ponsky TA, Rothenberg SS, Tsao K, Ostlie DJ, St Peter SD, Holcomb III GW. Thoracoscopy in children: is a chest tube necessary? J Laparoendosc Adv Surg Tech A. 2009;19 Suppl 1:S23–25.
4. Ponsky TA, Rothenberg SS. Thoracoscopic lung biopsy in infants and children with endoloops allows smaller trocar sites and discreet biopsies. J Laparoendosc Adv Surg Tech A. 2008;18:120–2.
5. Dinwiddie R, Sharief N, Crawford O. Idiopathic interstitial pneumonitis in children: a national survey in the United Kingdom and Ireland. Pediatr Pulmonol. 2002;34:23–9.
6. Fan LL, Langston C. Pediatric interstitial lung disease: children are not small adults. Am J Respir Crit Care Med. 2002;165:1466–7.
7. Langston C, Dishop MK. Infant lung biopsy: clarifying the pathologic spectrum. Pathol Int. 2004;54:s419–21.
8. Fan LL, Mullen AL, Brugman SM, Inscore SC, Parks DP, White CW. Clinical spectrum of chronic interstitial lung disease in children. J Pediatr. 1992;121:867–72.

9. Fan LL, Kozinetz CA. Factors influencing survival in children with chronic interstitial lung disease. Am J Respir Crit Care Med. 1997;156:939–42.

10. Fan LL, Kozinetz CA, Deterding RR, Brugman SM. Evaluation of a diagnostic approach to pediatric interstitial lung disease. Pediatrics. 1998;101:82–5.

11. Brody AS. Imaging considerations: interstitial lung disease in children. Radiol Clin North Am. 2005;43:391–403.

12. Guillerman RP. Imaging of childhood interstitial lung disease. Pediatr Allergy Immunol Pulmonol. 2010;23:43–68.

13. Dishop MK. Diagnostic pathology of diffuse lung disease in children. Pediatr Allergy Immunol Pulmonol. 2010;23:69–85.

14. Popler J, Wagner BD, Accurso F, et al. Airway cytokine profiles in children's interstitial lung diseases. Am J Respir Crit Care Med. 2010;181:A3316.

15. Deterding RR, Wolfson A, Harris JK, Walker JJ, Accurso FJ. Aptamer proteomic analysis of bronchoalveolar lavage fluid yields different protein signatures from children with children's interstitial lund disease, cystic fibrosis and disease controls. Am J Respir Crit Care Med. 2010;181:A6722.

16. ATS Patient Education Series. What is interstitial lung disease in children? Am J Respir Crit Care Med. 2010;181:P1–2.

17. Sen P, Thakur N, Stockton DW, Langston C, Bejjani BA. Expanding the phenotype of alveolar capillary dysplasia (ACD). J Pediatr. 2004;145:646–51.

18. Licht C, Schickendantz S, Sreeram N, et al. Prolonged survival in alveolar capillary dysplasia syndrome. Eur J Pediatr. 2004;163:181–2.

19. Stankiewicz P, Sen P, Bhatt SS, et al. Genomic and genic deletions of the FOX gene cluster on 16q24.1 and inactivating mutations of FOXF1 cause alveolar capillary dysplasia and other malformations. Am J Hum Genet. 2009;84:780–91.

20. Eulmesekian P, Cutz E, Parvez B, Bohn D, Adatia I. Alveolar capillary dysplasia: a six-year single center experience. J Perinat Med. 2005;33:347–52.

21. Garmany TH, Wambach JA, Heins HB, et al. Population and disease-based prevalence of the common mutations associated with surfactant deficiency. Pediatr Res. 2008;63:645–9.

22. Cole FS, Hamvas A, Rubinstein P, et al. Population-based estimates of surfactant protein B deficiency. Pediatrics. 2000;105:538–41.

23. Gower WA, Popler J, Hamvas A, Deterding R, Nogee LM. Clinical improvement in infants with ILD due to mutations in the surfactant protein C gene (SFTPC). Am J Respir Crit Care Med. 2010;181:A6733.

24. Rosen DM, Waltz DA. Hydroxychloroquine and surfactant protein C deficiency. N Engl J Med. 2005;352:207–8.

25. Karjalainen MK, Haataja R, Hallman M. Haplotype analysis of ABCA3: association with respiratory distress in very premature infants. Ann Med. 2008;40:56–65.

26. Clement A, Corvol H, Epaud R, Feldman D, Fauroux B. Dramatic improvement by macrolides in surfactant deficiency with ABCA3 mutation. Am J Respir Crit Care Med. 2009;179:A3011.

27. Doan ML, Guillerman RP, Dishop MK, et al. Clinical, radiological and pathological features of ABCA3 mutations in children. Thorax. 2008;63:366–73.

28. Guillot L, Carre A, Szinnai G, et al. NKX2-1 mutations leading to surfactant protein promoter dysregulation cause interstitial lung disease in "Brain-Lung-Thyroid Syndrome". Hum Mutat. 2010;31:E1146–62.

29. Iwatani N, Mabe H, Devriendt K, Kodama M, Miike T. Deletion of NKX2.1 gene encoding thyroid transcription factor-1 in two siblings with hypothyroidism and respiratory failure. J Pediatr. 2000;137:272–6.

30. Deterding R, Dishop MK, Uchida DA, et al. Thyroid transcription factor 1 gene abnormalities: an under recognized cause of children's interstitial lung disease. Am J Respir Crit Care Med. 2010;181:A6725.

31. Galambos C, Levy H, Cannon CL, et al. Pulmonary pathology in thyroid transcription factor-1 deficiency syndrome. Am J Respir Crit Care Med. 2010;182:549–54.

32. Willemsen MA, Breedveld GJ, Wouda S, et al. Brain-thyroid-lung syndrome: a patient with a severe multi-system disorder due to a de novo mutation in the thyroid transcription factor 1 gene. Eur J Pediatr. 2005;164:28–30.

33. Kerby GS, Wilcox SL, Hay TC, et al. Infant pulmonary function testing in chilren neuroendocrine cell hyperplasia with and without lung biopsy. Am J Respir Crit Care Med. 2009;179:A3671.

34. Deterding RR, Pye C, Fan LL, Langston C. Persistent tachypnea of infancy is associated with neuroendocrine cell hyperplasia. Pediatr Pulmonol. 2005;40:157–65.

35. Popler J, Young LR, Deterding RR. Beyond infancy: persistence of chronic lung disease in neusroendocrine cell hyperplasia of infancy (NEHI). Am J Respir Crit Care Med. 2010;181:A6721.

36. Brody AS, Guillerman RP, Hay TC, et al. Neuroendocrine cell hyperplasia of infancy: diagnosis with high-resolution CT. AJR Am J Roentgenol. 2010;194:238–44.

37. Popler J, Gower WA, Mogayzel Jr PJ, et al. Familial neuroendocrine cell hyperplasia of infancy. Pediatr Pulmonol. 2010;45:749–55.

38. Bramson RT, Cleveland R, Blickman JG, Kinane TB. Radiographic appearance of follicular bronchitis in children. AJR Am J Roentgenol. 1996;166:1447–50.

39. Canakis AM, Cutz E, Manson D, O'Brodovich H. Pulmonary interstitial glycogenosis: a new variant of neonatal interstitial lung disease. Am J Respir Crit Care Med. 2002;165:1557–65.

40. Onland W, Molenaar JJ, Leguit RJ, et al. Pulmonary interstitial glycogenosis in identical twins. Pediatr Pulmonol. 2005;40:362–6.

41. Castillo M, Vade A, Lim-Dunham JE, Masuda E, Massarani-Wafai R. Pulmonary interstitial glycogenosis in the setting of lung growth abnormality: radiographic and pathologic correlation. Pediatr Radiol. 2010;40:1562–5.

42. Langston C, Dishop MK. Diffuse lung disease in infancy: a proposed classification applied to 259 diagnostic biopsies. Pediatr Dev Pathol. 2009;12:421–37.

43. Clement A. Task force on chronic interstitial lung disease in immunocompetent children. Eur Respir J. 2004;24:686–97.

44. Smith KJ, Dishop MK, Fan LL, et al. Diagnosis of bronchiolitis obliterans with computed tomography in children. Pediatr Allergy Immunol Pulmonol. 2010;23:253–8.

45. Al-Ghanem S, Al-Jahdali H, Bamefleh H, Khan AN. Bronchiolitis obliterans organizing pneumonia: pathogenesis, clinical features, imaging and therapy review. Ann Thorac Med. 2008;3:67–75.

46. Fullmer JJ, Langston C, Dishop MK, Fan LL. Pulmonary capillaritis in children: a review of eight cases with comparison to other alveolar hemorrhage syndromes. J Pediatr. 2005;146:376–81.

47. Cleveland RH, Neish AS, Zurakowski D, Nichols DP, Wohl ME, Colin AA. Cystic fibrosis: predictors of accelerated

decline and distribution of disease in 230 patients. AJR Am J Roentgenol. 1998;171:1311–5.

48. Buckley RH. Pulmonary complications of primary immunodeficiencies. Paediatr Respir Rev. 2004;5(Suppl A): S225–33.

49. Bates CA, Ellison MC, Lynch DA, Cool CD, Brown KK, Routes JM. Granulomatous-lymphocytic lung disease shortens survival in common variable immunodeficiency. J Allergy Clin Immunol. 2004;114:415–21.

50. Thickett KM, Kumararatne DS, Banerjee AK, Dudley R, Stableforth DE. Common variable immune deficiency: respiratory manifestations, pulmonary function and high-resolution CT scan findings. QJM. 2002; 95:655–62.

51. Martinez Garcia MA, deRojas MD, Nauffal Manzur MD, et al. Respiratory disorders in common variable immunodeficiency. Respir Med. 2001;95:191–5.

52. Blankenberg FG, Robbins RC, Stoot JH, et al. Radionuclide imaging of acute lung transplant rejection with annexin V. Chest. 2000;117:834–40.

53. Pickhardt PJ, Siegel MJ, Hayashi RJ, Kelly M. Posttransplantation lymphoproliferative disorder in children: clinical, histopathologic, and imaging features. Radiology. 2000;217:16–25.

54. Barker PM, Esther Jr CR, Fordham LA, Maygarden SJ, Funkhouser WK. Primary pulmonary lymphangiectasia in infancy and childhood. Eur Respir J. 2004;24:413–9.

55. Esther Jr CR, Barker PM. Pulmonary lymphangiectasia: diagnosis and clinical course. Pediatr Pulmonol. 2004;38:308–13.

Abnormal Venous Drainage

9

Sanjay P. Prabhu, Edward Y. Lee, and Annabelle Quizon

CONTENTS

Sanjay P. Prabhu, MBBS, FRCR (✉)
Department of Radiology, Children's Hospital Boston
and Harvard Medical School, 300 Longwood Avenue,
Boston, MA, USA
e-mail: Sanjay.Prabhu@Childrens.harvard.edu

Edward Y. Lee
Division of Thoracic Imaging, Department of Radiology and
Medicine, Pulmonary Division, Children's Hospital Boston,
300 Longwood Avenue, Boston, MA 02115, USA

Annabelle Quizon, MD
Department of Pediatrics, Division of Pediatric Pulmonology,
University of Miami/Miller School of Medicine, Batchelor
Children's Research Institute, 1580 NW 10th Avenue,
Miami, FL 33136, USA

9.1 Pulmonary Venous Anomalies

Sanjay P. Prabhu and Edward Y. Lee

Congenital pulmonary venous anomalies, which arise from abnormal embryonic venous development, occur in a diverse spectrum in the pediatric population. Although echocardiography with pulsed Doppler remains the initial investigation of choice in

R.H. Cleveland (ed.), *Imaging in Pediatric Pulmonology*,
DOI 10.1007/978-1-4419-5872-3_9, © Springer Science+Business Media, LLC 2012

evaluation of the pulmonary venous developmental anomalies particularly in infants and young children, noninvasive imaging studies such as Magnetic Resonance Imaging (MRI) and Multidetector Computed Tomography (MDCT) are currently playing increasing roles in the initial diagnosis and further characterization of this group of disorders. In this chapter, we will review (1) embryology; (2) epidemiology; (3) anatomy; (4) clinical presentation; (5) preoperative imaging evaluation; (6) management; and (7) postoperative imaging evaluation of congenital pulmonary venous anomalies in the pediatric population.

9.1.1 Embryology of Congenital Pulmonary Venous Anomalies

A brief overview of the development of the pulmonary veins is a prerequisite to optimal understanding and ability to correctly classify various types of pulmonary venous anomalies.

Near the end of the fourth week of gestation, the primordial lung buds are surrounded by the splanchnic plexus. Multiple small connections exist between the splanchnic plexus and the umbilicovitelline and cardinal venous systems. But there is no direct connection to the heart at this stage. At this time, a single embryonic pulmonary vein develops as an outgrowth of the posterior left atrial wall, just to the left of the developing septum primum. This vein subsequently connects with veins of the developing lung buds and establishes a connection between the pulmonary venous plexus and the sinoatrial portion of the heart.

Historically, there is controversy with regard to the exact site of development of the common pulmonary vein. Some authors believe the common pulmonary vein originates from an evagination in the sinoatrial region of the heart [1]. Others believe that the common pulmonary vein results from a confluence of vessels emerging from the pulmonary plexus [2]. According to a third theory, the common pulmonary vein is formed by the confluence of capillaries growing into the mesocardium, located between the lung buds and the heart. Nevertheless, it is generally accepted that, by the end of the first month of gestation, the common pulmonary vein can be identified as a vessel draining the pulmonary plexus and

entering the sinoatrial portion of the heart. The site of entry is above the junction of the left and right horns of the sinus venosus and to the left of the developing septum primum [3]. The two right-sided pulmonary veins develop first and the left sided drainage enters the left atrium through a single trunk that eventually bifurcates to form two veins [4].

During further development, the common pulmonary vein becomes incorporated into the left atrium, forming the large smooth-walled part of the atrium at term. Consequently, the individual pulmonary veins connect separately and directly to the left atrium [4].

In summary, one common vein initially enters the left atrium and at the end of development, four separate major pulmonary veins (i.e., right and left superior and inferior pulmonary veins) enter the atrium as the branches are incorporated into the expanding atrial wall.

9.1.2 Epidemiology of Congenital Pulmonary Venous Anomalies

Total anomalous pulmonary venous return is a rare and heterogeneous cardiac anomaly that comprises 1.5–2.6% of congenital heart diseases [5, 6]. The prevalence of partial anomalous pulmonary venous connection (PAPVC) is approximately 0.6% in anatomic specimens [2]. This is less than the number gleaned from clinical studies, which suggests that some patients with PAPVC are not recognized during life. The most common type of PAPVC is to the right superior vena cava (SVC), and the second most common is to the right atrium.

Pulmonary vein stenosis is primarily an acquired disorder that occurs in approximately 2/100,000 children under the age of 2 years [7]. In most series from large centers, an average of two or three cases per year is identified that require treatment [8]. Preterm birth is associated with the development of pulmonary vein stenosis [7]. Pulmonary vein stenosis in the adult population is even rarer, and the small number of reported cases has often been associated with mediastinal processes such as neoplasms, fibrosing mediastinitis or as a complication of radiofrequency ablation procedures around the pulmonary veins [9].

9.1.3 Normal Anatomy of Congenital Pulmonary Venous Anomalies

Normal Anatomy of Pulmonary Veins

Normally, there are four separate pulmonary veins draining into the left atrium (1) right superior; (2) right inferior; (3) left superior; and (4) left inferior. The upper lobe pulmonary veins lie anterior to their respective pulmonary arteries. The left upper lobe vein enters the left atrium just posterior to the orifice of the left atrial appendage. The right upper lobe vein enters the left atrium immediately posterior to the entrance of the superior vena cava into the right atrium. The left lower lobe pulmonary vein courses anterior to the descending thoracic aorta before entering the left posterior aspect of the LA. The right lower lobe vein drains into the right posteroinferior aspect of the LA (Fig. 9.1).

Abnormalities of Pulmonary Veins

In anatomic terms, congenital pulmonary venous anomalies may be categorized as: (1) anomalous connections; (2) anomalous drainage with normal connections; (3) pulmonary vein stenosis; and (4) abnormal numbers of pulmonary veins.

Anomalous Pulmonary Venous Connections

In this condition, one or more of the pulmonary veins may connect anomalously to one or more of the systemic veins. Total anomalous pulmonary venous connection (TAPVC) encompasses a group of anomalies in which the pulmonary veins connect directly to the systemic venous circulation via persistent splanchnic connections (Fig. 9.2). The most common classification system described by Darling et al. consists of four types: supracardiac, cardiac, infracardiac, and mixed. If one or more, but not all, of the veins connect anomalously, the term PAPVC is currently used.

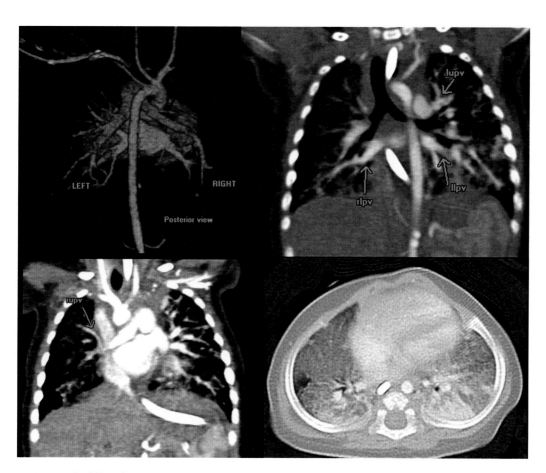

Fig. 9.1. Five-month-old boy, former 28-week gestation infant. Normal pulmonary venous anatomy but with a markedly narrowed right upper lobe pulmonary vein which is moderately to severely stenotic just proximal to the confluence. Lungs are abnormal secondary to chronic lung disease related to prematurity

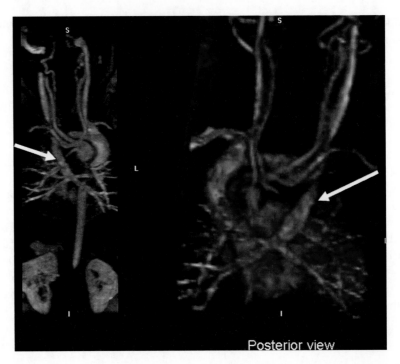

Fig. 9.2. MR angiography (MRA) in a 5-month-old boy with total anomalous venous connection: All four pulmonary veins are patent joining in the midline to a confluence, which extends to a right vertical vein (*arrow*), which continues to the innominate vein to left superior vena cava to a dilated structure that connects to the right side of a common atrial chamber

Anomalous Drainage with Normal Connections

Normal pulmonary venous connections with abnormal drainage can also exist. This may occur in conditions like a common atrium with complete absence of the interatrial septum or due to malposition of the septum primum. In this situation, pulmonary veins connect normally into the posterior wall of the atrium between the right and left horns of the sinus venosus, but absence of the interatrial septum or malposition of the septum primum results in anomalous pulmonary venous drainage into the morphologic right atrium (Fig. 9.3).

Pulmonary Vein Stenosis

Stenosis in one or more of the pulmonary veins or in the common pulmonary vein may occur either focally as a discrete shelf or as a longer segment of narrowing at the junction of the pulmonary vein to the left atrium that extends slightly into the pulmonary vein, or as diffuse hypoplasia of the pulmonary veins (Fig. 9.4). Veins with normal connections may exhibit stenoses, varying from stenosis of one or more of the individual pulmonary veins to cor triatriatum. These result in varying degrees of obstruction to pulmonary venous return to the left atrium. Anomalously connected veins may also be stenotic, with reduction of venous return to the right atrium.

Primary pulmonary vein stenosis without history of prior surgery or catheterization is thought to result from abnormal incorporation of the common pulmonary vein into the left atrium in the later stages of cardiac development. Pulmonary vein stenosis with no discernible preceding or concomitant cause of stenosis has been termed *congenital*. However, except in the small group of patients with diffusely hypoplastic pulmonary veins, the term *primary* pulmonary vein stenosis is preferred. The importance of making this distinction is that it is becoming more apparent that the *primary* form of the disease is often progressive and may not even be evident at birth and therefore not strictly *congenital*. Some authors believe that the rapidity of progression with no evidence of inflammation in many patients suggests an underlying neoproliferative process. This hypothesis is based on presence of apparently proliferative *myofibroblastic* cells that have been found in a small number of autopsy specimens [10]. These cells show features of both myocytes and fibroblasts, consistent with a myofibroblast cell type. In other parts of the body, these types of cells retain the ability to differentiate into either myocytes or fibroblasts. Trials using antiproliferation therapy are currently underway to evaluate whether radiation or chemotherapy might affect growth of these cells in patients with pulmonary vein stenosis. It is also not yet clear whether

these cell types may be more prevalent in the pulmonary veins of some patients and respond with excessive proliferation after a traumatic insult such as surgery or radiofrequency ablation.

Abnormal Numbers of Pulmonary Veins

Normally, there are four separate pulmonary veins; two on either side. The variations of pulmonary vein numbers include presence of a single vein on either side or all pulmonary veins entering a common pulmonary vein draining into the left atrium. A single left pulmonary vein is found more frequently than a single right [2]. A single common pulmonary vein, usually without stenosis, occurs almost exclusively in cases of visceral heterotaxy with asplenia. It is also possible to have an increased number of normally connecting pulmonary veins [2]. A fourth or even a fifth vein on one side has been reported as a rare finding. Abnormal numbers of pulmonary veins are not associated with any physiological problems.

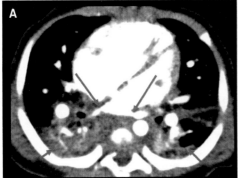

Fig. 9.3. Oblique maximum intensity projection of an MRA depicting a case of Cor triatriatum: The right lower pulmonary vein (*curved arrow*), left upper pulmonary vein (*arrowhead*) and left lower pulmonary vein (not seen on this image) join a pulmonary venous chamber (*straight arrow*) that had two egresses; one to the supramitral portion of the left atrium and one through a sinus venosus defect

9.1.4   Clinical Presentation of Congenital Pulmonary Venous Anomalies

Total Anomalous Pulmonary Venous Connection

A number of anatomic patterns of total anomalous PV connection can result from persistence of splanchnic venous connections at almost any point in the cardinal or umbilicovitelline venous systems [11, 12].

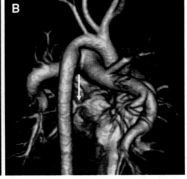

Fig. 9.4. (**a**) Axial CT performed with intravenous contrast in a 4-month old boy who presented with bilateral inferior pulmonary vein stenoses. Image shows markedly narrowed bilateral inferior pulmonary veins (*long arrows*). Also noted are marked lung parenchymal changes (*short arrows*) due to pulmonary vein stenoses. (**b**) Posterior view of the 3D volume-rendered image shows markedly narrowed short segment pulmonary vein stenosis (*arrow*). 3D volume-rendered image is helpful for evaluation of the location of extent of the narrowing

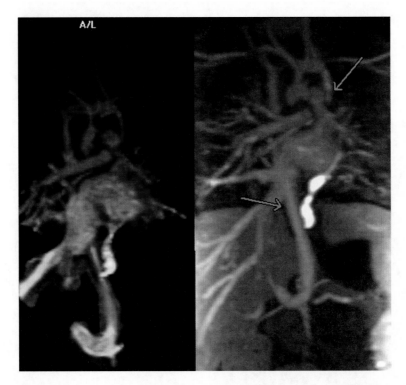

Fig. 9.5. MR angiography (MRA) in a 7-day-old girl with mixed total anomalous pulmonary venous connection. The right upper and right lower pulmonary veins drain infra-diaphragmatically via a vertical vein (*arrow*) which courses inferiorly, behind the right atrium, and leftward past the midline to connect with a dilated left portal vein. This pathway is without discrete obstruction. A right middle and two left pulmonary veins drain to a small confluence posterior to the left atrium. This confluence is decompressed via a second vertical vein flowing inferiorly to connect with a different branch of the left portal vein. This vertical vein has a discrete narrowing within the liver. The umbilical venous catheter tip is located at this narrowing and may be contributing to the obstruction

This wide anatomical spectrum of TAPVC results in a variety of physiological and clinical presentation in postnatal life (Fig. 9.5), ranging from right-to-left shunts with mild cyanosis to pulmonary edema. Obstruction of the PV pathway is the most important predictor of adverse outcome and the tendency for PV obstruction in the infracardiac type of TAPVC is well-described, particularly in cases where infracardiac connections prevent the ductus venosus from bypassing the liver [13].

The overall natural history of TAPVC is poor, with up to 50% mortality in the first 3 months of life and a median survival of approximately 2 months. Therefore, early surgical repair is currently recommended, even before the onset of clinical symptoms and irrespective of anatomic subtype. Results of TAPVC repair in infancy have markedly improved in recent years.

Partial Anomalous Pulmonary Venous Connection

Symptoms related to partial pulmonary venous return are uncommon in childhood, but some dyspnea may occur on exertion. A small right-to-left shunt may exist, depending on the location of the partial pulmonary venous return. The number of patients presenting with cyanosis increases during adult life as a result of changes in the pulmonary vascular bed, pulmonary hypertension, and increasing right-to-left shunt. Anomalous connection of a single pulmonary vein does not manifest clinically. If all except one of the veins connect anomalously, the clinical features mimic those of TAPVC. This is termed *subtotal TAPVC*. If all the veins of one lung connect anomalously, clinical symptoms will result.

The age of presentation and severity of clinical symptoms in pediatric patients with pulmonary vein stenosis depends largely on the number of pulmonary veins involved and the severity of obstruction to each pulmonary vein. Most patients present in the first few months to years of life with significant respiratory symptoms. They have recurrent pneumonia and tachypnea. In later stages, signs related to pulmonary hypertension become prominent. Widespread or localized pulmonary edema may develop, and the degree and distribution of edema depends on whether single or more pulmonary veins are involved. Hemoptysis is a prominent symptom, especially in older patients. Evaluation for stenotic pulmonary veins is indicated in any young patient with severe pulmonary hypertension.

Pulmonary Vein Stenosis

Pulmonary vein stenosis may occur as a secondary event in the pediatric age group, most often after surgical correction of anomalous pulmonary venous connection. Most series report clinically significant stenosis postoperatively in 10% of patients after repair of total anomalous pulmonary venous return [12]. The site of obstruction may be at the anastomotic site of the pulmonary venous confluence to the left atrium or may occur further into the central pulmonary veins. Cases of pulmonary vein stenosis have been described after cardiovascular surgical procedures for lesions not in proximity to the pulmonary veins [14].

Associated Cardiac Defects and Syndromes

Although PAPVR can present as an isolated structural abnormality, it commonly occurs with other cardiac abnormalities, most often an atrial septal defect (ASD). PAPVC or drainage has been seen in association with other congenital cardiac defects and syndromes. Most notably, patients with visceral heterotaxy and polysplenia have a high incidence of PAPVD secondary to malposition of the septum primum, and patients with asplenia have a high incidence of TAPVC. An increased incidence of PAPVC has been reported in association with Turner and Noonan syndromes. A rare but clinically important association is that of anomalous pulmonary venous connections with tetralogy of Fallot [15].

Pulmonary vein stenosis occurs in the setting of various congenital heart diseases, the most common being patent ductus arteriosus and atrial, ventricular,

and atrioventricular septal defects. Further, pulmonary vein stenosis is common after repair of TAPVC in patients with heterotaxy syndrome, may be diagnosed after infancy and is associated with poor outcomes [16].

Venolobar Syndrome

Special mention must be made in this context of the *scimitar syndrome*, which is a congenital anomaly affecting the right lung and the cardiovascular system (Fig. 9.6). It is also called the *congenital venolobar syndrome* and *hypogenetic lung syndrome*. The complete form of this syndrome consists of ipsilateral anomalous pulmonary drainage of part or all of the right pulmonary venous flow into the inferior vena cava, right lung hypoplasia, dextrocardia, hypoplasia or other malformation of the right branch pulmonary artery, and anomalous systemic arterial supply to the lower lobe of the right lung from the subdiaphragmatic aorta or its main branches [17]. The other features that may be seen include abnormal systemic blood flow to the right lung, abnormal bronchial anatomy, abnormal diaphragm, hemivertebrae, and anomalies of the genitourinary tract. Although most cases of scimitar syndrome are right-sided, rare cases have been reported involving the left side [18]. The three forms of this syndrome include the infantile form (with a large shunt between the abnormal artery that supplies the lower lobe of the right lung and the subdiaphragmatic aorta, sometimes called a sequestration), adult form (with a small shunt between the right pulmonary veins and IVC), and a third type with additional cardiac and extracardiac malformations [19].

Pulmonary Veno-Occlusive Disease

A brief note may be relevant here regarding the term pulmonary veno-occlusive disease (PVOD). Previously, this term was used to refer to subgroups of patients with pulmonary venous stenoses. Currently, this entity is classified as a subgroup of pulmonary arterial hypertension (Figs. 9.7 and 9.8). It can be either idiopathic or as a complication of other conditions including bone marrow transplantation, connective tissue disease, pulmonary Langerhans cell histiocytosis, and sarcoidosis. The clinical presentation, genetic associations, and hemodynamics of PVOD is similar to pulmonary arterial hypertension. The diagnosis of this entity may be made from high-resolution CT in the presence of centrilobular opacities,

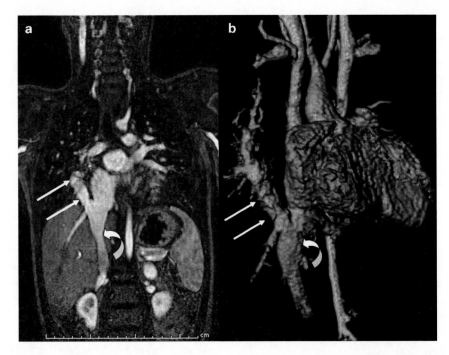

Fig. 9.6. (a) Coronal 2D image and (b) 3D reconstruction of MR angiogram demonstrate a large abnormal pulmonary vein (*straight arrows*) draining into the inferior vena cava (*curved arrow*) in a 5-year-old boy, characteristic of Scimitar syndrome

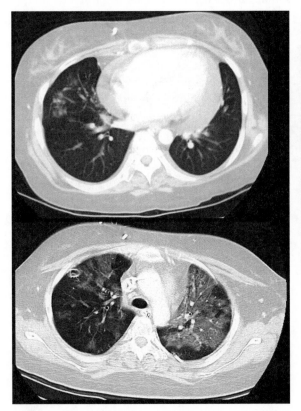

Fig. 9.7. Seventeen-year-old girl with aplastic anemia status-post bone marrow transplantation 6 months prior to admission with chest pain. (a) A chest CT performed on day 1 shows ill-defined nodular pattern that was initially interpreted as fungal infection. (b) On day 9, this developed into a widespread ground-glass pattern with septal lines. Biopsy was suggestive of pulmonary veno-occlusive disease characterized by fibrous obstruction of a septal vein and preseptal venules with pulmonary hemorrhage

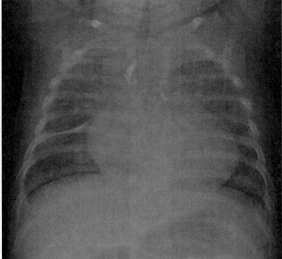

Fig. 9.8. Plain radiograph of an infant with pulmonary atresia, intact ventricular septum and right ventricular-dependent coronary circulation with left coronary stenoses, who presented 2 months after a modified Blalock Taussig shunt and PDA ligation. The radiographic findings are similar to cardiac failure, but the relative asymmetric vascularity and the patchy opacification of the lungs in the clinical context of prior surgery and congenital heart disease might suggest the presence of pulmonary vein stenosis. On further investigation, the child was found to have left upper and lower lobe pulmonary vein stenoses

septal lines, and lymphadenopathy in the appropriate clinical setting. Alveolar hemorrhage may be a feature of this condition [20].

9.1.5 Preoperative Evaluation of Congenital Pulmonary Venous Anomalies

Chest Radiography

In some instances of undiagnosed diffuse pulmonary venous obstruction, the signs and symptoms will be nonspecific leading to a conundrum of whether the clinical problem is primarily pulmonary or cardiovascular. A CXR in this setting will often merely suggest a nonspecific interstitial prominence. In these situations, an index of suspicion for venous obstructive disease should be entertained.

Echocardiography and Catheter Angiography

Two-dimensional (2D) echocardiography with color Doppler is usually the initial study of choice for evaluating the pulmonary veins particularly infants and young children. Although, pulmonary venous obstruction, intracardiac defects, and functional variables are often well-assessed by echocardiography, the pulmonary veins cannot be identified and followed to its entry into the atria in all patients. Conventional angiography is still regarded as the gold standard to confirm the diagnosis after echocardiography. However, there are inherent risks of this invasive procedure technique especially in young infants and children whose vessels are smaller and weaker than adults.

MRI and MDCT

MRI and MDCT angiography can accurately define pulmonary venous connections in a vast majority of patients and presently, assuming a role of noninvasive modalities of choice for presurgical assessment of anomalous pulmonary venous connections in children. Magnetic resonance imaging and MR angiography (MRA) can accurately demonstrate the abnormalities of pulmonary veins better than cardiac angiography and echocardiography. The best images for pulmonary vein evaluation are obtained using a phased-array cardiac coil. Use of black blood

and bright blood images may be obtained without IV contrast material [6]. Gradient-recalled echo (GRE) and 2D balanced steady-state free precession (SSFP) pulse sequences used to evaluate anatomy of the cardiac chambers and valvular function can also be used to evaluate the central pulmonary veins and the left atrium. In our institution, we use respiratory-triggered ECG-gated free breathing three-dimensional (3D) balanced SSFP pulse sequences that acquire near-isotropic volumetric data set that we then reformat in the various planes to define the pulmonary venous anatomy.

Post gadolinium MR angiography (MRA) is also a useful technique. To obtain the best results, gadolinium-based contrast material is injected by hand or power-injected at a rate of 1–2 mL/s using double dose contrast medium (0.2 mmol/kg). Scans are obtained in the arterial and venous phases with multiple breath-holds or during quiet breathing using a non-ECG-gated 3D spoiled gradient recall echo imaging. After reviewing individual source images, multiplanar 2D reformats and 3D maximum-intensity-projection (MIP) or volume-rendered images are obtained to depict the pulmonary venous anatomy optimally.

Velocity-encoded phase contrast images perpendicular to the orientation to the vein are used to quantify the flow through the veins.

MDCT has the ability to demonstrate the vascular structures peripheral to the heart in the thorax exquisitely. Axial and 3D reconstructed images can define anomalous pulmonary venous structures with accuracy rates approaching 100%. The downsides of MDCT are the need for ionizing radiation and the requirement for iodinated contrast material, which may affect renal function. It is imperative that bolus timing is optimal to ensure a diagnostic study with good opacification of pulmonary venous structures. We reserve MDCT for imaging pulmonary venous structures in patients who are incompletely evaluated by echocardiography and who cannot undergo an MRI examination.

Thin section isotropic axial and multiplanar reformats are obtained along with 3D volume-rendered images. Nonionic low-osmolality (or iso-osmolar) iodinated contrast material (<2.0 mL/kg up to a maximum of 100–150 mL maximum volume) is administered intravenously using a power injector at injection rates between 1 and 5 mL/s, depending on patient weight and size of the intravenous catheter. We prefer hand injection of contrast material in infants and small children with small caliber venous access.

In the evaluation of PAPVC, dual anomalous pulmonary venous drainage, and cor triatriatum in older patients, an initial test bolus may be used to optimize contrast opacification of the pulmonary venous system. For patients with suspected TAPVC as well as for small children, we image immediately after the injection of contrast material at our institution with visual triggering when contrast maximally opacifies the left ventricle. We do not recommend cardiac gating for the evaluation of the pulmonary veins structures, although it is suggested by some authors that gating can be used in cases of cor triatriatum, central pulmonary vein hypoplasia, or stenosis.

Preoperative Evaluation of the Scimitar (Venolobar) Syndrome

Imaging studies form the mainstay of diagnosis of the Scimitar syndrome. A combination of chest radiography, echocardiography, CT, and/or MRI may be used in various combinations. On the plain radiograph, the characteristic appearance of the pulmonary vein descending along the right cardiac border resembles a Turkish sword or scimitar, thereby lending the name to the syndrome. Visualization of the vein may be difficult if it is small or obscured by the cardiac contour. The small hemithorax, bronchial anomalies, and pulmonary vein are delineated optimally on CT. The entrance of the anomalous vein into the inferior vena cava may be visible on echocardiography with Doppler. In the past decade, cine MR imaging and contrast-enhanced MRA has been used extensively in the evaluation of these patients as this allows optimal excellent visualization of pulmonary vasculature and also helps determine the hemodynamic significance of the anomalous pulmonary venous drainage [21].

Preoperative Evaluation of Pulmonary Vein Stenosis

Pulsed Doppler echocardiography is considered the first-line imaging tool in the evaluation of patients suspected of having congenital PVS (Fig. 9.9). Normal pulmonary venous flow into the atrium is laminar and triphasic. In cases of primary pulmonary vein stenosis, a high-velocity, continuous turbulent flow pattern is detected throughout systole and diastole, highest near the vein orifice. Diagnosis can be difficult and delayed in cases of total obstruction

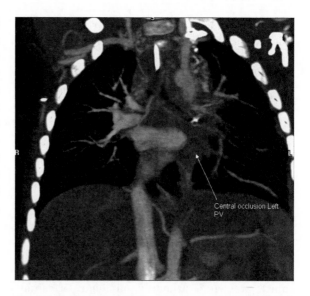

Fig. 9.9. Ten-month-old girl with history of hypoplastic left heart syndrome. Status post stage I Norwood consisting of Stansel anastomosis, and bidirectional Glenn. Pulmonary vein stenosis treated with sutureless repair. Small caliber peripheral left upper lobe and left lower lobe pulmonary veins with completely atretic central segment. Diffuse mediastinal soft tissue induration with multiple serpiginous enhancing structures consistent with venous collateralization

and when there is reduced flow due to pulmonary hypertension. Echocardiography is unable to assess the intrapulmonary venous stenosis due to its inherent inability to penetrate the aerated lung.

Therefore, there is a need for a noninvasive second line test either to confirm echocardiographic and/or clinical findings or define the exact anatomy. Although conventional angiography is still considered the gold standard for this purpose, MRI and CT can be used as noninvasive techniques.

MDCT has been described as a useful investigation in diagnosis and evaluation of primary PVS in children in few studies [22]. Diagnosing pulmonary vein stenosis early and obtaining accurate anatomical detail including the exact nature of the stenosis or atresia are invaluable in planning management.

MDCT angiography with multiplanar and 3D volume reformats allows detailed visualization of pulmonary venous drainage into the left atrium. Since MDCT examination can be typically completed within a few seconds in infants and children, it is possible to avoid intubating and anesthetizing the child for the procedure. Our own experience and the results of a few studies in the literature on this topic demonstrate that visualization of the pulmonary veins is possible even in young patients in most cases on MDCT angiography and optimal evaluation of pulmonary vein stenosis can be made in most cases. Postprocessing with multiplanar and 3D reformats aids in increasing the sensitivity and specificity of the exam. Spatial relationships of the narrowed and/or tortuous vessels with neighboring nonvascular structures are well-defined on CT.

Conventional catheter angiography is currently reserved for infants and children in whom pulmonary pressure measurement is considered necessary or a percutaneous treatment is being considered. Following ALARA (As Low As Reasonably Achievable), we recommend low kilovoltage (80 kV in neonates and infants) and non-gated acquisitions with optimized settings to reduce the radiation dose in the pediatric population.

Magnetic resonance imaging can provide excellent tomographic and 3D views of the pulmonary veins with the use of contrast-enhanced multiphase MRA acquisition. It may show abnormalities of the flow patterns in the pulmonary veins and pulmonary arteries. But its use is limited by the relatively longer scan times, sensitivity to motion and arrhythmias, and the requirement of general anesthesia in young children.

The use of radionuclide studies to quantitate pulmonary flow allows fairly accurate determination of flow distribution between the lungs and must be considered as part of the preoperative workup in patients with pulmonary stenosis and also as part of the post-treatment follow-up.

Value of Imaging in Deciding Therapy

The value of cross-sectional imaging is especially important in cases where it is unclear from the clinical history and echocardiography findings whether the pulmonary stenosis is primary or secondary. For example, the presence of pulmonary changes of lung disease related to prematurity in a child with pulmonary vein stenosis suggests an acquired or secondary process. Similarly, the presence of diffuse intrapulmonary venous stenoses indicates a primary process. This differentiation between the primary and secondary type is important as the prognosis for the acquired type is considered better and the therapeutic approach is also modified accordingly.

9.1.6 Management of Congenital Pulmonary Venous Anomalies

Total and Partial Anomalous Pulmonary Venous Connections and Drainage

Medical Therapy

Children with total anomalous pulmonary venous connection (TAPVC) with obstruction present immediately after birth with severe cyanosis and poor systemic perfusion and therefore need emergent treatment. Initial resuscitation measures instituted include sedation, assisted ventilation, high flow oxygen, prostaglandin infusion, and bicarbonate therapy. These are temporizing measures aimed at stabilizing the clinical condition of the patient and optimizing the preoperative state prior to surgical repair, which is currently the standard of care in this population. In neonates or young infants with unobstructed TAPVC, mild inotropic support, diuresis, and low level oxygen therapy are instituted to treat right ventricular failure, hypoxia, and congestive heart failure. As the patients with PAPVC are most commonly asymptomatic, treatment is initially required prior to surgical correction only in a small number of children who have arrhythmias or right heart failure.

Surgical Therapy

A number of techniques have been tried to surgically repair partial and total pulmonary venous drainage. Surgical correction is aimed at creating unobstructed venous flow into the left sided heart chambers. Associated anomalies like an ASD may be treated during the same procedure.

PAPVC is usually corrected surgically using patch repair of the anomalous vein to the atrium in most cases without complication. To correct supracardiac TAPVC, the vertical vein is ligated next to its connection to the systemic vein and the pulmonary venous confluence is identified. An incision is created in the pulmonary venous confluence and joined up with a similar incision in the posterior wall of left atrium extending into the atrial appendage. The aim is to create a large unobstructed anastomosis between the left atrium and the pulmonary venous confluence. The use of fine sutures decreases the potential for hyperplasia of the intimal lining, which can cause postrepair stenosis.

To correct cardiac TAPVC, the coronary sinus is unroofed by an incision between the coronary sinus and the foramen ovale, thus creating a large ASD. The pulmonary vein ostia are identified through the coronary sinus and its connection with the venous confluence. A patch is used to reconstruct the atrial septum. The end result of the procedure allows the pulmonary venous drainage to flow through the unroofed coronary sinus into the left atrium.

Treatment principles for infracardiac TAPVC is similar to that described for supracardiac TAPVC.

Mixed type of anomalous pulmonary venous drainage is corrected on an individual basis, depending on the exact nature and site of the abnormal venous connections. Surgical correction of mixed TAPVC depends on the exact anatomy and site of pulmonary venous connections. A combination of these procedures is required for the other types of TAPVC to successfully direct pulmonary venous blood to the left atrium.

The outcomes in treatment of TAPVC are still poor, even in the hands of experienced surgeons, primarily due to the poor hemodynamic and metabolic state at presentation. Even in those patients who undergo a successful first procedure, a repeat surgical procedure may be required in up to 15%. Further, every repeat procedure carries an increasingly poor prognosis, and there is a high incidence of pulmonary vein stenosis in these patients following surgical repair.

The technique of *sutureless marsupialization* has been used to treat pulmonary vein stenosis that develops following surgical correction of anomalous pulmonary venous drainage. More recently, this technique is being tried to correct primary venous anomalies as well.

Pulmonary Vein Stenosis

The outcome of pediatric patients with pulmonary vein stenosis is relatively poor and prognostication in these cases must be guarded. In the absence of treatment, patients with stenosis of three or four pulmonary veins have progressive disease in the vast majority of cases and long-term survival is rare [23]. The terminal stage of illness in these patients is characterized by pulmonary hypertensive crises and may be complicated by concomitant infection or hemoptysis. Patients with only one or two pulmonary veins involved have a significantly more benign course.

With the advances in cross-sectional imaging, there has been a recent increase in the early diagnoses of relatively asymptomatic children with milder forms of pulmonary vein stenosis. The natural history of the mild forms of pulmonary vein stenosis in these less symptomatic children needs to be studied in long-term studies.

The overall outcomes of both primary and secondary types of pulmonary vein stenosis have been similar, with similar techniques employed to treat both types [8, 24, 25]. Recurrence of pulmonary vein stenosis after repair of anomalous pulmonary venous return occurs in up to 10% of patients and this can prove to be a significant complication in patients with single-ventricle physiology [12]. Patients with stenosis of one or two veins and less marked stenosis have a better prognosis. When progressive pulmonary vein stenosis is unilateral, the patient may survive, even when there is no discernible flow to the affected lung on lung perfusion studies. Some patients need pneumonectomy to control hemoptysis.

The approaches to treating pulmonary vein stenosis can be broadly divided into three groups (1) surgical repair; (2) catheter based approaches (balloon dilatation or stenting); and (3) lung transplantation.

The currently accepted surgical technique employed in the surgical repair of pulmonary vein stenosis relies on minimizing trauma to the veins. The rationale behind this approach is that this may decrease the stimulus for recurrent growth of obstructive myofibroblastic tissue at the vein orifice. The technique is called *sutureless marsupialization*, wherein the pericardium around the pulmonary veins is attached to the left atrium and application of sutures is avoided along the cut edges of the pulmonary veins. This is now considered the best approach and early experience suggests that sutureless marsupialization may lead to better results compared to anastomosis following resection of stenotic segments and or patch insertion along the stenotic veins [26]. However, prognosis must be guarded, as even with the current advances in sutureless repair, up to 50% of patients may either need a second surgical procedure or die within 5 years of initial treatment [27].

Catheter based approaches have been tried with limited success in patients with pulmonary vein stenosis [28]. Although high pressure balloon dilatation appears to lead to an immediate angiographic response, recurrent stenosis occurs in the vast majority of patients. Cutting balloons have been found to be useful in cases with resistant stenoses. In our institution, catheter angioplasty is often complementary to surgery. Further, catheter angioplasty can be potentially repeated a number of times. The outcome of stents has been universally poor with high occurrence of restenosis. Stent placement in a young child is technically challenging and even if stents are successfully deployed, subsequent surgical treatment approaches in these patients become limited. Intraoperative stent placement has been tried in a few patients and repeated stent dilation to relatively diameters >8 mm have resulted in some outcome improvement [29].

Lung transplantation is an option in patients with marked pulmonary hypertension and progressive pulmonary vein stenosis. Early studies have indicated favorable short-term results in patients with pulmonary vein stenoses undergoing bilateral sequential lung transplantations, but longer-term studies have not yet been carried out in this population [8, 30]. In addition to these therapies, there is an ongoing search for agents that may help inhibit proliferation of myofibroblastic activity in the cases with progressive diffuse disease.

9.1.7 Postoperative Imaging Evaluation of Congenital Pulmonary Venous Anomalies

As described above, the complications following surgical treatment of anomalous pulmonary venous connections and pulmonary vein stenosis are primarily due to development of restenosis at the site of anastomosis. In a small number of patients with total anomalous pulmonary venous drainage, a diffuse stenotic process involving the entire length of the pulmonary veins including their intrapulmonary course may occur and may progress to almost complete vein occlusion. The prognosis in these cases, especially with bilateral involvement is poor. Transthoracic echocardiography is the first investigation in these patients. Presence of turbulence at the anastomotic site is the main diagnostic feature of restenosis. However, the echocardiogram may be limited in a number of cases (e.g., following an intracardiac patch baffle).

Both contrast-enhanced CT angiography and multiple phase acquisition contrast-enhanced MR angiography with multiplanar reconstructions and volume-rendered imaging are used for postoperative

evaluation of patients with anomalous pulmonary venous drainage and pulmonary vein stenosis. CT is particularly useful in cases where the echocardiogram is inconclusive, when MRI is either contraindicated or cannot be performed due to need for sedation, and also in cases of diffuse restenosis to assess the intrapulmonary involvement and help assess the need for and to plan future diagnostic catheterization [31].

MRI may also be used to evaluate for restenosis following surgery and may be augmented by performing phase contrast imaging perpendicular to the plane of the vein just proximal to the veno-atrial junction [32]. Repaired veins usually show a greater diastolic flow component than normal veins, and often contain an abnormal downward deflection wave in the early systolic phase [33]. These findings are considered related to the decreased compliance of the left atrium due to either scar formation at the site of atrial incision or presence of patch graft material in the atrial wall.

As described in the previous section, radionuclide lung perfusion studies allow fairly accurate determination of flow distribution and help determine the efficacy of treatment measures instituted.

9.1.8 Conclusion

In this chapter, we have reviewed the embryology, epidemiology, anatomy, clinical presentation, preoperative imaging evaluation, management, and postoperative imaging evaluation of congenital pulmonary venous anomalies in the pediatric population.

9.2 Lymphatic Disorders of the Lung

Annabelle Quizon

Disorders of the lymphatic system encompass a number of entities that may lead to chronic and serious pulmonary disease and manifest with a range of clinical presentations. Congenital errors in lymphatic development are rare and their diagnoses and management are difficult.

9.2.1 Review of Embryonic Development of the Lymphatic System

The lymphatic system begins to develop by the end of the sixth embryonic week. By the eighth week, six primary lymph sacs emerge as buds from the adjacent developing veins. The lymphatic vessels develop in a manner similar to that of the blood vessels and join the primitive lymph sacs. By the ninth week of gestation, there are two large lymphatic vessels (the right and left thoracic ducts) that subsequently merge to form the thoracic duct. Failure of the many connections to form between the embryonic lymphatic channels results in congenital malformations of the lymphatic system, alteration in lymphatic drainage, and development of lymphatic disease [34].

9.2.2 Classification

Clinically, disorders of the lymphatic system occur in a variety of clinical settings. For the pediatric age group in particular, congenital errors of lymphatic development can lead to primary pulmonary lymphatic disorders such as lymphangiomas, lymphangiectasis, lymphangiomatosis, and lymphatic dysplasia syndrome. Many of these disorders are diagnosed in infancy and childhood. Table 9.1 is a detailed classification of congenital abnormalities of the lymphatic system based on Faul et al. [35], which modified an earlier classification by Hillard et al. [36]. The former reference will be cited extensively in this chapter.

9.2.3 Clinical Presentation

Lymphangiomas

Lymphangiomas are focal benign proliferations of well differentiated lymphatic tissue that present as multicystic or spongelike accumulations and subdivided into three pathologic categories (1) lymphangioma simplex (capillary hemangiomas), which are cutaneous lesions unrelated to internal lymphangiomas. (2) cavernous lymphangiomas, which insinuate themselves into surrounding structures. (3) cystic lymphangiomas (cystic hygromas), which are large, well circumscribed multiloculated growth with a fibrous capsule. Mulliken et al., have used

different nomenclature, correlating lymphangiomas with microcystic lymphatic malformations, and cystic hygromas with the macrocystic type; combined forms can exist [37]. Histologically, these are composed of vascular spaces filled with eosinophilic, protein-rich fluid with walls of variable thickness and composed of abnormally formed smooth and skeletal muscular elements. Acquired or secondary lymphangiomas develop in areas of chronic lymphatic obstruction related to surgery, chronic infection, or radiation.

Most of these anomalies appear in the first 2 years of life and present as swelling in the head, neck, or axilla. Approximately, 10% extend into the mediastinum and are equally distributed into the anterior, middle, and posterior compartments [38]. Intrapulmonary lymphangiomas are rare [39]. Thoracic lymphangiomas are usually asymptomatic. When

Table 9.1. Disorders of the lymphatic system

Lymphangioma
Capillary
Cavernous
Cystic
Lymphangiectasis
Primary (congenital)
Secondary
Lymphangiomatosis
Single organ system involvement (e.g., diffuse pulmonary lymphangiomatosis)
Mulitple organ system involvement
Lymphatic dysplasia syndrome
Primary lymphedema
Lymphedema congenital
Lymphedema precox
Lymphedema tarda
Idiopathic effusion(s)
Pleural
Pericardial
Peritoneal
Yellow nail syndrome
Congenital chylothorax
Lymphatic injury (secondary chylous effusions and lymphedema)
Lymphangioma, acquired progressive
Lymphangiosarcoma
Lymphatic abnormalities combined with other tissue disorders
Lymphangioleiomyomatosis
Hemangiolymphangiomas
Lymphangiolipoma

From Faul et al. [36], with permission.

symptoms develop, they reflect a mass effect on vital structures and depending on the affected organ, manifest as cough, dyspnea, stridor, hemoptysis, Horner's syndrome, dysphagia, superior vena cava syndrome, constrictive pericarditis, phrenic nerve palsy, or of symptoms related to secondary infection of the lymphangioma [40, 41]. Chylous pleural and pericardial effusions may develop [42]. Lymphangiomas can also occur sporadically in various parenchymal organs including the gastrointestinal tract, spleen, liver, and bone; intra-abdominal lymphangiomas are rare [43].

Typical lymphatic malformations cause no serious threat of morbidity or death. Nuchal cystic hygromas diagnosed in utero, may have a poor prognosis when associated with Turner syndrome and fetal hydrops [44, 45]. It is not uncommon for a previously stable lymphatic malformation to suddenly enlarge, usually from acute bleeding into one or several cysts. This may relate to recognized trauma to the region of the malformation. Less commonly, the malformation may become infected and enlarge.

Lymphangiectasis

Lymphangiectasis refers to pathologic dilatation of lymphatics. It results from failure of pulmonary interstitial connective tissues to regress leading to dilatation of pulmonary lymphatic capillaries as in primary pulmonary lymphangiectasis. Secondary lymphangiectasis can occur as a result of disturbance of effective lymphatic drainage from surgery, radiation, infection, or trauma. It may also be associated with pulmonary venous obstruction or congenital cardiac defects (e.g., total anomalous pulmonary venous return or hypoplastic left heart syndromes) that result in increased lymphatic circulation [46]. Primary pulmonary lymphangiectasis has been traditionally viewed as often fatal in early life; with a mortality rate close to 100% in the newborn presenting with respiratory distress. Secondary lymphangiectasis can present with respiratory distress at any age. A number of congenital and genetic diseases have been associated with pulmonary lymphangiectasis such as Noonan, Ullrich-Turner, Ehlers-Danlos, and Down syndromes [47].

A number of retrospective reviews of patients who survive infancy or with postneonatal onset revealed that prognosis may not be as dismal as previously viewed [48, 49] and that respiratory symptoms such as wheezing, cough, increased work of breathing, and frequency of pneumonia improved over time [50].

Lymphangiomatosis

This condition is associated with diffuse proliferation of lymphatics with a particular pattern of visceral involvement and progressive course. It is frequently associated with other lymphatic abnormalities and involves multiple organs with a predilection for thoracic and neck involvement. Diffuse pulmonary lymphangiomatosis involves both lungs without extrathoracic lymphatic abnormalities. Lymphangiomatosis can present at birth to adulthood and most frequently presents in late childhood. A majority have bony involvement. Chylous effusions are common and chylopericardium and chylous ascites may occur [51]. Patients may present with hemoptysis, wheezing, protein losing enteropathy, peripheral lymphedema, hemihypertrophy, lymphopenia, and disseminated intravascular coagulation. In general, prognosis is poor and primarily determined by the progression of pulmonary dysfunction; neurological deficits have also been reported from involvement of the cervical vertebrae and impact on prognosis [52].

Lymphatic Dysplasia Syndrome

This term includes primary (idiopathic) lymphedema syndromes, congenital chylothorax, idiopathic effusions, and the yellow nail syndrome. The latter is a triad of idiopathic pleural effusions, lymphedema and dystrophic nails and is most likely to present in adulthood. Lymphatic dysplasia syndrome encompasses effusions of the pericardium, pleura, peritoneum, and lymphedema without any identifiable cause and in the absence of other lymphatic disorders such as lymphangiomas, lymphangiectasis, or lymphangiomatosis [53, 54]. Abnormal lymphatic development has been associated with clinical syndromes with different inheritance patterns such as achondrogenesis type 1, Turner syndrome, Noonan's syndrome, familial Milroy lymphedema, and congenital chylothorax [43].

In neonates, most chylous effusions are congenital and may be due to (1) an obstruction of the lymphatic drainage from the pleural cavity, (2) thoracic duct atresia, or (3) congenital fistulas [34]. In older children and adults, they result from infection, malignancy, or trauma. Congenital chylothorax has a variable prognosis depending on gestational age at birth, presence of other congenital abnormalities, and severity of pulmonary hypoplasia.

9.2.4 Diagnosis

The diagnosis of lymphatic disorders is based primarily on the suggestive history and findings on physical examination. Imaging techniques are key in delineating anatomic and physiologic derangements of the lymphatic system. The utility of a lung biopsy has been addressed primarily in helping to distinguish pulmonary lymphangiectasis from other forms of lung disease such as interstitial emphysema. Many refrain from biopsy as there is a risk of ongoing chylothorax at the time of lung biopsy from refractory leakage of lymph fluid from the incision site and there are no definitive criteria as to when this procedure should be performed [55, 56].

Imaging

Plain chest radiographs may show bilateral pulmonary hyperinflation and a reticulonodular pattern throughout the lung fields (Fig. 9.10a) and occasional fluid-filled cystic areas representing aerated distal bronchi or alveolar ducts as in pulmonary lymphangiectasia. In generalized lymphangiomatosis, chest radiography may reveal an effusion and also shows reticular nodular shadowing throughout both lungs. The ribs, cervical spine, and humerus, when involved, show multiple lytic areas. Chest radiographs also confirm pleural effusions when present in lymphatic disorders.

Conventional oil-contrast lymphography has been the mainstay for lymphatic imaging; however, the emergence of computed tomography (CT) and magnetic resonance (MR) imaging has superseded the use of lymphography. Improvements in direct lymphatic studies have enabled high-resolution imaging of peripheral lymphatic vessels and studies on lymphatic flow dynamics with lymphangioscintigraphy.

Lymphangioscintigraphy has replaced the conventional oil-contrast lymphography as standard of reference [57]. It allows high-resolution imaging of peripheral lymphatic vessels and provides insight

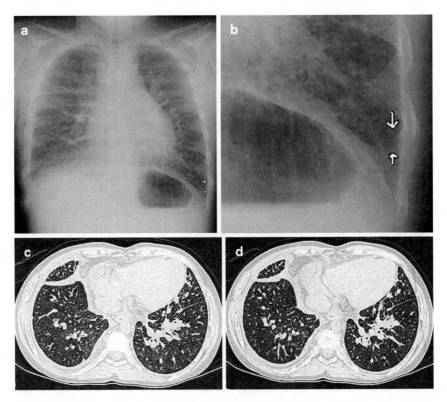

Fig. 9.10. (a) CXR, in this 17-year-old girl with Noonan's syndrome and pulmonary lymphangiectasis, reveals a diffuse coarse interstitial process and Kerley b lines (subpleural intralobular thickening) (*arrows*). There is a small right pleural effusion. As is usual for lymphangiectasis and lymphangiomatosis, these findings are nonspecific. (b) This coned image of the costopherenic sulcus from fig a, more clearly demonstrates the Kerly b lines. (c, d) CT findings are equally nonspecific, with variable indicators of interstitial lung disease, in this case, subpleural septal thickening and a mild mosaic profusion pattern. There is bronchial wall thickening and a right pleural effusion. There is incidental bibasilar dependent minor atelectasis

into lymphatic flow dynamics. It is useful in patients with known or suspected lymphatic circulatory disorders in terms of (1) confirming the diagnosis and delineating the pathogenesis and evolution of lymphedema, (2) helping evaluate lymphatic truncal anatomy and radiotracer transport, (3) useful in evaluating the efficacy of various treatment options designed to facilitate lymph flow or reduce lymph formation. It is noninvasive in that it only requires intradermal injection of tracer (usually Tc-99^m albumin) into web space of the foot or hand. It is also repeatable and does not adversely affect lymphatic vascular endothelium. Given the limited treatment

options especially for lymphedema, lymphatic imaging has not been utilized routinely and reliance on clinical history and physical examination has been emphasized.

Computerized tomography (Fig. 9.10b, c) and magnetic resonance imaging have been used for examining lymph nodes for size rather than architecture. It has been postulated that CT may show dilated subcutaneous lymphatics, although this is rarely if ever the case. Like CT, MR imaging may theoretically show pathologic dermal lymphatic vessels without added contrast material as well as more proximal lymph nodes and obstructing masses; it also allows visualization of the retroperitoneal ectatic lymphatic trunks and allows access for lymphatic truncal obliteration in the management of lymphangiectasia or lymphangiomas syndromes. Lymphangiomatous malformations may be demonstrated by ultrasonography particularly for evaluation of lymphangiomas which present as multiple complex septations in a fluid-filled mass.

Specific Diagnostic Modalities

For lymphangiomas, plain films (Fig. 9.11a), ultrasound (Fig. 9.11b), computerized tomography (Fig. 9.12) and magnetic resonance imaging (Fig. 9.13) have been used to determine the number and extent of lesions. For these lesions, accurate anatomic localization is important because the diagnosis is made postoperatively by means of histopathologic examination of the resected tissue. Lymphangiomatous malformations may be demonstrated by ultrasound

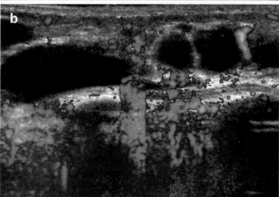

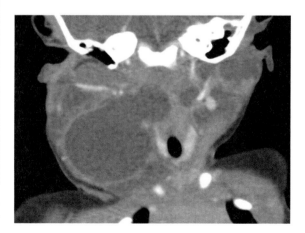

Fig. 9.11. (a) Portable AP chest X-ray shows a fullness of the left aspect of the neck with a soft tissue mass in the left upper mediastinum with left apical pleural thickening. The constellation of findings is suggestive of a lymphatic malformation. (b) Ultrasound of the neck mass reveals a multicystic mass with no flow within the cysts, consistent with the suspected lymphatic malformation

Fig. 9.12. Coronal reconstruction of a contrast enhanced CT in a child with a bilateral lymphatic malformation of the neck. The walls of the cystic spaces enhance with contrast while the centers do not

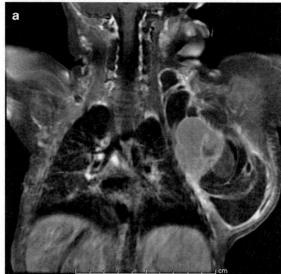

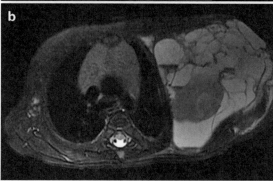

Fig. 9.13. (a) Coronal MRI, TI fat sat contrast enhanced image from a child with a large lymphatic malformation of the neck and left chest wall. The cyst walls enhance with contrast. The lymph containing cysts are of low signal intensity. The higher signal intensity of some cysts indicates blood within the cysts on this TI weighted image. (b) Cross-sectional T2 MRI of the chest wall component of the malformation reveals the low signal of the cyst walls with bright signal from the lymph containing cysts and low signal from the cysts containing blood. Note the lymph/blood fluid level in one of the medially, anteriorly placed cysts

with the typical pattern of multiple complex septations in a fluid-filled mass [43]. CT shows the anatomical distribution and dimensions of the mass and their relationship to other organs. Most lymphangiomas appear as cystic masses of low attenuation value with or without septations; some of the septae show enhancement after a bolus injection of contrast material [58]. The advantages of MRI include more conclusive demonstration of cystic components, better demonstration of invasion of adjacent structures, and improved surgical planning with coronal or sagittal imaging planes [59, 60].

In pulmonary lymphangiectasis, chest X-ray may show marked hyperinflation with interstitial infiltrates that may be localized or diffuse [50] (Fig. 9.10a). Unilateral or bilateral pleural effusions may also be found. MRI may show cystic lesions and abnormal lymphatic vessels. High-resolution CT may demonstrate extensive bilateral septal and peribronchovascular interstitial thickening, areas of ground-glass attenuation and bilateral pleural effusions [61] (Fig. 9.10b). Lymphangiography shows abnormally dilated lymphatics with obstructive changes and collateral channels in the retroperitoneal, mediastinal, and cervical lymphatic system [62]. In generalized lymphangiomatosis, chest radiography confirms pleural effusion and also shows reticular nodular shadowing throughout both lungs [52]. The ribs, cervical spine, and humerus, when involved, may show multiple lytic areas. The combination of lytic bone lesions and chylothorax is an important diagnostic clue; diagnosis is sometimes made by bone biopsy. CT and MRI demonstrate generalized cystic lesions in parenchymal organs, lytic bone lesions and diffuse thickening of pulmonary interstitium and mesenteries [63]. Specifically with regard to chest CT findings, the combination of septal thickening (presumably related to dilated lymph vessels or veins in the interlobular septa of the lung) and pleural effusion or diffuse mediastinal infiltration strongly suggest lymphangiomatosis. Moreover, ground-glass opacities are also demonstrated, and due to thickening of vascular structures within the alveolar interstitium [64]. Lymphangiography shows multiple lesions of the thoracic duct, dilated lymphatic channels, and lymphangiomas throughout the bones and lungs. Lymphangioscintigraphy helps delineate lymphatic flow and relation between normal and abnormal lymphatics [65]. Lung biopsy demonstrates anastomosing endothelial lined spaces along pulmonary lymphatic routes accompanied by asymmetrically spaced bundles of spindle cells.

Chylous effusions in congenital chylothorax have typical appearance and biochemical characteristics. The fluid is clear or serous but typically is milky after introduction of feedings. It is characterized by protein content greater than 30 g/L, triglycerides greater than 110 mg/dL after fat-containing feedings are started, and presence of chylomicrons. Lymphocytes predominate (greater than 90% of total cell count) and microbiologic cultures are sterile. In the lymphatic dysplasia syndrome, lymphangiography and lymphoscintigraphy allow an anatomic and functional assessment of lymphatic transport and demonstration of regional lymph nodes [42].

9.2.5 Management

Surgical excision or sclerosis is the treatment of choice for lymphangiomas. Surgical excision prevents complications from compression of vital structures by the lymphangioma. Complete resection however may be technically difficult since the lymphangiomas may be enmeshed in blood vessels, airways, and mediastinal organs. Sclerotherapy is not beneficial in the management of recurrent disease. Risk factors for recurrence include location (with the highest recurrence rate in the head) size, and complexity of lesions [66].

Conservative management is indicated for lymphangiectasis which include low fat, high protein diet with medium chain triglyceride (MCT) in order to decrease lymph production. Repeated aspirations of lymph accumulation in the pleural space may also be needed to relieve respiratory distress.

Conservative management with MCT and high protein diet to control lymph accumulation has also been implemented for the management of lymphangiomatosis. If lymph continues to accumulate, drainage of pleural fluid is done to decrease symptoms resulting from compressive effects. Given the potential for this lesion to grow and compress adjacent structures and high rates of recurrence with surgical resection, therapy is oftentimes palliative and if this fails, surgical or chemical pleurodesis can be considered [52]. Imaging modalities such as CT and MR may guide sclerotherapy and for postprocedure follow up.

Postnatal management of congenital chylothorax can be conservative and surgical. The goal of conservative management is to minimize chyle formation and to maintain adequate nutrition and may include (1) intermittent drainage of the chylous effusion by thoracentesis or continuous drainage by chest tube placement, (2) diet consisting of MCT, (3) respiratory support to improve oxygenation and ventilation, (4) octreotide infusion [67, 68]. Octreotide is a somatostatin analogue that decreases lymphatic flow through a reduction in gastric, intestinal, and pancreatic secretions or by decreasing hepatic venous pressure and splanchnic blood flow [69]. Conservative management is attempted for a few weeks and many cases resolve over time. Surgical options when conservative management fails, and pleural drainage cannot be discontinued include (1) thoracic duct ligation, (2) placement of pleuroperitoneal shunt to divert fluid to the peritoneal space, (3) pleurodesis to promote pleural adhesion, and (4) pleurectomy which involves stripping of the pleura and pericardium from lung apex to diaphragm [70]. Some patients may present with recurrent pulmonary infections due to loss of lymphocytes and proteins (including IgG) into the pleural space, such patients may require antibiotics or replacement immunoglobulin therapy. Familiarity with the therapeutic options along with appropriate timing of surgical intervention is important in preventing the complications of malnutrition and infection from persistent loss of chyle [71].

The cause of primary lymphedema cannot be treated; thus management is conservative and supportive and consists of external support, gravity, and massage. Volume-reducing surgery and lymphatic microsurgery have also been reported [72].

References

1. Neill CA. Development of the pulmonary veins; with reference to the embryology of anomalies of pulmonary venous return. Pediatrics. 1956;18(6):880–7.
2. Healey Jr JE. An anatomic survey of anomalous pulmonary veins: their clinical significance. J Thorac Surg. 1952;23(5):433–44.
3. Streeter GL. Developmental horizons in human embryos; a review of the histogenesis of cartilage and bone. Contrib Embryol. 1949;33(213–221):149–68.
4. Webb S, Kanani M, Anderson RH, et al. Development of the human pulmonary vein and its incorporation in the morphologically left atrium. Cardiol Young. 2001;11(6):632–42.
5. Delisle G, Ando M, Calder AL, et al. Total anomalous pulmonary venous connection: report of 93 autopsied cases with emphasis on diagnostic and surgical considerations. Am Heart J. 1976;91(1):99–122.
6. Ucar T, Fitoz S, Tutar E, et al. Diagnostic tools in the preoperative evaluation of children with anomalous pulmonary venous connections. Int J Cardiovasc Imaging. 2008;24(2):229–35.
7. Drossner DM, Kim DW, Maher KO, et al. Pulmonary vein stenosis: prematurity and associated conditions. Pediatrics. 2008;122(3):e656–61.
8. Latson LA, Prieto LR. Congenital and acquired pulmonary vein stenosis. Circulation. 2007;115(1):103–8.
9. Saad EB, Marrouche NF, Saad CP, et al. Pulmonary vein stenosis after catheter ablation of atrial fibrillation: emergence of a new clinical syndrome. Ann Intern Med. 2003;138(8):634–8.
10. Sadr IM, Tan PE, Kieran MW, et al. Mechanism of pulmonary vein stenosis in infants with normally connected veins. Am J Cardiol. 2000;86(5):577–9. A10.
11. Michielon G, Di Donato RM, Pasquini L, et al. Total anomalous pulmonary venous connection: long-term appraisal with evolving technical solutions. Eur J Cardiothorac Surg. 2002;22(2):184–91.
12. Hancock Friesen CL, Zurakowski D, Thiagarajan RR, et al. Total anomalous pulmonary venous connection: an analysis

of current management strategies in a single institution. Ann Thorac Surg. 2005;79(2):596–606. discussion 596–606.

13. van Son JA, Hambsch J, Kinzel P, et al. Urgency of operation in infracardiac total anomalous pulmonary venous connection. Ann Thorac Surg. 2000;70(1):128–30.

14. Ussia G, Marasini M, Zannini L, et al. Acquired pulmonary vein obstruction after open-heart surgery. Eur J Cardiothorac Surg. 2002;22(3):465–7.

15. Redington AN, Raine J, Shinebourne EA, et al. Tetralogy of Fallot with anomalous pulmonary venous connections: a rare but clinically important association. Br Heart J. 1990;64(5):325–8.

16. Foerster SR, Gauvreau K, McElhinney DB, et al. Importance of totally anomalous pulmonary venous connection and postoperative pulmonary vein stenosis in outcomes of heterotaxy syndrome. Pediatr Cardiol. 2008;29(3):536–44.

17. Berrocal T, Madrid C, Novo S, et al. Congenital anomalies of the tracheobronchial tree, lung, and mediastinum: embryology, radiology, and pathology. Radiographics. 2004;24(1):e17.

18. Hubbard AM, Adzick NS, Crombleholme TM, et al. Congenital chest lesions: diagnosis and characterization with prenatal MR imaging. Radiology. 1999;212(1):43–8.

19. Husain AN, Hessel RG. Neonatal pulmonary hypoplasia: an autopsy study of 25 cases. Pediatr Pathol. 1993;13(4):475–84.

20. Montani D, Price LC, Dormuller P, et al. Pulmonary veno-occlusive disease. Eur Respir J. 2009;33(1):189–200.

21. Henk CB, Prokesch R, Grampp S, et al. Scimitar syndrome: MR assessment of hemodynamic significance. J Comput Assist Tomogr. 1997;21(4):628–30.

22. Ou P, Marini D, Celermajer DS, et al. Non-invasive assessment of congenital pulmonary vein stenosis in children using cardiac-non-gated CT with 64-slice technology. Eur J Radiol. 2009;70(3):595–9.

23. Breinholt JP, Hawkins JA, Minich LA, et al. Pulmonary vein stenosis with normal connection: associated cardiac abnormalities and variable outcome. Ann Thorac Surg. 1999;68(1):164–8.

24. Devaney EJ, Chang AC, Ohye RG, et al. Management of congenital and acquired pulmonary vein stenosis. Ann Thorac Surg. 2006;81(3):992–5. discussion 995–6.

25. van Son JA, Danielson GK, Puga FJ, et al. Repair of congenital and acquired pulmonary vein stenosis. Ann Thorac Surg. 1995;60(1):144–50.

26. Lacour-Gayet F, Rey C, Planche C. Pulmonary vein stenosis. Description of a sutureless surgical procedure using the pericardium in situ. Arch Mal Coeur Vaiss. 1996;89(5):633–6.

27. Yun TJ, Coles JG, Konstantinov IE, et al. Conventional and sutureless techniques for management of the pulmonary veins: evolution of indications from postrepair pulmonary vein stenosis to primary pulmonary vein anomalies. J Thorac Cardiovasc Surg. 2005;129(1):167–74.

28. Lock JE, Bass JL, Castaneda-Zuniga W, et al. Dilation angioplasty of congenital or operative narrowings of venous channels. Circulation. 1984;70(3):457–64.

29. Ungerleider RM, Johnston TA, O'Laughlin MP, et al. Intraoperative stents to rehabilitate severely stenotic pulmonary vessels. Ann Thorac Surg. 2001;71(2):476–81.

30. Mendeloff EN, Spray TL, Huddleston CB, et al. Lung transplantation for congenital pulmonary vein stenosis. Ann Thorac Surg. 1995;60(4):903–6. discussion 907.

31. Kasahara H, Aeba R, Tanami Y, Yozu R. Multislice computed tomography is useful for evaluating partial anoma-

lous pulmonary venous connection. J Cardiothorac Surg. 2010;5:40.

32. Grosse-Wortmann L, Al-Otay A, Goo HW, et al. Anatomical and functional evaluation of pulmonary veins in children by magnetic resonance imaging. J Am Coll Cardiol. 2007;49(9):993–1002.

33. Valsangiacomo ER, Barrea C, Macgowan CK, et al. Phase-contrast MR assessment of pulmonary venous blood flow in children with surgically repaired pulmonary veins. Pediatr Radiol. 2003;33(9):607–13.

34. Gaede C, Trotter C. Congenital chylothorax. Neonatal Radiol. 2006;25:371–81.

35. Hillard RI, McKendry JB, Philips MH. Congenital abnormalities of the lymphatic system: embryology and pathogenesis. Pediatrics. 1990;86:988–94.

36. Faul JL, Berry GJ, Colby TV, Ruoss SJ, Walter MB, Rosen GD, et al. State of the art: thoracic lymphangiomas, lymphangiectasis, lymphagiomatosis, and lymphatic dysplasia syndrome. Am J Respir Crit Care Med. 2000;161:1037–46.

37. Mulliken JB, Fishman SJ, Burrows PE. Vascular malformations. Curr Prob Surg. 2000;37(8):520–76.

38. Brown LR, Reiman HM, Rosenow EC, Glovicki PM, Divertie MB. Intrathoracic lymphangioma. Mayo Clin. 1986;61:882–92.

39. Drut R, Mosca HH. Intrapulmonary cystic lymphangioma. Pediatr Pulmonol. 1996;22:204–6.

40. Papsin BC, Evans JNG. Isolated laryngeal lymphangioma: a rare cause of airway obstruction in infants. J Laryngol Otol. 1996;110:969–72.

41. Wright CC, Cohen DM, Vegunta RK, Davis JT, King DR. Intrathoracic cystic hygroma: a report of three cases. J Pediatr Surg. 1996;31:1430–2.

42. Hancock BJ, St. Vil D, Luks FI, diLorenzo M, Blanchard H. Complications of lymphangiomas in children. J Pediatr Surg. 1992;27:220–6.

43. Levine C. Primary disorders of the lymphatic vessels – a unified concept. J Pediatr Surgery. 1989;24(3):233–40.

44. Zadvinski DP, Benson MT, Kerr HH, Mancuso AA, Cacciarelli AA, Madrazo BL, et al. Congenital malformations of the cervico-thoracic lymphatic system: embryology and pathogenesis. Radiographics. 1992;12:1175–89.

45. Langer JC, Fitzgerald PG, Desa D, Filly RA, Golbus MS, Adzick S, et al. Cervical cystic hygroma in the fetus: clinical spectrum and outcome. J Pediatr Surg. 1990;25(1):58–62.

46. France NE, Brown RJK. Congenital pulmonary lymphangiectasis. Arch Dis Child. 1971;46:528–32.

47. Noonan JA, Walkers LR, Reeves JT. Congenital pulmonary lymphangiectasia. Arch Pediatr Adol Med. 1970;120:314–9.

48. Barker PM, Esther CR, Fordham LA, Maygarden SJ, Funkhouser WK. Primary pulmonary lymphangiectasis in infancy and childhood. Eur Respir J. 2004;24:413–9.

49. Chung CJ, Fordham LA, Barker P, Cooper LL. Children with congenital pulmonary lymphangiectasis: after infancy. Am J Radiol. 1999;173:1583–8.

50. Bouchard S, DiLorenzo M, Youssef S, Simard P, Lapierre JG. Pulmonary lymphangiectasia revisited. J Pediatr Surgery. 2000;35(5):796–800.

51. Dunkelman H, Sharief N, Berman L, Ninan T. Generalized lymphangiomatosis with chylothorax. Arch Dis Child. 1989;64:1058–60.

52. Shah AR, Dinwiddie R, Woolf D, Ramani R, Higgins JNP, Matthew DJ. Generalized lymphangiomatosis and chy-

lothorax in the pediatric age group. Pediatr Pulmonol. 1992;14:126–30.

53. Smeltzer DM, Stickler GB, Fleming RE. Primary lymphatic dysplasia in children: chylothorax, chylous ascites, and generalized lymphatic dysplasia. Eur J Pediatr. 2004;145:286–92.

54. Hen J, Dolan TF. Late-onset lymphedema complicated by pericardial effusion, cardiac tamponade, and pleural effusions. Arch Pediatr Adolesc Med. 1981;135:380–1.

55. Esther CR, Barker PM. Pulmonary lymphangiectasia: diagnosis and clinical course. Pediatr Pulmonol. 2004;38:308–13.

56. Dempsey EM, Sant'Anna GM, Williams RL, Brouillette RT. Congenital pulmonary lymphangiectasia presenting as nonimmune fetal hydrops and severe respiratory distress at birth: not uniformly fatal. Pediatr Pulmonol. 2005;40:270–4.

57. Witte CL, Witte MH, Unger EC, Williams WH, Bernas MJ, NcNeill GC, et al. Advances in imaging of lymph flow disorders. Radiographics. 2000;20:1697–719.

58. Caro PA, Mahboubi S, Faerber EN. Computed tomography in the diagnosis of lymphangiomas in infants and children. Clin Imaging. 1991;15:41–6.

59. Shaffer K, Rosado-de-Christenson ML, Patz EF, Young S, Farver CF. Thoracic lymphangioma in adults: CT and MR imaging features. Amer J Roentgen. 1994;162:283–9.

60. Siegel MJ, Glazer HS, St. Amour TE, Rosenthal DD. Lymphangiomas in children: MR imaging. Radiology. 1989;170:467–70.

61. Nobre LF, Muller NL, deSouza AS, Marchiori E, Souza IV. Congenital pulmonary lymphangiectasia: CT and pathologic findings. J Thorac Imaging. 2004;19:56–9.

62. Jang HJ, Lee KS, Han J. Intravascular lymphomatosis of the lung: radiologic findings. J Comput Assist Tomogr. 1998;22:427–9.

63. Wunderbaldinger P, Paya K, Partik B, Turetschek K, Hormann M, Horcher E, et al. CT and MR imaging of generalized cystic lymphangiomatosis in pediatric patients. Amer J Radiol. 2000;174:827–32.

64. Lynch DA, Hay T, Newell JD, Divgi VD, Fan LL. Pediatric diffuse lung diseases: diagnosis and classification using high-resolution CT. Amer J Radiol. 1999;173:713–8.

65. Piu MH, Yueh TC. Lymphoscintigraphy in chyluria, chyloperitoneum and chylothorax. J Nucl Med. 1998;39:1292–6.

66. Alqahtani L, Nguyen T, Flageole H, Shaw K, Laberge JM. 25 years' experience with lymphangioma in children. J Pediatr Surg. 1999;34:1164–8.

67. Beghetti M, LaScala G, Belli D, Bugmann P, Kalangas A, LeCoultre C. Etiology and management of pediatric chylothorax. J Pediatr. 2000;136:653–8.

68. Buttiker V, Fanconi S, Burger R. Chylothorax in children: guidelines for diagnosis and management. Chest. 1999;116:682–7.

69. Stajich GV, Ashworth L. Octreotide. Neonatal Netw. 2006;25:365–9.

70. Wolff AB, Silen ML, Kokoska ER, Rodgers BM. Treatment of refractory chylothorax with externalized pleuroperitoneal shunts in children. Ann Thorac Surg. 1999;68:1053–7.

71. Valentine VG, Raffin TA. The management of chylothorax. Chest. 1992;102:586–91.

72. Rockson SG, Miller LT, Senie R, Brennan MJ, Casley-Smith JR, Foldi E, et al. American cancer society lymphedema workshop. Workshop III: diagnosis and management of lymphedema. Cancer. 1998;83:2882–5.

Pulmonary Hypertension in Infants and Children   10

GULRAIZ CHAUDRY AND EDWARD Y. LEE

CONTENTS

GULRAIZ CHAUDRY, MBChB, MRCP, FRCR (✉)
Department of Radiology, Children's Hospital Boston,
Harvard Medical School, Boston, MA, USA
e-mail: Gulraiz.Chaudry@childrens.harvard.edu

EDWARD Y. LEE, MD, MPH
Division of Thoracic Imaging, Department of Radiology and
Medicine, Pulmonary Division, Children's Hospital Boston,
Harvard Medical School,
Boston, MA, USA

Pulmonary hypertension (PHT) is a condition defined by a mean pulmonary arterial pressure (PAP) of 25 mmHg or greater at rest and 30 mmHg or greater during exercise. PHT can be idiopathic or associated with a wide spectrum of etiological factors and conditions in the pediatric population [1], often resulting in diagnostic and therapeutic challenges. Due to recent advances in treatment which have markedly decreased the mortality and morbidity in pediatric patients with PHT [2], early and correct diagnosis is particularly essential in optimally managing children with PHT.

In this chapter, we address the clinical presentation and the methods of evaluation of PHT in the pediatric population. Unique underlying pathophysiological processes and characteristic diagnostic study findings in idiopathic pulmonary arterial hypertension (IPAH) and common conditions typically associated with PHT in infants and children are also highlighted.

10.1   Clinical Presentation of Pulmonary Hypertension

Pediatric patients with PHT usually present with clinical symptoms which are often non-specific. In addition, clinical symptoms somewhat differ between infants (<1 year old) and children. While infants typically present with failure to thrive, irritability and

R.H. Cleveland (ed.), *Imaging in Pediatric Pulmonology*,
DOI 10.1007/978-1-4419-5872-3_10, © Springer Science+Business Media, LLC 2012

cyanotic spells with exertion, children usually present with chest pain, exertional dyspnea or syncope [3]. On physical examination, common findings in pediatric patients with PHT include: (1) left parasternal heave caused by the right ventricular enlargement, detected by placing the heel of the hand over the left parasternal region; (2) a prolonged P2 with paradoxical splitting of the second heart sound on auscultation; and (3) a murmur due to pulmonary regurgitation. Clinical signs of right-sided cardiac failure such as hepatomegaly or peripheral edema are uncommon in children.

10.2 Evaluation of Pulmonary Hypertension

The overarching goal of evaluation in pediatric patients with PHT is to establish the diagnosis of PHT and determine the underlying cause [4]. For infants and children with clinical suspicion of underlying PHT, initial diagnostic evaluation typically consists of chest radiographs (CXR), electrocardiogram (ECG) and echocardiography. Based upon findings on these studies, further evaluation can be performed with advanced diagnostic studies including: (1) a 6-minute walk test, (2) cardiac catheterization, (3) computed tomography (CT), (4) ventilation-perfusion scan (V/Q scan) and (5) magnetic resonance imaging/angiography (MRI/MRA).

10.2.1 Initial Evaluation

Chest Radiographs (CXR)

Two views (posteroanterior and lateral views) of CXR are typically the first diagnostic imaging modality for evaluating infants and children with suspected PHT. The advantages of CXR in the evaluation of PHT include its widespread availability, relative low cost and easy acquisition. However, associated ionizing radiation exposure is an important disadvantage particularly in the pediatric population. The most common chest radiographic imaging findings in children with PHT of any cause include: (1) enlargement of the main and hilar pulmonary arteries, (2) tapering of the peripheral

pulmonary arteries and (3) right ventricular enlargement associated with loss of the retrosternal air space on the lateral view [5]. The CXR can also demonstrate lung parenchymal disease in some patients with PHT.

Electrocardiogram (ECG)

The ECG in pediatric patients with PHT typically demonstrates right-sided cardiac strain associated with right ventricular hypertrophy and right axis deviation [5].

Echocardiography

Transthoracic echocardiography can be helpful in evaluating pediatric patients with PHT by demonstrating: (1) left-sided cardiac disease; (2) valvular abnormalities, especially tricuspid regurgitation which is known to be present in the majority of children with PHT [1]; and (3) intracardiac shunting (e.g., atrial septal defect, ventricular septal defect [VSD]). Estimation of right ventricular systolic pressure (RVSP) by Doppler interrogation has also been shown to correlate well with pressures measured at catheterization [5].

10.2.2 Advanced Evaluation

Six-Minute Walk Test

A 6-minute walk test is a type of pulmonary function test in which the distance a patient can walk over a 6-min period is measured, usually including pulse oximetry. In children (>6 years) with PHT who can follow the direction of a 6-minute walk test, this allows objective assessment of the degree of dyspnea [1]. In addition, gas exchange capabilities can be evaluated with diffusing lung capacity for carbon monoxide (DLCO). The functional status is then classified according to the NYHA/WHO classification, with no limitation of physical activity seen in class I to patients unable to carry out any physical activity in class IV [6]. A 6-minute walk test combined with functional classification can play an important role in the initial evaluation, assessment of early response to treatment and response assessment following completion of therapy.

Cardiac Catheterization

Cardiac catheterization, which can directly measure the PAP, remains the gold standard for diagnosis of PHT in the pediatric population. In addition to PAP measurement, cardiac catheterization can also provide important information (regarding pulmonary capillary wedge pressure and pulmonary venous return) which can be used to determine the underlying etiology of PHT [6]. Furthermore, catheterization can also be used to guide therapy by determining the response to selective pulmonary vasodilators.

Advanced Radiological Imaging Studies

In children diagnosed with PHT by cardiac catheterization or suspected of having PHT based on CXR and other evaluation studies, advanced imaging studies can be performed to determine the underlying cause. These include computed tomography, ventilation-perfusion scan and magnetic resonance imaging/angiography. The choice of specific advanced imaging studies and their characteristic imaging findings will be discussed in detail under the discussion sections of idiopathic PHT and individual conditions associated with PHT.

10.3 Pulmonary Arterial Hypertension

10.3.1 Idiopathic Pulmonary Arterial Hypertension

IPAH is a diagnosis of exclusion when PHT occurs without identifiable underlying cause. Histologically, medial hypertrophy of pulmonary arterioles is commonly seen in children with IPAH without fixed changes (such as intimal fibrosis and plexiform lesions) typically seen in adult patients with IPAH [7]. Although the exact incidence of IPAH is currently not known, particularly in the pediatric population, it is estimated to be 1–2 cases per million in all ages [3]. Despite the current uncertainty of the true incidence of IPAH, it is important to recognize that the incidence of IPAH in the pediatric population may be higher than it has been recognized in the past due to the increased awareness of IPAH in recent years [8]. This presumed higher incidence of IPAH, coupled with the recent advances in therapy for IPAH, underscore the importance of early and correct diagnosis of IPAH. With the improved therapy for IPAH in recent years, the 3-year survival rate now reaches as high as 94% at 1 year and 84% at 3 years after the initial diagnosis [9], up significantly from the abysmal prognosis of mean survival time of less than 1 year in the past [8].

CXR, ECG and echocardiography are typically used in the initial evaluation of pediatric patients with IPAH. Common findings of these evaluation tests are included in the section of initial evaluation of PHT. Once the diagnosis of IPAH is suspected on the basis of these initial investigations, CT can provide further information on both pulmonary and extrapulmonary abnormalities associated with IPAH. With recent advances in CT technology, particularly with MDCT providing high resolution images in a faster scanning time with 2D and 3D image reconstruction capability, CT is assuming an important role in evaluating IPAH in infants and children. A combined CT angiography protocol (which can provide detailed information of pulmonary vessels) and high resolution technique (for lung parenchymal evaluation) should be utilized for complete evaluation of both pulmonary and extrapulmonary (e.g., vascular) abnormalities associated with IPAH. With a higher row MDCT (>16 MDCT) with very thin collimation (0.5–1.0 mm), diagnostic quality of thin section CT images is almost equal to high resolution CT images, with the added benefit of viewing in the transverse, sagittal or coronal planes.

The most common extrapulmonary (vascular) finding in IPAH is central pulmonary artery enlargement (Fig. 10.1). Distal main pulmonary artery exceeding the diameter of the ascending aorta has a specificity and positive predictive value of greater than 90% for PHT [10]. In addition, the ratio of the diameter of the right and left pulmonary arteries to their respective mainstem bronchi is invariably greater than 1:1, with a mean of 2:1 [11]. In some children, a peripheral vasculopathy is also identified, characterized by small tortuous vessels extending to the periphery (Fig. 10.2) [11]. The cause of this finding remains unknown, but possible etiologies include neovascularization or enlarged collateral vessels. Right-sided cardiac enlargement is also seen in the majority of these children (Fig. 10.3) [11]. In contrast, other extrapulmonary findings described in adults with IPAH, such as pericardial thickening and mural calcific deposits, are not commonly recognized in pediatric patients with IPAH [11].

The most common pulmonary parenchymal finding in infants and children with IPAH is the presence

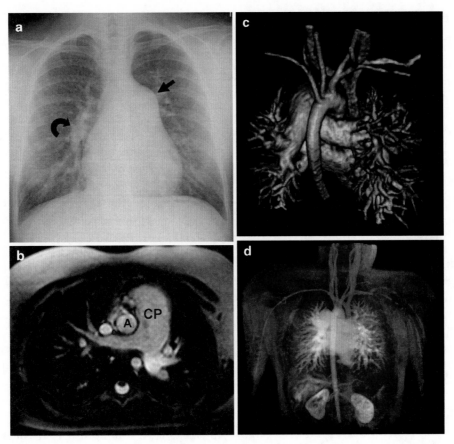

Fig. 10.1. Ten-year-old boy with idiopathic pulmonary hypertension (PHT) who initially presented with exertional dyspnea. (**a**) Frontal chest radiograph shows marked enlarged central (*arrow*) and main (*curved arrow*) pulmonary arteries. Also noted is mild cardiomegaly. (**b**) Axial T1 weighted MR image demonstrates an enlarged central pulmonary artery (CP). *A* aorta. (**c**) Posterior view of the 3D volume rendered image of the vascular structures shows enlarged central pulmonary artery, main pulmonary arteries, and segmental pulmonary arteries. (**d**) Posterior view of the 3D volume rendered image of the MRA shows the entire thoracic vascular structures

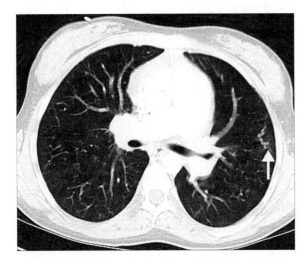

Fig. 10.2. Sixteen-year-old girl with idiopathic PHT presenting with shortness of breath. Axial lung window CT image demonstrates enlarged and tortuous peripheral pulmonary vessels (*arrow*)

of well-defined centrilobular opacities (Figs. 10.3d and 10.4). However, this finding is also frequently seen in veno-occlusive disorder (VOD) and thromboembolic disease [12, 13]. Inhomogeneous ground-glass opacification and focal areas of hyperlucency are also frequently noted, but septal thickening is less common and extensive than that seen in VOD (Figs. 10.5 and 10.6) [11].

In addition to evaluating pulmonary and extra-pulmonary findings associated with IPAH, CT is also helpful in identifying other conditions (e.g., thromboembolic and veno-occlusive disease) associated with PHT in infants and children.

Other radiological imaging studies currently available, including MRI and V/Q scan, have inherent limitations for evaluating IPAH in the pediatric population. However, a reported finding in pediatric patients with IPAH includes delayed contrast

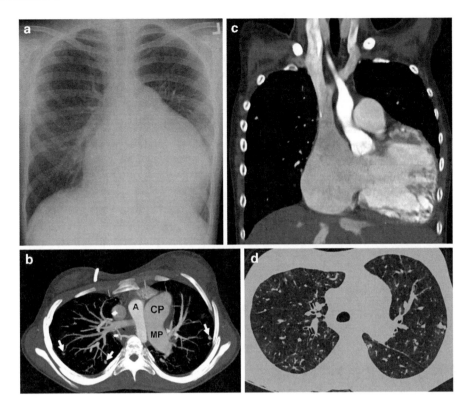

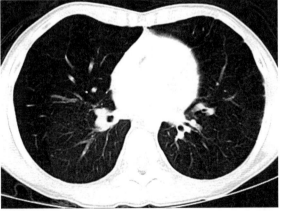

Fig. 10.3. Sixteen-year-old girl with idiopathic PHT who initially presented with syncope and chest pain. (**a**) Frontal chest radiograph demonstrates a markedly enlarged heart and aortopulmonary window region. (**b**) Enhanced axial maximum intensity projection image shows markedly enlarged central pulmonary artery (CP) and main pulmonary artery (MP). Also noted is development of small, enlarged, and tortuous vessels (*arrows*) within the periphery of the lungs. *A* aorta. (**c**) Coronal multiplanar image demonstrates a markedly enlarged right atrium and right ventricle. (**d**) High resolution axial lung image demonstrates relatively well-defined centrilobular opacities associated with areas of inhomogeneous ground-glass opacification

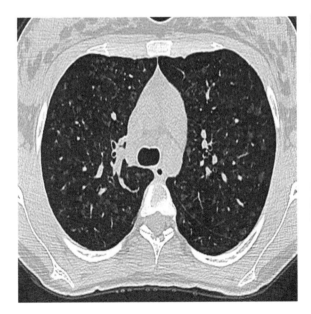

Fig. 10.4. Fifteen-year-old girl with idiopathic pulmonary arterial hypertension presenting with dyspnea and chest pain. High resolution axial lung image demonstrates diffuse centrilobular opacities bilaterally

Fig. 10.5. Ten-year-old girl with idiopathic PHT who initially presented with syncope and shortness of breath. Axial lung window CT image demonstrates geographic areas of ground-glass opacification and hyperlucency

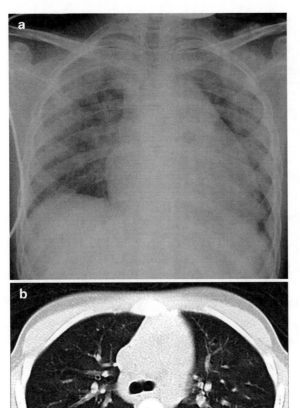

Fig. 10.6. Nine-year-old girl with idiopathic PHT who presented with chest pain. (**a**) Frontal chest radiograph shows mild diffuse opacities in both lungs. (**b**) Axial CT lung window image shows diffuse areas of both ground-glass opacification surrounded by hyperlucency. In comparison to Fig. 10.3, these lung findings are more diffuse and symmetric

enhancement of the myocardium at the junction of the free wall of the right ventricle and the interventricular septum on MRI. This delayed contrast enhancement has been shown to be inversely related to right ventricular systolic function [14]. The main role of scintigraphy in the assessment of IPAH is the exclusion of possible underlying thromboembolic disease. Although there are no specific findings of IPAH on ventilation-perfusion scanning [15], it has been shown that non-specific non-segmental patchy defect in perfusion with normal ventilation is the most common V/Q scan finding (Fig. 10.7) [16]. This finding is thought to be secondary to asymmetric vasoconstriction and occlusion of the pulmonary arterioles. In addition, quantitative assessment of these perfusion irregularities may also be useful in the assessment of severity of the disease [15].

Once the diagnosis of IPAH is established and treatment is initiated, follow-up imaging evaluation is primarily performed with ECG and echocardiography, including measurement of right ventricular pressures. Due to its relatively invasive nature, catheterization is seldom performed in pediatric patients with IPAH once diagnosis is made based on less invasive studies such as CT. However, catheterization with pulmonary vasodilator testing is useful for evaluating vascular responsiveness. Unfortunately, it has been reported that there is a wide variability of the results from catheterization with pulmonary vasodilator testing without accurate predictive factors, limiting its clinical utility [3].

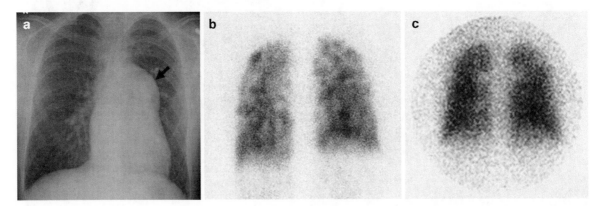

Fig. 10.7. Thirteen-year-old boy with a known idiopathic PHT who present with a shortness of breath and decreasing oxygen saturation. V/Q scan was obtained for evaluation of possible pulmonary embolism. (**a**) Frontal chest radiograph shows a markedly enlarged central pulmonary artery (*arrow*) and cardiomegaly. (**b**) Posterior view of perfusion image demonstrates diffusely patchy inhomogeneous uptake of tracer bilaterally compatible with innumerable subsegmental perfusion defects. (**c**) Posterior view of ventilation image shows relatively homogeneous tracer uptake without definite correlating matched ventilation and perfusion defects

10.3.2 Conditions Associated with Pulmonary Arterial Hypertension

It has long been recognized that a wide spectrum of conditions may be associated with pulmonary vascular disease that share similar clinical, pathological and imaging features with IPAH. These were previously termed *secondary pulmonary hypertension*, a potentially problematic nomenclature as it included conditions with pulmonary venous hypertension and altered respiratory function [4]. Thus in the revised Venice classification, the term associated with pulmonary arterial hypertension (APAH) was devised to describe pulmonary arterial hypertension associated with other conditions and risk factors. There is a wide spectrum of conditions associated with PAH as listed in Table 10.1 and several key conditions associated with PAH in pediatric population are reviewed in the following sections.

Congenital Systemic to Pulmonary Shunts

Infants and children with PAH secondary to congenital systemic to pulmonary shunts are a very heterogeneous group with regard to the underlying defect, as well as the timing and severity of PHT. Vicktor Eisenmenger published his report of pulmonary vascular disease associated with *congenital defects of the ventricular septum* in 1897. Eisenmenger syndrome was then further elucidated by Wood [17] and has come to encompass all systemic to pulmonary shunts that result in PHT and subsequent reversal or bidirectional shunt flow [4]. The low pulmonary vascular resistance and increased blood flow have a detrimental effect on the vascular bed, with suspected damage to the endothelial cells caused by shear stress [4]. Eventually, irreversible PHT develops with subsequent reversal of flow across the shunt and cyanosis. The histopathologic changes in the pulmonary vessels are identical to those seen in IPAH.

The likelihood of developing Eisenmenger syndrome depends on the location and size of the defect and the degree of the shunt [4]. Pediatric patients with a non-restrictive left-to-right shunt at the post-tricuspid level will develop irreversible hypertension in over half of the cases and present in early childhood [18]. Examples of such conditions include large VSDs, atrioventricular septal defects (AVSD) and patent ductus arteriosus (PDA). In contrast, only 10–20% of patients with a hemodynamically significant pre-tricuspid level lesion, such as an atrial septal defect, will develop PAH and generally not until the third or fourth decade [18]. The size of the defect is

Table 10.1. Classification of pulmonary hypertension (based on the Venice 2003 clinical classification)

1. Pulmonary arterial hypertension
   - Idiopathic (IPAH)
   - Familial (FIPAH)
   - Associated with (APAH)
     - Connective tissue disease
     - Congenital systemic to pulmonary shunts
     - Portal hypertension
     - HIV
     - Drugs and toxins
     - Other
   - Associated with significant venous or capillary involvement
     - Pulmonary veno-occlusive disease (PVOD)
     - Pulmonary capillary hemangiomatosis (PCH)
   - Persistent pulmonary hypertension of the newborn (PPHN)
2. Pulmonary hypertension associated with left heart diseases
   - Left-sided atrial or ventricular disease
   - Left-sided valvular heart disease
3. Pulmonary hypertension associated with respiratory disease or hypoxia
   - Chronic obstructive pulmonary disease
   - Interstitial lung disease
   - Sleep disordered breathing
   - Alveolar hypoventilation disorders
   - High altitude
   - Developmental abnormalities
4. Pulmonary hypertension due to chronic thrombotic and/or embolic disease
5. Miscellaneous

another critical factor in the development of PAH. While 3% of patients with a VSD less than 1.5 cm will develop PAH, this increases to 50% if the defect is greater than 1.5 cm [4].

If detected early and the shunt closed, the PAH initially appears to be reversible [18]. Even without correction, patients with Eisenemenger syndrome appear to have a much longer life expectancy, up to the seventh decade, compared with 2.8 years in children with IPAH [19]. However, great variability exists and a small subgroup of patients will continue to deteriorate even after correction of the defect [1]. This is believed to be due to the fact that there is a certain point of no return, following which pulmonary vascular remodeling will progress even after closure of the defect [18].

A further subgroup of children present with severe PHT early in life, associated with a cardiac defect with only mild hemodynamic effects [1, 18]. In these children, PAH due to another cause, such as IPAH, should be suspected and investigated accordingly.

A high index of suspicion is required for an early and timely diagnosis of a left-to-right shunt, which can allow closure of the defect prior to the development of irreversible pulmonary vascular changes. There may be evidence of left-to-right shunting on the CXR prior to the development of PHT characterized by increased pulmonary vascularity in a noncyanotic child (Fig. 10.8). The most common location of the shunt is within the interventricular septum. A large VSD may show evidence of pulmonary artery enlargement associated with left ventricular hypertrophy. In contrast, pulmonary artery enlargement is uncommon in pediatric patients with an ASD, and cardiomegaly, if any, is predominantly right sided. Increased pulmonary vascularity in an infant should raise the suspicion of a PDA or an AVSD. The aorta is often enlarged in the former condition, while commonly, there is evidence of congestive cardiac failure in children with an AVSD. Once the pulmonary vascular resistance has increased, the typical changes of PAH described earlier are seen. However, in Eisenmenger syndrome, small nodular opacities, corresponding to neovascularity, appear to be much more common [20]. Intrapulmonary hemorrhage, also relatively common, may appear as focal areas of opacification [20].

The CT imaging findings of PAH in pediatric patients with congenital systemic to pulmonary shunts are similar to those seen in IPAH. However, in adults, several studies have highlighted some important differences in CT appearances in Eisenmenger vs. isolated IPAH. In particular, pulmonary neovascularity, characterized by peripheral serpiginous vessels, appears to be much more common in patients with Eisenmenger physiology [20, 21]. This is particularly the case with post-tricuspid defects. Lobular ground-glass opacity, which may be related to hemorrhage or dilated capillary networks, is also more frequently seen in these patients (Fig. 10.9) [20, 22]. Enlarged bronchial artery collaterals are often identified in both groups, but are more common in Eisenmenger syndrome [21]. Extrapulmonary findings that are particularly suggestive of Eisenmenger syndrome include aneurysmal dilatation of the pulmonary arteries and proximal pulmonary artery thrombosis [22].

MRI of the heart and great vessels can readily identify the anatomic defect and quantify the magnitude of the shunt. However, MR imaging of congenital heart disease is an extensive topic and outside of the scope of this chapter.

Scintigraphy is rarely performed in this setting as the other imaging modalities can accurately establish the diagnosis. However, it can be useful in excluding thromboembolic disease and will often identify a hemodynamically significant shunt [23].

Most importantly, the key investigation in these infants and children is transthoracic or transesophageal echocardiography. This will generally define the size and location of the defect as well as the magnitude of the associated shunt. In addition, it provides an estimate of right ventricular and pulmonary artery systolic pressure. In cases of suspected irreversible hypertension, cardiac catheterization with vasodilator testing may be required prior to initiation of medical therapy.

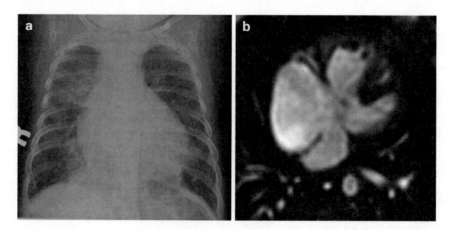

Fig. 10.8. A newborn girl with PHT secondary to atrioventricular defect. (**a**) Frontal chest radiograph shows increased pulmonary vascularity and cardiomegaly. (**b**) Axial T1 MR image demonstrates an atrioventricular septal defect

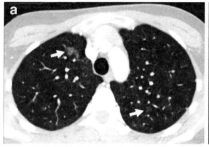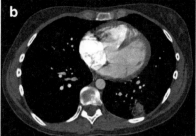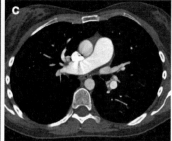

Fig. 10.9. Twenty-nine-year-old female with Eisenmenger's physiology who presented with PHT. (a) Axial lung window image shows areas of somewhat nodular and lobular ground-glass opacities (*arrows*). (b) Contrast enhanced axial CT image demonstrates ventricular defect. Focal opacification consistent with an area of pulmonary hemorrhage is also noted in the left lower lobe. (c) Contrast enhanced axial CT image shows an enlarged central pulmonary artery

10.3.3 Conditions Associated with Significant Venous or Capillary Involvement

Pulmonary Veno-Occlusive Disease

Pulmonary veno-occlusive disease (PVOD) is a rare cause of PHT. It preferentially affects the post-capillary vasculature with fibrous obliteration of the pulmonary venous system [24]. The disease affects all ages with no sex predilection in the pediatric age group [25].

The clinical presentation is essentially the same as IPAH. However, differentiation from IPAH is critical, as vasodilator therapy, while effective for IPAH, can result in potentially fatal pulmonary edema in patients with PVOD [13]. Histological examination in PVOD demonstrates obliteration of venous lamina by fibrous tissue, particularly within the veins in the intralobular septa [24]. In this setting, pulmonary arteriolar dilatation induced by vasodilators significantly increases capillary hydrostatic pressure, with development of pulmonary edema [13].

Open surgical biopsy remains the only definitive method of diagnosing PVOD, but is often contraindicated due to the fragile clinical and hemodynamic status of these patients. Imaging, therefore, plays a critical role in early and correct diagnosis. The CXR findings reflect the PHT and post-capillary venous congestion [26]. Therefore, enlarged central pulmonary arteries with rapid tapering are seen in conjunction with increased interstitial markings, including Kerley B lines [26]. Absence of left-sided heart disease is also an important finding on CXR indicated by normal cardiac contours and size of pulmonary veins.

In recent years, several published studies have demonstrated that CT, in particular high resolution CT, can be helpful in distinguishing PVOD from IPAH [11, 13, 24, 27]. While centrilobular opacities are more commonly seen in PVOD, these are also the most frequent intrapulmonary findings in IPAH [11, 13]. However, interlobular septal thickening is much more common and extensive in PVOD than in IPAH [13, 24]. Ground-glass opacity is also frequently seen and progresses from centrilobular to panlobular as the VOD worsens [13]. Of the extrapulmonary findings, the most specific imaging findings appear to be mediastinal lymphadenopathy in the absence of evidence for underlying chronic thromboembolic disease (CTED) or left-sided heart disease [13]. As with IPAH, central pulmonary artery and right-sided cardiac enlargement is identified, in the setting of normally sized left atrium and ventricle [26]. Pleural and pericardial effusions also appear to be non-specific and are seen in both conditions [13]. Ventilation-perfusion scans in PVOD are very variable in appearance, ranging from normal to multiple mismatched perfusion defects [26].

Pulmonary Capillary Hemangiomatosis

Due to the similarities in clinical, pathological and imaging features between PVOD and pulmonary capillary hemangiomatosis (PCH), in the most recent classification, these have been included in the same group [4]. Both conditions have similarly associated risk factors, such as systemic lupus erythematosis and scleroderma, but PCH has been reported much less frequently than PVOD [26]. It is characterized pathologically by atypical proliferation of capillaries along both sides of the alveolar wall [28]. As this proliferation fills the alveolar septa, it compromises the gas exchange mechanism [29]. PCH occurs in a wide age range of patients (2–70 years) and is associated with rapid clinical deterioration [30]. Clinical presentation is similar to that of PVOD, with the exception that hemoptysis is much more common, reported in up to 30% of patients [28]. Laboratory testing may reveal thrombocytopenia, particularly in children [29].

On CXR, in addition to the typical findings of PHT, there is a diffuse bilateral reticulonodular pattern [29]. In contrast to PVOD, septal lines and pleural effusions are not commonly seen [26]. The CT findings in this condition are often characteristic. Central pulmonary enlargement is consistently accompanied by poorly defined centrilobular nodules of ground-glass density, mixed with lobular ground-glass opacification [26, 28–30]. In contrast to PVOD, septal thickening is much less prominent and may be nodular in PCH [28, 29]. Although V/Q scintigraphy may demonstrate a non-homogeneous pattern with radioisotope uptake in areas of capillary proliferation [31], it is usually not helpful as results varying from normal to high probability have been reported [26, 30, 32].

10.3.4 Persistent Pulmonary Hypertension of the Newborn

At birth, pulmonary vascular resistance decreases rapidly which is initiated by expansion of the lungs, increased oxygenation and increased nitric oxide, PGI2 and bradykinin [33]. Over the course of 1 month, there is progressive remodeling of the airways with connective tissue deposition and smooth muscle maturation [34]. PPHN is a result of failure of normal pulmonary vascular relaxation at or shortly after birth [33]. It is characterized by high pulmonary vascular resistance, right to left shunting and severe hypoxemia [3]. Histologically, there is evidence of hyperplasia of the vascular smooth muscle combined with increased extracellular matrix deposition [35]. Persistent pulmonary hypertension of the newborn (PPHN) is frequently associated with perinatal stress (e.g., hypoglycemia, hypotension) and pulmonary parenchymal abnormalities, such as meconium aspiration, pneumonia and congenital lung anomalies [3, 36]. Although fatal in some cases, in the vast majority, PPHN is transient with complete resolution [1].

There are no specific imaging findings of PPHN. However, CXR often shows the underlying etiology of PPHN. Meconium aspiration is the most common cause of PPHN in the United States. On CXR, meconium aspiration is characterized by coarse opacities in the affected lungs associated with hyperinflation and often pneumothorax (i.e., air leaks). Profound hypoxemia with clear lungs may reflect idiopathic (or *black-lung*) PPHN [37], named due to its CXR findings of clear, hyperlucent lungs. This is most common in term and near-term (34-week gestation) newborns.

PPHN should be differentiated from alveolar capillary dysplasia, a rare, likely congenital, disorder of pulmonary vascular development characterized by severe hypoxemia and PHT refractory to treatment in the newborn. There is a high incidence of associated congenital anomalies, particularly of the gastrointestinal tract such as a malrotation [38]. These infants present on the first day of life and the condition is universally fatal in the first few weeks [39].

10.4 Pulmonary Hypertension Associated with Left Heart Diseases

Left heart disease in pediatric patients is primarily associated with congenital heart disease. This includes conditions such as hypoplastic left heart syndrome and mitral stenosis [40, 41]. Similar findings can also be seen in partial (Scimitar) and total anomalous pulmonary venous connection [42, 43]. The end result in all these conditions is the elevated left atrial pressure associated with subsequent pulmonary venous hypertension. This, in turn, often causes intimal fibrosis and medial hypertrophy of the arterioles resulting in increased PAPs [44]. However, pathologically, there is no evidence of plexiform lesions in these children, resulting in a significant degree of reversibility of the PAH following surgical correction of the cardiac abnormality [41]. The CXR and CT findings in the lungs can be very similar to PVOD, but with associated abnormalities in heart contour and configuration. The diagnosis is usually readily established by echocardiography.

10.5 Pulmonary Hypertension Associated with Respiratory Disease or Hypoxia

Alveolar hypoxia, by inducing pulmonary vasoconstriction, can reflexively result in elevated pulmonary pressures. If chronic, this typically results in pulmonary vascular remodeling and PHT [45]. Remodeling results in medial thickening in muscular arterioles and muscularization of previously non-muscular arterioles [46]. Although CXR has been the first-line imaging modality of initial investigation, high resolution CT is currently the investigation of choice for evaluating chronic lung disease. Contrast-enhanced MDCT scan will also demonstrate the vascular anatomy. In addition, ventilation-perfusion scans may be useful in the assessment of regional lung function.

10.5.1 Bronchopulmonary Dysplasia

Bronchopulmonary dysplasia (BPD) is a chronic lung disease of infancy characterized by the abnormal development of inflamed and scarred lung tissues, resulting from mechanical ventilation and oxygen therapy. Originally described by Northway in 1967, in the pre-surfactant era, this was seen in infants who underwent prolonged high pressure ventilation with elevated oxygen concentrations. With the advent of surfactant and advancement in ventilation techniques, this is now predominantly seen in premature neonates of low birth weight. Consistent with the changing demographic pattern, the pathological changes seen in current cases of BPD are also substantially different. The classic progressive stages commonly seen with acute lung injury have now given way to findings consistent with impaired alveolar and vascular growth [47]. Prominent pathological features include alveolar simplification with decreased growth of the capillary bed.

In addition to the previously described changes seen with PHT, the CXR may also demonstrate hyper-expansion, interstitial opacities and focal emphysema (Fig. 10.10) [48]. The lung findings tend to improve with age. HRCT demonstrates multifocal hyperlucent areas, linear opacities radiating from the periphery, and triangular subpleural opacities. The areas of low attenuation on CT are larger than a pulmonary segment and may reflect obstructive emphysema caused by destruction of small airways and arrest of acinar development [49, 50]. Large airway changes may also be noted with tracheo-broncho-malacia and decreased broncho-arterial diameter [49]. Thus in the setting of PHT, the broncho-arterial diameter should be interpreted with caution.

10.5.2 Cystic Fibrosis and Bronchiectasis

PHT can be identified in up to a half of adolescents and young adults with cystic fibrosis (CF). PHT is particularly common in children with low peripheral oxygen saturation at rest [51]. Often subclinical, this is associated with thickening of the right ventricular wall on echocardiography [51]. Radiographic and CT findings of CF are discussed in detail elsewhere in this book, but evidence of PHT in the setting of upper lobe predominant bronchial wall thickening, bronchiectasis and "tree-in-bud" opacities representing superimposed bronchiolitis should strongly suggest the diagnosis of PHT associated with cystic fibrosis (Fig. 10.11).

10.5.3 Congenital Diaphragmatic Hernia

CDH is the most common developmental abnormality associated with PHT [1]. Bilateral pulmonary

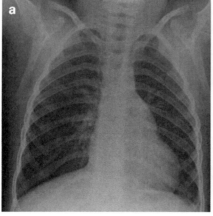
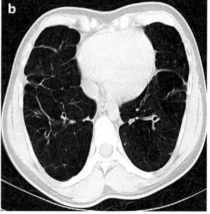

Fig. 10.10. Eight-year-old boy with prior history of prematurity and bronchopulmonary dysplasia presenting with PHT. (**a**) Frontal chest radiograph shows enlarged central pulmonary artery. Mild hyperlucency is also noted within the bilateral lower lobes. (**b**) Axial lung window image demonstrates marked lung parenchymal damage characterized by the areas of coarse parenchymal thickening and air-trapping

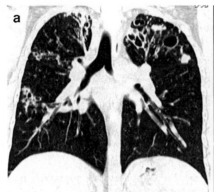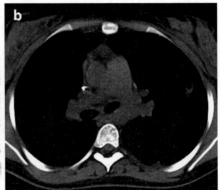

Fig. 10.11. Seventeen-year-old girl with PHT secondary to underlying lung disease (cystic fibrosis). (**a**) Coronal lung window image demonstrates advanced lung changes secondary to the patient's known cystic fibrosis characterized by bilateral upper lobe predominant bronchiectasis. (**b**) Axial non-enhanced CT image shows the enlarged central pulmonary artery

hypoplasia occurs early in fetal life with arrest of preacinar airway branching resulting in markedly decreased number of alveoli [52]. There is a similar arrest of the pulmonary vascular tree at 12–14 weeks of gestational age, with decreased cross-sectional area of the vascular bed and increased thickness of the muscular walls of the arterioles [53]. The PHT often abates in the first few weeks after birth, but can persist and is associated with a significantly increased mortality [54].

The diagnosis of CDH is usually straight forward and often identified on pre-natal imaging studies including pre-natal ultrasound and MRI. Characteristic post-natal CXR findings include mediastinal shift with bowel loops seen in the affected pleural cavity. Post-repair radiographs demonstrate resolution of the mediastinal shift with more marked hypoplasia of the ipsilateral lung. Similar findings are demonstrated on CT. Ventilation-perfusion scanning initially demonstrate decreased ventilation and perfusion in the affected ipsilateral lung. With increasing age, the ventilation normalizes but decreased perfusion persists, consistent with poor development of the pulmonary vascular tree [52].

<h2>10.6   Pulmonary Hypertension Due to Chronic Thrombotic and/or Embolic Disease</h2>

This is a very uncommon cause of PHT in children [1]. Historically, the incidence of pulmonary embolism (PE) was believed to be much lower in children than in adults, in part because of a protective mechanism which decreases thromboembolism in children [55–58]. The incidence of deep venous thrombosis (DVT) and PE is greatest in adolescents and infants less than 1 year of age, but still only accounts for 0.05–0.07 events per 10,000 children [55,59]. However, in the hospital-based population, the incidence rises to 5.3 events per 10,000 hospital admissions. Much of this higher incidence is due to DVT/PE related to central venous lines. This accounts for almost 90% of embolic events in neonates and 60% in older children [55, 60]. Other less common risk factors for thromboembolic disease in children include cancer, cardiac disease, surgery, sickle cell disease and tumor emboli.

There is currently limited data on PHT associated with CTED in the pediatric population. In adults, in the vast majority of cases in which the patient survives a pulmonary embolic event, the thrombus is resorbed by fibrinolysis. However, in 0.1–0.4% of cases, the emboli evolve to an organized clot [61]. Contributing to the PHT is propagation of thrombus due to slow flow upstream from an occluded artery. In addition, there also appears to be a vasculopathy, similar to that seen in IPAH, in the unobstructed segments of the lung [61]. Histologically, medial hypertrophy, intimal thickening and plexiform lesion have all been identified [62].

Clinically, the patient may remain asymptomatic for many years, the so-called *honeymoon period*. Following obliteration of 60% of the pulmonary vascular bed, progressive dyspnea typically develops [63].

Pulmonary angiography with right heart catheterization remains the gold standard investigation, providing a diagnosis as well as essential information on MPAP [64]. The aim of the investigation in CTED-related PHT is not only to establish the diagnosis but also to assess whether the hypertension is in proportion to the degree of vascular obstruction. Disproportionately high PHTN implies a significant degree of arteritis, with the condition less likely to respond to endarterectomy.

With the rapid advancement in MDCT technology in recent years, PE can now be identified to the sixth-order branches and is generally the investigation of choice in both the pediatric population and adults [65, 66]. Recently, there has also been growing interest in the use of MRI for evaluation of PE. It has been reported that MR angiography can be useful for evaluation of PE by demonstrating: (1) the visualization of pulmonary vessels to the subsegmental level; (2) the identification of the wedge-shaped lung parenchymal defects on MR perfusion sequences; and (3) the display of the extent of right heart impairment on cine MR sequences [63]. Scintigraphic ventilation-perfusion scans show large segmental, often bilateral, perfusion defects associated with PE with normal ventilation.

10.7 Miscellaneous

10.7.1 Hemoglobinopathies

PHT is a well-documented sequela of sickle cell disease and accounts for 3% of the mortality [4]. Elevated PAPs have been reported in almost half of children with sickle cell disease [67]. Historically, shear stress from the deformed erythrocytes passing through the pulmonary microvasculature has been proposed as the underlying cause of vascular injury. However, epidemiological evidence now suggests that hemolysis is the key factor in development of PHTN in sickle cell disease patients. The hemoglobin and arginase enzyme released from the hemolytic process produce a state of vascular proliferation and inflammatory stress [68] inducing a vasculopathy similar to that seen in IPAH, including the formation of plexiform lesions. In children, as in adults, the risk of developing PHTN appears to be related to the degree of hemolysis [67]. Co-existing underlying pulmonary disease such as asthma and obstructive sleep apnea also appear to play a contributing factor.

Transthoracic echocardiography plays a key role in diagnosis of elevated pressures and secondary

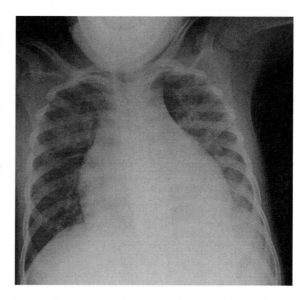

Fig. 10.12. Nine-year-old boy with known sickle cell disease who presents with shortness of breath and PHT. Frontal chest radiograph shows markedly enlarged heart and areas of mild patchy parenchymal opacities (worst in the left lower lobe) and surrounding lucencies in both lungs

cardiac changes. A V/Q scan is also usually performed to exclude CTED, a potentially treatable cause of PHTN which can occur in patients with sickle cell disease [69]. The CXR has a low overall sensitivity, but may indicate findings consistent with PHT in association with parenchymal disease and loss of volume consistent with fibrosis (Fig. 10.12). Fibrosis is better assessed on HRCT, characterized by predominantly basal interlobular septal thickening, traction bronchiectasis and architectural distortion.

PHT has been described in virtually all hemoglobinopathies, especially beta-thalassemia [70]. The exact mechanism remains unclear, although chronic tissue hypoxia and hemolysis have been advocated as potential causes [70, 71]. The risk also appears to be elevated by splenectomy. This may be due to platelet activation resulting in microthrombi in the pulmonary vasculature or increased hemolysis due to the lack of removal of senescent cells [70]. The imaging appearances are generally non-specific.

10.8 Treatments

For IPAH, treatments may include:

- *Inhaled oxygen* to help raise the levels of oxygen in the bloodstream.

- *Nitric oxide* (NO) to help reduce the resistance in the lung blood vessels and improve heart function.
- *Calcium-channel blockers* to relieve constriction in the pulmonary arteries and improve the heart's ability to pump blood.
- *Intravenous prostacyclin, Flolan,* to help open up constricted lung blood vessels and reduce high blood pressure in the lungs.
- *Endothelin antagonists, prostacyclin analogs and phosphodiesterase inhibitors* to reduce high blood pressure in the lungs.
- *Anticoagulants* to prevent blood clots in the lungs.
- *Diuretics* to help kidneys eliminate water.
- *Digoxin* to help support the ability of the heart to pump the blood.
- *Lung transplantation* for patients who do not respond to medication—a single-lung, double-lung or heart-lung transplant may be recommended.

For conditions associated with pulmonary arterial hypertension, treating the underlying disease or defect may have significant benefit. Use of many of the treatments listed above, in conjunction with treatment for the associated cause of the disease, may help ease the effects of PHT.

References

1. Haworth SG. The management of pulmonary hypertension in children. Arch Dis Child. 2008;93:620–5.
2. Rosenzweig EB, Barst RJ. Pulmonary arterial hypertension in children: a medical update. Curr Opin Pediatr. 2008;20:288–93.
3. Rosenzweig EB, Widlitz AC, Barst RJ. Pulmonary arterial hypertension in children. Pediatr Pulmonol. 2004;38:2–22.
4. Simonneau G, Galie N, Rubin LJ, et al. Clinical classification of pulmonary hypertension. J Am Coll Cardiol. 2004;43:5S–12.
5. LaRaia AV, Waxman AB. Pulmonary arterial hypertension: evaluation and management. South Med J. 2007;100:393–9.
6. Gabbay E, Reed A, Williams TJ. Assessment and treatment of pulmonary arterial hypertension: an Australian perspective in 2006. Intern Med J. 2007;37:38–48.
7. Rosenzweig EB, Barst RJ. Idiopathic pulmonary arterial hypertension in children. Curr Opin Pediatr. 2005;17:372–80.
8. Widlitz A, Barst RJ. Pulmonary arterial hypertension in children. Eur Respir J. 2003;21:155–76.
9. Lammers AE, Hislop AA, Flynn Y, et al. Epoprostenol treatment in children with severe pulmonary hypertension. Heart. 2007;93:739–43.
10. Ng CS, Wells AU, Padley SP. A CT sign of chronic pulmonary arterial hypertension: the ratio of main pulmonary artery to aortic diameter. J Thorac Imaging. 1999;14:270–8.
11. Chaudry G, MacDonald C, Adatia I, et al. CT of the chest in the evaluation of idiopathic pulmonary arterial hypertension in children. Pediatr Radiol. 2007;37:345–50.
12. King MA, Ysrael M, Bergin CJ. Chronic thromboembolic pulmonary hypertension: CT findings. AJR Am J Roentgenol. 1998;170:955–60.
13. Resten A, Maitre S, Humbert M, et al. Pulmonary hypertension: CT of the chest in pulmonary venoocclusive disease. AJR Am J Roentgenol. 2004;183:65–70.
14. McCann GP, Gan CT, Beek AM, et al. Extent of MRI delayed enhancement of myocardial mass is related to right ventricular dysfunction in pulmonary artery hypertension. AJR Am J Roentgenol. 2007;188:349–55.
15. Fukuchi K, Hayashida K, Nakanishi N, et al. Quantitative analysis of lung perfusion in patients with primary pulmonary hypertension. J Nucl Med. 2002;43:757–61.
16. Ogawa Y, Nishimura T, Hayashida K, et al. Perfusion lung scintigraphy in primary pulmonary hypertension. Br J Radiol. 1993;66:677–80.
17. Wood P. The Eisenmenger syndrome or pulmonary hypertension with reversed central shunt. I. Br Med J. 1958;2:701–9.
18. van Albada ME, Berger RM. Pulmonary arterial hypertension in congenital cardiac disease – the need for refinement of the Evian-Venice classification. Cardiol Young. 2008;18:10–7.
19. Daliento L, Somerville J, Presbitero P, et al. Eisenmenger syndrome. Factors relating to deterioration and death. Eur Heart J. 1998;19:1845–55.
20. Sheehan R, Perloff JK, Fishbein MC, et al. Pulmonary neovascularity: a distinctive radiographic finding in Eisenmenger syndrome. Circulation. 2005;112:2778–85.
21. Griffin N, Allen D, Wort J, et al. Eisenmenger syndrome and idiopathic pulmonary arterial hypertension: do parenchymal lung changes reflect aetiology? Clin Radiol. 2007;62:587–95.
22. Perloff JK, Hart EM, Greaves SM, et al. Proximal pulmonary arterial and intrapulmonary radiologic features of Eisenmenger syndrome and primary pulmonary hypertension. Am J Cardiol. 2003;92:182–7.
23. Sun SS, Tsai MK, Yang CH, et al. Atrial septal defect with Eisenmenger's syndrome confirmed by Tc-99m MAA scintigraphy. Clin Nucl Med. 2002;27:219–20.
24. Ozsoyoglu AA, Swartz J, Farver CF, et al. High-resolution computed tomographic imaging and pathologic features of pulmonary veno-occlusive disease: a review of three patients. Curr Probl Diagn Radiol. 2006;35:219–23.
25. Holcomb Jr BW, Loyd JE, Ely EW, et al. Pulmonary venoocclusive disease: a case series and new observations. Chest. 2000;118:1671–9.
26. Frazier AA, Franks TJ, Mohammed TL, et al. From the Archives of the AFIP: pulmonary veno-occlusive disease and pulmonary capillary hemangiomatosis. Radiographics. 2007;27:867–82.
27. Engelke C, Schaefer-Prokop C, Schirg E, et al. High-resolution CT and CT angiography of peripheral pulmonary vascular disorders. Radiographics. 2002;22:739–64.
28. Lippert JL, White CS, Cameron EW, et al. Pulmonary capillary hemangiomatosis: radiographic appearance. J Thorac Imaging. 1998;13:49–51.
29. El-Gabaly M, Farver CF, Budev MA, et al. Pulmonary capillary hemangiomatosis imaging findings and literature update. J Comput Assist Tomogr. 2007;31:608–10.
30. Ito K, Ichiki T, Ohi K, et al. Pulmonary capillary hemangiomatosis with severe pulmonary hypertension. Circ J. 2003;67:793–5.
31. Rush C, Langleben D, Schlesinger RD, et al. Lung scintigraphy in pulmonary capillary hemangiomatosis. A rare

disorder causing primary pulmonary hypertension. Clin Nucl Med. 1991;16:913–7.

32. Almagro P, Julia J, Sanjaume M, et al. Pulmonary capillary hemangiomatosis associated with primary pulmonary hypertension: report of 2 new cases and review of 35 cases from the literature. Medicine (Baltimore). 2002;81:417–24.

33. Dakshinamurti S. Pathophysiologic mechanisms of persistent pulmonary hypertension of the newborn. Pediatr Pulmonol. 2005;39:492–503.

34. Allen K, Haworth SG. Human postnatal pulmonary arterial remodeling. Ultrastructural studies of smooth muscle cell and connective tissue maturation. Lab Invest. 1988;59:702–9.

35. McLeod KA, Gerlis LM, Williams GJ. Morphology of the elastic pulmonary arteries in pulmonary hypertension: a quantitative study. Cardiol Young. 1999;9:364–70.

36. Atkinson JB, Ford EG, Kitagawa H, et al. Persistent pulmonary hypertension complicating cystic adenomatoid malformation in neonates. J Pediatr Surg. 1992;27:54–6.

37. Farrow KN, Fliman P, Steinhorn RH. The diseases treated with ECMO: focus on PPHN. Semin Perinatol. 2005;29:8–14.

38. Antao B, Samuel M, Kiely E, et al. Congenital alveolar capillary dysplasia and associated gastrointestinal anomalies. Fetal Pediatr Pathol. 2006;25:137–45.

39. Roy PG, Patel P, Vayalakkad A, et al. Alveolar capillary dysplasia presenting as pneumothorax: a case report and review of literature. Pediatr Surg Int. 2007;23:915–7.

40. Bardo DM, Frankel DG, Applegate KE, et al. Hypoplastic left heart syndrome. Radiographics. 2001;21:705–17.

41. Endo M, Yamaki S, Ohmi M, et al. Pulmonary vascular changes induced by congenital obstruction of pulmonary venous return. Ann Thorac Surg. 2000;69:193–7.

42. Gudjonsson U, Brown JW. Scimitar syndrome. Semin Thorac Cardiovasc Surg Pediatr Card Surg Annu. 2006;56–62.

43. Yamaki S, Tsunemoto M, Shimada M, et al. Quantitative analysis of pulmonary vascular disease in total anomalous pulmonary venous connection in sixty infants. J Thorac Cardiovasc Surg. 1992;104:728–35.

44. Yamaki S, Endo M, Takahashi T. Different grades of medial hypertrophy and intimal changes in small pulmonary arteries among various types of congenital heart disease with pulmonary hypertension. Tohoku J Exp Med. 1997;182:83–91.

45. Ghofrani HA, Voswinckel R, Reichenberger F, et al. Hypoxia- and non-hypoxia-related pulmonary hypertension – established and new therapies. Cardiovasc Res. 2006;72:30–40.

46. Howell K, Ooi H, Preston R, et al. Structural basis of hypoxic pulmonary hypertension: the modifying effect of chronic hypercapnia. Exp Physiol. 2004;89:66–72.

47. Stenmark KR, Abman SH. Lung vascular development: implications for the pathogenesis of bronchopulmonary dysplasia. Annu Rev Physiol. 2005;67:623–61.

48. Griscom NT, Wheeler WB, Sweezey NB, et al. Bronchopulmonary dysplasia: radiographic appearance in middle childhood. Radiology. 1989;171:811–4.

49. Howling SJ, Northway Jr WH, Hansell DM, et al. Pulmonary sequelae of bronchopulmonary dysplasia survivors: high-resolution CT findings. AJR Am J Roentgenol. 2000;174:1323–6.

50. Husain AN, Siddiqui NH, Stocker JT. Pathology of arrested acinar development in postsurfactant bronchopulmonary dysplasia. Hum Pathol. 1998;29:710–7.

51. Rovedder PM, Ziegler B, Pinotti AF, et al. Prevalence of pulmonary hypertension evaluated by Doppler echocardiography in a population of adolescent and adult patients with cystic fibrosis. J Bras Pneumol. 2008;34:83–90.

52. Keller RL. Antenatal and postnatal lung and vascular anatomic and functional studies in congenital diaphragmatic hernia: implications for clinical management. Am J Med Genet C Semin Med Genet. 2007;145C:184–200.

53. Kitagawa M, Hislop A, Boyden EA, et al. Lung hypoplasia in congenital diaphragmatic hernia. A quantitative study of airway, artery, and alveolar development. Br J Surg. 1971;58:342–6.

54. Dillon PW, Cilley RE, Mauger D, et al. The relationship of pulmonary artery pressure and survival in congenital diaphragmatic hernia. J Pediatr Surg. 2004;39:307–12. discussion 307–12.

55. Andrew M, David M, Adams M, et al. Venous thromboembolic complications (VTE) in children: first analyses of the Canadian Registry of VTE. Blood. 1994;83:1251–7.

56. Anton N, Massicotte MP. Venous thromboembolism in pediatrics. Semin Vasc Med. 2001;1:111–22.

57. Babyn PS, Gahunia HK, Massicotte P. Pulmonary thromboembolism in children. Pediatr Radiol. 2005;35:258–74.

58. Chan AK, Deveber G, Monagle P, et al. Venous thrombosis in children. J Thromb Haemost. 2003;1:1443–55.

59. Revel-Vilk S, Massicotte P. Thromboembolic diseases of childhood. Blood Rev. 2003;17:1–6.

60. Schmidt B, Andrew M. Neonatal thrombosis: report of a prospective Canadian and international registry. Pediatrics. 1995;96:939–43.

61. Dartevelle P, Fadel E, Mussot S, et al. Chronic thromboembolic pulmonary hypertension. Eur Respir J. 2004;23:637–48.

62. Moser KM, Bloor CM. Pulmonary vascular lesions occurring in patients with chronic major vessel thromboembolic pulmonary hypertension. Chest. 1993;103:685–92.

63. Kreitner KF, Kunz RP, Ley S, et al. Chronic thromboembolic pulmonary hypertension – assessment by magnetic resonance imaging. Eur Radiol. 2007;17:11–21.

64. Auger WR, Kim NH, Kerr KM, et al. Chronic thromboembolic pulmonary hypertension. Clin Chest Med. 2007;28:255–69. x.

65. Kritsaneepaiboon S, Lee EY, Zurakowoski D, et al. MDCT pulmonary angiography evaluation of pulmonary embolism in children. AJR Am J Roentgenol. 2009;192(5): 1246–52.

66. Schoepf UJ. Diagnosing pulmonary embolism: time to rewrite the textbooks. Int J Cardiovasc Imaging. 2005;21: 155–63.

67. Onyekwere OC, Campbell A, Teshome M, et al. Pulmonary hypertension in children and adolescents with sickle cell disease. Pediatr Cardiol. 2008;29:309–12.

68. Machado RF. Sickle cell anemia-associated pulmonary arterial hypertension. J Bras Pneumol. 2007;33:583–91.

69. Machado RF, Gladwin MT. Chronic sickle cell lung disease: new insights into the diagnosis, pathogenesis and treatment of pulmonary hypertension. Br J Haematol. 2005;129:449–64.

70. Barnett CF, Hsue PY, Machado RF. Pulmonary hypertension: an increasingly recognized complication of hereditary hemolytic anemias and HIV infection. JAMA. 2008;299:324–31.

71. Aessopos A, Farmakis D. Pulmonary hypertension in beta-thalassemia. Ann N Y Acad Sci. 2005;1054:342–9.

Focal Lung Disease

11

Jeanne S. Chow, Ellen M. Chung, Andrew A. Colin,
Robert H. Cleveland, and Gregory S. Sawicki

CONTENTS

Jeanne S. Chow, MD (✉)
Department of Radiology, Children's Hospital Boston,
Harvard Medical School, Boston, MA, USA
e-mail: jeanne.chow@childrens.harvard.edu

Ellen M. Chung, MD
Department of Radiology and Radiological Sciences,
Uniformed Services University of the Health Sciences,
Bethesda, MD, USA

Andrew A. Colin, MD
Miller School of Medicine, University of Miami, Miami, FL, USA

Robert H. Cleveland, MD
Department of Radiology, Harvard Medical School,
Boston, MA, USA

Departments of Radiology and Medicine, Division of Respiratory
Diseases, Children's Hospital Boston,
Boston, MA, USA

Gregory S. Sawicki, MD, MPH
Department of Pediatrics, Division of Respiratory Diseases,
Children's Hospital Boston, Harvard Medical School,
Boston, MA, USA

R.H. Cleveland (ed.), *Imaging in Pediatric Pulmonology*,
DOI 10.1007/978-1-4419-5872-3_11, © Springer Science+Business Media, LLC 2012

11.1 The Imaging of Pediatric Pneumonia

Jeanne S. Chow

Among the most common infections in children are those affecting the lower respiratory tract, lower respiratory tract infections (LRTIs). Most frequently, this involves viral or bacterial pneumonia. Worldwide, more than two million children die of pneumonia annually, predominately in developing countries [1]. Mortality is extremely rare in the United States and other parts of the developed world. In the United States, there has been a dramatic drop in mortality from pneumonia between 1939 and 1996 due to improved access to health care for poor children and the introduction of penicillin. In 1996, 800 deaths in children younger than 15 years of age were reported from pneumonia in the United States [2–4]. However, respiratory infections remain a major cause of morbidity in the United States. Children experience 6–8 acute respiratory illnesses per year [5].

Even in the most optimal circumstances, however, pediatric pneumonia is often difficult to diagnose. Patient history, physical findings, and laboratory results can all be elusive. Children with pneumonia do not necessarily present with the signs and symptoms typically associated with adult LRTI such as fever, cough, wheezing, tachypnea, and retractions. On physical examination, an accurate diagnosis may be further delayed by nonspecific complaints such as malaise, fever, and abdominal pain.

In addition, most clinicians attempt to distinguish bacterial pneumonias from viral pneumonia since bacterial pneumonias are treated with antibiotics and viral pneumonias are typically treated symptomatically. Unfortunately, signs and symptoms used to distinguish *typical* bacterial pneumonias from *atypical* viral or mycoplasmal pneumonias in adults do not reliably distinguish the two pneumonias in infants and young children [6–8].

At present, no laboratory test can accurately diagnose pneumonia or differentiate bacterial from nonbacterial pneumonia. Among diagnostically relevant laboratory values, C-reactive protein level, which measures the concentration of a protein in serum and the absolute neutrophil count which signals an increase in infection-fighting white blood cells, when elevated, are reliable indicators of acute infection and are clinically useful in distinguishing typical and atypical pneumonias [9–13].

One of the most common indications of imaging children arises from the need to evaluate suspected cases of LRTIs [14]. In this setting, chest radiographs are the most specific test to evaluate for pneumonia [15–17] and aid significantly in reaching diagnosis and in treating respiratory illnesses [18, 19].

This chapter concentrates on the plain film radiographic manifestations of community-acquired lower respiratory tract illnesses in immunocompetent children who have developed beyond the neonatal period (>30 days). In this chapter, the term *pneumonia* describes LRTI and inflammation [17].

11.1.1 Epidemiology of Lower Respiratory Tract Infections

Viruses are the most common cause of upper and LRTIs in children of all ages in the United States. They account for 65% of all pediatric pneumonias and for more than 90% of pneumonias in children under two [20, 21]. Bacteria account for 5–10% of childhood pneumonias [21]. The single most common agent that produces pneumonia in childhood is *Mycoplasma pneumoniae*. *Mycoplasma* is a microorganism that, unlike a virus, does not need a host cell; and unlike a bacterium, does not have a cell wall [22].

In the United States, the most common viral pathogen is respiratory syncytial virus (RSV); this virus is responsible for at least 60% of severe LRTIs in children under the age of 5 [23]. Other common viral causes of LRTIs are influenza, types A and B, and parainfluenza, types 1 and 3. Adenoviruses and Enteroviruses are other pathogens that are less common and/or more difficult to diagnose [3, 5, 24, 25].

One of the most predictive indicators of pediatric pneumonia is age [26]. The etiology of pneumonia may also be traced seasonally and by the symptom complex that presents in individual patients [5]. Certain viruses and bacteria, for example, are known to have higher prevalence rates in different age distributions – a largely unexplained phenomenon. For example, RSV, parainfluenza virus, influenza, and adenovirus account for most LRTIs in infants and toddlers (1–24 months) [6, 8, 27–29]. Among preschool-aged children (2–5 years), these same viruses remain the most common cause of pneumonia; although viruses account for a smaller percentage of pneumonias than in the infant and toddler population [26]. *Pneumococcus* is the most common cause of bacterial pneumonia in preschool-aged children [3]. Among school-aged children (6–18 years), *M. pneumoniae*, *Streptococcus pneumoniae*, and *Chlamydia pneumoniae* (TWAR) are common pathogens for pneumonia. *Mycoplasma* causes approximately 30% of respiratory infections in school-aged children (6–18 years). *C. pneumoniae* is another common cause of pneumonia in elementary school-age children, causing 15–18% of community-acquired pneumonia among children aged 3–12 years. Most infections are mild or asymptomatic with only 10% of cases resulting in clinically apparent pneumonia [30].

S. pneumoniae and Haemophilus influenzae (H. influenza) have been implicated as common causes of bacterial pneumonia in children from infancy to early elementary school-age [20]. However, the exact prevalence of these two pathogens is unknown because these organisms commonly live in the upper respiratory tract in asymptomatic individuals. The only way to truly isolate the organisms is to isolate them from the blood or pleural spaces by means of thoracentesis or directly from the lung through percutaneous aspiration [20]. Finally, with the introduction of a heptavalent conjugated pneumococcal vaccine (PCV7, Prevanar) in 2000, and the widespread use of the H. influenza Type b (Hib) vaccine, the overall degree of invasive disease [31] has decreased; although the exact prevalence of S. pneumoniae and H. influenza have not been restudied [32].

11.1.2 Pathophysiology of Childhood Pneumonia with Radiographic Correlation

Infectious agents reach the lower respiratory tract through aspiration, hematogenous seeding of the lungs, and direct spread from extrapulmonary sites. The most common cause of pneumonia is from inhalation of airborne organisms or aspiration of infected secretions or gastric material. Less commonly, infections are carried by the blood stream to the lungs through the pulmonary vasculature such as during diffuse blood infection (sepsis) or through infected thrombi. Infections from the mediastinum, chest wall, abdomen, and neck can also spread directly to the lungs.

The respiratory *tree* is composed of branching airways that terminate at the alveoli, the final gas exchange units between the outside world and the cells. The branching begins in the center of the chest at the hilum and extends peripherally. There are between 10 and 22 generations of branching airways before gas exchange occurs, with the largest airways called bronchi and the smaller airways called bronchioles. As the child grows, the length of the airways grow; but not the number. The airways complete their branching in fetal life at about the 16th week of gestation. The alveoli begin to mature at about the

29th week of gestation, and continue to proliferate and mature until approximately 8 years of age [25]. Grossly, a normal right lung is divided into three lobes; the right upper lobe, right middle lobe, and right lower lobe. The left lung is divided into the upper and lower lobes. The lobes are composed of segments. Lobes are separated from each other by fissures.

The inhaled or aspirated microorganisms giving rise to pneumonia cause distinctly different inflammatory reaction in the lungs; these differences, in turn, lead to three main distinctive pathologic patterns: interstitial pneumonia, lobar pneumonia, and lobular pneumonia (bronchopneumonia). The radiographic findings of pneumonia closely follow the pathologic processes.

Because viruses are the most common cause of childhood LRTIs, its pathologic process and radiographic manifestations will be described first. Interstitial pneumonia is the typical pathologic description of viral infection in the lungs. Although there is some variation in the microscopic reaction produced in the lung by the various viruses, they produce generally similar pathological and radiographic patterns. Viruses infect the epithelial cells lining of the small- and medium-sized airways causing destruction of the ciliated columnar epithelial cells, goblet cells, and mucus glands. The cell destruction triggers an inflammatory reaction that produces edematous bronchial walls infiltrated with mononuclear lymphocytic cells. The resulting sloughed cells, lymphocytic infiltrate, debris, and peribronchial edema cause occlusion of the small- and medium-sized airways. Thus, the pathologic hallmarks of viral pneumonia are peribronchial edema and occlusion of smaller airways.

On a frontal radiograph of the chest, normal appearing small- and medium-sized airways are best seen near the hilum. The airways branch from the center to the periphery and are normally invisible in the outer one third of the lungs. When the branching airways are seen on end, they appear as well-defined circles and are similar in diameter to the adjacent pulmonary artery (Fig. 11.1). Peribronchial edema causes irregularity and thickening of the normally sharply defined walls; this is described as peribronchial cuffing (Fig. 11.2). The relatively abundant overlapping thickened bronchioles near the hilum can give the appearance of enhanced linear soft tissue at the hilum or hilar enlargement (Fig. 11.3a). Occlusion of small airways causes both atelectasis and hyperinflation and both effects may occur simultaneously

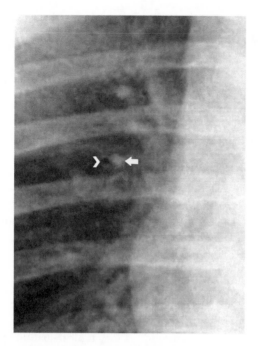

Fig. 11.1. This magnified AP view of the chest demonstrates a normal appearing bronchus (*arrowhead*) and artery (*arrow*) on end. Notice how the edges of the bronchus are sharp and well defined

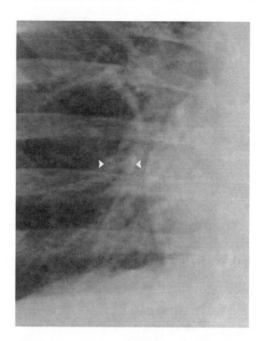

Fig. 11.2. This magnified view of the chest of an 8 month infant with severe respiratory distress demonstrates the radiographic finding of peribronchial cuffing. The margins of the bronchus (*arrowheads*) are thickened and irregular compared to the normal example (Fig. 11.1)

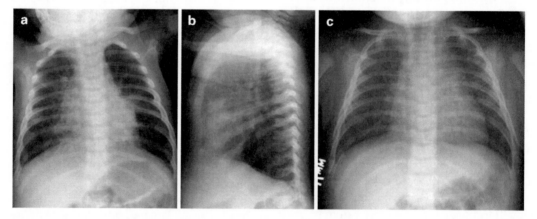

Fig. 11.3. This is a 2-month-old girl with cough and coarse breath sounds. (**a**) AP view of the chest demonstrates coarse linear opacities radiating from the hilum consistent with peribronchial thickening. The (**b**) lateral radiograph demonstrates flattening of the hemidiaphragms (as does the AP view) and anterior bowing of the sternum, signs of hyperinflation. These findings are consistent with classical viral pneumonia. No microbial etiology was found. (**c**) Several weeks later, her radiographs had returned to normal

(Fig. 11.3b). Although it may be difficult to differentiate atelectasis from an infiltrate, there are distinguishing characteristics. Atelectasis causes focal volume loss which may be recognized as bowing of fissures toward the opacified segment of lung. With subsegmental atelectasis, there may be a linear margin to the opacification which cannot be attributed to a fissure. Also, frequently subsegmental atelectasis is often more clearly seen on either the frontal or lateral image than on the other. On frontal CXR, with pectus excavatum, there frequently will be obscuration of the right heart border with no lung abnormality demonstrated on lateral projection. Without the presence of the pectus deformity, this would suggest right middle lobe atelectasis.

The effect of small- and medium-sized airway occlusion is especially dramatic in infants and young children, especially in 18 months old and younger.

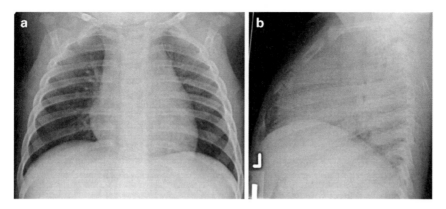

Fig. 11.4. Normal (**a**) AP and (**b**) lateral radiographs of an infant demonstrate that the anterior ribs curve downward relative to the posterior ribs and that the hemidiaphragms are curved on both the AP and lateral views

Children are more susceptible to airway narrowing than adults because the diameter of their airways is smaller, mucus production is greater, and collateral pathways of aeration such as the channels of Lambert (bronchoalveolar channels) and pores of Kohn (intraalveolar pores) are poorly developed. These pathways, which allow collateral air drift between airspaces, become fully developed at approximately 8 years of age. One of the causes of air trapping is tachypnea; air trapping is one of the most sensitive indicators of LRTIs in young children [33, 34].

Thus the radiographic appearance of increased lung volumes, especially intermingled with areas of subsegmental atelectasis and peribronchial cuffing, offers compelling diagnostic evidence of viral LRTIs in young children [17]. Because young children are unable to follow commands regarding breath holds, images of their lungs, especially when they are not crying, are used to assess total lung volume. In older children (18 months of age) and adults with larger airways and mature collateral pathways of aeration, hyperinflation is no longer a useful tool in diagnosing viral pneumonia. In addition, older children and adults can follow the command to hold their breath at maximum inspiration requested during routine radiographs.

The shape of the chest wall and the orientation of the diaphragm changes to accommodate increasing lung volume and these changes can be clearly seen on radiographs. Normally, the anterior ribs are angled inferiorly relative to the posterior ribs (Fig. 11.4). As the chest expands to meet increasing lung capacity, the anterior ribs rise and become relatively horizontally oriented. Each hemidiaphragm is normally curved, with the apex of the curvature near the junction of the medial and middle thirds of each hemidiaphragm. As lung volume increases, the diaphragm flattens and the apex of the diaphragm becomes positioned

anteriorly. Flattening of the hemidiaphragms is especially easy to visualize on the lateral view radiograph. If accessory muscles of respiration are being used as a sign of severe respiratory distress, the upper sternum is bowed outwardly and this can be visualized on the lateral view of a chest radiograph (Fig. 11.5).

The classical pathological description for bacterial pneumonia, specifically Streptococcal pneumonia, is lobar consolidation. Unlike viruses, bacteria infect the alveoli. The inflammatory response initiated by the bacteria cause the normally aerated alveoli to become filled with fluid, cells, and inflammatory reactors. The bacteria also injure the alveolar walls so that the fluid and inflammation can easily spread to adjacent alveoli. Fully developed channels of Lambert and pores of Kohn also contribute to the spread of infection to nearby alveoli and groups of alveoli called lobules. The lumina of the bronchioles in the affected areas may be filled with inflammatory exudates, but not to the same degree as in viral infections. Moreover, the bronchial walls and interstitial tissues generally do not become inflamed, as the infection primarily affects the alveoli. Radiographically, the normally dark aerated lung becomes opacified with cells, cellular debris, and fluid, initially spreading from adjacent alveoli and lobules to encompass lung segments, and eventually to the entire lobe (Fig. 11.6). The branching airways remain relatively aerated and appear lucent, in contrast to the adjacent opacified lung parenchyma. This appearance, referred to as an air bronchogram, is one of the radiographic hallmarks of pneumonia. However, air bronchograms will also be seen in some cases of atelectasis when the larger airways remain air filled, as in compressive atelectasis.

Complete lobar consolidation is uncommon in children, probably because of underdeveloped channels of collateral airflow. The radiographic findings of classical lobar pneumonia will be discussed briefly

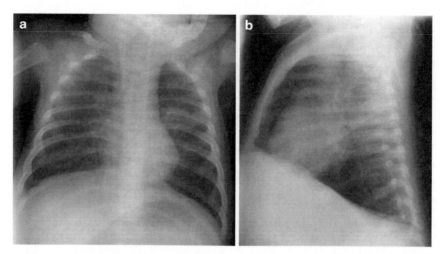

Fig. 11.5. The radiographs of this 4-month-old girl with tachypnea and fever show the typical manifestations of children with viral lower respiratory tract illness. Lungs are hyperinflated as evidenced by bilateral hyperlucent lungs, flattened hemidiaphragms, and anterior bowing of the sternum. There is a mild atelectasis in both perihilar regions. No microbial organism could be determined. (**a**) PA, (**b**) lateral projections

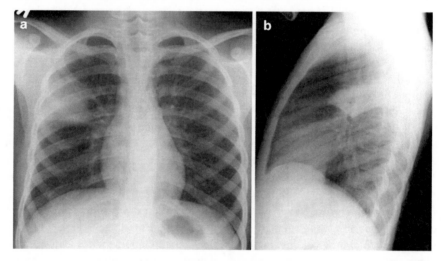

Fig. 11.6. (**a**) PA and (**b**) lateral radiographs in a teenager demonstrate a dense consolidation in the right upper lobe abutting the major and minor fissures. Sputum cultures grew *Pneumococcus* and the patient became well on penicillin therapy

here. More in-depth discussion and descriptions can be found in other textbooks of radiology [35], pediatric imaging [36], and chest imaging [37–39].

In diagnosing lobar pneumonias, radiographic findings that show that airspace opacity is space occupying such as mediastinal shift away from the opacity and bowing of the fissures away from the infiltrate, are important in distinguishing pneumonia from atelectasis, which causes volume loss. When an airspace consolidation abuts a fissure or is defined by a segment, the border of the opacity will be straight. By contrast, opacities involving the central portions of the lobes or segments will have more irregular borders. Infections which irritate the pleural surface are associated with pleural effusion. When an airspace opacity (e.g., lobar pneumonia) abuts a soft tissue structure, such as the mediastinum or diaphragm, the normal borders of the soft tissue structure blends in imperceptibly with the pneumonia. The addition of the lateral view to the frontal view is essential for accurately localizing airspace disease, as it provides three-dimensional information.

Lung infection by *M. pneumoniae*, as well as other bacteria including *Staphylococcus aureus* and gram negative bacteria, presents a pathological pattern characteristic of bronchopneumonia or lobular pneumonia. The initial infection and injury occurs at the terminal and respiratory bronchioles and spreads to the peribronchial alveoli. The alveoli then become filled with fluid and inflammatory cells and the reaction spreads to adjacent alveoli and acini. Peribronchial edema, interstitial thickening, small airway occlusion, and lobar consolidation may all occur [22]. Thus, the radiographic pattern of bronchopneumonia may be a composite of the findings seen in interstitial pneumonia and lobar pneumonia.

The radiological manifestations of certain LRTIs are peculiar to children. In children younger than 8 years of age whose collateral pathways of circulation have not yet developed, some bacterial pneumonias are round and may mimic a mass. In a patient with a corresponding clinical history, a round mass in the chest should be considered pneumonia; and, in fact,

when the illness presents in this way, it is typically called *round* pneumonia (Fig. 11.7) [40]. Round pneumonia has a predilection for the lower lobes. The most common pathogen of round pneumonia is *S. pneumoniae* [41, 42]. Occasionally, lung cysts, called pneumatoceles, develop as a result of severe staphylococcal infections, but have also been reported in cases of *S. pneumoniae*, *H. Influenzae*, and *Escherichia coli* [21]. Pneumatoceles are thin-walled, air-containing cavities that develop rapidly within the first week of infection (Fig. 11.8). Necrosis of the walls of small airways allows air to dissect into the interstitium causing these focal air collections. If pneumatoceles rupture into the pleural space, a pneumothorax may occur. Pneumatoceles typically resolve within 3 weeks.

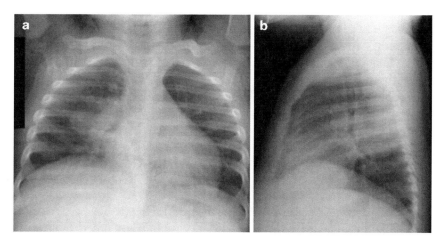

Fig. 11.7. (a) Frontal and (b) lateral radiographs of the chest in a 9-month-old girl with a 3 week history of cough and fever (102°F) demonstrate a round mass-like opacity in the superior segment of the right lower lobe. After antibiotic therapy, the mass resolved and the chest radiograph returned to normal

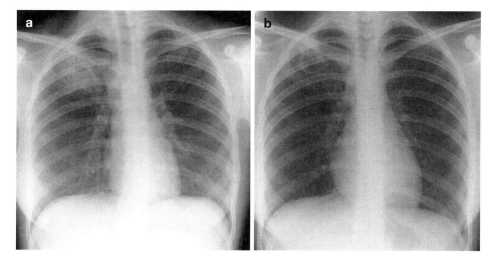

Fig. 11.8. This 14-year-old girl presented with a fever of 104°F, cough, and right upper chest pain. (a) Initial radiograph demonstrates right upper lobe opacity with an air-fluid level, consistent with a lung abscess. Sputum cultures revealed *Staphylococcus aureus*. (b) A film 1 week later shows that the abscess develops into a thin-walled lucent structure, a pneumatocele

11.1.3 The Usefulness of Chest Imaging in Diagnosing and Imaging Pneumonia

Despite the three distinct pathological and radiographic patterns of pneumonia, radiographic findings in pneumonia are very broad, and the usefulness of chest radiographs in diagnosing pneumonia is controversial.

At best, the level of diagnostic certainty provided by radiological findings is quite high with respect to LRTI [17, 43–45]. Among young children, the most common cause of pneumonia is viral. In these patients, when a pattern of hyperinflation or uneven aeration and bronchial wall thickening is observed; its etiology is most likely viral. By contrast, older children, who have mature, adult-like airways and collateral pathways of air drift, lobar consolidations that may develop are most likely bacterial in origin [43, 46, 47]. Radiographs are very useful in diagnosing LRTIs at these two extremes of the pediatric spectrum.

However, many studies have shown that the radiographic patterns of pneumonias caused by different infectious agents overlap, making the findings on chest radiographs unreliable for predicting the etiology of pneumonia [10, 44, 46, 48–50]. For example, while RSV most commonly presents with the typical *viral pattern* characterized by hyperinflation, peribronchial cuffing, and perihilar infiltrates [51]; patients admitted to the hospital for adenovirus most often have lobar consolidation and pleural effusions, findings that are classically described for bacterial pneumonias [49]. As mentioned previously, *Mycobacterium* is the most common cause of pneumonia in school-aged children. Because *Mycobacterium* infects both the epithelial lining of the bronchioles and the alveoli, the radiographic pattern is mixed with the radiographic findings of both the alveolar or interstitial patterns [5, 6, 22]. In addition, viral infections may be superimposed by bacterial infections, and a mixed radiographic pattern may reflect this.

Interobserver variation also affects diagnosis of an abnormal chest radiograph. Poor interobserver agreement and false negative errors further complicate the use of plain films in distinguishing bacterial and viral causes of pneumonia [10, 48]. This is especially true in young infants whose hyperinflation and interstitial abnormalities tend to be interpreted more subjectively [52]. The interobserver agreement in normal radiographs is much better than radiographs of pneumonia [53].

Not surprisingly, the *if and when* of ordering chest radiographs in the initial assessment of patients with suspected LRTIs remains controversial. In most cases of uncomplicated community-acquired pediatric pneumonia, imaging is not needed for initial diagnosis. Moreover, because LRTIs are routinely diagnosed and treated based on clinical findings, the addition of radiographs generally will not aid in diagnosis or result in more responsive treatment plans; nor is there any evidence that plain films will affect or hasten recovery [54]. For this reason, The World Health Organization does not recommend chest radiography in the management of acute LRTIs in children of developing countries [55]. Likewise, the British Thoracic Society and the American National Guideline Clearinghouse do not advise routine radiographs for children suspected to have community-acquired pneumonia [55, 56]. Despite these recommendations, in countries where radiographic imaging is readily available, respiratory tract infections remain one of the most common indications for imaging [14].

Perhaps chest radiographs are most useful in determining the diagnosis and affecting the management of children with suspected LRTIs when the clinical findings are ambiguous, failing to distinguish typical bacterial from atypical pneumonias [19, 56]. In suspected cases of LRTI, the purpose of a chest radiograph is to distinguish bacterial pneumonias from viral pneumonias and thereby distinguish which patients need antibiotic therapy. Chest radiography, in these circumstances, is generally useful. Only a small percentage of children with bacterial pneumonia have the clinical and radiographic appearance of lower viral respiratory infections [19]. Thus, the high negative predictive value of radiography in excluding bacterial pneumonia is valuable in distinguishing those with bacterial pneumonia who should be treated with antibiotics from those with viral pneumonia who can be treated more expectantly [14].

Routine follow-up chest radiographs are not needed in childhood community-acquired pneumonia if the child has a clinically uneventful recovery [46, 57]. Previously, healthy children with community-acquired pneumonia who have complete clinical resolution have normal chest radiographs 2–3 months after the initial infection. Prior to 3 months after the initial infection, radiographic abnormalities may still be present even if the infection is adequately treated [18]. Thus, follow-up chest radiographs sooner than 2–3 months may give the mistaken impression of a lingering infection where one does not exist.

However, chest radiographs are indicated in children with persistent or worsening signs of pneumonia, particularly in circumstances where there may be complications of pneumonia, or underlying problems such as a retained foreign body, congenital lung malformation, or atypical infections. In children with recurrent infections in the same location where an underlying congenital cause is suspected, the patient should be imaged during a well period.

Radiographs in patients with the clinical and radiographic picture of bacterial pneumonia can also help predict short-term mortality. Radiographs are very sensitive in detecting pleural effusions. As little as 50 cc of pleural fluid can be detected on a lateral radiograph [58]. Pneumonias associated with pleural effusions have a higher short-term mortality than pneumonias without effusions (Fig. 11.9) [59].

It is debatable whether children under 5 years of age with leukocytosis (>20,000/mm³) and fever (temperature greater than 39°C), but without signs of respiratory illness, should have chest radiographs to find occult pneumonias [56]. Chest radiographs have been shown to reveal occult pneumonias in 26% children without respiratory symptoms, but with high fever and an increased white blood cell count [60]. Although it is common practice in some institutions to obtain chest radiographs in all febrile infants, only those with respiratory symptoms are likely to have radiographic pneumonia [61]. Pneumonia is found in only 6% of febrile infants without respiratory symptoms [62, 63].

A final consideration on the use of imaging studies to diagnose and treat pneumonia is the harmful effect of radiation on children. Devices emitting ionizing radiation such as X-ray machines and computed tomography should be operated under the ALARA ("As Low As Reasonably Achievable") principle [64]. Radiation exposure should be minimized in children because it is well known that for the same dose, children are more susceptible to radiation effects than adults. The 1 year old *lifetime* cancer mortality rate from radiation is higher than in adults by an entire order of magnitude [65]. Children incur a far greater effective dose of radiation when undergoing CT than plain radiographs or fluoroscopy.

Traditionally, both frontal and lateral views have been considered standard views for evaluating the chest in children with pneumonia. The frontal radiograph is fundamental in creating a global picture of the chest. Most radiographic abnormalities can be visualized on this single view. The addition of the lateral view confirms the findings on the frontal radiograph, and helps to locate any abnormalities in three dimensions. The lateral view also is more sensitive than the frontal view in detecting left lower lobe abnormalities in the retrocardiac region and in the pleural space [58], and in detecting hyperinflation [17]. Two views have been shown to increase conspicuity of pneumonia compared to one view [66]. However, others have shown that the addition of a lateral radiograph did not improve sensitivity or specificity in the diagnosis of pneumonia [67]. The lateral radiograph more than doubles the dose of radiation per study of the chest. The radiation risks associated with the lateral radiograph as well as the costs that are incurred from ordering an additional study should be weighed against its usefulness in diagnosing pneumonia.

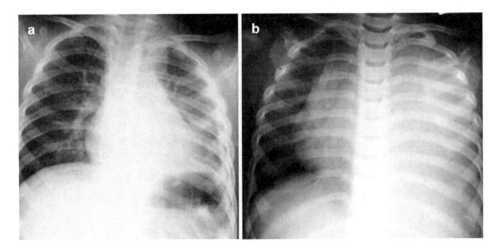

Fig. 11.9. Two frontal radiographs in an 18-month-old boy show progression of a left lower lobe pneumonia. (**a**) The initial image shows a left lower lobe pneumonia and small effusion. (**b**) Three days later, the entire left lung is opacified. A chest tube was required to drain the left empyema and the patient was hospitalized for 3 weeks

Because computed tomography (CT) delivers a much greater radiation dose than plain film, CT is reserved for only the most serious cases of pneumonia for which potential surgical intervention may be necessary or in cases of necrotizing pneumonia/empyema (see Sect. 11.6). Like radiographs, CT is of limited value in determining the microbial etiology of pneumonia [68] and should not be used to initially diagnose pneumonia. Even after optimizing techniques to reduce the dose of radiation in children, a chest CT delivers considerably more radiation than chest radiographs. Computed tomography is very helpful in better understanding complicated pneumonia, including cases of empyema, abscess or pulmonary cavitation, and bronchopulmonary fistula, complications which may require surgical or radiological intervention (Fig. 11.10) [69, 70]. Computed tomography and magnetic resonance imaging (MRI) are also helpful in diagnosing underlying developmental anomalies which may be causing recurrent pneumonias in the same location. (Developmental anomalies are discussed in detail in Sects. 11.2 and 11.3.) Ultrasound, by contrast, delivers no ionizing radiation and is useful in evaluating pleural effusions, a common complication of pneumonia [71]. Ultrasound, however, cannot be used to diagnose or distinguish different types of pneumonia (Fig. 11.11).

An important look alike of focal or multifocal alveolar or bacterial pneumonia occurs in sickle cell disease. The condition, referred to as acute chest syndrome presents with alveolar inflitrates and often a pleural effusion [72]. Although this may, and sometimes does, represent pneumonia, it frequently represents venular thrombosis and pre-infraction (Fig. 11.12).

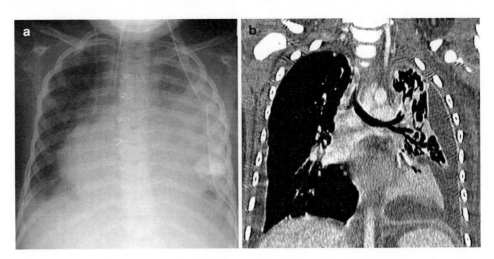

Fig. 11.10. This 3-year-old female with a history of repaired Tetrology of Fallot presented with high fever and left chest pain. Multiple radiographs demonstrated a left lower lobe pneumonia and pleural effusion. (**a**) Despite left chest tube placement, the left effusion persisted. (**b**) Chest CT with coronal reconstructions better delineates the left empyema and cavitation of the left upper lobe and lingula

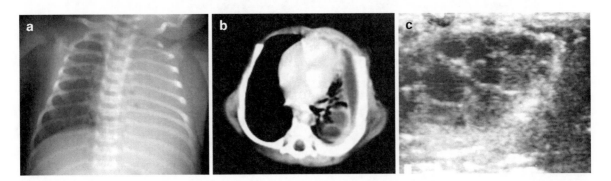

Fig. 11.11. One-month-old boy who developed fever and poor feeding. (**a**) The chest radiograph demonstrates near complete opacification of the left hemithorax. (**b**) Computed tomography was useful in showing a left lower lobe pneumonia complicated by liquification/cavitation and empyema. (**c**) An ultrasound shows that the empyema is very complex with many internal septations. Thoracentesis revealed *Pneumococcus*

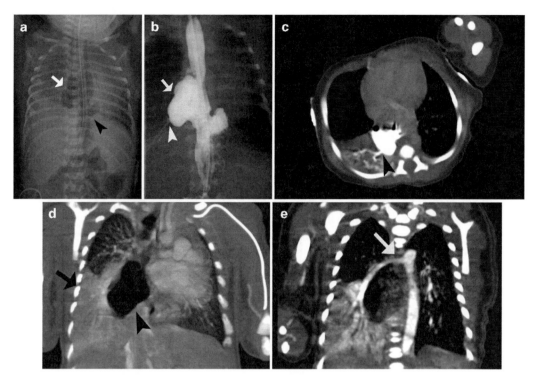

Fig. 11.12. Bronchopulmonary foregut malformation with systemic arterial supply and bronchial connection to GI tract in a 3-day-old baby boy. (**a**) AP radiograph of the chest shows dense opacification of right lower lobe silhouetting the right hemidiaphragm. There is also right lateral pleural effusion. An air-filled cystic structure is seen in the medial right hemithorax (*arrow*). Additionally there appears to be a hiatus hernia (*arrowhead*). (**b**) Esophagram shows the right medial lucent cystic lesion fills directly from the esophagus (*arrow*) and the subdiaphragmatic stomach is small. Also seen is filling of a distal branching structure extending to the right lower lobe opacity (*arrowhead*). (**c**) Axial CT image obtained after the esophagram without additional contrast shows that the branching structure is consistent with a bronchus communicating via the cystic structure with the esophagus (*arrow head*). (**d**) Coronal reformation of chest CT performed after intravenous iodinated contrast reveals enhancing mass peripherally in lower right hemithorax (*arrow*) and medial air-filled cystic structure (*arrow head*). (**e**) Coronal reformation of CT angiogram showing large artery coursing from the upper descending aorta to right lower lobe sequestration (*arrow*)

In summary, community-acquired pneumonias of all etiologies are generally diagnosed without the need of chest radiographs. Radiography is helpful in cases where the initial clinical diagnosis is unclear; in eliciting the cause of recurrent pneumonias; or in evaluating pneumonias that do not resolve clinically despite treatment. Because computed tomography delivers a relatively high dose of ionizing radiation, CT is reserved for evaluating complicated pneumonias that may require surgical intervention or in cases of necrotizing pneumonia/empyema.

11.1.4 Summary

Lower respiratory tract illness is a common affliction affecting thousands of children in the United States and around the world. Across the globe, an estimated two million children die from pneumonia and pneumonia-related illnesses each year; with developing countries bearing the brunt of this loss. In developed countries, lower respiratory tract illnesses are a significant source of morbidity.

However, even in countries where access to health care for children is readily available, accurately diagnosing pediatric pneumonia remains difficult as there is no single accurate test to diagnose pneumonia or to distinguish typical from atypical pneumonias. In cases where diagnosis is especially elusive, radiology plays an important diagnostic role.

Yet even in the most straightforward of circumstances, diagnosis of pediatric pneumonia is often complicated and challenging. Because pediatric airways are not yet fully developed, lower respiratory tract illnesses typically present quite differently in children than in adults. These differences are especially evident in comparing the various pathologic and radiologic manifestations of the illness. In addition to LRTI profiles that generally correspond to age, the clinical and radiological differences between bacterial and nonbacterial pneumonia are also difficult to discern in many instances. Although imaging children with community-acquired pneumonia is generally not recommended; radiographs are useful in cases where the diagnosis of pneumonia is elusive, and where the study may help distinguish typical from atypical pneumonia. And while computed tomography and follow-up radiographs after unremarkable recovery from infection are rarely ordered, additional imaging is helpful in evaluating complicated pneumonias, including those with unusual underlying causes, or those that have resisted conventional treatment and may require surgical intervention.

11.2 Pulmonary Cysts

Ellen M. Chung

Pulmonary cysts seen on plain chest radiographs as completely or partially air-filled, round masses may be of congenital, infectious/inflammatory, traumatic, or neoplastic in origin. Many of these lesions are discussed in greater detail elsewhere in the text, but are briefly discussed here in an approach to the differential diagnosis of lucent pulmonary cysts. The differential diagnosis can be refined based on the age of the patient and distribution within the lungs (unilateral vs. bilateral), as well as the clinical presentation and the presence of other findings such as nodules or wedge-shaped opacities. In neonates or young infants, unilateral findings most often represent bronchopulmonary foregut malformations, while bilateral involvement suggests chronic lung disease of prematurity (Table 11.1). Young children most commonly present with symptoms of infection with or without an underlying congenital anomaly. A solitary lesion suggests a congenital anomaly or bacterial infection in a previously healthy child. If findings are bilateral, a systemic disease should be considered. Langerhans histiocytosis and cystic fibrosis are bilateral upper lung zone predominant diseases early on, while septic emboli involve the lower lobes preferentially. The presence of nodules and cysts suggests conditions such as Langerhans cell histiocytosis

Table 11.1. Cystic lesions in neonate or young infant

Unilateral
Congenital malformations
Pulmonary
CPAM
Extralobar pulmonary sequestration
Congenital lobar emphysema
Diaphragm
Congenital diaphragmatic hernia
Bilateral
Chronic lung disease of prematurity
Persistent pulmonary interstitial emphysema

Table 11.2. Cystic lesions in children

Unilateral
Infection
Complicated pneumonia – abscess, cavitary necrosis, pneumatocele
Intralobar pulmonary sequestration
Hydatid disease
Trauma – contusion/laceration – pneumatocele
Neoplasm – pleuropulmonary blastoma, type I
Bilateral
Infectious/inflammatory
Cystic fibrosis/bronchiectasis
Septic emboli
Nonbacterial infections – fungi, mycobacteria, opportunistic organisms
Vasculitides
Hydrocarbon pneumonitis – pneumatocele
Neoplastic/proliferative
Laryngotracheal (juvenile) papillomatosis
Langerhans cell histiocytosis
Metastatic disease
Syndrome associated
Lymphangioleiomyomatosis with or without tuberous sclerosis
Proteus syndrome
Neurofibromatosis type I
Marfan syndrome

(LCH), Wegener granulomatosis, cystic fibrosis, and papillomatosis. The presence of wedge-shaped opacities suggests a vascular etiology as in Wegener granulomatosis or septic emboli (Table 11.2).

11.2.1 Neonate or Young Infant

Unilateral Lesions

Congenital Malformations

Congenital malformations are unilateral and most often discovered prenatally or in a neonate with respiratory distress. Some present later with symptoms suggesting recurrent infection.

The congenital pulmonary airway malformation (CPAM), previously referred to as congenital cystic adenomatoid malformation (CCAM), consists of cysts that are fluid-filled in utero. These communicate with the tracheobronchial tree via an abnormal bronchus and after birth the fluid in the cysts progressively clears and is replaced by air. Most often CPAM's consist of one large cyst surrounded by several smaller cysts (type 1) or of multiple smaller cysts of fairly uniform size (type 2). There is no lobar predilection. CPAM's generally do not have a systemic arterial supply, unless they are associated with an adjacent sequestration [73]. The main differential consideration for type 1 CPAM is type 1 pleuropulmonary blastoma (PPB) as these two entities are radiographically indistinguishable [74].

Pulmonary sequestrations are masses with systemic arterial supply and no connection to the tracheobronchial tree. Extralobar sequestrations have their own pleural investment and may be outside the lung, while intralobar sequestrations are contained in the same pleura as the adjacent normal lung. Extralobar sequestrations are definitely congenital, but intralobar sequestrations may be congenital or acquired. Intralobar sequestrations are found with increasing frequency with increased use of prenatal imaging, so at least in some cases, they are congenital [75, 76]. Sequestrations may be discovered prenatally or may present in the neonatal period with respiratory distress or later in infancy or childhood with a history of recurrent infections. They are usually solid or solid and cystic, but not generally air-filled unless they are associated with an adjacent CPAM [73] or an abnormal communication with the GI tract (Fig. 11.12) [75, 76]. These most commonly are found near the diaphragm in the lower lobe region, more commonly on the left. Extralobar sequestrations may also be within or below the diaphragm and may mimic an adrenal mass, especially on prenatal imaging [77].

Congenital lobar emphysema (CLE), or congenital lobar hyperinflation, is an overexpanded lobe sometimes caused by narrowing or compression of the bronchus. These often present in the neonatal period due to progressive respiratory distress. The lobe is fluid-filled at birth and the fluid is slow to clear due to bronchial obstruction. The fluid is slowly replaced by air, but the lobe becomes overinflated due to a check valve mechanism of the bronchial obstruction, causing progressive compression of the adjacent lobes. There is a predilection for the upper lobes, left greater than right, and the right middle lobe [78]. Even when large, the air collection often conforms to the basic configuration of the lobe. Polyalveolar lobe is similar in its macroscopic appearance, distribution, and behavior. However rather than associated with overexpanded alveoli, polyalveolar lobe has an increase number of normally inflated alveoli.

The differential diagnosis in the neonate of fluid-filled cysts that become air-filled includes congenital diaphragmatic hernia. These are most often on the left and they typically contain bowel. The distended bowel loops cause mass effect on the developing lung in utero causing pulmonary hypoplasia. At birth, the bowel contains fluid which is gradually replaced by air. Herniation of abdominal contents into the chest may cause deviation of NG tubes or umbilical catheters on radiographs.

Persistent Pulmonary Interstitial Emphysema

Pulmonary interstitial emphysema (PIE) develops as a complication of barotrauma from positive pressure ventilation and is usually, but not exclusively, encountered in premature neonates with surfactant deficiency. Rupture of alveoli results in dissection of air into the interstitium. For patients who survive, the interstitial air is usually resorbed, but the air may collect in an expanding radiolucent cyst termed *localized* or persistent PIE. Although the PIE is bilateral, persistent collections are most often unilateral [79]. On plain radiographs and CT, persistent PIE appears as hyperexpanded collections of thin-walled cysts. CT shows the characteristic appearance of linear and punctate densities within the cyst, the so-called *line-and-dot* pattern, which is thought to represent air in the interstitium surrounding the bronchovascular bundles [79, 80] (Fig. 11.13). It is important to distinguish these from congenital pulmonary malformations which are treated surgically, as lesions of persistent pulmonary emphysema are at least initially managed conservatively.

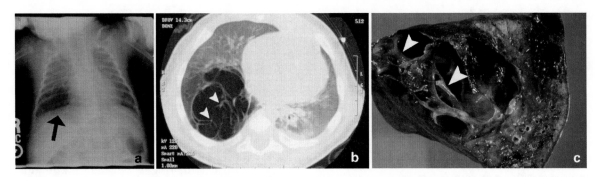

Fig. 11.13. Persistent pulmonary interstitial emphysema in 14-month-old ex-27 week premature infant found to have a persistent lucent lesion at right base at age 3 months. (**a**) PA radiograph of the chest shows a lucent cyst at the right base (*arrow*). (**b**) CT image demonstrates a multilocular air-filled cyst with thin walls and septa. Line-and-dot pattern is seen (*arrowheads*) reflecting air collections surrounding bronchovascular bundles. (**c**) Photograph of the gross resected specimen reveals large air-filled cysts surrounding bronchovascular bundles (*arrowheads*)

Bilateral Disease

Chronic Lung Disease of Prematurity (Bronchopulmonary Dysplasia)

In this age group, the most common cause of bilateral lung disease is chronic lung disease of prematurity, which usually occurs in premature neonates as the sequela of surfactant deficient disease, but may also occur in term or near-term infants with persistent pulmonary hypertension or meconium aspiration. The etiology is not fully understood, but barotrauma from positive pressure ventilation and oxygen toxicity is implicated. Chronic lung disease does not cause cyst formation and the classic *bubbly* appearance of Stage III bronchopulmonary dysplasia (BPD) described by Northway is not commonly seen today; however, after the third week of life, findings of atelectasis and fibrosis, appear adjacent to areas of hyperlucency and air trapping and the juxtaposition of these may suggest a cystic appearance. Chest radiography is relatively insensitive to the late findings of chronic lung disease and does not correlate well with results of lung function studies. CT is abnormal in almost all survivors [81, 82].

Table 11.3. Lucent lung and lung segments

Both lungs (air trapping)
Bronchiolitis
Hyperventilation
Asthma
Chronic lung disease
One lung
Obstruction
Hypoplasia/absence
Bronchiolitis obliterans
Post op CDH
Contralateral increased opacity
Effusion
Asymmetric pulmonary edema
Asymmetric soft tissues
Pneumothorax
Poland' syndrome
Rotation
Lung segments
Congenital lobar emphysema (CLE)
Bronchial obstruction
Chronic lung disease of prematurity (CLD)
Peripheral pulmonary artery stenosis (PPS)

11.2.2   Child

In children, infection is the most common cause of pulmonary disease. Bacterial infections are generally unilateral. Atypical infections, infections that occur in patients with underlying predisposing conditions, and inflammatory conditions are likely to involve both lungs. Rare primary neoplasms of the lung are unilateral, while metastases are bilateral (Table 11.3).

Unilateral Lesions

Complicated Pneumonia

Complicated pneumonia, while less common than in the past, is still a frequent cause of cystic lesions of the lung in young children. These children are quite ill with productive cough, fever, and tachypnea progressing to respiratory distress despite adequate oral

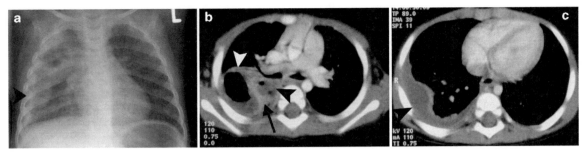

Fig. 11.14. Complicated pneumonia in a 22-month-old girl with fever and tachypnea due to complicated pneumonia. (**a**) PA radiograph shows round, soft tissue density masses containing air and adjacent pleural thickening (*arrowhead*) on the right. (**b**) CT image of the chest after intravenous administration of iodinated contrast material demonstrates fluid- and air-filled cavities in the right lung (*arrowheads*). Note that the surrounding lung parenchyma enhances indicating viable, consolidated tissue as opposed to necrotic lung (*arrow*). (**c**) A CT image inferior to (**b**) shows adjacent non-dependent pleural fluid (*arrowhead*) consistent with empyema

antibiotic therapy. Pneumonia beyond the neonatal period is usually unilateral and lobar, but can be complicated by the development of abscess or cavitary necrosis. Both are more easily detected on CT than on plain film. They are fluid-filled but may also contain air. With contrast-enhanced CT, the uncompromised, consolidated lung surrounding an abscess cavity enhances diffusely, while the parenchyma surrounding a necrotic cavity does not enhance [83]. In either case, an adjacent empyema is common (Fig. 11.14). The most common causative agent is *Pneumococcus* in healthy children and *S. aureus* in immunocompromised children. The differential diagnosis includes an infected congenital cystic malformation. History of severe acute illness, prior normal chest radiograph, and near complete resolution of the radiographic abnormalities after 40 days support a diagnosis of complicated pneumonia, as opposed to infected congenital cyst.

Staph and strep pneumonia can also be associated with pneumatocele formation as the infection resolves. Pneumatoceles are thought to result from alveolar rupture into inflamed interstitium, which traps the air in a collection. The improving clinical status of the patient favors a diagnosis of pneumatocele over abscess formation. Pneumatoceles can also develop in tuberculous infection, hydrocarbon pneumonitis, LCH, and pulmonary contusion/laceration.

Hydatid Disease

Hydatid disease, or echinococcosis, is a parasitic infection caused by *Echinococcus granulosus* or *Echinococcus multilocularis*. The disease is prevalent in shepherding regions. Humans contract the infection through contact with the definitive host, usually dogs, or by consuming contaminated food or water. Sheep or cattle serve as the intermediate host. Infection of the lung generally manifests as one or more large, well-circumscribed cysts which are generally fluid-filled. If the lung cyst ruptures into the tracheobronchial tree, an air-fluid level develops (Fig. 11.15). The cyst membrane may be seen floating on top of the air-fluid level, producing the so-called *water lily* sign. The liver is another commonly involved organ and liver cysts may be seen on chest CT [84, 85].

Congenital Malformations

Some bronchopulmonary foregut malformations are more likely to be discovered after infancy. First, intralobar sequestration can be associated with clinical and pathologic features of chronic or recurrent infection/inflammation, an observation that, along with the fact that patients tended to present after infancy, has led to controversy regarding whether intralobar sequestration is a congenital lesion or rather acquired as the sequela of chronic infection, with shunting of blood flow from the pulmonary to the systemic supply. The question remains whether the infection causes part of the normal lung to be sequestered or whether the infection is secondary to an underlying congenital malformation [76]. In young children as in neonates, the sequestration generally appears as a solid or solid and cystic mass in one of the lower lobes, more often on the left. Air may be seen in the cysts perhaps as a result of infection. All sequestrations have systemic arterial supply, usually from the descending or upper abdominal aorta.

Second, bronchogenic cyst may be diagnosed prenatally or later in infancy or childhood either incidentally or with respiratory distress or dysphagia. These are well-defined, typically unilocular cysts with very thin or imperceptible walls and homogenous fluid

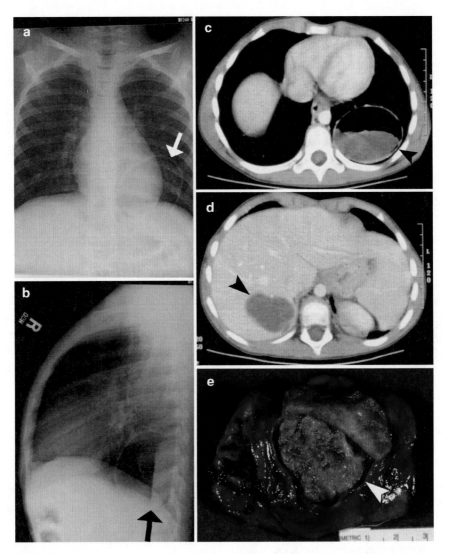

Fig. 11.15. Hydatid disease in a 7-year-old boy from Kosovo. (**a**) PA radiograph shows large well-circumscribed, thin-walled, lucent cyst on the left (*arrow*). (**b**) Cross-table lateral radiograph reveals a meniscus in this cyst in the left lower lobe (*arrow*). (**c**) CT image following intravenous administration of iodinated contrast again shows the thin-walled, air-filled cyst with meniscus. There is also a small inverted crescent of air behind the fluid density (*arrowhead*). (**d**) A CT image inferior to (**c**) demonstrates a cyst in the liver, a common site of disease. (**e**) Photograph of resected gross specimen shows the cyst with the roof retracted (*arrowhead*)

content. The fluid has the attenuation of proteinaceous fluid on CT. They appear solid on chest radiographs unless infected, when they may contain some air.

Finally, bronchial atresia is usually asymptomatic and often diagnosed serendipitously in older children or young adults. In contrast to CLE, which is often caused by bronchial compression or stenosis, bronchial atresia has no check valve mechanism but rather complete obstruction of the bronchus. As a result, air reaches the lung parenchyma beyond the atresia via collateral drift only, so that the segment or lobe does not become large enough to cause mass effect. There is mild hyperlucency of the involved segment or lobe which may suggest the diagnosis. Additionally, the bronchus beyond the atretic segment is dilated and mucoid secretions may become trapped within, forming an ovoid, tubular, or branching density. The dilated distal bronchus may also contain air and appear as a cystic lucency on radiographs (Fig. 11.16).

Trauma

Pulmonary laceration or contusion from blunt trauma can produce an air-filled cyst or pseudocyst. Contusions appear as peripheral nonsegmental, dense opacities in the posterior or posteromedial lung. They are frequently crescentic in configuration and a thin zone of subpleural sparing is a specific finding on CT [86]. Hemothorax or hemopneumothorax are also commonly seen with trauma. Adjacent rib fractures may also be present but are less common than in adults. Lacerations appear as opacities with areas of cavitation, which may contain air-fluid levels [87]. Also, as contusions resolve, pneumatoceles may develop within them.

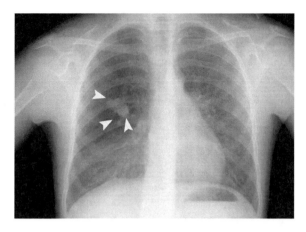

Fig. 11.16. Fourteen-year-old boy with bronchial atresia found incidentally. PA chest radiograph shows soft tissue- and air-attenuation round structures that appear to branch (*arrowheads*). Additionally, the surrounding lung is hyperlucent and exerts mild mass effect on adjacent lung

Pleuropulmonary Blastoma, Type 1

Primary neoplasms of the lung are rare, but the most common of these is the childhood form of PPB, a blastemal tumor similar to Wilms tumor. PPBs are usually large, solitary, solid masses, but the purely cystic form (type 1) may be indistinguishable on imaging from congenital cystic lesions, especially CPAM (Fig. 11.17). The additional findings of mediastinal shift and surrounding opacity favor the diagnosis of PPB [74]. Type 1 PPBs tends to occur in younger patients than the other types with a peak incidence at age 10 months of age. They also have a better prognosis for long-term survival than the other types. If they recur after treatment, they tend to recur as a more aggressive subtype. Children with PPB are at increased risk of other childhood tumors [88].

Bilateral Disease

Cystic Fibrosis (CF)/Bronchiectasis

Patients with cystic fibrosis may have cystic-appearing lesions due to abscesses, cystic or saccular bronchiectasis, and/or bullae. CF patients have additional findings of bilateral diffuse lung disease with hyperinflation and linear and patchy, confluent opacities. These changes

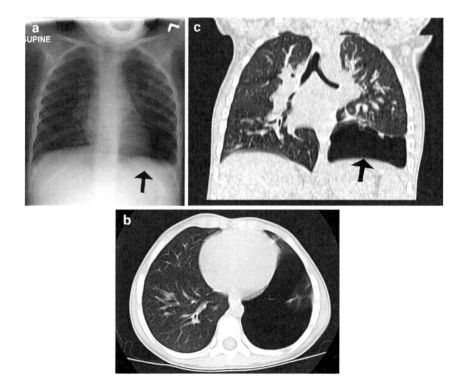

Fig. 11.17. Pleuropulmonary blastoma (PPB), type 1 in a 3-year-old boy. (**a**) PA radiograph shows solitary lucent cyst at left base (*arrow*). (**b, c**) Axial CT image and coronal reformation show large thin-walled cyst at left base (*arrow*), which is indistinguishable from a large cyst CPAM

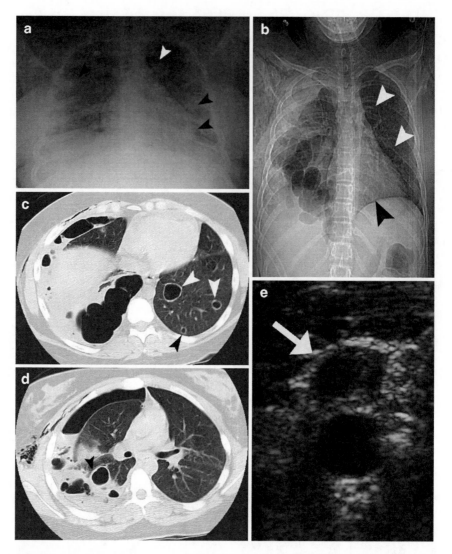

Fig. 11.18. Septic emboli in a 16-year-old girl with recent history of sore throat and fever. Blood cultures were positive for *Fusobacterium necrophorum*. (**a**) Initial PA chest radiograph shows ill-defined, rounded opacities (*arrowheads*), and right peripheral pleural based opacity consistent with pleural fluid. (**b**) Scout image from CT obtained 6 days later shows thin-walled lucent cysts on the left (*arrowheads*) and multiple air-filled cavi-ties on the right with a chest tube. (**c**) CT image displayed in pul-monary window demonstrates thin-walled intraparenchymal cysts on the left (*arrowheads*). The air collections on the right are loculated in the pleural space. (**d**) CT image superior to (**c**), shows an intraparenchymal cyst on the right with thicker wall and adja-cent airspace opacity (*arrowhead*). (**e**) Ultrasound image demon-strates thrombosis of the left internal jugular vein (*arrow*)

may be initially upper lobe predominant. Hilar and paratracheal adenopathy are common. Additionally, 10% of CF patients also have findings of allergic bronchopulmonary aspergillosis (ABPA). Bullae may rupture, leading to intractable pneumothorax. CF is a multisystem disease and findings of paranasal sinus disease, fatty liver and/or pancreas, and bowel obstruc-tion may also be noted on radiographs or CT.

Other less common causes of bronchiectasis include asthma with ABPA, recurrent aspiration pneumonia (usually in patients with neuromuscular disorder), chronic aspirated foreign body, congenital immunode-ficiency disorder (e.g., chronic granulomatous disease

of childhood), HIV/AIDS, and Immotile Cilia Syndrome, which may feature situs inversus totalis (Kartagener Syndrome). Bronchiectasis is best evaluated with HRCT, which may reveal thick or beaded bronchial walls, bron-chial diameter greater than that of the adjacent artery (signet ring appearance), and lack of distal tapering. Distal air trapping may also be seen.

Septic Pulmonary Emboli

Septic emboli typically appear as cavitary nodules which are bilateral and involve the lower lungs. Such children are acutely ill and septic. The margins of the nodules may be ill-defined and feeding vessels are

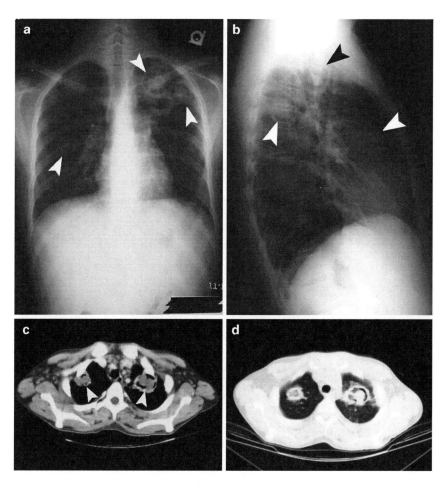

Fig. 11.19. Mucormycosis with fungus balls in 14-year-old boy on chemotherapy for ALL. (**a, b**) Plain radiographs show multiple bilateral upper lobe cysts filled with soft tissue attenuation masses. (*arrow heads*) (**c, d**) CT images following intravenous contrast administration show an air-filled cyst with thick, ill-defined walls containing a fungus ball on the *left* (*arrow head*). On the *right* (*arrow head*), a large cavitary nodule is seen

often noted. Air bronchograms may be seen within the nodules. The additional finding of peripheral wedge-shaped opacities suggests the diagnosis. Imaging often reveals the source of the infection such as a central venous catheter, cardiac valve vegetation, abscess, or jugular vein thrombosis due to pharyngitis (Lemierre Syndrome) [89] (Fig. 11.18). A situation as seen with Lemierre Syndrome may also rarely be encountered with septic thrombosis of other veins remove from the head and neck.

Atypical Infections

Nonbacterial infections can produce pulmonary nodules or confluent consolidations, which may cavitate. These include fungal infections, such as *Aspergillus* (nodules may be surrounded by a ground glass halo), mucormycosis, blastomycosis, and coccidioidomycosis. These may form fungus balls within air-filled cavities (Fig. 11.19). Other considerations include opportunistic infections such as nocardiosis and candidiasis. Pneumocystis pneumonia, atypical mycobacterial infections, and lymphocytic interstitial pneumonitis in patients with HIV infection can also be associated with cyst formation [90].

In childhood tuberculosis, partially air-filled cavities can form via several different mechanisms. First, postprimary TB may be seen in older children in the typical upper lobe distribution commonly seen in adults. Second, in young or immunocompromised children, progressive endobronchial spread caused by rupture of the liquefied Ghon focus into a bronchus can lead to development of bilateral, multiple, and small cavitary lesions. Third, in children under 3 years of age, mediastinal adenopathy is a prominent manifestation of the infection. Secondary bronchial

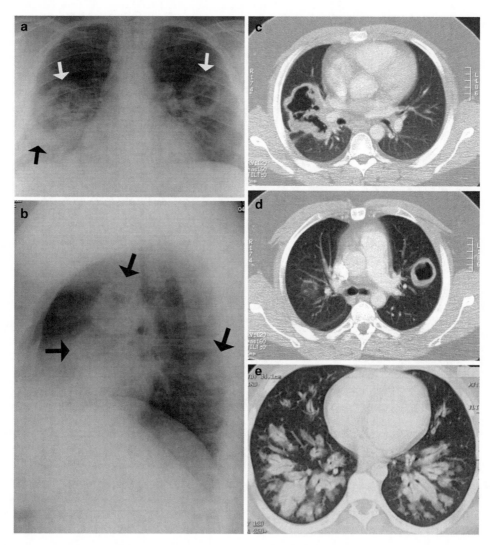

Fig. 11.20. Wegener granulomatosis in a 23-year-old man diagnosed 9 years prior. (**a**) PA and (**b**) lateral radiographs reveal bilateral cavitary round masses (*arrows*). (**c, d**) CT images obtained after intravenous iodinated contrast and dis-played in lung windows demonstrate bilateral thick air-filled masses with thick, irregular walls. (**e**) CT image in a 14-year-old boy with Wegener granulomatosis shows nodular opacities containing air bronchograms

obstruction by enlarged lymph nodes can lead to caseous liquefaction distal to the obstruction. The cavity is thick-walled with an air-fluid level and surrounding dense consolidation [91]. Finally, pneumatocele may form in the recovery phase of the disease.

Hydrocarbon Pneumonitis

Due to their low viscosity, ingestion of hydrocarbons such as lighter fluid, wood polish, gasoline, and kerosene typically leads to aspiration of these chemicals, which destroys surfactant and causes severe pneumonitis. Affected young children will show radiographic abnormalities by 12–24 h, developing patchy then confluent airspace opacities in both medial lower lung zones. Pneumothorax and pneumomedi-

astinum may also be seen. Pneumatoceles may develop as the patient clinically improves. Resolution of radiographic abnormalities frequently lags behind rapid clinical improvement.

Vasculitides

Wegener granulomatosis is a small-vessel vasculitis that affects multiple organ systems including the lungs, kidneys, nasopharynx, and paranasal sinuses. The disease usually presents in the teenage years. Findings include pulmonary nodules and small masses, some of which are cavitary (Fig. 11.20). Plain radiographs in children frequently show multifocal, ill-defined interstitial, and airspace opacities [92]. On CT, nodules are the most common finding. Also

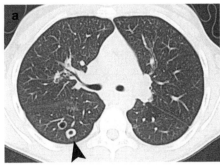 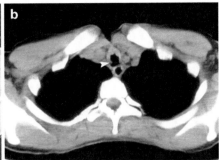

Fig. 11.21. Eleven year-old-girl with history of multiple surgical procedures for laryngotracheal papillomatosis. (**a**) CT image of the chest shows thin- and thick-walled pulmonary nodules (*arrowhead*). (**b**) CT image at the level of the trachea in another patient shows a small polypoid mass projecting from the wall of the trachea (*arrowhead*)

common are ground glass opacities and multifocal areas of airspace opacification [93, 94]. Vessels may be seen leading to the nodules and the margins of the nodules are often irregular or spiculated. Air bronchograms may be seen within the nodules (Fig. 11.20). Areas of consolidation are common and peripheral wedge-shaped opacities may also be seen. Diffuse pulmonary hemorrhage may occur [93, 95]. Additional findings of paranasal sinus disease may be noted.

Collagen vascular diseases may also involve the lung, but less frequently in children than in adults. Systemic sclerosis, or scleroderma, may cause large, thin-walled cysts in the upper lung zones in addition to peripheral interstitial fibrosis and ground glass opacities on high-resolution chest CT [96]. A dilated esophagus may also be observed.

Laryngotracheal (Juvenile) Papillomatosis

Laryngotracheal papillomatosis consists of lobulated or sessile benign cellular proliferations of the larynx or trachea thought to be related to human papilloma virus (HPV) infection acquired from the mother in the perinatal period. The peak age at diagnosis is almost 4 years. The lesions grow and recur necessitating multiple repeated surgical debulking procedures. These procedures are thought to facilitate endobronchial spread of the lesions to the lungs. The tumors appear as bilateral nodules, some of which are cavitary, with thick or thin walls. Occasionally, papillary lesions may be seen in the airway on CT (Fig. 11.21). Malignant degeneration to squamous cell carcinoma occurs in less than 2% of patients and should be suspected when a large mass develops. Even without malignant degeneration, pulmonary involvement carries a poor prognosis, as the tumors grow slowly but relentlessly and destroy adjacent lung [97].

Langerhans Cell Histiocytosis (LCH)

LCH is an idiopathic proliferative disorder of dendritic cells of the reticuloendothelial system. The disease may be localized to one organ system or disseminated. About 10% of children with localized or disseminated LCH have lung involvement at presentation [98]. In the lungs, peribronchiolar proliferations produce small nodules (1–10 mm) with irregular margins that often cavitate, forming thin- and thick-walled cysts best demonstrated on high-resolution chest CT [99, 100]. The earliest manifestation is interstitial prominence. Later nodules predominate and later yet, cystic changes prevail [101]. The disease predominantly involves the upper lungs symmetrically with sparing of the bases and pleural margins. The finding of nodules and cysts in this distribution on high-resolution chest CT in the appropriate clinical setting allows a confident diagnosis [100]. Lung volumes are normal to increased. Spontaneous pneumothorax occurs in about 10% of patients (Fig. 11.22). In younger children in whom the disease is more likely to be disseminated and aggressive, additional findings in other organ systems, such as lytic bone lesions or hepatosplenomegaly, may suggest the diagnosis (Fig. 11.23).

Metastatic Disease

Metastases are rarely cavitary. Squamous cell carcinoma commonly cavitates but is quite rare in children. Sarcomas, which are more common in children, may cavitate. These may also be associated with spontaneous pneumothorax. Metastatic angiosarcoma may rarely occur in children and may appear as multiple thin-walled cysts [102].

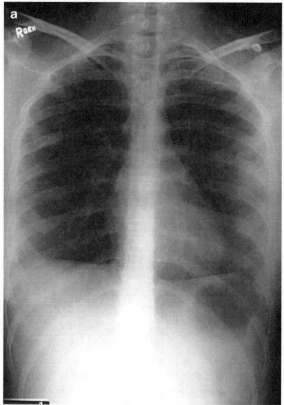

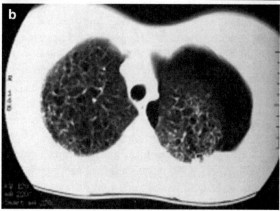

Fig. 11.22. Localized form of Langerhans cell histiocytosis in an 18-year-old male smoker. (**a**) PA radiograph shows upper lobe predominant interstitial lung disease. (**b**) CT image without contrast shows diffuse small lucent cysts throughout the upper lobes and a left spontaneous pneumothorax

Lung Disease Associated with Syndromes

Lymphangioleiomyomatosis (LAM) is a rare interstitial lung disease with thin-walled cysts, affecting almost exclusively women of child bearing age. The condition can be sporadic or associated with tuberous sclerosis. Patients most commonly present with progressive dyspnea. Cough and chest pain are also common complaints. Chest pain is due to spontane-

ous pneumothorax, which is found in about half of patients at presentation. Patients may also develop chylous effusion. Radiographs typically show hyperinflation and linear, reticular opacities, and apical sparing. Cysts may be visible on plain radiographs, particularly when the disease is severe. Pneumothorax and pleural effusion are also common findings (Fig. 11.24). On CT, thin-walled cysts are seen virtually in all patients. They are usually small (2–5 mm) and uniformly distributed throughout the parenchyma, although there may be relative sparing of the apices (Fig. 11.25). In severe disease, there are larger cysts, which may replace most of the parenchyma. High-resolution chest CT may demonstrate interlobular septal thickening. Nodules are generally not identified. Pleural effusion with an attenuation coefficient less than zero may also be observed. Extrapulmonary manifestations may be noted in patients with sporadic LAM as well as in tuberous sclerosis. Patients may have one or more renal angiomyolipomas, chylous ascites, and masses along the lymph node chains of the mediastinum, retroperitoneum, and pelvis. Patients with tuberous sclerosis may also have dermatologic manifestations, neurologic stigmata, renal cysts and angiomyolipomas, and cardiac rhabdomyomas (Fig. 11.25). The imaging differential diagnosis for pulmonary LAM includes LCH, but the latter is distinguished by the finding of nodules as well as cysts and a predilection for the upper lobes. Additionally, LCH occurs in males as well as females. Pneumothorax occurs in both LAM and LCH, but is more common in LAM. The natural history of sporadic LAM is usually progression to respiratory failure and cor pulmonale frequently requiring heart-lung transplant. Patients with LAM and tuberous sclerosis typically remain relatively asymptomatic for their lung disease [103].

Proteus Syndrome is a rare congenital hamartomatous disorder characterized by hemihyperplasia, decreased subcutaneous fat, palmar and plantar overgrowth, cutaneous and subcutaneous masses including vascular lesions, and kyphoscoliosis. Approximately 10% of patients may develop lung cysts consisting of hyperexpanded air spaces [104]. The cysts are usually large and multiple. The course of the lung disease is progressive and may require heart-lung transplant for survival [104].

Other congenital syndromes may also be associated with cystic changes in the lung. Patients with Down syndrome may have subpleural lung cysts, which are best detected with CT. A study of 25 patients

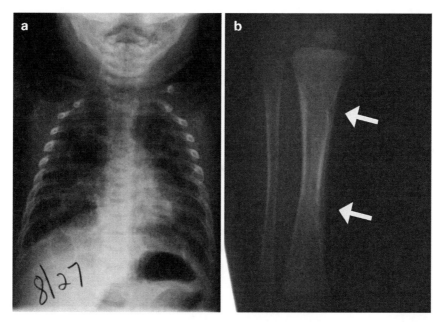

Fig. 11.23. Disseminated form of Langerhans cell histiocytosis in a 3-year-old boy involving the pulmonary and musculoskeletal systems. (a) PA chest radiograph shows extensive lucent cysts throughout both lungs. (b) AP radiograph of the right leg shows eccentric lucent lesions of the medial diaphysis of the tibia with adjacent periosteal thickening (*arrows*)

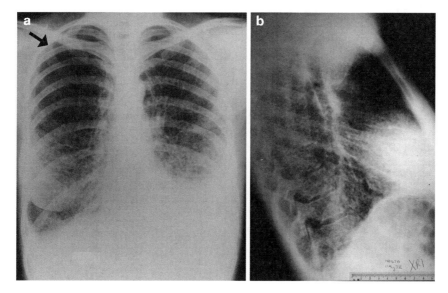

Fig. 11.24. Lymphangioleiomyomatosis in a 22-year-old woman with history of normal chest radiographs 2 years prior. (a) PA radiograph shows diffuse interstitial lung disease with small round lucent foci with apical sparing. Additional findings include right pneumothorax and bilateral effusions, which along with the age and gender of the patient suggest the diagnosis. (b) Lateral radiograph obtained 8 months prior shows to better advantage the diffuse reticular opacities and interposed small round lucencies. Note mild hyperinflation

revealed a prevalence of 36% [105]. They occur independent of congenital heart disease and may reflect reduced postnatal development of peripheral alveoli and peripheral airways [106]. These are most commonly found in the anteriomedial lungs and may also be found along fissures or surrounding bronchovascular bundles [105].

Patients with Neurofibromatosis type 1 typically have apical bullae and thin-walled cysts in their lungs, along with reticular disease and fibrosis. The pulmonary abnormalities are usually diagnosed in adulthood [107]. Additionally, Marfan syndrome may be associated with diffuse or apical bullous disease and cyst formation, particularly in males. Upper lobe

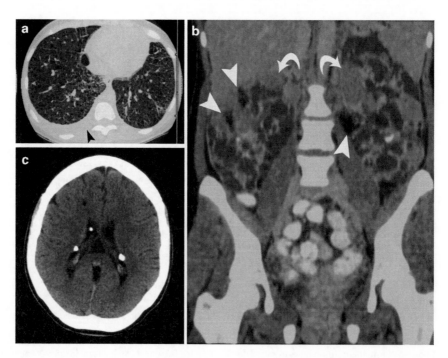

Fig. 11.25. Lymphangioleiomyomatosis in a 29-year-old woman with tuberous sclerosis. (**a**) HRCT image shows diffuse small cysts with imperceptible walls throughout both lungs. Note also the right pleural effusion (*arrowhead*). (**b**) Coronal reformation of CT scan performed following administration of intravenous iodinated contrast shows multiple fluid-attenuation cysts throughout both kidneys along with foci of fat-attenuation (*arrowheads*) and soft tissue attenuation (*curved arrows*) indicating angiomyolipomas. (**c**) CT image through the lateral ventricles of the brain reveals calcified subependymal nodules of tuberous sclerosis

fibrosis may also be seen. Patients often develop recurrent spontaneous pneumothorax (11%) and may present in adolescence [108].

In summary, lucent cystic lesions on imaging may be distinguished based on age at presentation and on the distribution of the findings in the lungs. Additional features, such as the presence of nodules or peripheral wedge-shaped opacities, and clinical signs and symptoms, such as fever and systemic illness or underlying chronic condition can further narrow the differential diagnosis.

11.3 Nodular Lung Disease

JEANNE S. CHOW AND ELLEN M. CHUNG

This section, which incorporates a conglomerate of different entities based on the common radiographic appearance of solitary or multiple pulmonary nodules, is divided into anomalies that tend to cause solitary nodules, and those that cause multiple nodules. Because developmental, infectious, inflammatory, hemorrhagic, and neoplastic disorders can all give the appearance of pulmonary nodules, many different disease entities will be touched upon or discussed in this chapter, or discussed elsewhere in this textbook in greater detail. Each section will describe the radiological or clinical traits of the various diseases characterized by pulmonary nodules.

A pulmonary nodule is a round opacity surrounded by normal lung tissue. Pulmonary nodules that arise close to the pleural surface may be difficult to distinguish from masses arising from the pleura or chest wall; however, an acute angle between the nodule and the chest wall suggests it may have originated from within the lung parenchyma. Radiographically, a *nodule* is defined as an opacity measuring 3 cm or smaller in size. *Masses* are defined as 3 cm or larger in size. In this chapter, the term nodule will be used more loosely and may include rounded opacities larger than 3 cm.

An *opacity* is a general radiographic term for any soft tissue density lesion in the lung. Unfortunately, radiographs cannot discern the composition of the opacity, whether fluid, blood, or cellular; and many entities that give rise to nodules may be comprised of a combination of these substances. Computed tomography (CT) and MRI are more specific in determining the composition of nodules. Nodules are also characterized by growth rate, margins, and various internal characteristics. Additional clinical history, physical examination, and laboratory tests are crucial in determining a differential or specific diagnosis for lung nodules. Finally, results from a percutaneous or open biopsy will provide a specific pathological diagnosis. Nuclear medicine studies, including PET, are not currently used to characterize pulmonary nodules but primarily to follow primary or metastatic tumors.

11.3.1 Solitary Pulmonary Nodules

Unlike the case in adults, a solitary pulmonary nodule in a child is generally not a harbinger of malignancy. In the absence of a known underlying malignancy, solitary pulmonary nodules in children are generally benign and congenital or infectious in nature. Primary pulmonary malignancies are extremely rare [109]. This section classifies solitary pulmonary nodules into congenital, infectious, neoplastic, and vascular causes.

Congenital

A variety of bronchopulmonary foregut malformations can give the appearance of a solitary nodule in the lung. Bronchopulmonary foregut malformations are discussed in greater detail elsewhere, but will be described briefly here as a cause of a solitary pulmonary nodule or mass.

Sequestration

Both intralobar and extralobar pulmonary sequestrations are lung masses formed by disorganized lung tissue with systemic arterial supply, but without a normal connection to the tracheal bronchial tree. Extralobar sequestration is surrounded by a separate pleural investment, whereas intralobar sequestration is included within the adjacent lung. Although extralobar sequestration is considered a congenital abnormality, the congenital or infectious etiology of intralobar sequestration is still debated [110]. These solitary, solid-appearing lesions typically occur in the lower lobes; but may rarely occur in other lobes, or in extrathoracic ectopic locations (extralobar sequestration only). Sequestration is diagnosed prenatally by US or MRI in 25% of cases and by 3 months of age in

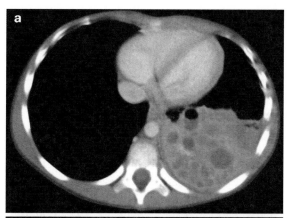
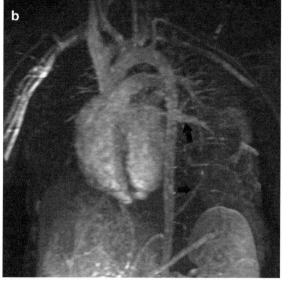

Fig. 11.26. (a) This 12-year-old child presented with signs of pneumonia and was found to have a complex left lower lobe mass with areas of fluid and enhancing septations by CT. (b) MRA shows two large feeding vessels arising from the aorta (*arrows*). Pathology after surgical resection proved intralobar sequestration

about 60% of cases [111]. Sequestrations found postnatally may be noted incidentally or as the cause of repeated pulmonary infections. Computed tomography, MRI, and US are all useful in demonstrating the characteristic systemic arterial vessel, which often arises from the aorta and supplies this lesion (Fig. 11.26) [112, 113]. Lesions are surgically resected to prevent further infection and for diagnosis.

Congenital Pulmonary Airway Malformation

CPAM, previously known as CCAM is a hamartomatous lung lesion composed of abnormal solid or cystic pulmonary tissue with an excess proliferation of bronchial structures. The five subtypes of CPAM occur in 1 in 5,000 live births [114]. CPAM is now the preferred term to CCAM because not all of the lesions are cystic or adenomatoid [114]. These lesions are often cystic and the appearance of the lung mass depends on the size of the cysts. Masses composed of a multitude of tiny cysts may appear solid, whereas those with larger cysts are readily distinguished as cystic on cross-sectional imaging; and when filled with air, are typically seen as lucent on plain radiographs [115]. Like sequestrations, many of these lesions are now diagnosed prenatally by ultrasound and MRI. However, large masses detected prenatally may regress and appear remarkably small at birth. Unlike sequestrations, most CPAMs receive their blood supply from the pulmonary circulation, but some are also supplied by systemic vasculature. There is growing evidence that sequestrations and CPAM are interrelated developmental abnormalities, as they often occur together [111]. Lesions are removed surgically to prevent infection, confirm diagnosis, and to prevent the very rare, but reported, transformation to pulmonary malignancy [116, 117].

Bronchogenic Cysts

Bronchogenic cysts are another type of bronchopulmonary foregut malformation that may appear as an intrapulmonary round nodule. These thin-walled cysts result from abnormal airway branching early in fetal gestation. Like the more commonly seen mediastinal bronchogenic cysts that are round, well-defined, and fluid-filled structures; pulmonary bronchogenic cysts are typically fluid-filled. However bronchogenic cysts complicated by infection or instrumentation may communicate with the bronchial tree and contain air in addition to fluid [118]. On plain radiograph, they appear solid, unless they contain air in addition to fluid. Computed tomography and MRI are helpful in showing that these radiographically solid-appearing lesions actually contain fluid (Fig. 11.27) [119].

Infectious

Infections are likely the most common cause of nodules in children.

Round Pneumonia

One of the most common causes of a pulmonary mass or a nodule in a child is bacterial pneumonia. In children younger than 8 years of age whose collateral pathways of circulation have not yet developed, some bacterial pneumonias appear round and may mimic a mass. However, unlike classical bacterial pneumonias, round pneumo-

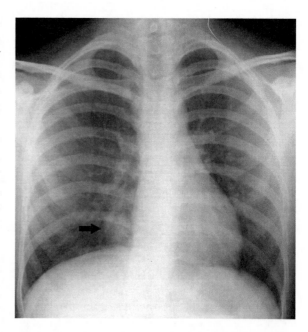

Fig. 11.27. This 11-year-old boy presented with a cough and was found to have a well-defined solitary right middle lobe pulmonary nodule in the right cardiophrenic angle (*arrow*). Surgical specimen after resection showed this to be a bronchogenic cyst

nias may not have air bronchograms and tend to resolve on follow-up imaging. They are most commonly found posteriorly [120]. In a patient with the appropriate clinical history, a round mass in the chest is most likely to be due to pneumonia (Fig. 11.28). The most common pathogen causing round pneumonia is *S. pneumoniae* [121, 122]. In cases where round pneumonia becomes necrotic and cavitates, an air-fluid level may be seen on upright views of the chest or by CT. Pneumonias are discussed more thoroughly in the section on pneumonia in this textbook.

Tuberculosis

Tuberculosis (TB) is an infection caused by any of the Mycobacterium complex mycobacteria (*Mycobacterium tuberculosis, Mycobacterium bovis, Mycobacterium africanum, Mycobacterium microti, and Mycobacterium canetti*). *M. tuberculosis* is the most common cause of this disease worldwide.

The lungs are the most commonly affected organ because most tuberculous infections are caused by aspiration or inhalation of the tubercle bacillus. From the lungs, the bacilli may spread hematogenously to infect any part of the body. Children appear to have a higher risk of developing extrapulmonary TB than adults [123]. Primary pulmonary tuberculosis occurs after a 2–10 week incubation period. The most classic

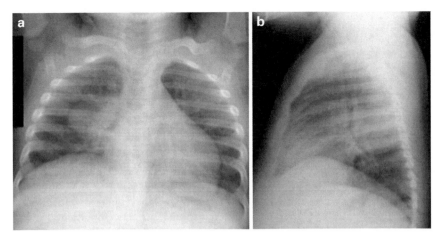

Fig. 11.28. Round pneumonia, (a) PA projection, (b) lateral projection

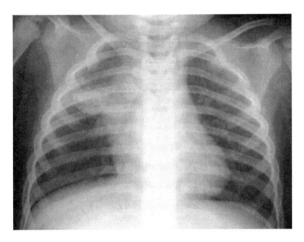

Fig. 11.29. This infant of a mother who died of tuberculosis presented with fever. Chest radiograph demonstrates a right upper lobe partially calcified opacity and right hilar and paratracheal adenopathy, consistent with primary tuberculosis

finding of primary pulmonary tuberculosis is the "primary complex," which consists of a solitary peripheral parenchymal opacity, resembling bacterial lobar pneumonia, and enlargement of mediastinal and regional lymph nodes (92%) (Fig. 11.29) [124, 125]. Lymphadenopathy is a more common finding in primary tuberculosis in children than parenchymal opacity [126]. If the pulmonary focus abuts or affects the pleura, pleural thickening and effusion often results. Patients may also present with signs of air trapping as the primary infection may affect the airway directly or surrounding hilar lymph nodes, causing airway obstruction [126, 127]. Six months following the initial formation of the primary lung infection, greater than 50% of the pulmonary opacities and lymph nodes calcify, thus creating the radio-

graphic findings of prior TB infection commonly seen in adults [128].

Miliary tuberculosis may develop within 6 months of the primary infection and results from hematogenous spread. The result is innumerable tiny nodules scattered throughout the lungs and other organs, particularly the liver and spleen [29].

Primary tuberculosis may be treated successfully, or may progress or recur as postprimary tuberculosis. Postprimary tuberculosis results from the growth of previously dormant bacilli in the apices of the lung. The reactivated lesions typically found in the apical and posterior segments of the upper lobes, are necrotic and often appear cavitary. The cavities have irregular thick walls readily seen on radiographs. Unlike primary tuberculosis, however, adenopathy is rare in postprimary TB. Reactivation tuberculosis is extremely uncommon in children, especially if the primary infection occurs before 2 years of age [130].

Fungal Infections and Certain Bacterial Infections That Resemble Fungi

Fungal infections can have a variety of appearances but, in general, mimic tuberculosis radiographically. Fungal infections and tuberculosis can be distinguished by history, clinical examination, skin, and laboratory tests. Most pulmonary fungal infections are caused by aspiration and are especially virulent in immunocompromised patients. Histoplasmosis, coccidiomycosis, and blastomycosis also cause pulmonary infections in immunocompetent hosts. Actinomycosis and *Nocardia*, two types of bacterial infections, are also discussed in this section as they mimic fungal infections.

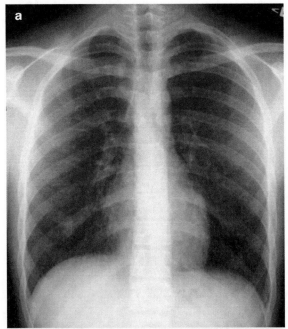

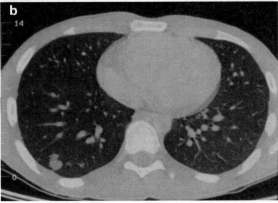

Fig. 11.30. This 16-year-old girl with a history of treated neuroblastoma presented with right chest pain. (**a**) Chest radiograph and (**b**) computed tomography revealed multiple bilateral pulmonary nodules, with the largest seen in the right lower lobe. Open biopsy of the right lower lobe nodule demonstrated histoplasmosis

Histoplasmosis is a fungal infection caused by inhaling *Histoplasma capsulatum*, a fungus endemic to the Ohio and Mississippi River valleys, spread by contaminated bird and bat feces. Ninety-five percent of patients are asymptomatic during the initial infection, and the radiographic manifestations are often not documented during this period because the disease is occult. Radiographic manifestations of remote infection include multiple calcified nodules in the lungs, liver, and spleen and are often found incidentally [131]. Chronic histoplasmosis may develop in patients with underlying lung disease, and like tuber-

culosis, presents as a cavitary mass in the lungs. Progressive disseminated histoplasmosis occurs in immunocompromised hosts and results from hematogenous spread of infection to anywhere in the body (Fig. 11.30) [132].

Coccidiomycosis, also called Valley Fever or desert rheumatism, is caused by aspiration of the *Coccidioides immitis* spores, a fungus endemic to California, Arizona, New Mexico and Texas. Blastomycosis is an infection caused by inhaling *Blastomyces dermatitidis*, a fungus commonly found in the soil. This fungus is distributed throughout the world and in the United States; it is endemic to Mississippi, Kentucky, Arkansas, and Wisconsin. Most cases of coccidiomycosis and blastomycosis are asymptomatic. On radiographs, chest abnormalities in acute and chronic infection mimic those seen in tuberculosis; although the adenopathy and effusions reported in 20% of adult cases have not been noted in neonates and infants [133, 134]. Approximately, 5% of patients with primary disease are left with chronic, residual lesions of the lung.

Cryptococcus neoformans is a fungus that causes infections primarily in immunocompromised patients, especially patients with AIDS [135]. The most common form of this fungus is found in aged pigeon droppings. The inhaled spores most commonly cause infections in the lungs and may spread hematogenously resulting in meningitis. The initial pulmonary infection often has the appearance of a bacterial pneumonia or of solitary or multiple pulmonary nodules. Nodules may cavitate. In chronic or treated pulmonary infections, lymph nodes may calcify [128].

Candida albicans, the most common cause of pulmonary candidiasis, results from inhalation or aspiration of this yeast, which normally colonizes the upper respiratory tract. Hematogenous infection may occur in patients who are immunocompromised, have a history of prolonged antibiotic therapy, or have indwelling catheters. Candidal infections acquired through aspiration appear as a focal opacity, similar to bacterial pneumonia, or as multiple nodules. Hematogenous candidiasis is characterized by microabscesses in the lungs, liver, spleen, and kidneys. In the lungs, these appear as tiny diffuse nodules [136, 138].

Infections caused by *Aspergillus fumigatus*, a ubiquitous mold, have a wide variety of appearances, which depend on the patient's immune status and the presence or absence of preexisting disease. The pulmonary disease is separated into four categories: ABPA, fungal balls or mycetomas, semi-invasive

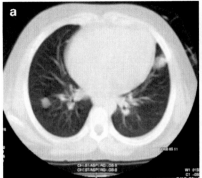
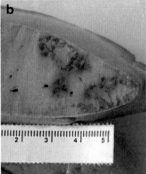
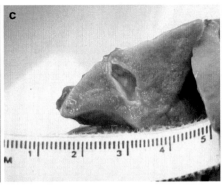

Fig. 11.31. This 7 year old with presumed immunodeficiency presented with 4 months of headache and was found to have a posterior fossa mass. Biopsy of the mass in the cerebellum revealed *Aspergillus*. (a) Chest CT performed for respiratory distress demonstrates bilateral pulmonary nodules, which at (b, c) autopsy, was found to be invasive aspergillosis

aspergillosis, and invasive aspergillosis. *Aspergillus* infections may present as solitary or multiple pulmonary nodules [138, 139].

ABPA is caused by a hypersensitivity reaction to *Aspergillus* colonizing the airways, occurring in 1–2% of patients with asthma and 7–9% of individuals with cystic fibrosis [140]. The classical appearance of finger-like, tubular densities radiating from the hilum represents central dilated bronchi filled with mucus. Mucus plugging also causes areas of atelectasis or consolidation radiating from the hilum peripherally. Smaller airway mucus plugging causes additional peripheral opacities to form. Findings are often bilateral. *Aspergillus* may parasitize a preexisting pulmonary cavity or cyst, forming a mycetoma or fungus ball. Thus, the finding of a known pulmonary cystic lucency that becomes opacified should raise the possibility of a superimposed fungal infection.

Invasive aspergillosis is a severe, rapidly progressive, often fatal infection that occurs in immunocompromised neutropenic patients. In these patients, *Aspergillus* aggressively invades the airways and blood vessels, causing airway obstruction or hemorrhage, both of which can give the appearance of bilateral diffuse pulmonary nodules (Fig. 11.31). Computed tomography shows that the borders of the nodules are poorly defined forming a *halo* around the nodule. As the patient's neutropenia and the infection begin to resolve, the nodule cavitates [141]. Semi-invasive aspergillosis occurs in mildly immunocompromised patients and is a less severe disease than invasive aspergillosis [142].

Actinomycosis is caused by an anaerobic organism that combines traits of bacteria and fungi. This is primarily an opportunistic infection that affects immunocompromised hosts. Chest wall invasion and enlarged lymph nodes, in addition to solitary or multiple pulmonary nodules, distinguish this infection from the others discussed in this section [143].

Nocardia is an infection most commonly caused by *Nocardia asteroides*, with a small minority caused by *Nocardia barsiliens* and *Nocardia farcinica*. Cavitation is a very common feature, both of consolidations and of multiple nodules [144, 145], which are manifestations of the pulmonary disease.

Hydatid Cyst

In the endemic sheep and cattle raising areas around the world, larvae from the tapeworm, *Echinococcus*, are swallowed and may disseminate hematogenously throughout the body. The most commonly affected organs are the liver and lungs. As the hydatid enlarges, a round well-circumscribed cyst forms in the lung parenchyma. Between 7 and 38% of patients with lung disease have multiple cysts. As the cysts enlarge, they may cause mass effect on adjacent bronchi with resulting atelectasis, or may erode into nearby structures. Up to 30% of lung cysts may be complicated by rupture into the pleural space or bronchus. CT is helpful in confirming the diagnosis and in better assessing complications (Fig. 11.32) [146].

Neoplastic

Tumors of the lung, both benign and malignant, are unusual in children. In a review of the files of the Armed Forces Institute of Pathology, over a 40-year period, 166 pulmonary tumors were found in patients 21 years of age or younger, and the ratio of benign to malignant tumors was 1:1.68. The most common tumor was the benign inflammatory pseudotumor,

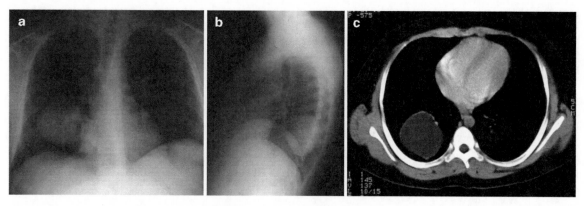

Fig. 11.32. This 7-year-old daughter of an Australian sheep farmer presented with fever and chills. (**a**) Frontal and (**b**) lateral radiographs demonstrate a well-circumscribed right lower lobe mass which was found to be primarily cystic on (**c**) CT. Surgical resection revealed a hydatid cyst

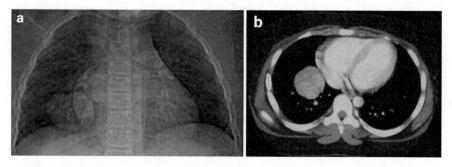

Fig. 11.33. This round well-circumscribed mass in the right lower lobe, well seen both on the CT (**a**) scout and (**b**) axial image was found to be an inflammatory pseudotumor after surgical resection

followed by three malignant tumors, bronchial adenoma, bronchogenic carcinoma, and mesenchymal tumors in order of frequency [114]. Some of these tumors are also discussed elsewhere in this textbook.

Inflammatory Pseudotumor

Inflammatory pseudotumor (inflammatory myofibroblastic tumor, plasma cell granuloma, histiocytoma, and xanthofibroma) is a distinctive, but controversial lesion, usually occurring during childhood [147]. Although rare, these are the most frequent primary lung tumors in childhood [109, 114] and are most commonly seen in older children. The masses are composed of fascicles of bland myofibroblastic cells admixed with a prominent inflammatory infiltrate consisting of lymphocytes, plasma cells, and eosinophils. This lesion has been variously termed plasma cell granuloma, inflammatory myofibroblastic tumor, histiocytoma, xanthofibroma, inflammatory myofibrohistiocytic proliferation, and inflammatory fibrosarcoma, reflecting divergent views concerning its pathogenesis and malignant potential.

Patients with pseudotumor typically present with respiratory symptoms, chiefly cough, chest pain, fever, or hemoptysis. On radiographs, the lesions are typically solitary, well-defined nodules, but they may be multiple (Fig. 11.33). They are most commonly found in the lung parenchyma, though these lesions have also been found within the bronchi and trachea [148, 149]. Tumors arising within the airway can cause obstruction and likely contribute to the high percentage of patients presenting with respiratory symptoms. These tumors can invade adjacent nonpulmonary structures including the mediastinum, heart, and pulmonary artery [150–152]. Lesions may partially calcify; this can be seen on radiography and computed tomography. The attenuation coefficient measured by CT is variable, however. Some lesions are uniform, while others are heterogeneous and demonstrate a variable amount of enhancement following the administration of intravenous contrast [153].

Inflammatory pseudotumors can cause secondary hypertrophic osteoarthropathy (HOA). HOA is a

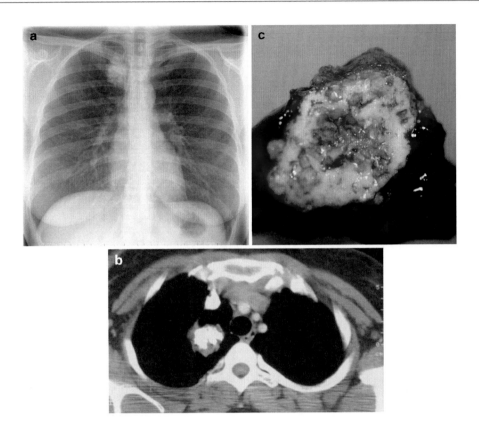

Fig. 11.34. (a) The frontal radiograph demonstrates a right upper lobe well-circumscribed mass with multiple calcifications. (b) Computed tomography confirms the large *popcorn* calcifications which are typical of hamartomas. (c) Pathology after surgical resection confirmed the diagnosis

clinical syndrome of clubbing of the fingers and toes, enlargement of the extremities, and painful swollen joints. Radiographs show symmetric periostitis, an inflammatory reaction of the bones, involving the radius and fibula and, to a lesser extent, the femur, humerus, metacarpals, and metatarsals. After the lesion is removed, the bone findings resolve [154, 155]. The treatment of pseudotumor is limited to complete resection [156].

Hamartoma

Pulmonary hamartomas are congenital tumors composed of normal lung tissue in abnormal proportions. These pulmonary masses, composed of pulmonary, bronchial, and cartilaginous elements, are usually found incidentally. They are most commonly located in the right lower lobe. Rarely are these tumors endobronchial. These well-defined lesions are smoothly marginated and lobular in contour. The additional presence of coarse, large "popcorn" shaped calcifications is clearly defined on plain film or computed tomography, which are helpful in making a confident diagnosis (see Fig. 11.34). These benign lesions may grow slowly over time [157]. They can become quite large and may even simulate chest tumors of extrapulmonary origin [158].

Because pulmonary hemangiomas and chondromas contain bronchial and other pulmonary elements, these too can be considered hamartomas [159]. Occasionally, hemangiomas may be multiple. Chondromas are usually solitary and nearly half calcify (Fig. 11.35). Chondromas occur in 76% of patients with Carney's Triad of pulmonary chondromas, gastric smooth muscle tumors, and extra-adrenal paragangliomas. In association with Carney's Triad, chondromas are often multiple [160]. Choristoma is another type of pulmonary tumor that consists of non-pulmonary as well as the pulmonary elements of hamartomas; but unlike hamartomas, these have no known growth potential. Confidently diagnosed hamartomas can be treated expectantly [161].

Bronchial Adenomas

Bronchial adenoma is the broad term for a group of malignant tumors arising from neuroendocrine cells in the lungs [162]. This group includes bronchial carcinoid, adenoid cystic carcinoma, and mucoepidermoid carcinoma; these lesions account for nearly

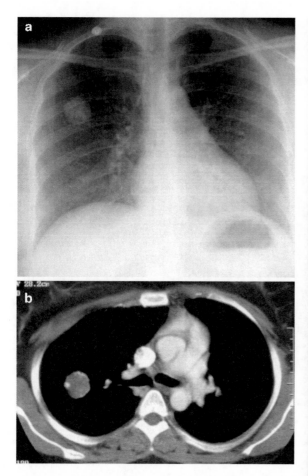

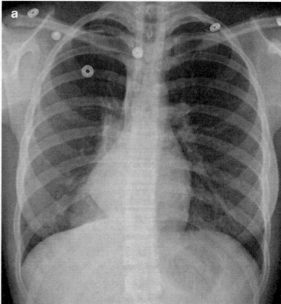

Fig. 11.35. A round well-circumscribed mass was seen on (**a**) routine preoperative chest radiograph. (**b**) Computed tomography reveals a solitary soft tissue mass with a coarse calcification in the periphery of the nodule. Surgical resection revealed a chondroma

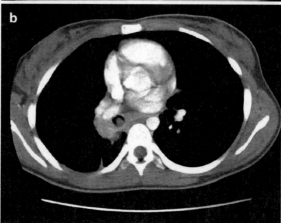

Fig. 11.36. This 15-year-old girl who presented with cough was found to have a right lower lobe opacity with sharp margins and volume loss on (**a**) CXR, findings consistent with atelectasis. (**b**) CT to further define the opacity demonstrates a well-circumscribed endobronchial mass with resultant right lower lobe atelectasis. At bronchoscopy, the patient was found to have an endobronchial carcinoid tumor

45% of primary malignant tumors of the lung [114]. Carcinoids comprise 80% of bronchial adenomas and are the most common primary malignant tumor of the lung in children and adolescents. They typically arise in the lobar bronchi and cause airway obstruction. On radiographs, these lesions may be detected as filling defects in large airways, but more commonly result in plain film findings of airway obstruction (i.e., air trapping, atelectasis, or postobstructive pneumonia). Computed tomography is very helpful in further defining the underlying endobronchial lesion revealed by the plain film findings or in further evaluating the clinical symptoms of airway obstruction (Fig. 11.36) [55]. Tumors are slow growing and rarely show malignant transformation. These tumors generally present as endobronchial lesions, but rarely may occur peripherally in the lung parenchyma as pulmonary nodules [164].

Bronchogenic Carcinoma

Unlike adults, bronchogenic carcinomas are relatively rare in childhood and account for 25% of the primary malignant tumors of the lung [114]. Tumors present as nodules and show very rapid growth and early metastases [165].

Primary Mesenchymal Tumors

Primary mesenchymal tumors or sarcomas of lungs are composed of primitive mesenchymal tissue and

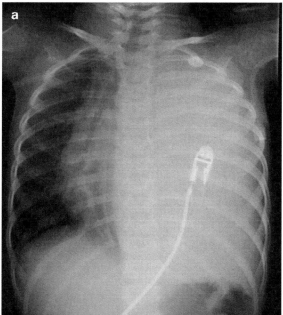

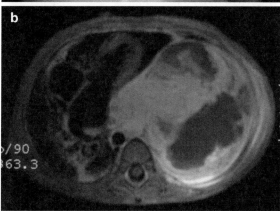

Fig. 11.37. This large heterogeneous mass which occupied the entire left hemithorax in this 1-year-old girl was found to be a PPB after surgical resection. (**a**) CXR, (**b**) CT

contain varying quantities of cartilage, skeletal and smooth muscle, and fibrous tissue. Sarcomas are named for the predominant tissue composition, including rhabdomyosarcoma, malignant mesenchymoma, leiomyosarcoma, fibrosarcoma, mesenchymal sarcoma, and Pleuropulmonary blastoma (PPB).

PPB, the largest subgroup of the mesenchymal tumors, is derived from primitive lung tissue, or pulmonary blastoma, and shares many features with Wilm's tumor, or nephroblastoma. Both tumors arise from primitive developmental tissue that normally regresses after birth. The presence of persistent, primitive pluripotent mesoderm is thought to be related to the development of malignancy [166]. Histologically, PPB and nephroblastoma are similar. Both are composed of a stroma of spindle cells and glandular elements. In addition,

PPB and cystic nephroma have been reported to occur synchronously in the same patients, providing further evidence of their close relationship [167]. This tumor is histologically different from a tumor of the same name, which occurs in adults.

These aggressive tumors often present as large pulmonary masses composed of a mixture of solid and cystic components. A variable appearance is seen on CT (Fig. 11.37). Some are solid and hemorrhagic, similar to nephroblastoma, while others are primarily cystic, mimicking CPAM [168]. Calcifications are uncommon, but have been reported on computed tomography [169]. Hilar lymph nodes are not typically enlarged. Because these tumors are so rare and often fatal, the usefulness of additional radiation or chemotherapy following surgical excision is unknown.

Vascular

Vascular lesions such as arteriovenous malformations or pulmonary vein (or venous) varices may give the appearance of a solitary or multiple pulmonary nodules in children (Fig. 11.38). Pulmonary arteriovenous malformations (PAVMs) are congenital anomalous connections between a pulmonary artery and veins. Occasionally, these develop following trauma. Associated clinical symptoms include hemoptysis, clubbing, cyanosis, and polycythemia [170]. Major complications include massive hemoptysis and paradoxical embolization to the brain resulting in either stroke or abscess. Two thirds of pulmonary AVMs are associated with Osler Weber Rendu syndrome, an autosomal dominant condition in which telangiectatic lesions involve the mucous membranes, skin, and lungs. In these patients, PAVMs are often multiple [171].

In contrast to arteriovenous fistulas, pulmonary varices typically cause no symptoms. These are abnormally dilated pulmonary veins that tend to have a smoother, more regular contour than PAVMs, and are most commonly solitary. The diagnosis of either type of vascular malformation can be made by angiography, MRI, or contrast-enhanced computed tomography, all of which will show a dilated vessel or tangle of vessels characteristic of the lesion [172–175].

11.3.2 Multiple Pulmonary Nodules

Multiple nodules are caused by processes that proliferate diffusely throughout the lungs. These processes may reach the lungs by aspiration or hematogenous

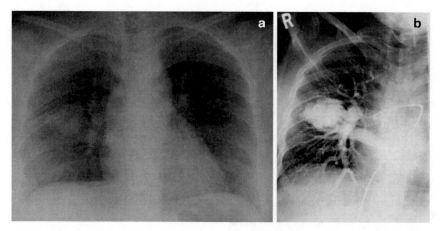

Fig. 11.38. This 15 year old presented with hemoptysis and was found to have a right parahilar pulmonary nodule on (**a**) CXR. (**b**) Angiography revealed a mass-like tangle of vessels forming an arteriovenous malformation

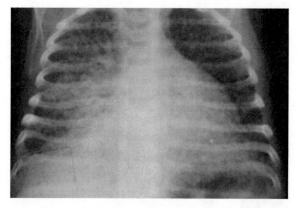

Fig. 11.39. This infant with tuberculosis has a typical radiograph of miliary tuberculosis. The radiographic image of bilateral diffuse tiny nodular densities resembles a snow storm

spread or may have a particular affinity for lung tissue. In addition, many of the disorders that cause diffuse pulmonary nodules are a part of multiorgan system disease, having manifestations in other organs as well. Infections and inflammatory disorders are the most common cause of multiple pulmonary nodules [109, 176]. Knowledge of the patient's clinical history is crucial in distinguishing the disparate causes of multiple nodules as the radiographic appearances often overlap. This section classifies multiple pulmonary nodules into infections, neoplasms, systemic autoimmune disease, and noninfectious inflammatory disorders.

Infections

Infections are one of the most common causes of multiple pulmonary nodules in children [176]. Many infections may also present as a solitary pulmonary nodule and were discussed in the prior section. Naturally, patients with immunodeficiency, either congenital or acquired, are more likely to have severe systemic and respiratory infections, both of which may lead to the appearance of bilateral pulmonary nodules.

Tuberculosis and Disseminated Fungal Infections

The classical description of hematogenously disseminated tuberculosis in the lung is miliary tuberculosis. The tiny, uniformly sized abscesses have the appearance of millet seeds, and are scattered diffusely throughout the lungs giving a "snowstorm" appearance to the lung parenchyma (Fig. 11.39). Miliary tuberculosis typically occurs within 6 months of the original infection, and is rare in children. Hematogenously disseminated fungal infections may cause diffuse bilateral pulmonary nodules. These nodules may be as small as those seen in miliary tuberculosis or larger. In treated or chronic tuberculosis and fungal infections, the nodules often calcify. The clinical and radiographic manifestations of tuberculosis and fungal infections are more thoroughly discussed earlier in Sect. 11.3.1.

Varicella and Measles

Pneumonia is a relatively rare complication of infections caused by the viruses, varicella-zoster and measles, in normal immunocompetent children. However, in those patients who are hospitalized for varicella, 17% of patients also have pneumonia [177]. Both viruses are more virulent in immunocompromised children and can cause pneumonia, meningitis, and hepatitis [178]. Children inoculated with the inactivated measles virus vaccine who are then exposed to a natural measles virus, rarely develop pneumonia [179].

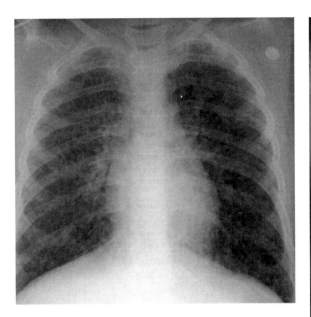

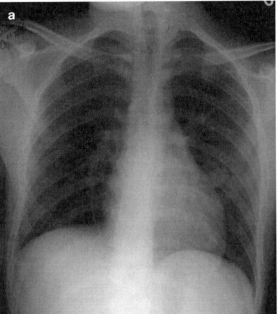

Fig. 11.40. This 9-year-old boy presented with a classical maculopapular rash of varicella and was admitted to the hospital for high fever and seizures. This frontal radiograph demonstrates diffuse bilateral small nodular densities characteristic of varicella pneumonia

Both measles and varicella pneumonias will also be heralded by typical rashes on the skin [180]; only rarely do these viral pneumonias occur without the tell-tale rash [181]. In the acute phase, the classic radiographic findings of both pneumonias are bilateral small pulmonary nodules and interstitial thickening (Fig. 11.40). Occasionally, the radiographic pattern resembles that of bronchopneumonia. Residual calcified nodules may remain after treatment [182]. Adenopathy is rare.

Septic Emboli

Infected thrombi that seed the lungs via the pulmonary arteries cause septic emboli. The most common predisposing factors include indwelling catheters, prosthetic heart valves [183], endocarditis, skin infections, and osteomyelitis [184]. In addition, children with bacterial pharyngitis may develop thrombophlebitis of the internal jugular vein (Lemierre syndrome). The most common complication of Lemierre syndrome is septic emboli to the lungs [185]. *S. aureus* and *S. pneumoniae* are the most common bacteria associated with septic emboli [186].

The appearance of septic emboli tends to evolve from well-defined, round, wedge-shaped or diffuse nodular opacities, measuring less than 2 cm to thick-walled cavities (Fig. 11.41). Septic emboli have a

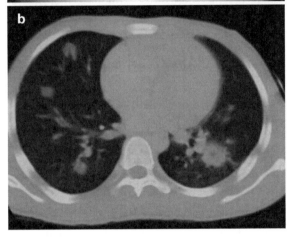

Fig. 11.41. This patient with thrombophlebitis of the internal jugular vein developed ill-defined bilateral nodular pulmonary opacities which were seen both on (**a**) chest X-ray and (**b**) CT. There is cavitation of the left posterior nodule. These nodules are consistent with septic emboli

predilection for the periphery and lower lobes of the lungs. A feeding vessel may be seen abutting (or leading to) the nodule, though this sign is not specific for septic emboli [187]. The frequently associated enlarged hilar and mediastinal lymph nodes are expected, as the emboli are due to the spread of an infection.

Plague

In certain areas where plague is endemic, such as Native American reservations in the Southwestern United States, patients with secondary pneumonic plague may have bilateral alveolar infiltrates or nodules on imaging studies. Hilar and mediastinal adenopathy and pleural effusions are frequently present as well. Patients with diffuse bilateral disease have a higher mortality rate than those with milder radiological findings [188].

Neoplasms

Metastases

Because primary lung cancers are so uncommon in children, lung metastases are the most common cause of malignant pulmonary nodules in children [1]. Most metastases are spread hematogenously, via the pulmonary arterial supply, but occasionally may spread via the lymphatics or the airways. The most common primary tumors that cause pulmonary metastases are Wilm's tumor and sarcomas [176]. A history of primary malignancy suggests the proper diagnosis. In rare instances, multiple pulmonary metastases will be the initial manifestation of an unknown malignancy.

Metastatic lesions, unlike infectious causes of multiple pulmonary nodules, tend to vary in size. Nodules are commonly spherical, well-defined, and located in the peripheral two thirds of the lungs. Certain metastases do have characteristic appearances. The metastases of osteogenic sarcoma can ossify, cavitate, and cause pneumothorax [189]. Thyroid metastases manifest with innumerable tiny nodules, mimicking the appearance of miliary tuberculosis. Unfortunately, the majority of pulmonary nodules caused by metastases cannot be distinguished from other causes of pulmonary nodules. In a patient with primary cancer other causes of and concern for metastases, computed tomography is much more sensitive than chest radiography for the detection of nodules, and is generally the means by which diagnosis is reached and follow-up is conducted.

Leukemia

Leukemia may present with diffuse bilateral nodular or interstitial infiltrates even before clinical disease is evident. Lung disease is most commonly seen in acute monocytic and myelogenous leukemias [190]; however, the most common cause of pulmonary nodules in children with leukemia is infection, often opportunistic, related to systemic neutropenia [191, 192]. Reactions or infections related to bone marrow transplantation, immunosuppression, and chemotherapy toxicity are other causes of pulmonary abnormalities in these children.

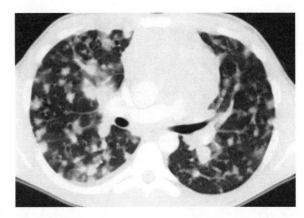

Fig. 11.42. These scattered ill-defined bilateral pulmonary nodules seen on computed tomography were found at the time of the patient's diagnosis of B cell lymphoma

Lymphoma

Neither Hodgkin's nor non-Hodgkin's lymphomas typically involve the lung. Only 12% of patients with Hodgkin's disease and 4% of patients with non-Hodgkin's lymphoma present with lung abnormalities [193]. Hodgkin's disease is always associated with mediastinal or hilar adenopathy; non-Hodgkin's lymphoma, by contrast, is characterized by parenchymal lung disease (Fig. 11.42). Primary disease may develop from lymphoid tissue and cause interlobular septal thickening, nodules, and pulmonary masses. Lung disease may be present at initial presentation, during relapse or both.

Papillomatosis

Recurrent respiratory papillomatosis (RRP) is a generally benign neoplasm caused by the human papilloma virus (HPV) transmitted from mother to infant during vaginal delivery. Papillomatosis is characterized by multiple warty excrescences composed of stratified squamous epithelium covering a fibrovascular stalk on the mucosal surface of the respiratory tract. Papillomas are the most common laryngeal tumors in children [194]. These are commonly recurrent throughout childhood, necessitating multiple procedures to remove them. Lung parenchymal involvement occurs in approximately 20% of cases [194]. Surgical procedures, intubation, or tracheostomy placement augment spread into the lung parenchyma. Once they reach the lungs, they find a rich vascular supply to support their growth. Continued growth and desquamation of the epithelium may lead to respiratory insufficiency or even death. Very rarely, malignant transformation to pulmonary carcinoma has been reported [195].

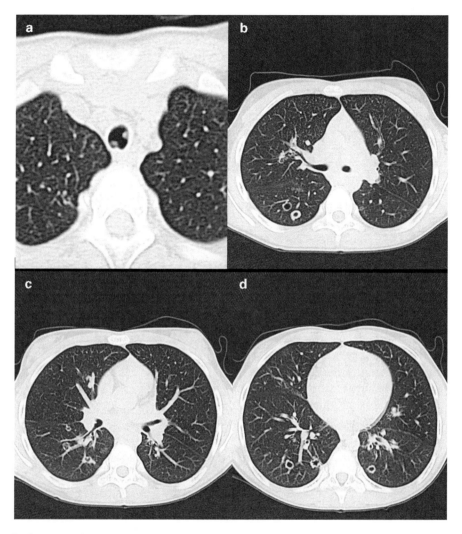

Fig. 11.43. Multiple computed tomography images (**a–d**) demonstrate multiple endotracheal soft tissue masses, as well is bilateral cavitary pulmonary nodules, typical for laryngotracheal papillomatosis

When the tumor spreads into the distal airway, the radiographic appearance depends on the site of involvement. Endobronchial tumors cause airway obstruction and atelectasis. Distal bronchiole and pulmonary lesions appear as multiple nodules, often with central cavitation in the dependent portions of the lower lobes (Fig. 11.43) [196]. Bronchiectasis may also be a sign of distal airway involvement and repeated infections due to chronic obstruction. Calcification is not a common feature [197, 198].

Systemic Autoimmune Diseases

Systemic autoimmune diseases include collagen vascular disease and the syndromes of pulmonary angiitis and granulomatosis. Because lymphocytic interstitial pneumonia (LIP) is associated with autoimmune disorders, it is also discussed in this section.

These diseases cause a variety of pulmonary parenchymal, airway, vascular, and pleural abnormalities. High-resolution computed tomography is a very useful adjunct to chest radiography for determining the extent of these pulmonary abnormalities [199]. These diseases are far more common in adults than children.

Collagen Vascular Diseases

Collagen vascular diseases are a subgroup of autoimmune connective tissue disorders, including juvenile idiopathic arthritis (JIA, previously referred to as juvenile rheumatoid arthritis), systemic lupus erythematous (SLE), progressive systemic sclerosis (scleroderma), dermatomyositis, polyarteritis nodosa, and mixed connective tissue disorders. All share common features including inflammation or fragility

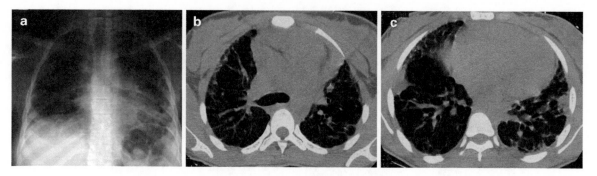

Fig. 11.44. The (**a**) CXR and (**b, c**) computed tomography images of this 16-year-old girl with scleroderma demonstrate low lung volumes due to pulmonary fibrosis and peripheral pulmonary opacities

of the connective tissues. Of all of the disorders, juvenile idiopathic arthritis (JIA) most commonly affects children. Intrathoracic disease is characterized by pleural effusions associated with lung disease (Fig. 11.44) [200]. By contrast, SLE and systemic sclerosis are more common in adults than in children and also is often associated with pleural effusions. SLE is particularly associated with pericardial effusions. This diverse group of collagen vascular diseases may cause various lung abnormalities, including hemorrhage due to vasculitis, usual interstitial pneumonia, nonspecific interstitial pneumonia, organizing pneumonia, diffuse alveolar damage, lymphoid interstitial pneumonia, bronchiectasis, bronchiolitis, and, ultimately, pulmonary fibrosis and hypertension. The radiographic manifestations of these several entities can resemble pulmonary nodules, as well as diffuse ground glass opacities and diffuse alveolar parenchymal opacities [201, 202]. Overall, collagen vascular diseases affect the lungs less frequently in children than adults. Pulmonary fibrosis, a common finding in adults, is uncommon in children.

Pulmonary Angiitis and Granulomatosis

There are five distinctive syndromes of pulmonary angiitis and granulomatosis: Wegener granulomatosis; allergic angiitis, and granulomatosis (AAG or Churg Strauss); necrotizing sarcoidal angiitis (NSA); bronchocentric granulomatosis, and lymphomatoid granulomatosis. These diseases cause necrosis of the small vessels anywhere in the body, including the lung, with resulting hemorrhage and granuloma formation [203, 209]. These rare diseases are most commonly seen in adults and only occasionally in children.

The classic triad of Wegener granulomatosis consists of necrotizing lesions in the upper respiratory tract, lower respiratory tract, and kidneys. A limited and much less common form involves only the lungs.

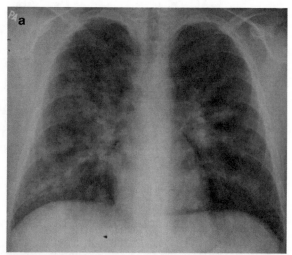

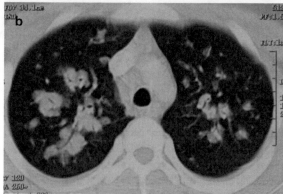

Fig. 11.45. This 14-year-old boy presented with fever, shortness of breath, and rising creatinine. (**a**) Chest radiograph demonstrates bilateral diffuse nodular opacities radiating from the hila. The nodules were confirmed by (**b**) CT. Thoracoscopic biopsy and further pathologic evaluation demonstrated findings consistent with Wegener's granulomatosis

The radiographic appearance of pulmonary hemorrhage includes bilateral solid or cavitary nodules and small masses (Fig. 11.45). Confluent areas of hemorrhage may give the appearance of segmental or lobar consolidation [205].

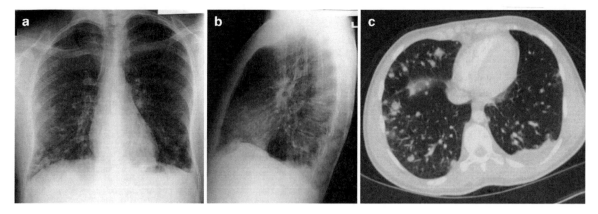

Fig. 11.46. This 16 year old who presented to the emergency room with nonproductive cough and fever had (**a**) PA and (**b**) lateral chest radiographs which demonstrated bilateral irregular pulmonary nodules and a left pleural effusion concerning for granulomatous disease. (**c**) Computed tomography confirmed the findings. A lung biopsy showed necrotizing sarcoid granulomatosis

Churg Strauss is a systemic disorder characterized by asthma, transient pulmonary opacities, hypereosinophilia, and systemic vasculitis. The first phase of the disease is characterized by asthma and rhinitis; the lungs often appear normal on radiographs. In the second phase of the disease, eosinophilic infiltration of the lungs is characterized by fleeting peripheral pulmonary opacities. In the third phase of the disease, vasculitis may produce areas of pulmonary hemorrhage. Thus, the second and third phases of the disease show distinctly different findings in the chest [206]. In addition, high-resolution CT shows thickening of the septal lines and bronchial walls, likely also representing eosinophilic infiltration [207]. Like Churg Strauss, bronchocentric granulomatosis is always associated with asthma, and may be associated with peripheral eosinophilia. Radiographic findings are varied and include bilateral pulmonary nodules, like the other entities in this group [203].

NSA is a variant of sarcoidosis that only involves the lungs; it is characterized by pulmonary vasculitis, granulomas, and pulmonary nodules on chest radiographs (Fig. 11.46). Hilar adenopathy occurs in up to 60% of patients. The nodules are typically up to one centimeter in diameter and often cavitate [203].

Lymphoid granulomatosis is another rare disease, considered an Epstein-Barr virus-mediated variant of B cell lymphoma. The lungs are the most common site of involvement, but the skin, central nervous system, kidneys, and liver are also commonly involved. On radiographs, lymphoid granulomatosis commonly shows bilateral nodules or occasionally migratory masses as well as pleural effusions. Thirty percent of the nodules or opacities cavitate [208].

Lymphocytic Interstitial Pneumonia

LIP is an uncommon syndrome which causes fever, cough, and dyspnea [209]. This disease is common among pediatric patients infected with the human immunodeficiency virus (HIV) type 1, and an AIDS-defining illness. In the era of aggressive use of anti-retroviral therapy, LIP has become very rare with HIV. LIP is also associated with other viruses, Epstein-Barr virus, and the human T cell leukemia virus (HTLV) type 1 [210], as well as autoimmune and lymphoproliferative disorders [211]. The radiographic findings of bilateral, mostly bibasilar, pulmonary nodules and opacities are due to dense interstitial accumulations of lymphocytes and plasma cells. The opacities may progress to cysts, honeycombing, and centrilobular nodules [212–214].

Inflammatory Noninfectious

Sarcoidosis

Sarcoidosis is an idiopathic inflammatory disorder in which non-necrotic, noncaseating granulomas comprised of epithelioid and multinucleate giant cells affect one or more organs. Childhood sarcoid is rare; there appear to be two different types [215]. Most patients diagnosed with sarcoidosis present as teenagers (<18) with a multisystem disease similar to that observed in the adult form. Pulmonary findings, similar to those noted in the adult form of the disease, typically mimic those of tuberculosis. Paratracheal and subcarinal lymph node enlargement are the two most common features of intrathoracic disease. Lung parenchymal abnormalities are less common and

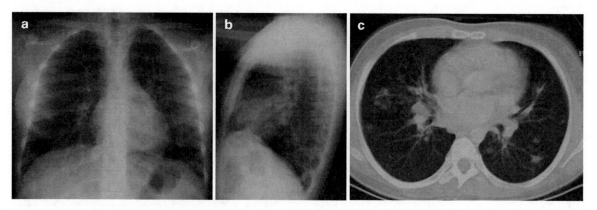

Fig. 11.47. This 20-year-old man with sarcoidosis has pulmonary nodules in the chest seen both by (**a**) frontal and (**b**) lateral radiographs and (**c**) computed tomography

may include widespread parenchymal opacities simulating bronchopneumonia or bilateral, diffuse reticulonodular densities (Fig. 11.47) [216, 217].

The second childhood form of sarcoid typically occurs in children less than 4 years of age, and is rarely associated with pulmonary abnormalities. These patients generally present with rash, uveitis, and arthritis/synovitis, a clinical presentation that can be confused with that of juvenile idiopathic arthritis [218].

Langerhans Cell Histiocytosis

LCH is also called Histiocytosis X. It represents a disease spectrum which previously has been described as three distinct illnesses but which now are recognized as points on a spectrum. The classic terminology included Letterer-Siwe disease, Hand-Schuller-Christian disease, and eosinophilic granuloma. LCH is caused by a proliferation of histiocytes called Langerhans cells. Letterer-Siwe disease is an aggressive, systemic disease that occurs in infants and young children, characterized by hepatosplenomegaly, lymphadenopathy, skin lesions, pancytopenia, and lung disease. Hand-Schuller-Christian disease is a milder form of the condition that occurs in older children and may present with the classic triad of exophthalmos, diabetes insipidus, and osteolytic lesions of the skull. Well-defined, lytic skeletal lesions are also common in this form of the disease. Finally, eosinophilic granuloma refers to disease affecting a single organ system, typically the skeleton or lungs, usually encountered in adolescents or adults.

Although all forms of LCH may involve the lungs, the lungs are affected in only approximately 10% cases involving children. Half of children with multisystem organ disease have lung involvement, usually interstitial lung disease, which may progress to fibrosis [219]. In cases of primary, pulmonary Langerhans cell histiocytosis (PLCH) with involvement limited to the lungs, teenagers and adults are primarily affected, with a greater incidence among smokers. The Langerhans cells form granulomas in the peribronchial and perivascular interstitial tissues. Radiographically, these granulomas appear as diffuse nodules and predominate at the lung apices. Over time, the nodules may cavitate and form cysts accompanied by fibrosis (Fig. 11.48) [220–222].

Pulmonary Alveolar Microlithiasis

This nodular lung disease is of unknown etiology, and is characterized by 1–3 mm-sized calcium phosphate microliths scattered throughout the lungs. Pathologically, microliths are present in the alveolar airspaces and along interlobular septa, bronchovascular bundles, and the pleura. This rare disease has a very typical radiographic pattern of small, calcified nodules, measuring approximately 1 mm in size, resembling sand; they are scattered diffusely throughout the lungs. On CT, the nodules can be seen in a backdrop of ground glass attenuation, a finding especially common in children [223–226]. Chronic disease seen in adults may result in pulmonary fibrosis and induce right heart failure. Although the cause is unknown, the disease is known to be familial and especially common in Turkey.

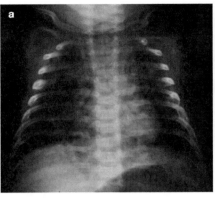

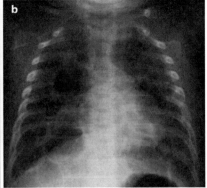

Fig. 11.48. This 3-month-old baby presented with fever and lethargy. (a) Initial chest radiograph demonstrates scattered pulmonary nodules. (b) Serial radiographs demonstrated progression to bilateral pulmonary cysts of varying sizes, findings typical for Langerhans cell histiocytosis

11.4 Hemoptysis

ANDREW A. COLIN

Bleeding from the airway (hemoptysis) in childhood is an infrequent occurrence that represents a large array of underlying pathologies. The source of the blood is frequently in the mouth or other upper airway structure, and because cough and vomiting are often contemporaneous, gastrointestinal bleeding may be mistaken as emanating from the airway.

11.4.1 Clinical Evaluation

Diffuse bleeding from the lung commonly referred to as pulmonary hemosiderosis in its complete presentation consists of a triad of hemoptysis, anemia, and diffuse alveolar infiltration (Fig. 11.49). The three elements rarely coexist, however, and thus, a fall in hematocrit with the onset of respiratory disease should suggest pulmonary bleeding. The presentation is variable and ranges from a fulminant onset with acute, occasionally fatal hemoptysis, to an insidious presentation, characterized by anemia, pallor, weakness, and poor weight gain. The hematological work-up includes markers of anemia and iron loss reflecting ongoing blood loss. Coagulation studies are important to rule out pulmonary hemorrhage from treatable cause.

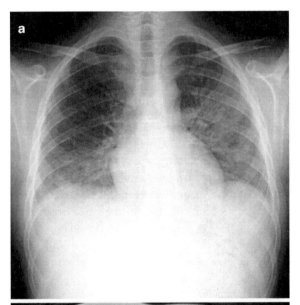

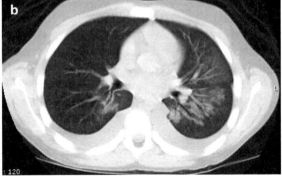

Fig. 11.49. Acute pulmonary hemorrhage. (a) CXR showing alveolar infiltrates superimposed on chronic interstitial disease. (b) CT also reveals alveolar and interstitial abnormalities, providing no increased specificity as to the cause of the alveolar infiltrates

Cardiac evaluation, including EKG and echocardiography, seeks evidence of pulmonary hypertension, myocarditis, mitral stenosis, pulmonary venous obstruction, and chronic left heart failure all of which can underlie cardiovascular etiologies for pulmonary bleeding. In the context of cardiovascular diseases pulmonary embolism, pulmonary veno-occlusive disease and pulmonary edema are rare presentations as well.

Once the origin of the bleeding from the lower airway is questioned, the investigation is guided by the radiographic image that directs the clinician toward a localized vs. diffuse process (see Sect. 11.4, Chap. 1). It is of note that localized large bleeds may represent complications of a systemic disease, and bronchiectases related to cystic fibrosis is the leading cause of hemoptysis in late childhood and adolescence. Infections such as pneumonia are uncommon reasons for bleeding but infections with tuberculosis are a leading cause and should be considered where clinically and epidemiologically relevant.

The clinician often uses bronchoscopy to establish the cause of hemoptysis. Direct inspection excludes bleeding sites in the nasopharynx, trachea and, bronchi, it also can detect bleeding masses in the airway, most notably carcinoid tumor. Bronchoalveolar lavage (BAL) also obtained with the flexible bronchoscope can detect active alveolar bleeding, or show iron laden macrophages, as evidence of recent bleeding. BAL cultures help identify infections. Occasionally, endoscopy of the gastrointestinal tract is used to exclude GI bleeding in which aspiration of blood leads to a spurious diagnosis of pulmonary hemorrhage.

Once bleeding has been localized to the lung parenchyma, a lung biopsy may be needed to establish the etiology. Lung histology may reveal specific conditions such as pulmonary veno-occlusive disease, infectious causes, and most importantly vasculitic lesions of various types indicating the presence of multisystem diseases. Immunofluorescence studies can reveal deposits of immunoglobulin and complement along the basement membrane which point to the diagnosis of Goodpasture's syndrome. Electron microscopy may reveal breaks along the capillary endothelial lining.

11.4.2 Broad Classification of Conditions

Classifications of conditions associated with diffuse pulmonary hemorrhage have been attempted. Although these are helpful for a methodological approach to the pursuit of a diagnosis, it is important to point out that only rarely can a pediatric patient be classified into a well-defined nosologic entity. In most cases the diagnosis remains primary pulmonary hemosiderosis (PPH), lumping a variety of conditions that elude definition and have variable and unpredictable prognoses. Some of these patients declare themselves over time to have multisystem diseases, and chronic or recurrent bleeding into the lung can be associated with the development of pulmonary fibrosis. It is therefore important to follow these patients by regular radiographs and pulmonary function testing. In this broad group an emerging subpopulation are infants who present with serious, occasionally recurrent, and potentially fatal bleeding. Such episodes may be clustered regionally suggesting infectious or environmental etiologies (for a while Stachybotrys chartarum, a fungus, was considered an important etiology), and recently some cases raised the possibility of von Willebrand Disease as a possible underlying etiology.

An important if uncommon group of etiologies for hemoptysis is lumped under the term Pulmonary-Renal Syndromes. In these diseases, the lung and kidney have the major involvement while other organ systems are variably affected. The leading diagnoses are: (1) Goodpasture's Syndrome, an immune complex disease that affects almost exclusively the kidneys and lungs. (2) SLE which often affects multiple organs. The bleeding in these two conditions is related to a vasculitic process. (3) Wegener's Granulomatosis, and (4) Microscopic Polyangiitis. These two conditions are closely related, and in both the hemoptysis may be due to cavitary lesions in the lungs. Extremely rare cases of lung bleeding have been associated with renal complications of Henoch-Schonlein Purpura (HSP). The specific diagnosis of this important series of diseases relies on an immune work-up and ultimately on tissue diagnosis from renal or lung biopsy.

Two curious associations with lung bleeding are milk protein allergy in infancy, often referred to as Heiner's syndrome. The other is a series of case reports of hemoptysis with celiac disease. In both conditions, a putative underlying immune mechanism is assumed; for the former the diagnosis is reliant on identification of milk precipitins but the strength of the association has been questioned, for the latter the underlying mechanism remains elusive.

Radiographic abnormalities are not specific and vary from minimal fleeting infiltrates to massive parenchymal involvement (Fig. 11.49), and may change in the

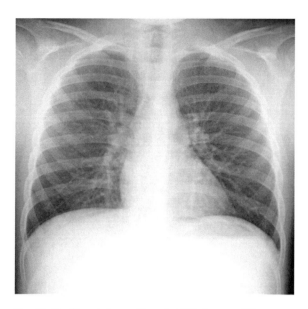

Fig. 11.50. Chronic hemosiderosis. CXR shows a diffuse non-specific interstitial process

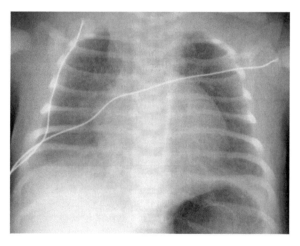

Fig. 11.51. Chronic hemosiderosis. CXR shows a diffuse interstitial prominence with an almost airspace like quality most notable in right perihilar region and right lower lobe

individual patient with recurrent bleeding. In patients with small frequent episodes of bleeding the radiographs may reflect chronic diffuse interstitial involvement (Fig. 11.50) and may change only minimally with an acute episode of bleeding. CT scan appears to offer no better specificity. MRI of the lung may prove more useful in defining the presence of blood, showing decreased signal on the T2-weighted images.

However, there are few causes of focal alveolar opacification which resolve rapidly, within hours or 1–2 days. These most commonly include atelectasis, asymmetric pulmonary edema, and aspiration of your own blood. With focal pulmonary hemorrhage, the specific site of primary bleeding will remain

abnormal for several days. Other areas of aspirated blood, however will resolve as the blood is cleared from the acini and airway. On occasion, the interstitial process of chronic hemosiderosis on CXR will have a hazy blurred appearance almost suggestive of an alveolar filling process (Fig. 11.51).

11.5 Hyperlucent Lung and Lung Segments

ROBERT H. CLEVELAND

There are many causes of overinflation of the lungs and increased lucency. This may affect all of both lungs, all of one lung or scattered segments of one or both lungs. These observations may be easily recognized from CXR or require dynamic imaging such as chest fluoroscopy or inspiratory/expiratory CT.

11.5.1 Diffuse Air Trapping

Diffuse air trapping may be perceived as bilateral hyperlucent lungs. Air trapping is best confirmed by flattening of the diaphragms on all concurrent images. If even one image fails to reveal flattened diaphragms, then there is not air trapping. Counting the level of the hemidiaphragms in relation to the ribs may help, but this is complicated by variable degrees of lordotic projection which accompanies portable imaging. If rib/diaphragm relationship is used for assessment, the relationship of the anterior ribs is more reliable than the posterior ribs. The anterior rib ends are half as far from the dome of the diaphragms than the posterior ribs and therefore are affected by half as much by beam angle variance. There should be 6–6.5 right anterior ribs in the midclavicular line above the hemidiaphragm in a normally inflated child's chest. As in the adult, there should be ten posterior ribs above the hemidiaphragm. Be aware however, that many young children, around ages 5–7 years, when asked to take a deep breath will take it as a challenge! This may produce high lung volumes and suggest air trapping.

In children under 18 months of age, diffuse air trapping is most commonly encountered with acute lower airway viral infections (bronchiolitis). There may be accompanying bronchial wall thickening and

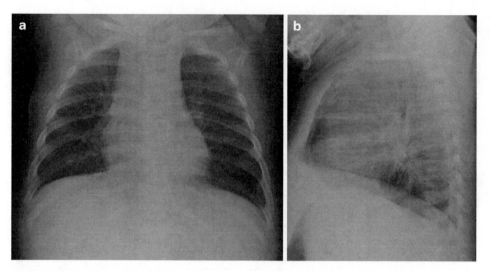

Fig. 11.52. The chest radiograph on this infant with RSV positive bronchiolitis reveals diffuse air trapping. The flattening of the diaphragm is the most reliable indicator of overinflation. There is also multifocal subsegmental atelectasis and diffuse bronchial wall thickening. (**a**) PA projection (**b**) Lateral projection

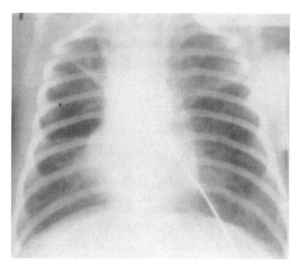

Fig. 11.53. Bronchopulmonary dysplasia

atelectasis, but the hallmark of the disease is air trapping (Fig. 11.52) (see Chap. 6).

Also in children under 18 months of age, hyperventilation (the normal rate varies by age, sex, and activity) will cause increase in lung volume and eventually hyperinflation. With increased respiratory rate in children of this age, the inspiratory constant exceeds the expiratory constant leading to breathing just below peak inspiratory volume, and hence the high lung volume. The cause of the hyperventilation is irrelevant.

Children of any age with reactive airway disease or asthma, when experiencing an acute attack, will potentially have hyperinflated lungs. The CXR may mimic a baby's with bronchiolitis (Fig. 11.52) (see Chap. 14).

A former premature with chronic lung disease (CLD) of prematurity, also known as BPD, may at some point in the evolution of their lung pathology present with diffusely overinflated, hyperlucent lungs. More commonly, however, the lungs will be irregularly inflated, with multifocal areas of hyperinflation alternating with areas of atelectasis or fibrosis (Fig. 11.53) (see Chap. 7).

11.5.2   Unilateral Hyperlucent Lung

The most common difficulty when encountering a unilaterally hyperlucent lung is to determine if the hyperlucent lung is overinflated or the other lung underinflated. Corollary finding may provide the clue, or dynamic imaging may be required. If dynamic imaging is employed, fluoroscopy has several advantages. It is readily available and requires no sedation or anesthesia. In fact it is important to have the child awake and actively breathing or crying to best assess through a full and dynamic range of lung volumes. The brief fluoroscopy required exposes the child to less irradiation than inspiratory/expiratory CT, adhering to the ALARA concept of *imaging gently* [227, 228].

In toddlers and older children who are of an age capable of placing objects in their mouths and then aspirating them, an airway foreign body may produce either atelectasis or air trapping. In either case,

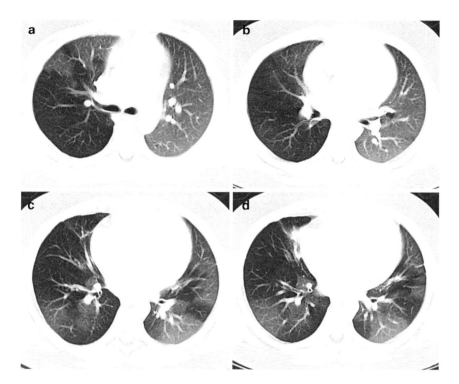

Fig. 11.54. CT of bonchiolitis obliterans presents with accentuated hyperlucent oligemic segments of lung, usually worse in one lung with associated mild to moderate bronchiectasis. (**a**–**d**) represent images at discontiguous levels from cranial to caudal

a careful assessment for an airway foreign body is required. Fluoroscopy is preferred over decubitus images, as the commonly encountered oblique projection of the decubitus images makes comparison of lung volumes potentially inaccurate (see Chap. 6). Evaluation for a lucent foreign body may be greatly enhanced by CT, with or without *virtual bronchoscopy*. Extrinsic bronchial compression, as from a mass or vascular structure, if severe, may cause altered inflation. Rarely an intrinsic airway obstruction may be encountered, such as a tuberculoma.

Children may be born with a hypoplastic or absent lung. With hypoplasia, the abnormal small lung is usually hyperlucent. This may be a part of a syndrome, such as venolobar or scimitar syndrome. In that specific instance, the abnormal, usually right upper lobe, anomalously draining pulmonary vein, should be recognized as a vertically oriented vessel coursing to the diaphragm through the smaller hyperlucent lung (see Chap. 6). With any cause of unilateral lung hypoplasia, the smaller lung should be relatively hyperlucent. The hypoplastic lung is hyperlucent partially because its vasculature in diminished. An additional, related observation is that the pulmonary vasculature of the normal lung is increased. This abnormally prominent vasculature of the normal lung may be the most obvious clue to the contralateral hypoplasia. Acquired

under inflation, unless present for an extended period of time, should not have recognizably asymmetric pulmonary vasculature.

Bronchiolitis obliterans, also known as Swyer James syndrome or McLeod syndrome usually occurs after viral infection, although it can also arise from a bacterial or parasitic infection (i.e., *Mycoplasma*). In adults, bronchiolitis obliterans is characterized by unilateral hyperlucent small volume lung; but in children, by an overexpanded hyperlucent lung, a discrepancy explained by diminished lung growth following onset of the disease. While air trapping is initially evident on imaging, proportionately less growth results in reduced lung volume compared to the more normal lung. In addition, it has been established that many cases of bronchiolitis obliterans feature diffuse and irregularly affected lungs. Specifically, on CT both lungs may show abnormalities, including bronchiectasis, but one lung typically dominates (Fig. 11.54) (see Chap. 6).

Children born with diaphragmatic hernia will usually have hypoplasia of the ipsilateral lung. If the amount of herniated bowel is large, the resultant shift of the mediastinum may cause hypoplasia of the contralateral lung. However even in the latter case, the ipsilateral lung will be more profoundly affected. Following repair of the hernia, the lungs will continue to develop with increase in volume of the hypoplastic lung. However, in most cases, the ipsilateral lung will remain smaller, more lucent, and with relatively diminished vasculature than the lung opposite to the side of the hernia. A clue to this diagnosis, postoperatively, is that the smaller, lucent lung is associated with a hemidiaphragm that is lower and flatter than the other. This is the result of the tension involved in plicating the diaphragmatic defect (see Sect. 5.3).

One lung may seem hyperlucent because the other hemithorax is of increased opacity. This most commonly occurs when there is a pleural effusion or thickening. If the thickening is dominantly posterior or anterior, its presence may not be readily apparent on frontal projection radiographs. If the image is acquired with the patient supine, a relatively small effusion may be most easily appreciated as an apical cap, greater in degree than on the opposite side (see Chap. 12).

Asymmetric pulmonary edema may cause one lung to be more opaque than the other. In children, especially those with a history of complex congenital heart disease, this may be related to asymmetric pulmonary vasculature. Main branch pulmonary artery stenosis may be severe enough to cause decreased arterial flow on the affected side and "protect" that side from developing high output pulmonary edema. Likewise central pulmonary venous obstruction may raise the baseline venous pressure to above oncotic pressure and cause pulmonary edema or predispose to edema when left atrial pressure increases above baseline. Asymmetric lymphatic flow may be associated with asymmetric pulmonary lymphedema. Any of these situations may be a component of the congenital abnormality or acquired as a postoperative condition. In children, as adults, if the patient is left for a protracted period in a dominantly decubitus position, the dependent side can develop pulmonary edema.

Asymmetric increased size of the chest wall soft tissues can cause the affected side to be more opaque and therefore the other seem hyperlucent. This may occur with hemihypertrophy (congenital or acquired) or extensive chest wall masses such as lymphatic malformations or plexiform neurofibroma.

One lung may seem hyperlucent because of issues affecting that side other than the lung. This commonly is seen if the image is acquired in mild degrees of rotation. In small children, rotation may not be equal throughout the chest. On a perfectly straight frontal projection of the chest, not only should the medial ends of the clavicles be equidistant from the vertebral posterior spinous processes, but also the anterior ends of all pairs of ribs.

A subtle pneumothorax may be perceived as an increased lucency of the hemithorax. This is most common with supine imaging. In the supine position, the pleural edge of a small pneumothorax will be first encountered, medially adjacent to the inferior mediastinum or cardiac apex (see Chap. 12).

Asymmetric decreased size of the chest wall soft tissues can cause the affected side to be hyperlucent. This may be congenital, as in Poland's syndrome (decrease in chest wall musculature and rarely ribs, sometimes associated with hypoplasia/absence the radius or radial digits). The asymmetry may be acquired.

11.5.3   Hyperlucent Lung Segments

Possibly the most difficult observation is that of segmental hyperlucency. Confirmation often will require CT, frequently performed in inspiration and expiration. This is especially true for demonstrating the irregular air trapping associated with interstitial lung disease (see Chap. 8).

A common cause of markedly irregular aeration is chronic lung disease of prematurity, as discussed earlier. As the child grows older, this observation may abate or occasionally resolve (see Chap. 7).

Obstruction of a segmental or subsegmental bronchus may cause altered aeration of the lung distal to the obstruction. This may be encountered with mucous plugging, allergic bronchopulmonary aspergillosis (APBA) (see Chaps. 14 and 15), cast bronchitis (see Sect. 5.2), bronchial stenosis or atresia, foreign body, intrinsic obstruction (such as carcinoid tumors), or extrinsic compression (see Chap. 6).

Chronic lobar emphysema (CLE) may have some evidence of focal bronchial obstruction (in up to 50% of cases) that manifests itself as an overinflated, hyperlucent lobe. In at least half of cases, no such obstruction is encountered. In the first few days of life this may present with preferential trapping of fetal lung liquid in the abnormal lobe. This, in turn, produces an overinflated, opaque lobe, which slowly drains the fluid over ensuing days, subsequently becoming hyperlucent. The distribution of CLE is roughly 43% in the left upper lobe, 32% in the right middle lobe, 20% in the right upper lobe, and 5% in two lobes. With an overinflated hyperlucent lobe and associated mediastinal shift to the contralateral side, CLE may be mistaken as tension pneumothorax. When this occurs, CT is useful in visualizing the underlying, overinflated, and hyperlucent lung parenchyma (see Chap. 6).

Rarely peripheral pulmonary artery stenosis (PPS), with focally diminished pulmonary artery prominence, will be perceived as a focal hyperlucent lung segment. PPS may be seen as an isolated phenomena. It is encountered as a part of several conditions including congenital rubella, neurofibromatosis 1, Williams syndrome (congenital hypercalcemia), Ehlers-Danlos syndrome, and tetrology of Fallot (most commonly the left main pulmonary artery) [229].

11.6 Necrotizing Pneumonia

GREGORY S. SAWICKI

11.6.1 Epidemiology

Necrotizing pneumonia (NP) is becoming an increasingly recognized complication of community-acquired pneumonia in children. NP is also termed cavitary pneumonia or cavitatory necrosis, and has been associated with poor clinical outcomes in adults. Although NP has been recognized as a complication of pneumonia in adults for several decades, when initially described NP was thought to be extremely rare in children. In fact, the first case series of NP including four children was published in 1994 [230]. Subsequently there have been several additional case series of pediatric NP reported [231–237]. The incidence of NP appears to be increasing, similar to the observed rise in cases of complicated pneumonia overall [238]. Possible explanations for the increased incidence of NP include the emergence of particularly virulent microorganisms or simply the increased awareness and detection of this complication due to improved imaging techniques.

11.6.2 Pathophysiology and Microbiology of Necrotizing Pneumonia

The pathophysiology of NP is thought to be one of massive pulmonary gangrene and tissue liquefaction and necrosis secondary to bacterial infection and the resultant inflammatory response [239, 240]. The pathologic progression of pneumonia leads to resultant pulmonary parenchymal necrosis. The pathologic process is distinct from that of pulmonary abscess, in which bacterial infection leads to the development of a well-defined, often walled off, area of infection. The most common causative bacteria isolated in cases of NP is *S. pneumoniae* [230, 237, 240, 241], though other bacterial organisms including *S. aureus* (both methicillin-sensitive and methicillin-resistant strains), other *Streptococcus* species such as *Streptococcus millerei*, *M. pneumoniae*, *C. pneumoniae*, *Pseudomonas aeruginosa*, and *Fusobacterium* species have also been reported as pathogens leading to NP [242–245]. Aspiration pneumonia leading to anaerobic infection may also lead to the development of NP. In recent years, more virulent strains of methicillin-resistant *Staphylococcus aureus* (MRSA), particularly MRSA strains producing Panton-Valentine leukocidin (PVL) have emerged in the community and may be driving the increasing incidence of pediatric NP [246–248]. Coinfection with respiratory viruses such as influenza A, including the novel H1N1 strain, have recently been described in pediatric NP as well [249].

11.6.3 Clinical Presentation

In its initial stages, the clinical presentation of necrotizing pneumonia is indistinguishable from community-acquired pneumonia. As such, NP is often diagnosed late in children who present to medical attention following treatment failure of pneumonia with oral antibiotics. Symptoms often include prolonged high fevers, cough, sputum production, tachypnea, dyspnea, and anorexia. However, many children may simply present with persistent fevers despite seemingly adequate treatment for community-acquired pneumonia. Hypoxia may be present although many children with NP do not require oxygen supplementation. NP results in the development of a pleural effusion in up to 70% of cases [237] and thus may also present with resultant pleuritic chest pain. Physical exam findings are consistent with other complicated pneumonias with parapneumonic effusion. Common laboratory findings are an elevated white blood cell count and low hemoglobin and low serum albumin. If pleural fluid is analyzed, parameters are consistent with empyema, with elevated white blood cell counts, decreased pleural pH, elevated pleural LDH, and decreased pleural fluid glucose.

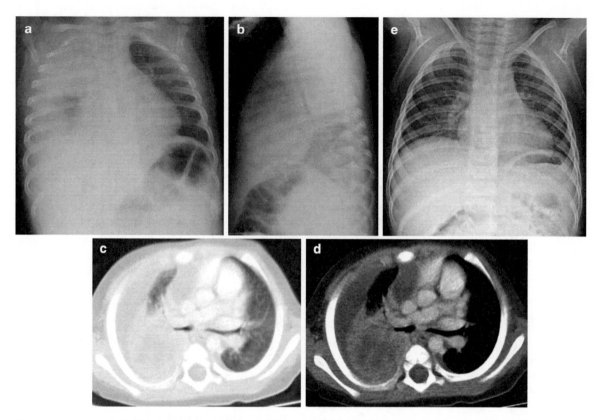

Fig. 11.55. (a) PA CXR shows a consolidation of the majority of the right lung and possible loculated pleural effusion. (b) The lateral image confirms significant opacification. Neither suggests cavitation. (c) CT (lung window) suggests irregular areas of non-enhancing tissue, representing necrotic areas, and surrounded by enhancing lung parenchyma. The necrotic areas have not yet drained their fluid and become air containing. There is a large partially located pleural effusion. (d) CT (mediastinal window) more clearly confirms areas of non-enhancing pulmonary necrosis with surrounding enhancing lung. The pleura are enhanced. (e) Follow-up PA CXR, 9.5 months following the image in (a), is essentially normal

11.6.4   Imaging of Necrotizing Pneumonia

Chest radiography, including PA, lateral, and, on occasion, decubitus views, constitute the initial imaging for diagnosis of NP [250]. The initial findings on CXR are variable. There may merely be an alveolar infiltrate. However, in many instances there will be an associated, ipsilateral pleural effusion, which may be free flowing or loculated. If free flowing, the concern for NP should be present. If the effusion is loculated (representing an organizing empyema), the presence NP should be highly suspected (see Chap. 12 for a description of CXR findings with loculated effusion) (Fig. 11.55). Often by the time of initial imaging, there will be air (or air and fluid) containing cystic areas noted by CXR. This may represent necrotic regions within the lung parenchyma, loculated collections within an empyema or both (Fig. 11.56). It is impossible to determine the location of these cystic areas by CXR alone. Therefore, even though the diagnosis of NP can be suspected by plain chest radiography, CT is necessary to clearly define the extent and nature of disease. CT should always be performed with contrast enhancement to clearly define the pleura and clarify the pleural or parenchymal location of cysts and potentially drainable pleural fluid (Fig. 11.56d). If characterization of the pleural process is required, usually prior to thoracostomy drainage, ultrasound can be employed to determine if the effusion is loculated (see Chap. 12) and, if so, where the largest drainable collections are located. Ultrasound-guided drainage of the effusion may also be employed. It is possible that NP is underdiagnosed as CT scans may not always be obtained in the management of prolonged, complicated courses of pneumonia. This is particularly true when a significant pleural effusion is present and assumed to be the reason for persistent symptoms.

Radiographic CT criteria for NP have been established and include the loss of normal pulmonary parenchymal architecture, the presence of multiple small air or fluid-filled cavities, and decreased parenchymal enhancement [250] (Figs. 11.55 and 11.56).

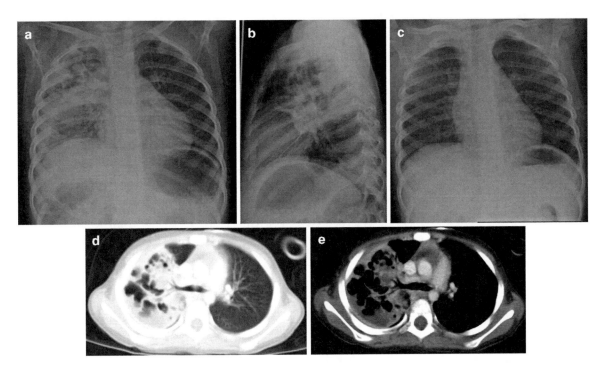

Fig. 11.56. (a) PA CXR shows multiple cavities in the upper right hemithorax. It is unclear whether these are in the lung or pleura. There is a moderate size pleural effusion, questionably partially loculated. (b) Lateral CXR confirms the PA image observations. (c) CT (lung window) confirms the cavities within the lung parenchyma with an effusion. (d) CT (mediastinal window) more clearly delineates the enhanced pleura separating the fluid in the pleural space and the air- and fluid-filled lung cysts. (e) Follow-up PA CXR, 3.5 months after the initial CXR (a), reveals almost complete clearing of the affected lung

CT scanning generally reveals segments of lung showing multiple areas of lung parenchyma containing air, air and fluid, or non-enhancing fluid surrounded by contrast enhancing lung parenchyma without a defined rim of enhancement. This is distinguished from pulmonary abscess in which CT imaging shows a well-defined enhancing rim outlining a single pulmonary cavity.

11.6.5 Management, Complications, and Long-Term Outcomes of Necrotizing Pneumonia

Since NP involves the presence of multiple fluid and subsequently air-filled cavities within the affected lung parenchyma, there is a heightened concern over the risk for developing a bronchopleural fistula (BPF), defined as a persistent air leak lasting over 48 h. In a small study of pediatric NP, five of the nine NP cases developed BPF following pleural intervention [251]. In a more recent larger series of cases, a smaller proportion of patients developed a fistula, and those that did develop a fistula had chest drains in place for over 7 days [237]. The observed decline may be attributed to awareness of the risk of a chest drain in the presence of NP, resulting in minimization of the drainage time. Therefore, it may be prudent to remove a pleural drain within 7 days of placement to decrease the risk of complication.

There have been no randomized trials of surgical intervention in pediatric NP, and in many cases conservative management with antibiotics, chest drainage, and intrapleural thrombolytics such as urokinase or tissue plasminogen activator (tPa) may be sufficient. Video-assisted thoracoscopic surgery (VATS) may be indicated in certain situations and may reduce hospital length of stay [252]. However, although several small studies have suggested lobar resection as therapy for NP [253–255], such surgery is not necessary and should be avoided. In spite of the CT evidence of extensive and severe lung damage, follow-up studies have shown significant normalization of the previously affected parenchyma [237, 256] (Figs. 11.55e and 11.56e). The capacity of the young lung for repair is remarkable in its completeness and rapidity. Despite the extensive radiographic abnormalities and significant short-term morbidity caused by NP, the long-term clinical and radiographic outcomes for patients seen in follow-up have been good. Clinical symptoms tend to resolve with therapy in 3–4 weeks time. Significant normalization of pulmonary parenchyma seen on CXR and CT also occurs within several months of acute illness. This pattern of improvement suggests the lung damage caused by NP in children is transient and that NP should be recognized as a severe, yet, self-limiting, and reversible disease.

References

1. Rudan I, Tomaskovic L, Boschi-Pinto C, Campbell H. Global estimate of the incidence of clinical pneumonia among children under five years of age. Bull World Health Organ. 2004;82:895–903.

2. Dowell SF, Kupronis BA, Zell ER, Shay DK. Mortality from pneumonia in children in the United States, 1939 through 1996. N Engl J Med. 2000;342:1399–407.

3. Gaston B. Pneumonia. Pediatr Rev. 2002;23:132–40.

4. Pandey MR, Daulaire NM, Starbuck ES, Houston RM, McPherson K. Reduction in total under-five mortality in western Nepal through community-based antimicrobial treatment of pneumonia. Lancet. 1991;338:993–7.

5. Glezen P, Denny FW. Epidemiology of acute lower respiratory disease in children. N Engl J Med. 1973;288:498–505.

6. Turner RB, Lande AE, Chase P, Hilton N, Weinberg D. Pneumonia in pediatric outpatients: cause and clinical manifestations. J Pediatr. 1987;111:194–200.

7. Ramsey BW, Marcuse EK, Foy HM, et al. Use of bacterial antigen detection in the diagnosis of pediatric lower respiratory tract infections. Pediatrics. 1986;78:1–9.

8. Paisley JW, Lauer BA, McIntosh K, Glode MP, Schachter J, Rumack C. Pathogens associated with acute lower respiratory tract infection in young children. Pediatr Infect Dis. 1984;3:14–9.

9. Ponka A, Sarna S. Differential diagnosis of viral, mycoplasmal and bacteraemic pneumococcal pneumonias on admission to hospital. Eur J Respir Dis. 1983;64:360–8.

10. McCarthy PL, Spiesel SZ, Stashwick CA, Ablow RC, Masters SJ, Dolan Jr TF. Radiographic findings and etiologic diagnosis in ambulatory childhood pneumonias. Clin Pediatr (Phila). 1981;20:686–91.

11. Nohynek H, Valkeila E, Leinonen M, Eskola J. Erythrocyte sedimentation rate, white blood cell count and serum C-reactive protein in assessing etiologic diagnosis of acute lower respiratory infections in children. Pediatr Infect Dis J. 1995;14:484–90.

12. Korppi M, Kroger L. C-reactive protein in viral and bacterial respiratory infection in children. Scand J Infect Dis. 1993;25:207–13.

13. Korppi M, Heiskanen-Kosma T, Leinonen M. White blood cells, C-reactive protein and erythrocyte sedimentation rate in pneumococcal pneumonia in children. Eur Respir J. 1997;10:1125–9.

14. Donnelly LF. Imaging in immunocompetent children who have pneumonia. Radiol Clin North Am. 2005;43:253–65.

15. Condon VR. Pneumonia in children. J Thorac Imaging. 1991;6:31–44.

16. Leventhal JM. Clinical predictors of pneumonia as a guide to ordering chest roentgenograms. Clin Pediatr (Phila). 1982;21:730–4.

17. Griscom NT, Wohl ME, Kirkpatrick Jr JA. Lower respiratory infections: how infants differ from adults. Radiol Clin North Am. 1978;16:367–87.

18. Grossman LK, Caplan SE. Clinical, laboratory, and radiological information in the diagnosis of pneumonia in children. Ann Emerg Med. 1988;17:43–6.

19. Alario AJ, McCarthy PL, Markowitz R, Kornguth P, Rosenfield N, Leventhal JM. Usefulness of chest radiographs in children with acute lower respiratory tract disease. J Pediatr. 1987;111:187–93.

20. Denny FW, Clyde Jr WA. Acute lower respiratory tract infections in nonhospitalized children. J Pediatr. 1986;108:635–46.

21. Effmann EL. Pulmonary infection. In: Kuhn JP, Slovis TH, Haller JO, editors. Caffey's pediatric diagnostic imaging. 10th ed. Philadelphia: Mosby; 2004. p. 992–1039.

22. Broughton RA. Infections due to *Mycoplasma pneumoniae* in childhood. Pediatr Infect Dis. 1986;5:71–85.

23. Dubois DB, Ray CG. Viral infections of the lower respiratory tract. In: Taussig LM, Landau LI, editors. Pediatric respiratory medicine. St. Louis: Mosby; 1999. p. 572–9.

24. Denny FW. Acute respiratory tract infections: general considerations. In: Taussig LM, Landau LI, editors. Pediatric respiratory medicine. St. Louis: Mosby; 1999. p. 556–72.

25. Bramson RT, Griscom NT, Cleveland RH. Interpretation of chest radiographs in infants with cough and fever. Radiology. 2005;236:22–9.

26. Jadavji T, Law B, Lebel MH, Kennedy WA, Gold R, Wang EE. A practical guide for the diagnosis and treatment of pediatric pneumonia. CMAJ. 1997;156:S703–11.

27. Murphy TF, Henderson FW, Clyde Jr WA, Collier AM, Denny FW. Pneumonia: an eleven-year study in a pediatric practice. Am J Epidemiol. 1981;113:12–21.

28. Wright AL, Taussig LM, Ray CG, Harrison HR, Holberg CJ. The Tucson Children's Respiratory Study. II. Lower respiratory tract illness in the first year of life. Am J Epidemiol. 1989;129:1232–46.

29. Claesson BA, Trollfors B, Brolin I, et al. Etiology of community-acquired pneumonia in children based on antibody responses to bacterial and viral antigens. Pediatr Infect Dis J. 1989;8:856–62.

30. Hammerschlag MR. Atypical pneumonias in children. Adv Pediatr Infect Dis. 1995;10:1–39.

31. Black SB, Shinefield HR, Ling S, et al. Effectiveness of heptavalent pneumococcal conjugate vaccine in children younger than five years of age for prevention of pneumonia. Pediatr Infect Dis J. 2002;21:810–5.

32. Heiskanen-Kosma T, Korppi M, Leinonen M. Serologically indicated pneumococcal pneumonia in children: a population-based study in primary care settings. APMIS. 2003;111:945–50.

33. WHO. The management of acute respiratory infections in children: practical guidelines for outpatient care. Geneva: World Health Organization; 1995.

34. Zukin DD, Hoffman JR, Cleveland RH, Kushner DC, Herman TE. Correlation of pulmonary signs and symptoms with chest radiographs in the pediatric age group. Ann Emerg Med. 1986;15:792–6.

35. Brant WE, Helms CA. Fundamentals of diagnostic radiology. Philadelphia: Williams & Wilkins; 1999.

36. Kuhn JP, Slovis TL, Haller JO. Caffey's pediatric diagnostic imaging. Philadelphia: Mosby; 2004.

37. Fraser RG, Muller NL, Colman NC, Pare JA. Fraser and Pare's diagnosis of disease of the chest. Philadelphia: Saunders; 1999.

38. Armstrong P, Wilson AG, Dee P, Hansel DM. Imaging of disease of the chest. St. Louis: Mosby; 1995.

39. Goodman LR. Felson's principles of chest roentgenology: a programmed text. Philadelphia: Saunders; 1999.

40. Kim YW, Donnelly LF. Round pneumonia: imaging findings in a large series of children. Pediatr Radiol. 2007;37: 1235–40.

41. Rose RW, Ward BH. Spherical pneumonias in children simulating pulmonary and mediastinal masses. Radiology. 1973;106:179–82.

42. Camargos PA, Ferreira CS. On round pneumonia in children. Pediatr Pulmonol. 1995;20:194–5.

43. McIntosh K. Community-acquired pneumonia in children. N Engl J Med. 2002;346:429–37.

44. Markowitz RI, Ruchelli E. Pneumonia in infants and children: radiological-pathological correlation. Semin Roentgenol. 1998;33:151–62.

45. Swischuk LE, Hayden Jr CK. Viral vs. bacterial pulmonary infections in children (is roentgenographic differentiation possible?). Pediatr Radiol. 1986;16:278–84.

46. Virkki R, Juven T, Rikalainen H, Svedstrom E, Mertsola J, Ruuskanen O. Differentiation of bacterial and viral pneumonia in children. Thorax. 2002;57:438–41.

47. Korppi M, Leinonen M, Koskela M, Makela PH, Launiala K. Bacterial coinfection in children hospitalized with respiratory syncytial virus infections. Pediatr Infect Dis J. 1989;8:687–92.

48. Courtoy I, Lande AE, Turner RB. Accuracy of radiographic differentiation of bacterial from nonbacterial pneumonia. Clin Pediatr (Phila). 1989;28:261–4.

49. Han BK, Son JA, Yoon HK, Lee SI. Epidemic adenoviral lower respiratory tract infection in pediatric patients: radiographic and clinical characteristics. AJR Am J Roentgenol. 1998;170:1077–80.

50. Wahlgren H, Mortensson W, Eriksson M, Finkel Y, Forsgren M. Radiographic patterns and viral studies in childhood pneumonia at various ages. Pediatr Radiol. 1995;25:627–30.

51. Kern S, Uhl M, Berner R, Schwoerer T, Langer M. Respiratory syncytial virus infection of the lower respiratory tract: radiological findings in 108 children. Eur Radiol. 2001;11:2581–4.

52. Kiekara O, Korppi M, Tanska S, Soimakallio S. Radiological diagnosis of pneumonia in children. Ann Med. 1996;28: 69–72.

53. Hopstaken RM, Witbraad T, van Engelshoven JM, Dinant GJ. Inter-observer variation in the interpretation of chest radiographs for pneumonia in community-acquired lower respiratory tract infections. Clin Radiol. 2004;59:743–52.

54. Swingler GH, Hussey GD, Zwarenstein M. Randomised controlled trial of clinical outcome after chest radiograph in ambulatory acute lower-respiratory infection in children. Lancet. 1998;351:404–8.

55. British Thoracic Society Standards of Care Committee. British Thoracic Society guidelines for the management of community acquired pneumonia in childhood. Thorax. 2002;57 Suppl 1:1–24.

56. Cincinatti Children's Hospital Medical Center. Evidence based care guideline: community acquired pneumonia in children 60 days through 17 years of age.

57. Wacogne I, Negrine RJ. Are follow up chest x ray examinations helpful in the management of children recovering from pneumonia? Arch Dis Child. 2003;88:457–8.

58. Blackmore CC, Black WC, Dallas RV, Crow HC. Pleural fluid volume estimation: a chest radiograph prediction rule. Acad Radiol. 1996;3:103–9.

59. Grafakou O, Moustaki M, Tsolia M, et al. Can chest X-ray predict pneumonia severity? Pediatr Pulmonol. 2004;38:465–9.

60. Bachur R, Perry H, Harper MB. Occult pneumonias: empiric chest radiographs in febrile children with leukocytosis. Ann Emerg Med. 1999;33:166–73.

61. Rosenberg DM, Maisels MJ. Chest radiographs in the evaluation of febrile infants under 3 months of age. Clin Pediatr (Phila). 2002;41:67.

62. Heulitt MJ, Ablow RC, Santos CC, O'Shea TM, Hilfer CL. Febrile infants less than 3 months old: value of chest radiography. Radiology. 1988;167:135–7.

63. Patterson RJ, Bisset III GS, Kirks DR, Vanness A. Chest radiographs in the evaluation of the febrile infant. AJR Am J Roentgenol. 1990;155:833–5.

64. Slovis TL. Children, computed tomography radiation dose, and the As Low As Reasonably Achievable (ALARA) concept. Pediatrics. 2003;112:971–2.

65. Brenner D, Elliston C, Hall E, Berdon W. Estimated risks of radiation-induced fatal cancer from pediatric CT. AJR Am J Roentgenol. 2001;176:289–96.

66. Ojutiku O, Haramati LB, Rakoff S, Sprayregen S. Radiology residents' on-call interpretation of chest radiographs for pneumonia. Acad Radiol. 2005;12:658–64.

67. Lynch T, Platt R, Gouin S, Larson C, Patenaude Y. Can we predict which children with clinically suspected pneumonia will have the presence of focal infiltrates on chest radiographs? Pediatrics. 2004;113:e186–9.

68. Reittner P, Ward S, Heyneman L, Johkoh T, Muller NL. Pneumonia: high-resolution CT findings in 114 patients. Eur Radiol. 2003;13:515–21.

69. Tan Kendrick AP, Ling H, Subramaniam R, Joseph VT. The value of early CT in complicated childhood pneumonia. Pediatr Radiol. 2002;32:16–21.

70. Kosucu P, Ahmetoglu A, Cay A, et al. Computed tomography evaluation of cavitary necrosis in complicated childhood pneumonia. Australas Radiol. 2004;48:318–23.

71. Ramnath RR, Heller RM, Ben-Ami T, et al. Implications of early sonographic evaluation of parapneumonic effusions in children with pneumonia. Pediatrics. 1998;101:68–71.

72. Martin L, Buonomo C. Peaiatr Radiol 1997;27:637–41.

73. Conran RM, Stocker JT. Extralobar sequestration with frequently associated congenital cystic adenomatoid malformation, type 2: report of 50 cases. Pediatr Dev Pathol. 1999;2(5):454–63.

74. Griffin N, Devaraj A, Goldstraw P, Bush A, Nicholson AG, Padley S. CT and histopathological correlation of congenital cystic pulmonary lesions: a common pathogenesis? Clin Radiol. 2008;63(9):995–1005.

75. Bratu I, Flageole H, Chen MF, Di Lorenzo M, Yazbeck S, Laberge JM. The multiple facets of pulmonary sequestration. J Pediatr Surg. 2001;36(5):784–90.

76. Newman B. Congenital bronchopulmonary foregut malformations: concepts and controversies. Pediatr Radiol. 2006;36(8):773–91.

77. Pumberger W, Moroder W, Wiesbauer P. Intraabdominal extralobar pulmonary sequestration exhibiting cystic adenomatoid malformation: prenatal diagnosis and characterization of a left suprarenal mass in the newborn. Abdom Imaging. 2001;26(1):28–31.

78. Mani H, Suarez E, Stocker JT. The morphologic spectrum of infantile lobar emphysema: a study of 33 cases. Paediatr Respir Rev. 2004;5(Suppl A):S313–20.

79. Donnelly LF, Lucaya J, Ozelame V, et al. CT findings and temporal course of persistent pulmonary interstitial emphysema in neonates: a multiinstitutional study. AJR Am J Roentgenol. 2003;180(4):1129–33.

80. Jabra AA, Fishman EK, Shehata BM, Perlman EJ. Localized persistent pulmonary interstitial emphysema: CT findings with radiographic-pathologic correlation. AJR Am J Roentgenol. 1997;169(5):1381–4.

81. Mahut B, De Blic J, Emond S, et al. Chest computed tomography findings in bronchopulmonary dysplasia and correlation with lung function. Arch Dis Child Fetal Neonatal Ed. 2007;92(6):F459–64.

82. Oppenheim C, Mamou-Mani T, Sayegh N, de Blic J, Scheinmann P, Lallemand D. Bronchopulmonary dysplasia: value of CT in identifying pulmonary sequelae. AJR Am J Roentgenol. 1994;163(1):169–72.

83. Donnelly LF, Klosterman LA. Cavitary necrosis complicating pneumonia in children: sequential findings on chest radiography. AJR Am J Roentgenol. 1998;171(1):253–6.

84. Erdem CZ, Erdem LO. Radiological characteristics of pulmonary hydatid disease in children: less common radiological appearances. Eur J Radiol. 2003;45(2):123–8.

85. Haliloglu M, Saatci I, Akhan O, Ozmen MN, Besim A. Spectrum of imaging findings in pediatric hydatid disease. AJR Am J Roentgenol. 1997;169(6):1627–31.

86. Donnelly LF, Klosterman LA. Subpleural sparing: a CT finding of lung contusion in children. Radiology. 1997; 204(2):385–7.

87. Manson D, Babyn PS, Palder S, Bergman K. CT of blunt chest trauma in children. Pediatr Radiol. 1993;23(1):1–5.

88. Priest JR, Watterson J, Strong L, et al. Pleuropulmonary blastoma: a marker for familial disease. J Pediatr. 1996;128(2):220–4.

89. Kuhlman JE, Fishman EK, Teigen C. Pulmonary septic emboli: diagnosis with CT. Radiology. 1990;174(1):211–3.

90. Pursner M, Haller JO, Berdon WE. Imaging features of *Mycobacterium avium*-intracellulare complex (MAC) in children with AIDS. Pediatr Radiol. 2000;30(6):426–9.

91. Griffith-Richards SB, Goussard P, Andronikou S, et al. Cavitating pulmonary tuberculosis in children: correlating radiology with pathogenesis. Pediatr Radiol. 2007;37(8): 798–804; quiz 48–9.

92. Wadsworth DT, Siegel MJ, Day DL. Wegener's granulomatosis in children: chest radiographic manifestations. AJR Am J Roentgenol. 1994;163(4):901–4.

93. Levine D, Akikusa J, Manson D, Silverman E, Schneider R. Chest CT findings in pediatric Wegener's granulomatosis. Pediatr Radiol. 2007;37(1):57–62.

94. Lohrmann C, Uhl M, Schaefer O, Ghanem N, Kotter E, Langer M. Serial high-resolution computed tomography imaging in patients with Wegener granulomatosis: differentiation between active inflammatory and chronic fibrotic lesions. Acta Radiol. 2005;46(5):484–91.

95. Kuhlman JE, Hruban RH, Fishman EK. Wegener granulomatosis: CT features of parenchymal lung disease. J Comput Assist Tomogr. 1991;15(6):948–52.

96. Seely JM, Jones LT, Wallace C, Sherry D, Effmann EL. Systemic sclerosis: using high-resolution CT to detect lung disease in children. AJR Am J Roentgenol. 1998;170(3):691–7.

97. Kramer SS, Wehunt WD, Stocker JT, Kashima H. Pulmonary manifestations of juvenile laryngotracheal papillomatosis. AJR Am J Roentgenol. 1985;144(4): 687–94.

98. Braier J, Chantada G, Rosso D, et al. Langerhans cell histiocytosis: retrospective evaluation of 123 patients at a single institution. Pediatr Hematol Oncol. 1999;16(5): 377–85.

99. Abbott GF, Rosado-de-Christenson ML, Franks TJ, Frazier AA, Galvin JR. From the archives of the AFIP: pulmonary Langerhans cell histiocytosis. Radiographics. 2004;24(3): 821–41.

100. Grenier P, Valeyre D, Cluzel P, Brauner MW, Lenoir S, Chastang C. Chronic diffuse interstitial lung disease: diagnostic value of chest radiography and high-resolution CT. Radiology. 1991;179(1):123–32.

101. Brauner MW, Grenier P, Mouelhi MM, Mompoint D, Lenoir S. Pulmonary histiocytosis X: evaluation with high-resolution CT. Radiology. 1989;172(1):255–8.

102. Tateishi U, Hasegawa T, Kusumoto M, et al. Metastatic angiosarcoma of the lung: spectrum of CT findings. AJR Am J Roentgenol. 2003;180(6):1671–4.

103. Abbott GF, Rosado-de-Christenson ML, Frazier AA, Franks TJ, Pugatch RD, Galvin JR. From the archives of the AFIP: lymphangioleiomyomatosis: radiologic-pathologic correlation. Radiographics. 2005;25(3):803–28.

104. Newman B, Urbach AH, Orenstein D, Dickman PS. Proteus syndrome: emphasis on the pulmonary manifestations. Pediatr Radiol. 1994;24(3):189–93.

105. Biko DM, Schwartz M, Anupindi SA, Altes TA. Subpleural lung cysts in Down syndrome: prevalence and association with coexisting diagnoses. Pediatr Radiol. 2008;38(3):280–4.

106. Gonzalez OR, Gomez IG, Recalde AL, Landing BH. Postnatal development of the cystic lung lesion of Down syndrome: suggestion that the cause is reduced formation of peripheral air spaces. Pediatr Pathol. 1991;11(4):623–33.

107. Zamora AC, Collard HR, Wolters PJ, Webb WR, King TE. Neurofibromatosis-associated lung disease: a case series and literature review. Eur Respir J. 2007;29(1):210–4.

108. Wood JR, Bellamy D, Child AH, Citron KM. Pulmonary disease in patients with Marfan syndrome. Thorax. 1984;39(10):780–4.

109. Cohen MC, Kaschula RO. Primary pulmonary tumors in childhood: a review of 31 years' experience and the literature. Pediatr Pulmonol. 1992;14:222–32.

110. Newman B. Congenital bronchopulmonary foregut malformations: concepts and controversies. Pediatr Radiol. 2006;36:773–91.

111. Conran RM, Stocker JT. Extralobar sequestration with frequently associated congenital cystic adenomatoid malformation, type 2: report of 50 cases. Pediatr Dev Pathol. 1999;2:454–63.

112. Hernanz-Schulman M, Stein SM, Neblett WW, et al. Pulmonary sequestration: diagnosis with color Doppler sonography and a new theory of associated hydrothorax. Radiology. 1991;180:817–21.

113. Winters WD, Effmann EL. Congenital masses of the lung: prenatal and postnatal imaging evaluation. J Thorac Imaging. 2001;16:196–206.

114. Stocker JE. The respiratory tract. In: Stocker JT, Dejner LP, editors. Pediatric pathology. 2nd ed. Philadelphia: Lippincott, Williams & Williams; 2001. p. 466–73.

115. Rosado-de-Christenson ML, Stocker JT. Congenital cystic adenomatoid malformation. Radiographics. 1991;11: 865–86.

116. Hedlund GL, Bisset III GS, Bove KE. Malignant neoplasms arising in cystic hamartomas of the lung in childhood. Radiology. 1989;173:77–9.

117. Tagge EP, Mulvihill D, Chandler JC, Richardson M, Uflacker R, Othersen HD. Childhood pleuropulmonary blastoma: caution against nonoperative management of

congenital lung cysts. J Pediatr Surg. 1996;31:187–9; discussion 190.

118. Berrocal T, Madrid C, Novo S, Gutierrez J, Arjonilla A, Gomez-Leon N. Congenital anomalies of the tracheobronchial tree, lung, and mediastinum: embryology, radiology, and pathology. Radiographics. 2004;24:e17.

119. McAdams HP, Kirejczyk WM, Rosado-de-Christenson ML, Matsumoto S. Bronchogenic cyst: imaging features with clinical and histopathologic correlation. Radiology. 2000;217:441–6.

120. Kim YW, Donnelly LF. Round pneumonia: imaging findings in a large series of children. Pediatr Radiol. 2007;37:1235–40.

121. Rose RW, Ward BH. Spherical pneumonias in children simulating pulmonary and mediastinal masses. Radiology. 1973;106:179–82.

122. Camargos PA, Ferreira CS. On round pneumonia in children. Pediatr Pulmonol. 1995;20:194–5.

123. Fonseca-Santos J. Tuberculosis in children. Eur J Radiol. 2005;55:202–8.

124. Rottenberg GT, Shaw P. Radiology of pulmonary tuberculosis. Br J Hosp Med. 1996;56:195–9.

125. McAdams HP, Erasmus J, Winter JA. Radiologic manifestations of pulmonary tuberculosis. Radiol Clin North Am. 1995;33:655–78.

126. Agrons GA, Markowitz RI, Kramer SS. Pulmonary tuberculosis in children. Semin Roentgenol. 1993;28:158–72.

127. Leung AN, Muller NL, Pineda PR, FitzGerald JM. Primary tuberculosis in childhood: radiographic manifestations. Radiology. 1992;182:87–91.

128. Effmann EL. Pulmonary infection. In: Kuhn JP, Slovis TH, Haller JO, editors. Caffey's pediatric diagnostic imaging. 10th ed. Philadelphia: Mosby; 2004. p. 992–1039.

129. McGuinness G, Naidich DP, Jagirdar J, Leitman B, McCauley DI. High resolution CT findings in miliary lung disease. J Comput Assist Tomogr. 1992;16:384–90.

130. Lamont AC, Cremin BJ, Pelteret RM. Radiological patterns of pulmonary tuberculosis in the paediatric age group. Pediatr Radiol. 1986;16:2–7.

131. Gurney JW, Conces DJ. Pulmonary histoplasmosis. Radiology. 1996;199:297–306.

132. Wheat LJ, Wass J, Norton J, Kohler RB, French ML. Cavitary histoplasmosis occurring during two large urban outbreaks. Analysis of clinical, epidemiologic, roentgenographic, and laboratory features. Medicine (Baltimore). 1984;63:201–9.

133. Child DD, Newell JD, Bjelland JC, Spark RP. Radiographic findings of pulmonary coccidioidomycosis in neonates and infants. AJR Am J Roentgenol. 1985;145:261–3.

134. Davies SF, Sarosi GA. Epidemiological and clinical features of pulmonary blastomycosis. Semin Respir Infect. 1997;12:206–18.

135. Chuck SL, Sande MA. Infections with *Cryptococcus neoformans* in the acquired immunodeficiency syndrome. N Engl J Med. 1989;321:794–9.

136. Buff SJ, McLelland R, Gallis HA, Matthay R, Putman CE. *Candida albicans* pneumonia: radiographic appearance. AJR Am J Roentgenol. 1982;138:645–8.

137. Kassner EG, Kauffman SL, Yoon JJ, Semiglia M, Kozinn PJ, Goldberg PL. Pulmonary candidiasis in infants: clinical, radiologic, and pathologic features. AJR Am J Roentgenol. 1981;137:707–16.

138. Aquino SL, Kee ST, Warnock ML, Gamsu G. Pulmonary aspergillosis: imaging findings with pathologic correlation. AJR Am J Roentgenol. 1994;163:811–5.

139. Logan PM, Primack SL, Miller RR, Muller NL. Invasive aspergillosis of the airways: radiographic, CT, and pathologic findings. Radiology. 1994;193:383–8.

140. Knutsen AP, Slavin RG. Allergic bronchopulmonary aspergillosis in patients with cystic fibrosis. Clin Rev Allergy. 1991;9:103–18.

141. Abramson S. The air crescent sign. Radiology. 2001;218: 230–2.

142. Gefter WB, Weingrad TR, Epstein DM, Ochs RH, Miller WT. "Semi-invasive" pulmonary aspergillosis: a new look at the spectrum of *Aspergillus* infections of the lung. Radiology. 1981;140:313–21.

143. Cheon JE, Im JG, Kim MY, Lee JS, Choi GM, Yeon KM. Thoracic actinomycosis: CT findings. Radiology. 1998;209:229–33.

144. Yoon HK, Im JG, Ahn JM, Han MC. Pulmonary nocardiosis: CT findings. J Comput Assist Tomogr. 1995;19:52–5.

145. Feigin DS. Nocardiosis of the lung: chest radiographic findings in 21 cases. Radiology. 1986;159:9–14.

146. Erdem CZ, Erdem LO. Radiological characteristics of pulmonary hydatid disease in children: less common radiological appearances. Eur J Radiol. 2003;45:123–8.

147. Hajjar WA, Ashour MH, Al-Rikabi AC. Endobronchial inflammatory pseudotumor of the lung. Saudi Med J. 2001;22:366–8.

148. Kim JH, Cho JH, Park MS, et al. Pulmonary inflammatory pseudotumor – a report of 28 cases. Korean J Intern Med. 2002;17:252–8.

149. Kim TS, Han J, Kim GY, Lee KS, Kim H, Kim J. Pulmonary inflammatory pseudotumor (inflammatory myofibroblastic tumor): CT features with pathologic correlation. J Comput Assist Tomogr. 2005;29:633–9.

150. Kim I, Kim WS, Yeon KM, Chi JG. Inflammatory pseudotumor of the lung manifesting as a posterior mediastinal mass. Pediatr Radiol. 1992;22:467–8.

151. Hedlund GL, Navoy JF, Galliani CA, Johnson Jr WH. Aggressive manifestations of inflammatory pulmonary pseudotumor in children. Pediatr Radiol. 1999;29:112–6.

152. Berman M, Georghiou GP, Schonfeld T, et al. Pulmonary inflammatory myofibroblastic tumor invading the left atrium. Ann Thorac Surg. 2003;76:601–3.

153. Agrons GA, Rosado-de-Christenson ML, Kirejczyk WM, Conran RM, Stocker JT. Pulmonary inflammatory pseudotumor: radiologic features. Radiology. 1998;206:511–8.

154. Mas Estelles F, Andres V, Vallcanera A, Muro D, Cortina H. Plasma cell granuloma of the lung in childhood: atypical radiologic findings and association with hypertrophic osteoarthropathy. Pediatr Radiol. 1995;25:369–72.

155. Pichler G, Eber E, Thalhammer G, Muntean W, Zach MS. Arthralgia and digital clubbing in a child: hypertrophic osteoarthropathy with inflammatory pseudotumour of the lung. Scand J Rheumatol. 2004;33:189–91.

156. Messineo A, Mognato G, D'Amore ES, Antoniello L, Guglielmi M, Cecchetto G. Inflammatory pseudotumors of the lung in children: conservative or aggressive approach? Med Pediatr Oncol. 1998;31:100–4.

157. Sagel SS, Ablow RC. Hamartoma: on occasion a rapidly growing tumor of the lung. Radiology. 1968;91:971–2.

158. Davies MR, Cywes S, Rode H. Cystic pulmonary hamartoma simulating posterolateral diaphragmatic hernia. S Afr Med J. 1979;56:947–50.

159. Meza MP, Newman B, Dickman PS, Towbin RB. Pediatric case of the day. Pulmonary mesenchymal cystic hamartoma. Radiographics. 1992;12:843–4.

160. Carney JA, Sheps SG, Go VL, Gordon H. The triad of gastric leiomyosarcoma, functioning extra-adrenal paraganglioma and pulmonary chondroma. N Engl J Med. 1977;296:1517–8.

161. Green D. Incidental findings computed tomography of the thorax. Semin Ultrasound CT MR. 2005;26:14–9.

162. Davila DG, Dunn WF, Tazelaar HD, Pairolero PC. Bronchial carcinoid tumors. Mayo Clin Proc. 1993;68:795–803.

163. Nessi R, Basso Ricci P, Basso Ricci S, Bosco M, Blanc M, Uslenghi C. Bronchial carcinoid tumors: radiologic observations in 49 cases. J Thorac Imaging. 1991;6:47–53.

164. Rosado de Christenson ML, Abbott GF, Kirejczyk WM, Galvin JR, Travis WD. Thoracic carcinoids: radiologic-pathologic correlation. Radiographics. 1999;19:707–36.

165. Shelley BE, Lorenzo RL. Primary squamous cell carcinoma of the lung in childhood. Pediatr Radiol. 1983;13:92–4.

166. Graham Jr JM, Boyle W, Troxell J, Cullity GJ, Sprague PL, Beckwith JB. Cystic hamartomata of lung and kidney: a spectrum of developmental abnormalities. Am J Med Genet. 1987;27:45–59.

167. Ishida Y, Kato K, Kigasawa H, Ohama Y, Ijiri R, Tanaka Y. Synchronous occurrence of pleuropulmonary blastoma and cystic nephroma: possible genetic link in cystic lesions of the lung and the kidney. Med Pediatr Oncol. 2000;35:85–7.

168. Senac Jr MO, Wood BP, Isaacs H, Weller M. Pulmonary blastoma: a rare childhood malignancy. Radiology. 1991;179:743–6.

169. Solomon A, Rubinstein ZJ, Rogoff M, Rozenman J, Urbach D. Pulmonary blastoma. Pediatr Radiol. 1982;12:148–9.

170. Mei-Zahav M, Letarte M, Faughnan ME, Abdalla SA, Cymerman U, MacLusky IB. Symptomatic children with hereditary hemorrhagic telangiectasia: a pediatric center experience. Arch Pediatr Adolesc Med. 2006;160:596–601.

171. McCue CM, Hartenberg M, Nance WE. Pulmonary arteriovenous malformations related to Rendu-Osler-Weber syndrome. Am J Med Genet. 1984;19:19–27.

172. Bartram O, Strickland B. Pulmonary varices. Proc R Soc Med. 1971;64:839.

173. Chilton SJ, Campbell JB. Pulmonary varix in early infancy: case report with 8-year follow up. Radiology. 1978;129:400.

174. Dinsmore BJ, Gefter WB, Hatabu H, Kressel HY. Pulmonary arteriovenous malformations: diagnosis by gradient-refocused MR imaging. J Comput Assist Tomogr. 1990;14:918–23.

175. Rankin S, Faling LJ, Pugatch RD. CT diagnosis of pulmonary arteriovenous malformations. J Comput Assist Tomogr. 1982;6:746–9.

176. Eggli KD, Newman B. Nodules, masses, and pseudomasses in the pediatric lung. Radiol Clin North Am. 1993;31:651–66.

177. Somekh E, Maharashak N, Shapira Y, Greenberg D, Dagan R. Hospitalization for primary varicella-zoster virus infection and its complications in patients from Southern Israel. Infection. 2000;28:200–4.

178. Saulsbury FT. Varicella pneumonia as the presenting manifestation of immunodeficiency. Clin Pediatr (Phila). 1991;30:555–8.

179. Mitnick J, Becker MH, Rothberg M, Genieser NB. Nodular residua of atypical measles pneumonia. AJR Am J Roentgenol. 1980;134:257–60.

180. Martin DB, Weiner LB, Nieburg PI, Blair DC. Atypical measles in adolescents and young adults. Ann Intern Med. 1979;90:877–81.

181. Markowitz LE, Chandler FW, Roldan EO, et al. Fatal measles pneumonia without rash in a child with AIDS. J Infect Dis. 1988;158:480–3.

182. Conte P, Heitzman ER, Markarian B. Viral pneumonia. Roentgen pathological correlations. Radiology. 1970;95:267–72.

183. Cook RJ, Ashton RW, Aughenbaugh GL, Ryu JH. Septic pulmonary embolism: presenting features and clinical course of 14 patients. Chest. 2005;128:162–6.

184. Gonzalez BE, Teruya J, Mahoney Jr DH, et al. Venous thrombosis associated with staphylococcal osteomyelitis in children. Pediatrics. 2006;117:1673–9.

185. Goldenberg NA, Knapp-Clevenger R, Hays T, Manco-Johnson MJ. Lemierre's and Lemierre's-like syndromes in children: survival and thromboembolic outcomes. Pediatrics. 2005;116:e543–8.

186. Wong KS, Lin TY, Huang YC, Hsia SH, Yang PH, Chu SM. Clinical and radiographic spectrum of septic pulmonary embolism. Arch Dis Child. 2002;87:312–5.

187. Dodd JD, Souza CA, Muller NL. High-resolution MDCT of pulmonary septic embolism: evaluation of the feeding vessel sign. AJR Am J Roentgenol. 2006;187:623–9.

188. Alsofrom DJ, Mettler Jr FA, Mann JM. Radiographic manifestations of plaque in New Mexico, 1975–1980. A review of 42 proved cases. Radiology. 1981;139:561–5.

189. Maile CW, Rodan BA, Godwin JD, Chen JT, Ravin CE. Calcification in pulmonary metastases. Br J Radiol. 1982;55:108–13.

190. Armstrong P, Dyer R, Alford BA, O'Hara M. Leukemic pulmonary infiltrates: rapid development mimicking pulmonary edema. AJR Am J Roentgenol. 1980;135:373–4.

191. Cohen M, Smith WL, Weetman R, Provisor A. Pulmonary pseudometastases in children with malignant tumors. Radiology. 1981;141:371–4.

192. Winer-Muram HT, Arheart KL, Jennings SG, Rubin SA, Kauffman WM, Slobod KS. Pulmonary complications in children with hematologic malignancies: accuracy of diagnosis with chest radiography and CT. Radiology. 1997;204:643–9.

193. Castellino RA, Bellani FF, Gasparini M, Musumeci R. Radiographic findings in previously untreated children with non-Hodgkin's lymphoma. Radiology. 1975;117:657–63.

194. Soldatski IL, Onufrieva EK, Steklov AM, Schepin NV. Tracheal, bronchial, and pulmonary papillomatosis in children. Laryngoscope. 2005;115:1848–54.

195. Simma B, Burger R, Uehlinger J, et al. Squamous-cell carcinoma arising in a non-irradiated child with recurrent respiratory papillomatosis. Eur J Pediatr. 1993;152:776–8.

196. Godwin JD, Webb WR, Savoca CJ, Gamsu G, Goodman PC. Multiple, thin-walled cystic lesions of the lung. AJR Am J Roentgenol. 1980;135:593–604.

197. Smith L, Gooding CA. Pulmonary involvement in laryngeal papillomatosis. Pediatr Radiol. 1974;2:161–6.

198. Kramer SS, Wehunt WD, Stocker JT, Kashima H. Pulmonary manifestations of juvenile laryngotracheal papillomatosis. AJR Am J Roentgenol. 1985;144:687–94.

199. Mayberry JP, Primack SL, Muller NL. Thoracic manifestations of systemic autoimmune diseases: radiographic and high-resolution CT findings. Radiographics. 2000;20:1623–35.

200. Yousefzadeh DK, Fishman PA. The triad of pneumonitis, pleuritis, and pericarditis in juvenile rheumatoid arthritis. Pediatr Radiol. 1979;8:147–50.
201. Tanaka N, Newell JD, Brown KK, Cool CD, Lynch DA. Collagen vascular disease-related lung disease: high-resolution computed tomography findings based on the pathologic classification. J Comput Assist Tomogr. 2004;28:351–60.
202. Ramirez RE, Glasier C, Kirks D, Shackelford GD, Locey M. Pulmonary hemorrhage associated with systemic lupus erythematosus in children. Radiology. 1984;152:409–12.
203. Frazier AA, Rosado-de-Christenson ML, Galvin JR, Fleming MV. Pulmonary angiitis and granulomatosis: radiologic-pathologic correlation. Radiographics. 1998;18:687–710; quiz 727.
204. Staples CA. Pulmonary angiitis and granulomatosis. Radiol Clin North Am. 1991;29:973–82.
205. Wadsworth DT, Siegel MJ, Day DL. Wegener's granulomatosis in children: chest radiographic manifestations. AJR Am J Roentgenol. 1994;163:901–4.
206. Abril A, Calamia KT, Cohen MD. The Churg Strauss syndrome (allergic granulomatous angiitis): review and update. Semin Arthritis Rheum. 2003;33:106–14.
207. Silva CI, Muller NL, Fujimoto K, Johkoh T, Ajzen SA, Churg A. Churg-Strauss syndrome: high resolution CT and pathologic findings. J Thorac Imaging. 2005;20:74–80.
208. Bolaman Z, Kadikoylu G, Polatli M, Barutca S, Culhaci N, Senturk T. Migratory nodules in the lung: lymphomatoid granulomatosis. Leuk Lymphoma. 2003;44:197–200.
209. Morris JC, Rosen MJ, Marchevsky A, Teirstein AS. Lymphocytic interstitial pneumonia in patients at risk for the acquired immune deficiency syndrome. Chest. 1987;91:63–7.
210. Nadal D, Caduff R, Frey E, et al. Non-Hodgkin's lymphoma in four children infected with the human immunodeficiency virus. Association with Epstein-Barr Virus and treatment. Cancer. 1994;73:224–30.
211. Houghton KM, Cabral DA, Petty RE, Tucker LB. Primary Sjogren's syndrome in dizygotic adolescent twins: one case with lymphocytic interstitial pneumonia. J Rheumatol. 2005;32:1603–6.
212. Marks MJ, Haney PJ, McDermott MP, White CS, Vennos AD. Thoracic disease in children with AIDS. Radiographics. 1996;16:1349–62.
213. Johkoh T, Ichikado K, Akira M, et al. Lymphocytic interstitial pneumonia: follow-up CT findings in 14 patients. J Thorac Imaging. 2000;15:162–7.
214. Becciolini V, Gudinchet F, Cheseaux JJ, Schnyder P. Lymphocytic interstitial pneumonia in children with AIDS: high-resolution CT findings. Eur Radiol. 2001;11:1015–20.
215. Shetty AK, Gedalia A. Sarcoidosis: a pediatric perspective. Clin Pediatr (Phila). 1998;37:707–17.
216. Merten DF, Kirks DR, Grossman H. Pulmonary sarcoidosis in childhood. AJR Am J Roentgenol. 1980;135:673–9.
217. Keesling CA, Frush DP, O'Hara SM, Fordham LA. Clinical and imaging manifestations of pediatric sarcoidosis. Acad Radiol. 1998;5:122–32.
218. Hafner R, Vogel P. Sarcoidosis of early onset. A challenge for the pediatric rheumatologist. Clin Exp Rheumatol. 1993;11:685–91.
219. Braier J, Chantada G, Rosso D, et al. Langerhans cell histiocytosis: retrospective evaluation of 123 patients at a single institution. Pediatr Hematol Oncol. 1999;16:377–85.
220. Abbott GF, Rosado-de-Christenson ML, Franks TJ, Frazier AA, Galvin JR. From the archives of the AFIP: pulmonary Langerhans cell histiocytosis. Radiographics. 2004;24(3):821–41.
221. Smets A, Mortele K, de Praeter G, Francois O, Benoit Y, Kunnen M. Pulmonary and mediastinal lesions in children with Langerhans cell histiocytosis. Pediatr Radiol. 1997;27:873–6.
222. Meyer JS, Harty MP, Mahboubi S, et al. Langerhans cell histiocytosis: presentation and evolution of radiologic findings with clinical correlation. Radiographics. 1995;15:1135–46.
223. Helbich TH, Wojnarovsky C, Wunderbaldinger P, Heinz-Peer G, Eichler I, Herold CJ. Pulmonary alveolar microlithiasis in children: radiographic and high-resolution CT findings. AJR Am J Roentgenol. 1997;168:63–5.
224. Sumikawa H, Johkoh T, Tomiyama N, et al. Pulmonary alveolar microlithiasis: CT and pathologic findings in 10 patients. Monaldi Arch Chest Dis. 2005;63:59–64.
225. Korn MA, Schurawitzki H, Klepetko W, Burghuber OC. Pulmonary alveolar microlithiasis: findings on high-resolution CT. AJR Am J Roentgenol. 1992;158:981–2.
226. Volle E, Kaufmann HJ. Pulmonary alveolar microlithiasis in pediatric patients – review of the world literature and two new observations. Pediatr Radiol. 1987;17:439–42.
227. The ALARA (As Low As Reasonably Achievable) Concept in Pediatric CT Intelligent Dose Reduction. Multidisciplinary conference organized by the Society of Pediatric Radiology. August 18–19, 2001. Pediatr Radiol. 2002;32:217–313.
228. Frush DP, Donnelly LF, Rosen NS. Computed tomography and radiation risks: what pediatric health care providers should know. Pediatrics. 2003;112:951–7.
229. Shah R, Cestone P, Mueller C. Congenital multiple peripheral pulmonary artery stenosis (pulmonary branch stenosis or supravalvular pulmonary stenosis). AJR Am J Roentgenol. 2000;175:856–7.
230. Kerem E, Bar Ziv Y, Rudenski B, Katz S, Kleid D, Branski D. Bacteremic necrotizing pneumococcal pneumonia in children. Am J Respir Crit Care Med. 1994;149:242–4.
231. Chen KC, Su YT, Lin WL, Chiu KC, Niu CK. Clinical analysis of necrotizing pneumonia in children: three-year experience in a single medical center. Acta Paediatr Taiwan. 2003;44:343–8.
232. Hacimustafaoglu M, Celebi S, Sarimehmet H, Gurpinar A, Ercan I. Necrotizing pneumonia in children. Acta Paediatr. 2004;93:1172–7.
233. McCarthy VP, Patamasucon P, Gaines T, Lucas MA. Necrotizing pneumococcal pneumonia in childhood. Pediatr Pulmonol. 1999;28:217–21.
234. Wong KS, Chiu CH, Yeow KM, Huang YC, Liu HP, Lin TY. Necrotising pneumonitis in children. Eur J Pediatr. 2000;159:684–8.
235. Schadeck T, Beckers D, Eucher P, deBilderling G, Tuerlinckx D, Bodart E. Necrotizing pneumonia in children: apropos 4 cases. Arch Pediatr. 2006;13:1209–14.
236. Ramphul N, Eastham KM, Freeman R, Eltringham G, Kearns AM, Leeming JP, et al. Cavitatory lung disease complicating empyema in children. Pediatr Pulmonol. 2006;41:750–3.
237. Sawicki GS, Lu FL, Valim C, Cleveland RC, Colin AA. Necrotizing pneumonia is increasingly detected as a complication of pneumonia in children. Eur Respir J. 2008;31(6):1285–91.

238. Schultz KD, Fan LL, Pinsky J, Ochoa L, Smith EO, Kaplan SL, et al. The changing face of pleural empyemas in children: epidemiology and management. Pediatrics. 2004;113:1735–40.

239. Curry CA, Fishman EK, Buckley JA. Pulmonary gangrene: radiologic and pathologic correlation. South Med J. 1999;91:957–60.

240. Hsieh YC, Hsiao CH, Tsao PN, Wang JY, Hsieh PR, Chiang BL, et al. Necrotizing pneumococcal pneumonia in children: the role of pulmonary gangrene. Pediatr Pulmonol. 2006;41:623–9.

241. Hsieh YC, Hsueh PR, Lu CY, Lee PI, Lee CY, Huang LM. Clinical manifestations and molecular epidemiology of necrotizing pneumonia and empyema caused by *Streptococcus pneumoniae* in children in Taiwan. Clin Infect Dis. 2004;38:830–5.

242. Oermann C, Sockrider MM, Langston C. Severe necrotizing pneumonitis in a child with *Mycoplasma pneumoniae* infection. Pediatr Pulmonol. 1997;24:61–5.

243. Wang RS, Wang SY, Hsieh KS, Chiou YH, Huang IF, Cheng MF, et al. Necrotizing pneumonitis caused by *Mycoplasma pneumoniae* in pediatric patients: report of five cases and review of literature. Pediatr Infect Dis J. 2004;23:564–7.

244. Cengiz AB, Kanra G, Caglar M, Kar A, Gucer S, Ince T. Fatal necrotizing pneumonia caused by group A streptococcus. J Paediatr Child Health. 2004;40:69–71.

245. Tsai MH, Huang YC, Chen CJ, Lin PY, Chang LY, Chiu CH, et al. Chlamydial pneumonia in children requiring hospitalization: effect of mixed infection on clinical outcome. J Microbiol Immunol Infect. 2005;38:117–22.

246. Gillet Y, Issartel B, Vanhems P, Lina G, Vandenesch F, Etienne J, et al. Severe staphylococcal pneumonia in children. Arch Pediatr. 2001;8 Suppl 4:742s–6.

247. Al-Tawfiq JA, Aldaabil RA. Community-acquired MRSA bacteremic necrotizing pneumonia in a patient with scrotal ulceration. J Infect. 2005;51:e241–3.

248. Labandeira-Rey M, Couzon F, Boisset S, Brown EL, Bes M, Benito Y, et al. *Staphylococcus aureus* Panton-Valentine leukocidin causes necrotizing pneumonia. Science. 2007;315(5815):1130–3.

249. Gilbert CR, Vipul K, Baram M. Novel H1N1 influenza A viral infection complicated by alveolar hemorrhage. Respir Care. 2010;55(5):623–5.

250. Hodina M, Hanquinet S, Cotting J, Schnyder P, Gudinchet F. Imaging of cavitary necrosis in complicated childhood pneumonia. Eur Radiol. 2002;12:391–6.

251. Hoffer FA, Bloom DA, Colin AA, Fishman SJ. Lung abscess versus necrotizing pneumonia: implications for interventional therapy. Pediatr Radiol. 1999;29:87–91.

252. Li ST, Gates RL. Primary operative management for pediatric empyema: decreases in hospital length of stay and charges in a national sample. Arch Pediatr Adolesc Med. 2008;162(1):44–8.

253. Ayed AK, Al-Rowayeh A. Lung resection in children for infectious pulmonary diseases. Pediatr Surg Int. 2005;21:604–8.

254. Eren S, Eren MN, Balci AE. Pneumonectomy in children for destroyed lung and the long-term consequences. J Thorac Cardiovasc Surg. 2003;126:574–81.

255. Kalfa N, Allal H, Lopez M, Counil FO, Forques D, Guibal MP, et al. An early thoracoscopic approach in necrotizing pneumonia in children: a report of three cases. J Laparoendosc Adv Surg Tech A. 2005;15:18–22.

256. Donnelly LF, Klosterman LA. Cavitary necrosis complicating pneumonia in children: sequential findings on chest radiography. AJR Am J Roentgenol. 1998;171:253–6.

Pleural Effusion and Pneumothorax

12

Efraim Sadot

The pleural space is bounded by two membranes. The visceral pleura covering the lung, and the parietal pleura covering the chest wall, mediastinum and the diaphragm. Protein-containing fluid, derives from the systemic circulation, resides in the pleural space and is continuously absorbed by the lymphatics of the parietal pleura. Sub-atmospheric pressure in the pleural space aids in mechanical coupling of lung inflation throughout the respiratory cycle. Development of the pleura is notable by the third week of gestation along with the pericardial and peritoneal spaces [1]. By 9 weeks of gestation, the pleural space becomes separated.

12.1 Pleural Effusion

The volume of normal pleural fluid is small and approximates 0.26 mL/kg body weight [2]. In the healthy pleura, about 10% of the volume is formed hourly and the same volume is absorbed to maintain steady state. Hydrostatic pressure opposed by counter balancing osmotic pressure with an average of approximately 12 cmH_2O drives pressure for the movement of liquid into the pleural space.

Pleural fluid originates from systemic vessels that feed the pleura and it is assumed that the parietal pleura is the major source for fluid formation [3]. Several mechanisms are suggested for fluid removal from the pleural space including re-absorption by mesothelial cells and passive flow of fluid into the low-pressure interstitial space of the lung. The most likely route of fluid removal is by lymphatic drainage via openings in the parietal portion of the pleural membrane, the stomata. Flow of lymphatic fluid is influenced both by contractility of the lymph vessels and by respiratory movements [4–6].

When balance between the entry and exit of fluid is disturbed, pleural effusion develops. Both mechanisms, increase in fluid entrance and decrease in fluid clearance, contribute to fluid accumulation [7]. Increase in fluid entry can be due to increase in fluid conductance through the pleura, elevated microvascular pressure (venous more than arterial), decrease in pleural pressure (as seen in significant atelectasis) and decrease in plasma oncotic pressure. Decrease in fluid clearance is usually the result of reduction in lymphatic drainage as listed in Table 12.1.

Efraim Sadot, MD(✉)
Dana Children's Hospital, Tel-Aviv Sourasky Medical Center,
6 Weizmann Street, Tel-Aviv, 64239, Israel
e-mail: efraims@tasmc.health.gov.il

R.H. Cleveland (ed.), *Imaging in Pediatric Pulmonology*,
DOI 10.1007/978-1-4419-5872-3_12, © Springer Science+Business Media, LLC 2012

Table 12.1. Factors altering pleural lymphatic drainage

Intrinsic	Extrinsic
Inflammation	Increase central venous pressure
Injury (e.g., iatrogenic during surgery, irradiation, etc.)	Pleural disease (pneumonia, malignancy) with decreased or blocked stomata
Congenital abnormality (e.g., lymphangiectasis)	Compression of the lymphatic vessels Decreased motion of the diaphragm (e.g., collapsed lung, diaphragmatic paralysis)

Table 12.2. Light's criteria to differentiate transudate from exudate

Protein ratio (pleural fluid/serum) less than 0.5
Lactic dehydrogenase (LDH) ratio (pleural fluid/serum) greater than 0.6
Pleural fluid LDH more than 2/3 the upper limit for serum

Normal pleural fluid is clear in appearance, slightly alkaline compared to serum, has low protein content (1–2 g/dL), 1,500–4,500 white blood cells per cubic millimeter, mostly monocytes. Glucose content is similar to that of plasma, and lactate dehydrogenase level is less than 50% of plasma [8]. Abnormal pleural fluid should be characterized in order to distinguish different pathophysiologic processes. The Light criteria assist in differentiating transudate from exudate (Table 12.2) [9]. When none of the criteria are met, fluid accumulation is likely transudate.

Fluid pH, glucose concentration, white cell count and differential, stains, cultures and specific serologic assays are additional tests that assist in characterizing the fluid nature. When pleural fluid sample is milky in appearance, or a question of chylothorax is raised (e.g., congenital or following surgical intervention), triglyceride level should be checked to ascertain if it is elevated above 110 mg/dL. When fluid is bloody with a hematocrit of greater than 50% that in blood, hemothorax is likely the diagnosis.

Empyema is the presence of purulent material consisting typically of neutrophils and fibrin in the pleural space. Nearly one-half of all children with bacterial pneumonia will develop parapneumonic effusions. Approximately 5% of the effusions complicating community-acquired pneumonia progress to empyema with an increase in the incidence of empyema over time [10]. Progression of a pleural effusion to empyema starts with the *exudative* phase, where most pleural effusions progress to and resolve with antibiotics alone [11, 12]. The *fibrinopurulent* phase is the next stage that starts when the pleural fluid becomes infected. White blood cells, mainly neutrophils, accumulate and fibrin deposition starts. The fluid becomes loculated, with decrease in pH and glucose concentration and increase in lactate dehydrogenase concentration. The most common pathogens in children are *Streptococcus pneumoniae*, *Staphylococcus aureus* and *Streptococcus pyogenes* [11, 13–15]. The *organization* step takes place when fibroblasts migrate into the fluid and form membranes. Complications of empyema include restriction of inspiration, bronchopleural fistula, bacteremia, pericarditis and pneumothorax. In addition to infected pleural effusion, two other conditions commonly will be associated with organizing effusions, hemothorax and malignant effusions (other than lymphoma).

12.2 Imaging Studies

It is important to recognize even a small pleural effusion as it will affect the differential diagnosis. In practice, this is most commonly relevant in differentiating bacterial pneumonia (may have an effusion) as opposed to viral infection (rarely has an effusion). In preterm neonates with respiratory distress, a small effusion suggests neonatal pneumonia or transient tachypnea as opposed to uncomplicated hyaline membrane disease.

Free pleural fluid will accumulate in the dependent area. In the upright patient, a small amount of pleural fluid will blunt the posterior costophrenic angle, often more apparent on a lateral chest X-ray (CXR) than on frontal projection (Fig. 12.1). With slightly larger effusions, a small amount of fluid will be noted in the lateral costophrenic angle (Fig. 12.2) and often the medial costophrenic angle. As more fluid accumulates, the entire outline of the diaphragm on the affected side may become obscured with fluid extending upward around the anterior, lateral and posterior thoracic walls, producing opacification of the lung base with a smooth tapering meniscus narrowing superiorly (Fig. 12.3).

In the supine position, small effusions will first be seen as an apical cap (Fig. 12.4) and then, as it enlarges, as blunting of the inferior medial costophrenic sulcus (Fig. 12.5) and subsequently the lateral costophrenic angle (Fig. 12.6). As it enlarges further, it will build up around the lung, and will extend into the fissures (Fig. 12.7) eventually causing

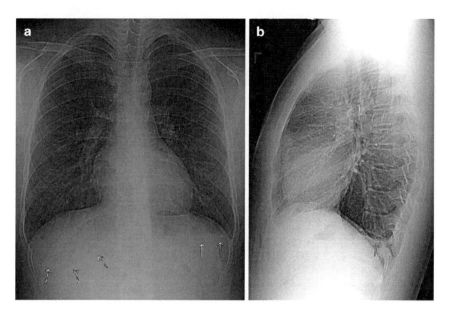

Fig. 12.1. (a) PA image: *Right arrows* indicate the normal posterior costophrenic margin. *Left arrows* point to the stomach air/fluid level. No clear effusion is noted. (b) Lateral image: *Arrows* indicate a small left sided pleural effusion, obscured by the gastric content on the PA image

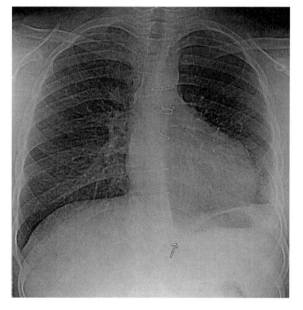

Fig. 12.2. A small effusion is noted in the lateral costophrenic angle, with a component in the inferior portion of the major fissure. The *arrow* indicates fluid in the medial costophrenic angle

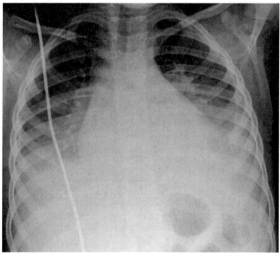

Fig. 12.3. There is a moderate effusion on the left extending up the lateral chest wall. A similarly distributed, smaller effusion is present on the right

the entire hemithorax to become opacified [16] (Fig. 12.8). Lateral decubitus film, while lying on the affected side, can help in differentiating between the presence of fluid and other reasons for opacification such as large pneumonia or pleural thickening (Figs. 12.3, 12.9). As little as 5 mL of pleural fluid can be detected with properly exposed decubitus radiographs [17]. When pleural fluid is loculated, the contour of the effusion may be irregular and not conform to gravitational forces. It will not change appreciably in distribution on decubitus imaging (Fig. 12.10). When the whole hemithorax is opacified, decubitus radiographs are of no use and ultrasonic examination or computed tomography (CT) should be

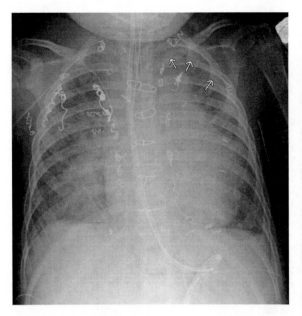

Fig. 12.4. *Arrows* indicate a small effusion extending over the left apex and somewhat laterally. A smaller effusion is also noted on the right

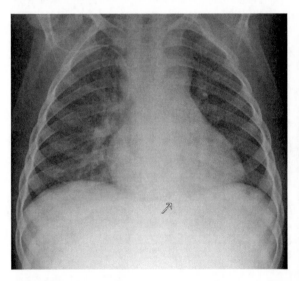

Fig. 12.5. *Arrow* indicates a small amount of fluid blunting the medial costophrenic angle

obtained. The advantages of ultrasound over CT are the ease and speed with which the study can be done and the absence of irradiation. Both have the ability to provide real-time guidance for thoracocentesis when required [18] (Fig. 12.11).

CT is the best study to visualize the pleural space [19, 20] (Fig. 12.12). CT differentiates parenchymal and pleural lesions, such as lung abscess and necrotizing pneumonia from an air fluid level due to empyema, and in addition CT has the ability to image the margins of the lesion well. When pulmonary embolism is suspected, CT angiography (CTA) is the study of choice with high sensitivity and specificity for proximal or segmental pulmonary artery involvement [21, 22].

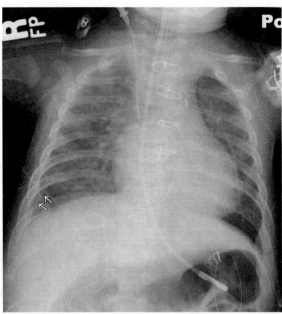

Fig. 12.6. There is blunting of the right lateral costophrenic angle with a small amount of fluid in the major fissure (*arrows*)

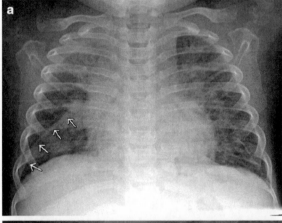

Fig. 12.7. (a) *Arrows* indicate a moderate amount of fluid in the right major fissure. (b) *Arrow* indicates a small amount of fluid in the minor fissure with effusions surrounding both lungs

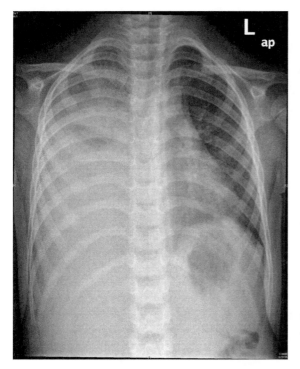

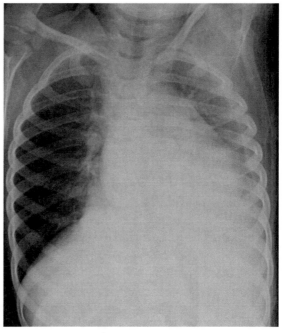

Fig. 12.8. There is almost complete opacification of the right hemithorax secondary to pneumonia and a large right effusion

Fig. 12.9. Free flowing effusion on supine is shown in Fig. 12.3. In this figure the left decubitus image reveals layering of the effusion dependently on the left. The right effusion has layered medially and is not convincingly seen

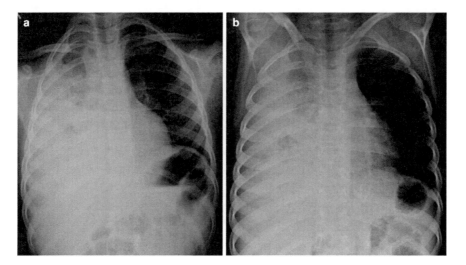

Fig. 12.10. Loculated pleural effusion on supine (a) and decubitus (b) images with no significant change in the configuration or distribution of the effusion

12.3 Exudative Pleural Effusions

Exudative pleural effusions are common and may develop as a result of infection, inflammation, injury or malignancy. They are all prone to becoming organized and loculated. Effusions caused by pus, blood or malignancy often become loculated. Once this occurs, it will no longer be free flowing. If an effusion is irregular in its configuration or is not dominantly in the dependent portion of the hemithorax, it is either partly or completely loculated (Fig. 12.10).

Parapneumonic effusion is an effusion associated with an infection of the lung with the spread of inflammation and infection to the pleural space. These effusions are becoming more common in the pediatric population with an increase in incidence that coincides with the rise in antibiotic resistant organisms [23–27]. It is more common to develop parapneu-

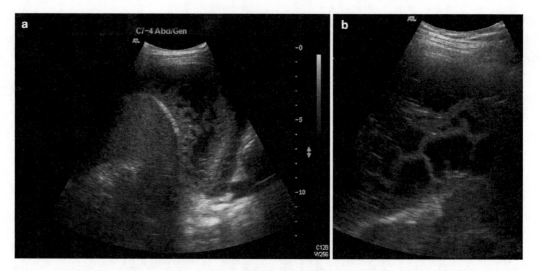

Fig. 12.11. Ultrasound of the chest demonstrating effusion with fine septae (a) and thick septae with loculated fluid compartments (b)

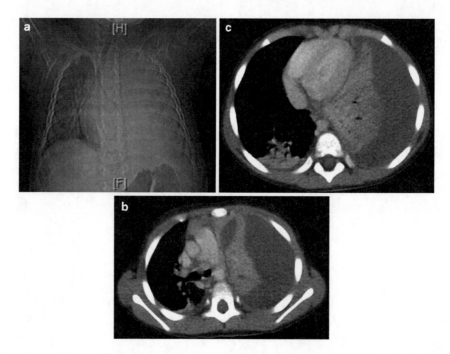

Fig. 12.12. CXR (a) and CT images (b, c) demonstrating a large left pleural effusion with significant deviation of the mediastinum to the right

monic effusions in winter and spring, twice as often than in the rest of the year [28, 29]. The most common presenting symptoms are persistent fever, tachypnea, cough, dyspnea, chest pain and decreased appetite [23, 28, 30, 31]. Usually, the child will not appear toxic, or in shock [32]. On exam, splinting towards the affected side could be noted; in addition, decrease in air entry and dullness to percussion are common findings.

Hypoalbuminemia, thrombocytosis and leukocytosis are characteristic [33]. Hyponatremia secondary to inappropriate antidiuretic hormone (SIADH)

secretion should be looked for. Chest radiograph will reveal the effusion and with large volume of pleural fluid; mediastinal shift can occur (Fig. 12.8).

Blood, sputum and pleural fluid, when available, should be sent for stains and cultures. Chest tube placement, intrapleural antifibrinolytic treatment, video-assisted thoracoscopic surgery (VATS) and pleurodesis are additional interventions to consider in cases of poor or no response to conventional antibiotic therapy.

In addition to pneumonia, there are other etiologies for exudative pleural effusions as previously discussed.

12.3.1 Pulmonary Embolism

Dyspnea and ipsilateral chest pain are the main symptoms and will go along with pleural effusion in approximately 80% of cases. Associated conditions are hemoglobinopathies, nephrotic syndrome and long bone fractures [34].

12.3.2 Pancreatitis

Cough, chest pain and dyspnea accompany symptoms of pancreatitis. Effusion is usually left sided in chronic cases, fluid is hemorrhagic and amylase content is elevated [35–37].

12.3.3 Uremia

Chest pain, fever, cough and pleural friction rub are common with uremia and resolve gradually with dialysis in most patients [38, 39].

12.3.4 Connective Tissue Disease

Pleural effusion is most commonly present in rheumatoid arthritis (RA) and systemic lupus erythematosus (SLE) among the connective tissue diseases. Immune complexes deposit in the pleural space and a consequent inflammatory response damages the pleural capillaries and causes capillary leak [40–42]. Pleurisy, dyspnea and fever are common complaints, although pleural effusion can be asymptomatic. Spontaneous resolution can occur in cases of RA. Corticosteroids are often required in SLE cases. Decortication is indicated in non-responsive cases to avoid severe pleural thickening and trapped lung [43–46]. In cases of drug-induced lupus, discontinuation of the offending medication is recommended [47].

12.3.5 Mediastinal Injury

Esophageal perforation can be associated with pleural effusion and be accompanied by chest pain, dyspnea, fever, subcutaneous emphysema and dysphagia.

Pleuritic chest pain, fever and dyspnea following cardiac injury are known as Dressler's syndrome and can develop within a few days to several months following injury [48–50].

12.3.6 Malignancy

Lymphoma is the most common childhood malignancy associated with pleural effusion [44]. In non-Hodgkin's lymphoma, effusion can be the presenting sign in contrast to Hodgkin's lymphoma where effusion is usually a late manifestation [51–53]. Large effusions are more common in non-Hodgkin's lymphoma. Leukemia, neuroblastoma, rhabdomyosarcoma, Ewing sarcoma and Wilm's tumor are occasionally associated with pleural effusions. Malignant effusion is usually unilateral. Most effusions will resolve with chemotherapy and irradiation. In refractory cases, pleurodesis is recommended [54].

12.3.7 Chylous Effusion

These are most commonly due to injury to the thoracic duct either from trauma or following cardiothoracic surgery [55]. In newborns with pleural effusion and no history of birth trauma, chylothorax is common. Chyle appears milky, but will have straw color appearance in malnourished patients and in newborns [56, 57]. Triglyceride content >110 mg/dl is diagnostic of chylothorax, whereas levels below 50 mg/dL make the diagnosis unlikely. Treatment includes drainage and nutritional support [58, 59]. However, if associated with pulmonary lymphangiectasia (which is usually not apparent), drainage may be prolonged leading to depletion of lymphocytes and hypoproteinemia. Therefore, drainage of a congenital chylous effusion should be approached cautiously.

12.3.8 Hemothorax

Collection of fluid in the pleural space with a hematocrit of at least 50% that of blood is considered as hemothorax [60]. The most common cause of hemothorax is trauma. Additional causes for hemothorax include erosion of a vessel by a central venous catheter, pulmonary infarction, rupture of a congenital vascular anomaly, bleeding diathesis and spontaneous rupture of an intrathoracic blood vessel. The radiographic evidence of the presence of blood in the pleural space will appear several hours after the bleed. Chest radiographs should be repeated in trauma cases particularly if the patient develops respiratory distress.

Management consists of drainage of the bloody fluid, allowing re-expansion of the collapsed lung, and treatment of the underlying problem.

12.4   Transudative Pleural Effusions

Transudative pleural effusions frequently accompany common disease states. The primary abnormality originates, usually, from an organ other than the pleura.

12.4.1   Congestive Heart Failure

Clearance of the pleural fluid is decreased with heart failure. On chest radiography, cardiomegally is apparent. Dyspnea on exertion and failure to gain weight will be additional clinical signs. The effusion tends to be right sided or bilateral. Interstitial and alveolar edema can often be seen. Pleural fluid meets transudate characteristics according to Light's criteria, but can have higher protein and LDH concentration under diuretic therapy [61]. Treatment includes afterload reduction with diuretics and inotrops.

12.4.2   Nephrotic Syndrome

Approximately 20% of nephrotic syndrome patients have a concomitant pleural effusion [62]. The accumulation of fluid is due to the combination of decreased plasma oncotic pressure and increase in hydrostatic pressure secondary to salt retention.

12.4.3   Peritoneal Dialysis

Pleural effusion is well documented in patients receiving continuous peritoneal dialysis. Fluid accu-

mulates in the right hemithorax in most cases and is due to flow of dialysate from the peritoneal cavity into the pleural cavity [63].

12.4.4   Fontan Procedure

The final operation for single ventricle palliative repair is the anastomosis of the inferior vena cava to the pulmonary vessels. In Fontan physiology, central venous hydrostatic pressure is elevated and can contribute to the development of pleural effusion. Reduction of the pulmonary vascular resistance pharmacologically is the initial treatment approach. In severe cases, pleuroperitoneal shunt or pleurodesis are optional treatments [64].

12.5   Pneumothorax

Pressure in the pleural space is lower than alveolar pressure and ambient pressure during the entire respiratory cycle. When communication develops between either an alveolus or through the chest wall, air will flow into the pleural space. The main physiologic results of a pneumothorax (PTX) are decrease in vital capacity and decline in the PaO_2 secondary to ventilation perfusion mismatch, shunts and alveolar hypoventilation [65].

Tension pneumothorax is present when intrapleural pressure exceeds the atmospheric pressure. Patients who develop tension pneumothorax commonly either are positive pressure ventilated (mechanical ventilation, bag mask ventilation) or have some type of one-way valve mechanism secondary to chest wall integrity defect, such as in penetrating trauma [66–68]. Causes of pneumothorax are listed in Table 12.3.

A small pneumothorax may be asymptomatic. Sudden chest pain and dyspnea are the two most common symptoms associated with the development of primary spontaneous pneumothorax. The pain is usually diffuse on the affected side of the chest with radiation to the ipsilateral shoulder. A non-productive cough is occasionally seen in association with pneumothorax.

Breath sounds and fremitus are diminished, hyperresonance with percussion is evident on the affected side. When tension pneumothorax develops, the patient will appear distressed, with tracheal/

Table 12.3. Causes for pneumothorax

Traumatic	Penetrating or blunt trauma
Airway disease	Asthma Cystic fibrosis
Interstitial lung disease	Langerhans' cell histiocytosis Sarcoidosis
Infectious	Bacterial Necrotizing pneumonia Pneumocystis jirovesi (carinii) Tuberculosis
Iatrogenic	Barotrauma Subclavian central venous catheter placement Laparoscopic procedures Airway procedures (intubation, bronchoscopy, etc.)
Congenital/familial	Marfan's syndrome Rheumatoid arthritis Homocystinuria Ehlers Danlos syndrome Polymyositis Dermatomyositis Alfa 1 antitrypsin deficiency Birt–Hogg–Dubé syndrome Subpleural cysts or blebs Congenital lung malformation (lobar emphysema, lung cyst, etc.)
Toxins	Cigarette smoking Marijuana smoking Cocaine snorting
Miscellaneous	Foreign body aspiration Catamenial pneumothorax Primary lung tumor Metastatic disease Irradiation

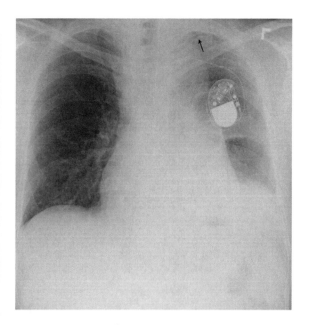

Fig. 12.13. Small left apical pneumothorax (*arrow*) with partially loculated hydropneumothorax noted elsewhere on the left

mediastinal deviation towards the contralateral side, congestion of the jugular veins, narrow pulse pressure and signs of shock. Subcutaneous emphysema can be extensive when air dissects into the mediastinum and the subcutaneous tissue. Chest radiograph can confirm even small volumes of intrapleural air in the upright position [69]. Outlining of the visceral pleura, hyperlucency and attenuation of vascular and lung markings on the affected side are typical findings (Fig. 12.13). Collapsed lung and flattening of the diaphragm can be additional findings on the ipsilateral side with large amount of intrapleural air, mediastinal and tracheal shift away from the affected side will be apparent when tension pneumothorax develops (Fig. 12.14).

Although on an upright chest radiograph, air first accumulates in the apical location, when the patient is supine, a small or even moderate-sized PTX may only be apparent as a *medial pneumothorax* [69] adjacent to the mediastinum (Fig. 12.15). As the PTX

enlarges, it may become apparent in the lateral costophrenic angle, then along the lateral chest and only finally, when moderately large, over the pulmonary apex. Commonly, a small medial PTX will be suggested when actually not present. Normal retinal physiology produces an edge enhancement along the junction of lung and mediastinum, which is perceived as a faint lucent line adjacent to the mediastinum, remarkably simulating a small medial PTX. A simple process will allow the observer to differentiate between this mock effect and a true PTX. An opaque object, such as a piece of paper, should be placed over the mediastinum, being careful not to cover the lucent line. If the lucent line disappears, it was a mock line (Fig. 12.16). If it remains, it is a PTX. When small pneumothorax is suspected, a lateral decubitus view, or cross table lateral view, will provide additional information [70] (Fig. 12.17). Of these two, the decubitus view is preferred as it does not suffer from potential obscuring of the PTX by superimposed mediastinum and contralateral hemithorax. A pneumomediastinum or pneumopericardium should affect both sides, roughly to the same degree. In young children with persistence of the thymus, pneumomediastinum may not dissect into the neck. If there is air underneath the thymus, and lifting it away from the heart, it is mediastinal air, not a PTX (Fig. 12.18). A pneumopericardium will never ascend above the level of the main branch pulmonary arteries. In the upright patient, estimation of

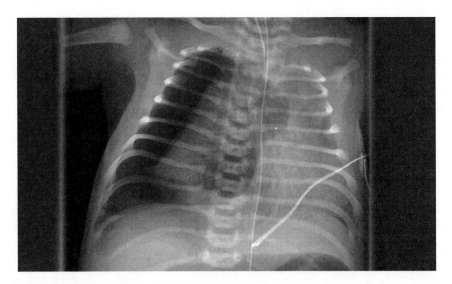

Fig. 12.14. Right tension pneumothorax

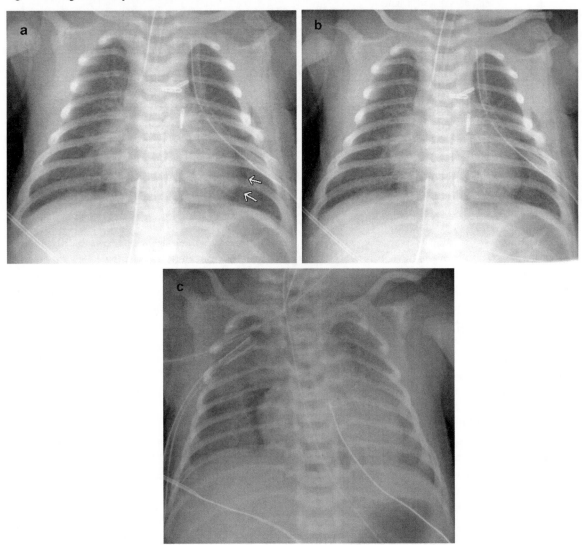

Fig. 12.15. Medial PTX. (**a**) The *arrows* indicate a relatively small left medial PTX, (**b**) same image as (**a**) but without the *arrows*, (**c**) a relatively large right medial PTX

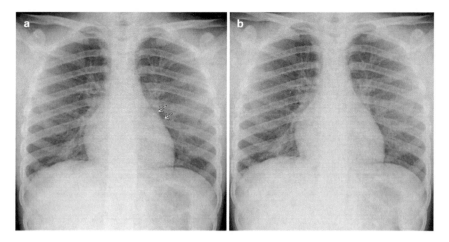

Fig. 12.16. (a) The *arrows* indicate a mock band adjacent to the left heart border. (b) Same image as (a) but without the *arrows*

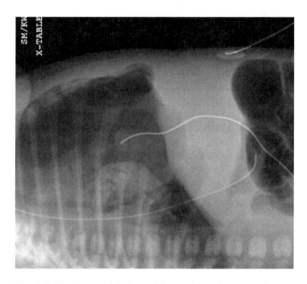

Fig. 12.17. Cross table lateral image showing a moderate-sized pneumothorax anteroinferiorly

the pneumothorax size has been suggested by Collins by taking the sum of the distance between the ribs and the visceral pleura in millimeters, at three levels: apical, midthoracic and base of the lung and dividing by three which will express the percent of pneumothorax [71]. Other methods [47, 72] have also been proposed. However, opposed to these somewhat complicated calculations, the British Thoracic Society guidelines define the size by measuring the distance between the chest wall to the visceral pleura. A distance of 2 cm or more is considered a large pneumothorax [72].

Large subpleural bullae, stomach herniation through a diaphragmatic defect (congenital or trau-matic), and skin folds are conditions that can mimic pneumothorax and should be looked for. The edge of a skin fold often is perceived as a thin line of increased density at the junction with the region of decreased density (i.e., the suspected pneumothorax).

The size of the pneumothorax will dictate management. Small asymptomatic cases can be observed for spontaneous re-absorption. Administrating 100% oxygen to the patient will accelerate the absorption of the pleural air [73].

Simple aspiration is indicated in cases with pneumothoraces greater than 15% in size and is successful in approximately 60% of cases [74]. When simple aspiration fails, tube thoracostomy is recommended, using small diameter chest tubes or pigtail catheters [72, 75, 76]. In addition, negative pressure by suction (-20 cmH$_2$O) should be administered until it becomes evident that no air exists in the pleural space and no ongoing air leak is present. Pleurodesis, stapling of blebs or pleural abrasion are indicated in cases of recurrent pneumothoraces or an ongoing air leak [77].

In cases of tension pneumothorax, a life-threatening situation, urgent needle application to the affected side in the second intercostal space at the midclavicular line should be performed. Immediate air evacuation will relieve the tension pneumothorax and allows time to perform thoracostomy safely.

Complications of thoracostomy include bleeding secondary to ruptured blood vessel and rarely infection of the pleural space. Re-expansion pulmonary edema is an additional possible complication.

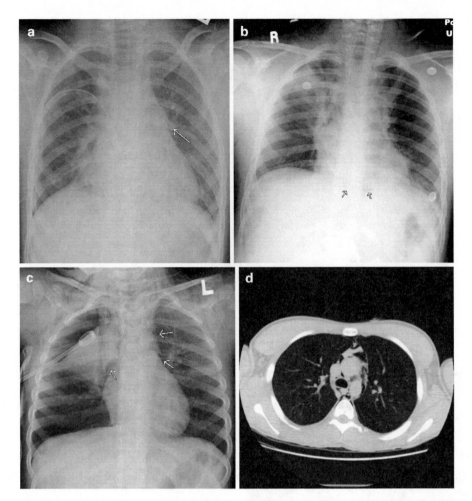

Fig. 12.18. (a) There is a pneumomediastinum seen only on the left. It is distinguished from a medial pneumothorax by the small amount of air lifting the left lobe of the thymus off the mediastinum (*arrow*). (b) In a different patient, there is a relatively large pneumomediastinum, with a larger right component. A small amount of air is noted beneath the heart (*arrows*). Air also has extended into the neck. A small right pneumothorax is present. (c) Portable AP CXR reveals air within the mediastinum (*upper arrow*) with both lobes of the thymus separated from the heart by air (*lower arrows*) (air separating the thymus from the heart occurs only with pneumomediastinum or pneumopericardium). Subcutaneous air is present within the neck. There is a moderately large right pneumothorax. (d) In another patient, CT easily shows an extensive pneumomediastinum with small left pneumothorax

12.6 Pneumoperitoneum

Free intraperitoneal air, with few exceptions, suggests bowel perforation, which may be life threatening. It may be the consequence of recent abdominal surgery and of no clinical concern. Occasionally, a pneumomediastinum or pneumothorax may lead to a *benign* pneumoperitoneum.

Since well-performed frontal chest radiographs include a portion of the upper abdomen, it is important to assess for free intraperitoneal air. This is especially true in patients at risk for bowel ischemia as in an intensive care setting.

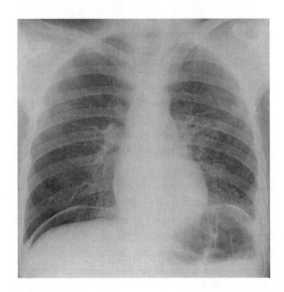

Fig. 12.19. Upright image with pneumoperitoneum noted under the right hemidiapharm

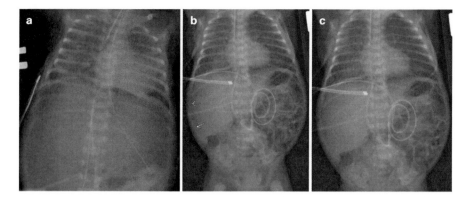

Fig. 12.20. (a) Supine image with a large pneumoperitoneum, (b) the lateral extent of this relatively subtle pneumoperitoneum is indicated by the *arrows*, (c) same image as (b) without the *arrows*

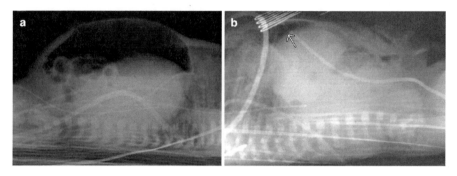

Fig. 12.21. (a, b) Cross table lateral image showing anteriorly placed pneumoperitoneum (*arrow*)

Identification of a pneumoperitoneum is simple on an upright image where the air outlines the inferior margin of the diaphragm (Fig. 12.19). In a supine patient, the manifestations of free intraperitoneal air may be much more difficult to perceive. Frequently, the only suggestion may be a subtle lucency over the abdomen with a faint margin defining the lateral peritoneal reflection (Fig. 12.20). If there are doubts concerning the observation, a cross table lateral image (Fig. 12.21) or right side down decubitus image should be performed.

References

1. Moore KL. The developing human. 2nd ed. Philadelphia: WB Saunders; 1977. p. 145–55.
2. Noppen M, De Waele M, Li R, et al. Volume and cellular content of normal pleural fluid in humans examined by pleural lavage. Am J Respir Crit Care Med. 2000;162:1023–6.
3. Staub NC, Wiener-Kronish JP, Albertine KH. Transport through the pleura: physiology of normal liquid and solute exchange in the pleural space. In: Chrétien J, Bignon J, Hirsch A, editors. The pleura in health and disease, Lung biology in health and disease, vol. 30. New York: Marcel Dekker; 1985. p. 169–93.
4. Negrini D, Ballard ST, Benoit JN. Contribution of lymphatic myogenic activity and respiratory movements to pleural lymph flow. J Appl Physiol. 1994;76:2267–74.
5. Wang PM. Lai-Fook ST. Upward flow of pleural liquid near lobar margins due to cardiogenic motion. J Appl Physiol. 1992;73:2314–9.
6. Miserocchi G, Pistolesi M, Miniati M, et al. Pleural liquid pressure gradients and intrapleural distribution of injected bolus. J Appl Physiol. 1984;56:526–32.
7. Broaddus VC. Weiner-Kronish JP, Berthiaume Y, Staub NC. Removal of pleural liquid and protein by lymphatics in awake sheep. J Appl Physiol. 1988;64:384–90.
8. Wang NS. Anatomy and physiology of the pleural space. Clin Chest Med. 1985;6:3–16.
9. Light RW, MacGregor MI, Luchsinger PC, et al. Pleural effusions: the diagnostic separation of transudates and exudates. Ann Intern Med. 1972;77:507–13.
10. Kilbane BJ, Reynolds SL. Emergency department management of community-acquired methicillin-resistant Staphylococcus aureus. Pediatr Emerg Care. 2008;24(2):109–14.
11. Buckingham SC, King MD, Miller ML. Incidence and etiologies of complicated parapneumonic effusions in children 1996 to 2001. Pediatr Infect Dis J. 2003;22(6):499–504.
12. Kuhn J. Caffey's pediatric diagnostic imaging. 10th ed. Philadelphia: Mosby; 2004.
13. Chonmaitree T, Powell KR. Parapneumonic pleural effusion and empyema in children. Review of a 19-year experience, 1962-1980. Clin Pediatr (Phila). 1983;22(6):414–9.

14. Freij BJ et al. Parapneumonic effusions and empyema in hospitalized children: a retrospective review of 227 cases. Pediatr Infect Dis. 1984;3(6):578–91.

15. Hardie W et al. Pneumococcal pleural empyemas in children. Clin Infect Dis. 1996;22(6):1057–63.

16. Rudikoff JC. Early detection of pleural fluid. Chest. 1980;77:109–11.

17. Moskowitz H, Platt RT, Schachar R, et al. Roentgen visualization of minute pleural effusion. Radiology. 1973;109:33–5.

18. Tsai T-H, Yang P-C. Ultrasound in the diagnosis and management of pleural disease. Curr Opin Pulm Med. 2003;9:282–90.

19. Davies CL, Gleeson FV. Diagnostic radiology. In: Light RW, Lee GYC, editors. Textbook of pleural diseases. London: Arnold; 2003. p. 210–37.

20. Kohan JM, Poe RH, Israel RH, et al. Value of chest ultrasonography versus decubitus roentgenography for thoracentesis. Am Rev Respir Dis. 1986;133:1124–6.

21. Remy-Jardin M, Remy J, Deschildre F, et al. Diagnosis of pulmonary embolism with spiral CT: comparison with pulmonary angiography and scintigraphy. Radiology. 1996;200:699–706.

22. MacDonald SL, Mayo JR. Computed tomography of acute pulmonary embolism. Semin Ultrasound CT MR. 2003;24:217–31.

23. Byington CL, Spencer LY, Johnson TA, et al. An epidemiological investigation of a sustained high rate of pediatric parapneumonic empyema: risk factors and microbiological association. Clin Infect Dis. 2002;34:434–40.

24. Rees JH, Spencer DA, Parikh D, Weller P. Increase in incidence of childhood empyema in West Midlands, UK. Lancet. 1997;349:402.

25. Playfor SD, Smyth AR, Stewart RJ. Increase in incidence of childhood empyema. Thorax. 1997;52:932.

26. Roxburgh CS, Youngson GG, Townend JA, Turner SW. Trends in pneumonia and empyema in Scottish children in the past 25 years. Arch Dis Child. 2008;93:316–8.

27. Schultz KD, Fan LL, Pinsky J, et al. The changing face of pleural empyemas in children: epidemiology and management. Pediatrics. 2004;113:1735–40.

28. Hardie W, Bokulic R, Garcia VF, et al. Pneumococcal pleural empyemas in children. Clin Infect Dis. 1996;22:1057–63.

29. Freij BJ, Kusmiesz H, Nelson JD, McCracken Jr GH. Parapneumonic effusions and empyema in hospitalized children: a retrospective review of 227 cases. Pediatr Infect Dis. 1984;3:578–91.

30. Balfour-Lynn IM, Abrahamson E, Cohen G, et al. BTS guidelines for the management of pleural infection in children. Thorax. 2005;60 Suppl 1:i1–21.

31. Rodgers BM, McGahren ED. Mediastinum and pleura. In: Oldham KT, Colombani PM, Foglia RP, Skinner MA, editors. Principles and practice of pediatric surgery. Philadelphia: Lippincott, Williams & Wilkins; 2005. p. 929–49.

32. Wheeler JG, Jacobs RF. Pleural effusions and empyema. In: Feigin RD, Cherry JD, Demmler GJ, Kaplan SL, editors. Textbook of pediatric infectious diseases. 5th ed. Philadelphia: Saunders; 2004. p. 320–30.

33. Wolach B, Morag H, Drucker M, Sadan N. Thrombocytosis after pneumonia with empyema and other bacterial infections in children. Pediatr Infect Dis J. 1990;9:718–21.

34. Bynum LJ, Wilson III JE. Characteristic of pleural effusions associated with pulmonary embolism. Arch Intern Med. 1976;136:159–62.

35. Light RW, Ball Jr WC. Glucose and amylase in pleural effusions. JAMA. 1973;225:257–9.

36. Rockey DC, Cello JP. Pancreaticopleural fistula: report of 7 patients and review of the literature. Medicine. 1990;69:332–44.

37. Lankisch PG, Droge M, Becher R. Pleural effusions: a new negative prognostic parameter for acute pancreatitis. Am J Gastroenterol. 1994;89:1849–51.

38. Berger HW, Rammohan G, Neff MS, et al. Uremic pleural effusion: a study in 14 patients on chronic dialysis. Ann Intern Med. 1975;82:362–4.

39. Rodelas R, Rakowski TA, Argy WP, et al. Fibrosing uremic pleuritis during hemodialysis. JAMA. 1980;243:2424–5.

40. Halla JT, Schrohenloher RE, Volanakis JE. Immune complexes and other laboratory features of pleural effusion. Ann Intern Med. 1980;92:748–52.

41. Koster FT, McGregor DD, Mackaness GB. The mediator of cellular immunity: II. Migration of immunologically committed lymphocytes into inflammatory exudates. J Exp Med. 1971;133:400–9.

42. Horler AR, Thompson M. The pleural and pulmonary complications of rheumatoid arthritis. Ann Intern Med. 1959;51:1179–203.

43. Walker WC, Wright V. Pulmonary lesions and rheumatoid arthritis. Medicine. 1968;47:501–19.

44. Sahn SA. State of the art: the pleura. Am Rev Respir Dis. 1988;138:184–234.

45. Yarbrough JW, Sealy WC, Miller JA. Thoracic surgical problems associated with rheumatoid arthritis. J Thorac Cardiovasc Surg. 1975;68:347–54.

46. Vargas FS, Milanez JR, Filomeno LT, et al. Intrapleural talc for the prevention of recurrence in benign or undiagnosed pleural effusions. Chest. 1994;106:1771–5.

47. Light RW. Pleural diseases. 4th ed. Baltimore: Lippincott, Williams & Wilkins; 2001.

48. Stelzner TJ, King Jr TE, Antony VB, Sahn SA. The pleuropulmonary manifestations of the postcardiac injury syndrome. Chest. 1983;84:383–7.

49. Bladergroen MR, Lowe JE, Postlethwait RW. Diagnosis and recommended management of esophageal perforation and rupture. Ann Thorac Surg. 1986;42:235–9.

50. Reeder LB, DeFilippi VJ, Ferguson MK. Current results of therapy for esophageal perforation. Am J Surg. 1995;169:615–7.

51. Castellino RA, Bellani FF, Gasparini M, Musumeci R. Radiographic findings in previously untreated children with non- Hodgkin's lymphoma. Radiology. 1975;117:657–63.

52. Celikoglu F, Teirstein AS, Krellenstein DJ, Strauchen JA. Pleural effusion in non Hodgkin's lymphoma. Chest. 1992;101:1357–60.

53. Fisher AMH, Kendall B, VanLeuven BD. Hodgkin's disease: a radiological survey. Clin Radiol. 1962;13:115–27.

54. Keller SM. Current and future therapy for malignant pleural effusion. Chest. 1993;103:63s–7.

55. Teba L, Dedhia HV, Bowen R, Alexander JC. Chylothorax review. Crit Care Med. 1985;13:49–52.

56. Chernick V, Reed MH. Pneumothorax and chylothorax in the neonatal period. J Pediatr. 1970;76:624–32.

57. Yancy WS, Spock A. Spontaneous neonatal pleural effusion. J Pediatr Surg. 1967;2:313–9.

58. Strausser JL, Flye MW. Management of non traumatic chylothorax. Ann Thorac Surg. 1981;31:520–6.

59. Rubin JW, Moore HV, Ellison RG. Chylothorax: therapeutic alternatives. Am Surgeon. 1977;43:292–7.

60. Light RW. Pleural diseases. Philadelphia: Lea & Febiger; 1990.

61. Romero-Candeira S, Fernandez C, Martin C, et al. Influence of diuretics on the concentration of proteins and other components of pleural transudates in patients with heart failure. Am J Med. 2001;110:681–6.

62. Cavina G, Vichi G. Radiological aspects of pleural effusions in medical nephropathy in children. Ann Radiol Diagn. 1958;31:163–202.

63. Nomoto Y, Suga T, Nakajima K, et al. Acute hydrothorax in continuous ambulatory peritoneal dialysis: a collaborative study of 161 centers. Am J Nephrol. 1989;9:363–7.

64. Sade RM, Wiles HB. Pleuroperitoneal shunt for persistent pleural drainage after Fontan procedure. J Thorac Cardiovasc Surg. 1990;100:621–3.

65. Norris RM, Jones JG, Bishop JM. Respiratory gas exchange in patients with spontaneous pneumothorax. Thorax. 1968;23:427–33.

66. Baumann MH. Non-spontaneous pneumothorax. In: Light RW, Lee YCG, editors. Textbook of pleural diseases. London: Arnold; 2003. p. 464–74.

67. Murphy DG, Sloan EP, Hart RG, et al. Tension pneumothorax associated with hyperbaric oxygen therapy. Am J Emerg Med. 1991;9:176–9.

68. Mainini SE, Johnson FE. Tension pneumothorax complicating small-caliber chest tube insertion. Chest. 1990;97:759–60.

69. Moskowitz PS, Griscom NT. The medial pneumothorax. Radiology. 1976;120:143–7.

70. Carr JJ, Reed CJ, Choplin RH, et al. Plain and computed radiography for detecting experimentally induced pneumothorax in cadavers: implications for detection in patients. Radiology. 1992;183:193–9.

71. Collins CD, Lopez A, Mathie A, et al. Quantification of pneumothorax size on chest radiographs using interpleural distances: regression analysis based on volume measurements from helical CT. AJR Am J Roentgenol. 1995;165:1127–30.

72. Henry M, Arnold T, Harvey J. BTS guidelines for the management of spontaneous pneumothorax. Thorax. 2003;58(Suppl II):II39–52.

73. Northfield TC. Oxygen therapy for spontaneous pneumothorax. Br Med J. 1971;4:86–8.

74. Light RW. Manual aspiration: the preferred method for managing primary spontaneous pneumothorax? Am J Respir Crit Care Med. 2002;165:1202–3.

75. Ponn RB, Silverman HJ, Federico JA. Outpatient chest tube management. Ann Thorac Surg. 1997;64:1437–40.

76. Liu CM, Hang LW, Chen WK, et al. Pigtail tube drainage in the treatment of spontaneous pneumothorax. Am J Emerg Med. 2003;21:241–4.

77. Yim AP, Ng CS. Thoracoscopy in the management of pneumothorax. Curr Opin Pulm Med. 2001;7:210–4.

Oncologic Disease

13

Benjamin A. Nelson, Edward Y. Lee, and Shashi H. Ranganath

CONTENTS

Benjamin A. Nelson, MD (✉)
Department of Pediatrics, Harvard University/Massachusetts General Hospital for Children, Boston, MA, USA
e-mail: banelson@partners.org

Edward Y. Lee, MD, MPH
Division of Thoracic Imaging, Department of Radiology and Medicine, Pulmonary Division, Children's Hospital Boston, Harvard Medical School, Boston, MA, USA
e-mail: Edward.Lee@childrens.harvard.edu

Shashi H. Ranganath, MD
Department of Pediatric Radiology, Children's Hospital Boston, Harvard Medical School, Boston, MA, USA

13.1 Pediatric Lung, Central Airway, and Chest Wall Neoplasm

Benjamin A. Nelson and Edward Y. Lee

Primary thoracic neoplasms in children can arise within the lung, central airway, or chest wall. Malignant lesions are much more common than benign processes. Metastatic tumors account for up to 80% of all lung tumors in children and more than 95% of the malignant ones. Due to the rarity and nonspecific presenting clinical symptoms of thoracic neoplasms in the pediatric population, a substantial delay in the diagnosis often occurs. Therefore, a high index of suspicion coupled with optimal imaging evaluation is of paramount importance in early and correct diagnosis. Early management can, in turn, result in decreased morbidity and mortality associated with lung, central airway, and chest wall neoplasms in pediatric patients. The prognosis of thoracic tumors in children varies depending on the malignant nature of the tumor, evidence of metastasis, and amenability to surgical excision. In this section, we discuss pediatric lung, central airway, and chest wall neoplasms including (1) clinical presentation; (2) practical approach to diagnosis; (3) histopathological characteristics; (4) imaging findings; and (5) patient outcome.

R.H. Cleveland (ed.), *Imaging in Pediatric Pulmonology*,
DOI 10.1007/978-1-4419-5872-3_13, © Springer Science+Business Media, LLC 2012

13.1.1 Clinical Presentation and Practical Approach to Diagnosis

There are many chief complaints and clinical presentations which ultimately lead to the discovery of a thoracic neoplasm. Since chest tumors are rare in the pediatric population, other more common diagnoses are often excluded before the actual diagnosis can be made. Frequently, tumors are inadvertently discovered when a patient undergoes an imaging study for some other unrelated complaint. Although history and physical examination can help to localize a mass, imaging is paramount in formulating a diagnostic and therapeutic plan.

More often than not children with thoracic neoplasms do not complain of symptoms commonly associated with neoplastic processes such as fever, weight loss, and fatigue. Therefore, when pediatric patients do not respond to conventional therapies, other rarer diagnoses must be considered. Cough is one of the most common chief complaints that a pediatrician will encounter in the office, which can be the presenting symptom of a malignancy. After excluding common causes of cough such as asthma, postnasal drip, and gastroesophageal reflux, other entities must be considered. If the child has difficulty gaining weight or has evidence of malabsorption, he/she might need a sweat test or genetic testing to exclude cystic fibrosis. If there is a history of recurrent infections, an immune workup, placing a PPD, or sending a sputum sample looking for routine bacteria, acid fast bacilli, and fungus may be warranted. Sinusitis can be difficult to diagnose in young children due to lack of specific symptoms. Pulmonary function tests (PFTs) may aid in the diagnosis of cough, but almost all patients with unexplained cough will need some form of an imaging study. A PA and lateral chest X-ray (CXR) can reveal a great deal of information including signs of a possible infection, aspiration, persistent atelectasis, lymphadenopathy, or even a chest mass. Lymphadenopathy can be secondary to infection, but could also be related to an underlying primary neoplasm and may be the only clue to a lymphoma. The chest drains into the supraclavicular nodes, so a thorough physical exam looking for lymphadenopathy is vital. External compression of the airway can be secondary to an enlarged lymph node or any type of mass in the thoracic cavity. CT scan is therefore warranted to obtain better visualization of the abnormality. A CT scan can often detect abnormalities that are not seen on a plain film, can better delineate the anatomy, and may

aid in determining a surgical approach for biopsy. Calcifications and lung parenchymal abnormalities are better elucidated via CT and, if present, may narrow the differential diagnosis. Magnetic resonance imaging (MRI), which is not associated with ionizing radiation exposure, has superior diagnostic capability when evaluating soft tissues. Therefore, MRI can be a valuable tool when evaluating certain abnormalities in the chest. Although imaging studies can often narrow the differential, biopsy is typically required for a definitive diagnosis.

Wheezing, stridor, and noisy breathing are chief complaints associated with common pediatric disorders such as asthma, gastroesophageal reflux, laryngomalacia, and tracheomalacia. However, children with endobronchial tumors may present in similar fashion. Therefore, it is crucial to do a thorough history and physical examination when assessing a patient with these common symptoms. A healthy, thriving child less than 1 year of age might need a very limited workup for noisy breathing. However, at the minimum, these children should have a CXR to ensure the symptoms are not secondary to a mass- or space-occupying lesion. In fact, one could argue that every child who wheezes for the first time should have a baseline CXR to rule out a mass in the thoracic cavity. For the child who has persistent noisy breathing, difficulty gaining weight, repeated respiratory infections, or anything else causing concern on history or physical examination, further workup is warranted. If the noisy breathing is associated with difficulty feeding or choking, then a barium swallow should be ordered to look for a vascular ring. If the child is old enough, a good place to start would be to obtain PFTs. PFTs can suggest a fixed intra- or extra-thoracic lesion. Total lung capacity and diffusing capacity of the lungs are also helpful when evaluating the patient. The next step in diagnosis is either a bronchoscopy to directly evaluate the airway, or a CT scan. Often this is determined by availability. A CT scan is often much easier to obtain, but has the disadvantage of exposing the child to radiation. A bronchoscopy allows assessment of the vocal cords for mobility and presence of any abnormal lesions which may be responsible for the clinical symptoms. Common diagnoses such as laryngomalacia and tracheomalacia can be ruled out during bronchoscopy by assessing the dynamic movement of the larynx and trachea. Bronchoalveolar lavage fluid is tested for signs of infection, aspiration, and malignancy. It is important to look for an external compression causing symptoms, such as an aberrant innominate artery, as well as any endobronchial lesions which may account for the presenting clinical symptoms. If there is evidence of external compression on the airway or if an endobronchial lesion is visualized, the next step must be a CT scan or MRI. A CT or MRI can sometimes suggest a specific diagnosis but almost always narrows the differential. Furthermore, the findings on imaging can demonstrate the extent of the lesion, and dictate which service is most appropriate to attempt biopsy and/or removal of the lesion.

Dyspnea on exertion is another common complaint seen in the pediatric office, and may be a clue to an underlying malignancy. It is important to take a careful cardiac history. After ruling out a cardiac problem, exercise-induced bronchoconstriction, vocal cord dysfunction, and deconditioning, other possible entities should be carefully considered. In this scenario, PFTs are quite helpful and some children will need a full cardiopulmonary exercise test to determine the etiology of their symptoms. A CXR may show a mass, persistent atelectasis, or lymphadenopathy which could all be signs of an underlying malignancy and would therefore necessitate further examination. Symptoms often become apparent only after the tumor has grown large enough to cause a mass effect.

Inquiring about systemic complaints on a thorough review of systems is crucial as the lungs or chest wall may not be the primary source of the malignancy. Lung metastases are much more common that primary lung tumors in children, and presenting symptoms are based on location. If the tumor load is large enough to replace parenchymal tissue, the patient will complain of dyspnea. Extension into the pleura causes pleuritic chest pain, and endobronchial metastases manifest as wheezing or hemoptysis. However, respiratory symptoms are often absent in patients with metastatic disease, making diagnosis that much more difficult. Sputum cytologic analysis or lung biopsy may ultimately be necessary to make an accurate diagnosis when evaluating patients with metastatic disease, but imaging studies are always required and a CXR is the first step. In fact, metastases are sometimes inadvertently picked up on a CXR obtained for other reasons. CT is more sensitive than a CXR in detecting pulmonary nodules, and when multiple nodules are seen, the clinician is obligated to look for a primary tumor. Common sites in this scenario would be bones, testicles, kidneys, or soft tissues. The child may need to be screened with a bone scan, testicular ultrasound, evaluation of the peripheral blood smear, or a PET scan.

13.1.2 Pediatric Lung Neoplasm

Primary Tumors

Benign

Inflammatory myofibroblastic tumor. Inflammatory myofibroblastic tumor (IMT), also known as inflammatory pseudotumor of the lung or plasma cell granuloma, is a benign tumor of unknown origin. It was first described in 1939 and was thought to arise as a reaction to a previous insult [1]. Although IMT has been traditionally considered as a benign lesion, recent molecular analysis has raised suspicions to the contrary. The WHO has currently defined this tumor as an intermediary neoplasm, characterized by a molecular rearrangement on chromosome locus 2p23 involving the tyrosine kinase receptor anaplastic lymphoma kinase (ALK), which is involved in other forms of malignancy [2]. This genetic rearrangement has been documented in some but not all IMTs.

IMT is the most common primary tumor of the lung in children less than 16 years of age [3]. It is estimated that IMTs account for approximately 20% of all primary lung tumors and 57% of all benign lesions [4]. They are typically slow growing neoplasms and show signs of both reactive and neoplastic components [5]. Clubbing can be a presenting sign and often disappears after surgical removal [3, 6]. Patients with IMT are usually asymptomatic due to its predilection for occurring in the periphery. However, the tumor can grow in size over a long period of time and eventually lead to symptoms such as cough, hemoptysis and dyspnea due to local invasion, and/or mass-effect on mediastinal structures. If allowed to grow substantially without treatment, IMTs can lead to significant morbidity as multiple deaths have been reported due to local invasion of this tumor [7–9]. IMTs are more likely to recur locally than to metastasize and there is a 14% recurrence rate [10], which is highly correlated to the presence of local invasion. On gross inspection, they are usually firm and white to yellow in color. Microscopically, IMT is characterized by a localized proliferation of plasma cells, lymphocytes, and eosinophils with Russell bodies and reticuloendothelial cells supported by a stroma of granulation tissue [3, 6, 11].

Radiologically, IMTs are most often solitary, found in the periphery, and range from 1 to 12 cm in size. They are typically heterogeneously enhancing soft

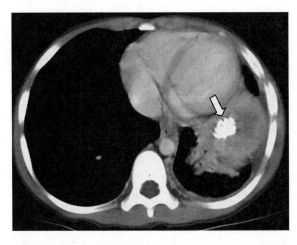

Fig. 13.1. Six-year-old girl presented with fever and abnormal chest radiographs. Enhanced axial CT image demonstrates a heterogeneously enhancing mass with associated chunky calcification (*arrow*) in the left lower lobe. Surgical pathology confirmed a diagnosis of inflammatory pseudotumor

tissue masses often with calcification (Fig. 13.1). They are round- or oval-shaped circumscribed masses that are described as "coin lesions" [3, 6]. The potential differential should include infectious processes, other neoplasms, and congenital malformations. There seems to be two types of IMT. The first is noninvasive, often asymptomatic, and easily removed by wedge resection. The second type is larger, invasive, occurs in younger patients with systemic symptoms of fever, fatigue, or weight loss, and often requires a lobectomy or pneumonectomy [11]. Complete surgical resection when possible is the treatment of choice and the overall prognosis is excellent.

Leiomyoma. A leiomyoma is a rare, benign, smooth muscle neoplasm which can present in the lung parenchyma or as an endobronchial lesion. Epstein–Barr virus is often associated with lymphoproliferative disorders in immunosuppressed children, but is also linked to the development of pulmonary leiomyomas in children with HIV, recipients of solid organ transplants, and those with primary immunodeficiencies. Clinical presentation in children with leiomyoma depends on location of the tumor. Endobronchial lesions may present with cough, hemoptysis, or repeated bouts of pneumonia, whereas peripheral lesions within the lung parenchyma may be asymptomatic [12]. Clubbing of the fingers may be the only presenting abnormality in children [13, 14]. Histologically, leiomyomas are composed of spindle-shaped cells and lack significant atypia and mitotic activity [12]. There is a spectrum from benign (leiomyoma) to malignant (leiomyosarcoma) morphology, and there is potential for regression with

modulation of immunosuppression [5]. Management of pediatric patients with leiomyoma is currently not well defined. However, benign tumors in noncritical locations may be observed, whereas endobronchial symptomatic lesions need to be removed by bronchoscopic resection or may even necessitate lobectomy or bronchial sleeve resection. Ultimately, management is tailored to the general clinical condition of the patient, the location of the tumor, and the effect of the tumor on the patient [15].

Congenital pulmonary myofibroblastic tumor. Congenital pulmonary myofibroblastic tumor (CPMT) is a very rare, congenital, benign lung tumor of the fetus and infant. It has been described under various terminologies, including massive congenital mesenchymal malformation of the lung, hamartoma of the lung, bronchopulmonary leiomyosarcoma, and primary bronchopulmonary fibrosarcoma (PBF) [16]. It is thought to arise from the pluripotent mesenchyme found around the developing bronchi at approximately 12 weeks gestation [5]. Children often present in utero or at birth with a unilateral lung mass with mediastinal shift resulting in polyhydramnios, hydrops, or immediate respiratory failure at delivery. Grossly, a large portion of the lung is enlarged and replaced by a firm rubbery mass. Due to its cellularity and mitotic activity, it was originally thought to be malignant in nature. However, all reported cases have behaved in a benign fashion; no cases have shown tumor recurrence or metastases [17]. Karyotyping may show complex rearrangements involving chromosomes 4, 8, and 10, which can help to differentiate this lesion from other similar smooth muscle tumors. Although the lesion is benign, the large size may result in respiratory or hemodynamic compromise necessitating surgical removal. One series reported a mortality rate of 55% [18]. With early resection, typically by pneumonectomy or lobectomy, long-term survival is expected [17].

Lipoblastoma. Lipoblastoma is a rare, benign, adipose tumor occurring exclusively in children. Eighty-eight percent of cases occur before the age of 3, and 40% before the first year of life [19]. Greater than 70% of all lipoblastomas arise in the superficial layers of the extremities; the rest are deeper and arise in the mediastinum, retroperitoneum, and the axilla [20]. Patients often present with rapidly growing asymptomatic masses; however, if involving the lung the patient may develop respiratory distress. Two forms of this tumor have been described: a well-circumscribed, encapsulated type occurring superficially (lipoblastoma), and a diffuse, infiltrating type occurring in deep soft tissues (lipoblastomatosis) [21, 22]. Histology reveals mature fat cells mixed with mesenchymal and immature fat cells. CT can often reveal the lipoid nature of the tumor, but cannot distinguish between other lesions made up of adipose tissue. Therefore, a biopsy is needed for a definitive diagnosis. The treatment for lipoblastomas is surgical resection, and the prognosis is excellent if complete surgical resection with clear margins can be achieved. Recurrence rates of 14–25% have been reported for infiltrating tumors where complete surgical resection was not possible [20, 23–25].

Hamartoma. A pulmonary hamartoma is a collection of disorganized tissues intrinsic to the lung with a peak incidence in the sixth decade. They are the most common benign pulmonary lesion in adults, and the second most common in children (18–23%) [7, 26]. It is composed of normal cells in an abnormal pattern; however, there is some evidence that it is actually a benign neoplasm [27]. In a Dutch series, the annual incidence was found to be 1:100,000. Patients ranged from 14 to 74 years of age with a mean of 51. 92% of tumors are parenchymal with 8% being endobronchial in location [27]. Patients with parenchymal lesions are often asymptomatic at diagnosis; however, if they are large enough they can cause respiratory distress. Endobronchial lesions often present with symptoms of obstruction such as cough, hemoptysis, and dyspnea on exertion. Pathology often reveals various mesenchymal components such as cartilage, fat, fibrous tissue, smooth muscle, and bone. Tumors with a single dominant component may be classified as a chondroma, fibroma, or lipoma depending on the mesenchymal component [5]. Hamartomas of the lung are usually seen on radiography as a round homogenous opacity in the periphery of the lung. Chest CT may show fat and "popcorn" calcifications which are pathognomatic for a hamartoma, but they are only seen in 10–25% of cases (Fig. 13.2) [28, 29]. Management consists of surgical resection and the prognosis is excellent; however, a 6.3 times increased risk of lung cancer has been described in patients with pulmonary hamartomas [30].

Malignant

Bronchogenic carcinoma. Primary lung carcinoma in children and adolescents is extremely rare, with 0.16% of all lung cancers occurring in the first decade and 0.7% in the second decade [31]. The overall incidence is hard to determine as reports are limited to

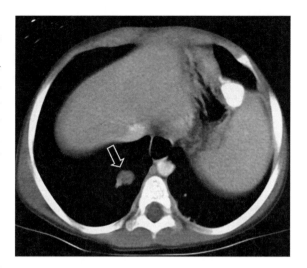

Fig. 13.2. Five-year-old boy with a history of Wilm's tumor. Right lower lobe lung mass (*arrow*) was detected on chest CT examination performed for evaluation of thoracic metastatic disease. Enhanced axial CT image demonstrates a round pulmonary mass with areas of low attenuation consistent with a fat component. Surgical pathology was consistent with a diagnosis of a pulmonary hamartoma

case reports and small series. Most cases in the literature of pediatric lung carcinoma describe undifferentiated carcinomas followed by adenocarcinoma and squamous cell carcinoma. Primary lung carcinoma in children is often aggressive with evidence of metastatic disease at the time of diagnosis, and carries an extremely high mortality rate of up to 90% [7, 26]. Symptoms include cough, chest pain, pneumonia, and hemoptysis. However, patients can also present with bone pain, weight loss, or anemia due to metastatic disease. Radiologically, bronchogenic carcinoma typically presents as a large heterogeneously enhancing mass often invading adjacent thoracic structures (Fig. 13.3). NUT midline carcinoma (NMC) is a poorly differentiated neoplasm which is most common in children and pursues a highly aggressive course, usually resulting in death within weeks of diagnosis [32–38]. Patients with NMCs may present with constitutional symptoms or symptoms due to local mass effect from the tumor [35, 36, 39]. This tumor is characterized by rearrangement of the *NUT* gene (*nu*clear protein in *t*estis) on chromosome 15q14 [32–38, 40]. In approximately two-thirds of cases, *NUT* (chromosome 15q14) is fused to the gene *BRD4* on chromosome 19p13.1, resulting in a novel *BRD4-NUT* fusion gene [33]. Such tumors have also been termed BRD4-NUT carcinoma or t(15;19) carcinoma. Anatomically, NMCs arise in or near the midline, most commonly in the head, neck, or

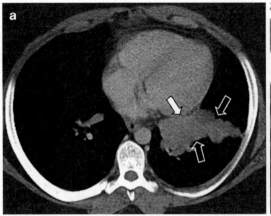

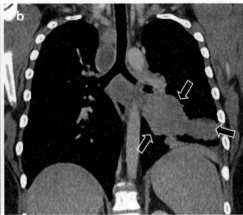

Fig. 13.3. Fifteen-year-old boy with bronchogeric carcinoma presented with weight loss and progressively worsening shortness of breath. (**a**) Enhanced axial CT image demonstrates a large heterogeneous mass (*arrows*) with irregular borders located in the left lower lobe and abutting the left heart border. (**b**) Enhanced coronal CT image better demonstrates the entire extent of the mass (*arrows*)

mediastinum, as poorly differentiated carcinomas with variable degrees of squamous differentiation [32]. On imaging studies, NMC is usually a heterogeneously enhancing mass located within the mediastinum (Fig. 13.4). CT is the imaging modality of choice and can alert the surgical pathologist to submit tissue for karyotype analysis. Surgical resection is the primary mode of therapy for bronchogenic carcinoma. Adjuvant therapy for local and disseminated disease utilizes both radio- and chemotherapy. Patients with disseminated disease at the time of diagnosis live on average less than 7 months [7].

Pleuropulmonary blastoma (Types I, II, III). Pleuropulmonary blastoma (PPB) is a rare, embryonal, mesenchymal neoplasm of the lung and pleura occurring almost exclusively in children [5, 41]. The actual incidence is unknown, but this is thought to be the most common malignant parenchymal tumor of childhood [42]. It is diagnosed mainly in infants and toddlers and rarely in those beyond 12 years of age. In the past, this specific entity had been referred to as an embryona of the lung, pulmonary blastoma, pulmonary sarcoma, embryonal sarcoma, and malignant mesenchymoma [42]. The tumor is thought to arise from pleuropulmonary germ cells and has been subclassified into three types based on gross morphological appearance. Type I tumors are exclusively cystic (Fig. 13.5), type II contain both cystic and solid material, whereas type III lesions are predominantly solid (Fig. 13.6). As in bronchogenic carcinoma, PPB has been reported to arise from congenital malformations of the lung, including Cystic a pulmonary airway malformation (CPAM), sequestrations, and

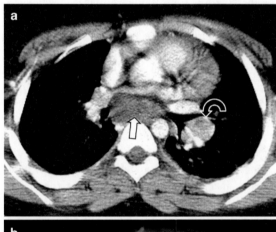

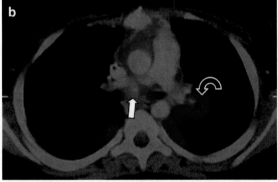

Fig. 13.4. Ten-year-old boy with NMC presented with multiple lower extremity arterial thromboses. Echocardiography showed a possible mediastinal mass and CT was subsequently performed for further evaluation. (**a**) Enhanced axial CT image demonstrates a heterogeneously enhancing mass (*arrow*) located behind the heart with mass effect upon the right inferior pulmonary vein. Also noted is left hilar lymphadenopathy (*curved arrow*). (**b**) Axial CT and PET fusion image shows an increased metabolism in the mediastinal mass (*arrow*) and left hilar lymphadenopathy (*curved arrow*)

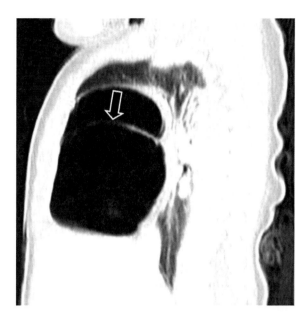

Fig. 13.5. Two-month-old boy presented with respiratory distress and abnormal chest radiographs. Sagittal lung window image shows a large cystic mass with internal septation (*arrow*) located in the right lung. Surgical pathology was consistent with type 1 pleuropulmonary blastoma (PPB)

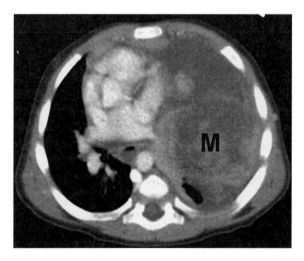

Fig. 13.6. One-month-old girl presented with weight loss and respiratory distress. Enhanced axial CT image demonstrates a large heterogeneously enhancing mass (M) located in the left hemithorax with mediastinal shift to the right side. Surgical pathology was consistent with type 3 PPB

bronchogenic cysts [43–46]. Patients with type I tumors present earlier than the other types with a mean age of 10 months compared to 34 and 44 months for types II and III, respectively [47]. Patients typically present with nonspecific respiratory symptoms, and spontaneous pneumothoraces have been described with cystic lesions. PPB may consist of

solitary or multiple lesions, and may even have a familial predisposition. They are often misdiagnosed as CPAM on imaging studies. Microscopically, these lesions are very similar to a CPAM in that PPBs have thin cyst walls lined by alveolar epithelium, but are distinguished by focal areas of hypercellularity and hypervascularity. Complete surgical resection is the goal for children with PPB. Resection with clear margins may be adequate for type I lesions, but adjuvant therapy is required for higher-grade lesions after surgical resection, and radiation is recommended for any residual disease [5, 41]. Metastases to the brain, bone, and liver are seen in up to 30% of patients with type II and III PPB. The outcome for children with PPB correlates with the grade. Type I lesions have an 83% long-term survival and cure rate whereas this goes down to only 42% for those with type II and II lesions [48].

Bronchoalveolar carcinoma. Bronchoalveolar carcinoma (BAC) is classified as a subset of lung adenocarcinoma but has a distinct clinical presentation, tumor biology, response to therapy, and prognosis compared with other subtypes of non-small-cell lung carcinoma. It is characterized by growth along alveolar septae without evidence of stromal, vascular, or pleural invasion [49]. BAC is much more common in adults than children. More than half of all patients with BAC are asymptomatic. Those who are symptomatic will complain of cough, sputum production, shortness of breath, weight loss, hemoptysis, and fever. Later stages of BAC are associated with a greater likelihood of symptoms. When the patient is symptomatic, the tumor usually has a rapidly progressive downhill course [50]. Spread of the tumor tends to occur via the airways, but lymphogenous and hematogenous dissemination may occur in 50–60% of cases [51–53].

BAC can be classified into mucinous and nonmucinous lesions with the former accounting for 80% of cases [53–55]. Mucinous BAC originate from columnar mucus-containing cells, whereas nonmucinous tumors arise from Clara cells or type 2 pneumocytes. The prognosis for mucinous BAC is worse than nonmucinous tumors with a 5-year survival rate of 26 vs. 72% [54, 55]. Surgical resection is the only potentially curative treatment.

CPAMs are rare lesions characterized by the presence of an abnormal mass of pulmonary tissue that appears immature and malformed and may show varying degrees of cystic change. CPAMs can host metaplastic mucous cells, primitive mesenchymal cells, and differentiated but poorly organized striated muscle fibers. Therefore, these congenital malformations are viewed as a predisposing condition for possible oncogenesis [56]. Both BAC and rhabdomyosarcoma (RMS) have been reported in association with CPAMs, which justifies prompt surgical removal after diagnosis.

Leiomyosarcoma. Leiomyosarcoma is a mesenchymal tumor with smooth muscle differentiation, and is very rare in children. The annual incidence is estimated to be less than 2 cases per ten million children [57]. Primary leiomyosarcoma of the lung may arise from the smooth muscle coat of the bronchial tree [58] or the vascular smooth muscle. The presenting symptoms are similar to those of bronchogenic carcinoma including cough, chest pain, pneumonia, or hemoptysis. As is the case in pulmonary leiomyomas, immunosuppression after solid organ transplant, congenital immune deficiencies, and HIV are all predisposing conditions to developing leiomyosarcomas in children [59]. Furthermore, there are documented reports linking Epstein–Barr virus with the development of this malignancy [59]. As with a leiomyoma, there is a potential for regression of this tumor with modulation of immunosuppression [5].

Histologically, the tumor is made up of interlacing bundles of elongated cells, showing in some cases many mitotic figures and occasional tumor giant cells. Nuclear atypia, necrosis, and hemorrhage distinguish leiomyosarcoma from both leiomyomas and the myofibroblastic tumors [5]. In spite of its anaplasia, this tumor has a much better prognosis than bronchogenic carcinoma. Metastases are uncommon, but if present occur late and usually spare the lymphatics [60]. Most primary lesions are solitary, whereas multiplicity suggests metastasis from another site. Treatment consists of local excision when possible as well as chemotherapy and radiation [61].

Primary bronchopulmonary fibrosarcoma. Primary bronchopulmonary fibrosarcoma (PBF) is an uncommon, mesenchymal tumor with less than 30 cases reported in the literature. They are low-grade tumors with a relatively good prognosis and should be regarded as the bronchopulmonary counterpart of the congenital-infantile fibrosarcoma of the soft tissues [62]. Patients with PBF typically present with cough, fever, chest pain, pneumonitis, and hemoptysis. Endobronchial and intraparenchymal tumors have both been described, with the former having a better prognosis, possibly due to earlier discovery

because of obstructive symptoms. Endobronchial lesions are usually of a lower histologic grade, show less mitotic activity, and have a more uniform pattern of growth than the intraparenchymal tumors [63]. Histologically, these tumors are highly cellular and made up of interlacing bundles of densely packed spindle cells. Radiologically, PBF is a markedly heterogeneously enhancing large mass which typically occupies almost the entire hemithorax (Fig. 13.7). Metastases are uncommon and occur in 7% of patients. In the absence of metastases, complete resection can be curative. Bronchoscopic removal of endobronchial lesions is discouraged due to the possibility of endobronchial extension. Radiation and chemotherapy are reserved for unresectable lesions. There is a mortality rate of 21% [62] associated with PBF, but 5-year survival rates can reach as high as 84% [64].

Congenital/infantile fibrosarcoma. Congenital fibrosarcoma most often occurs in children under 2 years of age, and almost half are present at birth. They most commonly affect the distal portions of the extremities, and most patients are asymptomatic other than a nontender swelling or mass. Fibrosarcoma is a tumor composed of anaplastic spindle-shaped

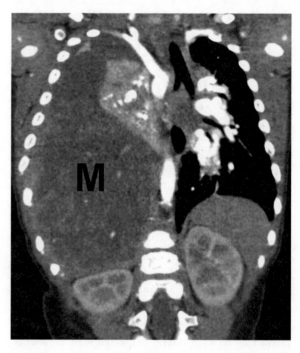

Fig. 13.7. Two-month-old boy presented with cough, fever, and hemoptysis. Enhanced coronal CT image demonstrates a large heterogeneously enhancing mass (M) almost completely occupying the right hemithorax (mass histologically confirmed as PBF)

cells that are arranged in a herringbone pattern. The degree of cellular differentiation and mitotic activity may be stratified into a specific grade, and then used to predict the clinical behavior of the tumor [65]. However, fibrous proliferations in infants and children are often difficult to evaluate because their histologic features do not always correlate with clinical behavior [66]. Congenital fibrosarcomas are rapidly growing tumors composed of immature-appearing spindle-shaped cells with high cellularity and mitotic activity. Despite these features, they have a relatively good prognosis, especially compared with the adult form of fibrosarcoma. Eight percent of patients will have evidence of metastases and there is an 84% associated 5-year survival rate [66]. Wide local excision is the treatment of choice with radiation and chemotherapy being reserved for recurrent or metastatic lesions.

13.1.3 Pediatric Metastatic Neoplasm

An overwhelming majority of lung tumors in the pediatric population are metastatic. Metastatic tumors account for 80% of all lung tumors in children and more than 95% of the malignant ones [4]. In children, it is extremely important to diagnose lung metastases at an early stage as early detection has important therapeutic and prognostic implications. Osteosarcoma and Wilms tumor are the most common malignancies to metastasize to the lungs. Since lung metastases are far more common than primary lung tumors, the clinician is obligated to look for a primary source when suspicious lesions are detected by imaging studies. Plain radiographs will often fail to detect a substantial number of thoracic metastases, as most metastatic lesions are pleural based, subpleural, or in the outer one-third of the lung which is more difficult to detect. Therefore, CT is the image of choice for completely evaluating metastatic thoracic disease in children. Metastases often appear as single or multiple circumscribed nodules, and preferentially involve the lower lobes [28]. The current indications for using CT for evaluating metastatic thoracic disease include (1) searching for occult metastases for diagnostic and therapeutic reasons; (2) further evaluation when conventional studies are limited for a complete evaluation; (3) preoperative evaluation; (4) evaluation of prognostic indicators; (5) CT-directed transthoracic thin-needle aspiration; and (6) radiation planning [67].

It is important to remember that no imaging modality has the ability to definitively distinguish between benign and malignant disease. Some metastatic lung nodules are excised in children for diagnostic purposes, but others are removed to achieve long-term survival and even cure [68]. Pulmonary metastasectomy is most common for osteosarcoma, but may also be beneficial in tumors resistant to chemotherapy and radiation. Surgical management of pulmonary metastases is uncommon and usually unnecessary for chemo- and radiosensitive tumors. However, when necessary, surgical resection of pulmonary metastases is always performed with a curative intent. In general, good surgical candidates meet all of the following criteria:

- Primary tumor diagnosis
- Primary tumor site adequately controlled or resected
- No other known extrapulmonary metastases (if additional metastases are present, they should be considered amenable to surgery or some other form of therapy)
- Good surgical candidates from the standpoint of cardiopulmonary and other comorbid conditions
- Location of metastatic lesion is such that it can be completely resected with reasonable preservation of the remaining normal lung

Wilms Tumor

Wilms tumor is the most common childhood abdominal malignancy. It affects the kidney and is successfully treated in over 90% of patients. Pulmonary metastases are found in 12–15% of patients at the time of diagnosis [69, 70]. Metastases are typically asymptomatic and detected by imaging such as plain radiographs or CT (Fig. 13.8). Patients with a favorable histology and lung metastases have a 75% 4-year survival rate [71]. Metastases from a Wilms' tumor tend to be more chemo- and radiosensitive, so there is a limited role for metastasectomy. However, suspicious pulmonary lesions in the setting of a Wilms' tumor should be biopsied as up to 33% will be negative for tumor [72]. Thus, a biopsy can spare the patient extra radiation.

Hepatoblastoma

Hepatoblastoma is the most common malignant hepatic tumor in children, although it is relatively uncommon compared with other solid tumors in the pediatric age group. It accounts for 79% of all liver tumors in children and almost two-thirds of primary malignant liver tumors in the pediatric age group. Children are most often diagnosed before 3 years of age with a median age of 1 year. Surgical techniques and adjuvant chemotherapy have markedly improved the prognosis of children with hepatoblastoma.

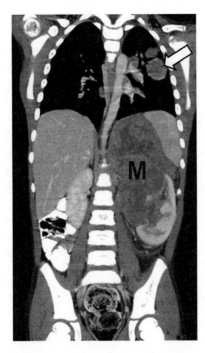

Fig. 13.8. Four-year-old girl with left flank pain and hematuria. Enhanced coronal CT image shows a large mass (M) arising from the left kidney and pulmonary metastasis (*arrow*). Surgical pathology of the left renal mass was consistent with Wilm's tumor

Complete surgical resection of the tumor at diagnosis, followed by adjuvant chemotherapy, is associated with 100% survival rates.

Although patients with hepatoblastoma are usually asymptomatic at diagnosis, approximately 40% of patients will have advanced disease and 20% will have pulmonary metastases. Surgical resection of pulmonary metastases is a preferred treatment option if local control of the primary tumor has been accomplished with preoperative chemotherapy and local resection [73]. Micrometastases at the time of diagnosis are treated by preoperative chemotherapy. Although the overall prognosis of patients with lung metastases is worse compared to those with localized involvement, metastasectomy may be curative with local control of the primary tumor (Fig. 13.9). The overall 5-year survival rate of patients with a positive CT scan and a negative CXR is 77% compared with 42% in patients who had positive findings on both CT and plain films [74].

Neuroblastoma

Neuroblastoma is the most common extracranial solid tumor in children accounting for 10% of all childhood cancers [75, 76]. It is an embryonal malignancy of the sympathetic nervous system arising from neuroblasts. Infants younger than 1 year of age have a good prognosis, even in the presence of metastatic disease; whereas older patients with metastatic disease fare poorly, even when treated with aggressive therapy. Infants more commonly present with thoracic and cervical tumors, whereas in older children neuroblastomas are more likely abdominal in location.

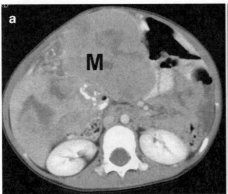
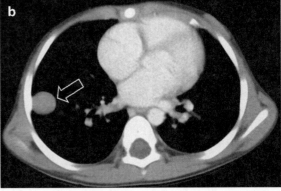

Fig. 13.9. Three-year-old girl presented with weight loss and a palpable right abdominal mass. Surgical pathology of the hepatic mass was consistent with hepatoblastoma. (**a**) Enhanced axial CT image of the upper abdomen shows a large heterogeneously enhancing (M) mass. (**b**) Enhanced axial CT image of the lung demonstrates a pulmonary mass (*arrow*) consistent with metastatic disease

Neuroblastoma can occur in the sympathetic ganglia in the chest wall in children. They manifest as palpable masses which may or may not be painful [61]. Prognosis is variable and depends on the patient's age, stage of disease, and histologic findings. Most patients present with signs and symptoms related to tumor growth.

Pulmonary involvement in neuroblastoma can result from direct extension, hematogenous, or lymphangetic spread. Most large studies report an incidence of pulmonary metastases to be 5% or less [77–79]. Neuroblastoma lung metastases occur when the tumor is widely disseminated and is a poor prognostic factor. Patients with lung metastases are found to have N-MYC amplification and an unfavorable histopathology. Furthermore, children with lung metastases have a lower event-free survival (EFS) as compared to all other patients with stage IV disease; 15 vs. 50%, respectively at 2 years after diagnosis [78].

A routine chest CT at the time of diagnosis is warranted to look for pulmonary metastases which can have a profound impact on prognosis. Due to the poor prognosis in patients with pulmonary metastases, pulmonary metastasectomy is not recommended. However, if there is concern about the nature of a pulmonary lesion after or during treatment, then a biopsy is warranted [80].

Osteosarcoma

Osteosarcoma is the third most common cancer in adolescence, occurring less frequently than lymphomas and brain tumors. It is thought to arise from a primitive mesenchymal bone-forming cell and is characterized by production of osteoid. The mainstay of therapy is removal of the lesion. Chemotherapy is also required to treat micrometastatic disease, which is present but not detectable in most patients at diagnosis.

Pulmonary metastases are found in approximately 10–15% of patients at the time of diagnosis [81]. They are usually asymptomatic and detected by imaging studies. The lung metastases are usually multiple, bilateral in over half the patients (Fig. 13.10), and calcified in 14% (Fig. 13.11) [82]. Both the number of nodules and number of lobes involved are significant predictors of survival. Each additional lobe that is affected signifies a 1.4 times increased risk of death. In patients with more than 3 nodules present at the time of diagnosis, the risk of death is 5.1 times greater [82]. Survival has been improved by metastasectomy

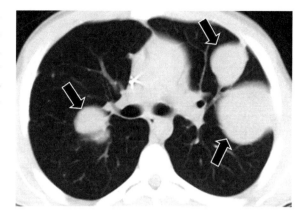

Fig. 13.10. Five-year-old boy with right femoral osteosarcoma. Lung window axial CT image shows multiple pulmonary nodules (*arrows*) consistent with metastatic disease

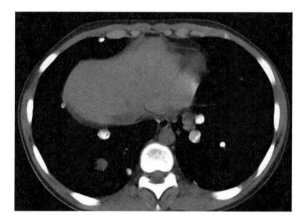

Fig. 13.11. Seventeen-year-old boy with metastatic osteosarcoma. Non-enhanced axial CT image demonstrates multiple calcified pulmonary nodules

which may require multiple thoracotomies. There is a 3-year survival rate of 45 vs. 5% with and without metastasectomy [68].

Ewing's Sarcoma

Ewing's sarcoma is the second most common primary osseous malignancy in childhood with an incidence of approximately 0.6 per million [83]. Twenty to twenty-five percent of patients with Ewing's sarcoma will present with stage IV metastases with one-third having only lung or pleural nodules [84, 85]. This tumor is generally sensitive to both chemotherapy as well as radiation. Surgical excision of metastatic lesions is mainly for diagnostic purposes and the role of metastasectomy is unclear.

Rhabdomyosarcoma

RMS is the most common soft tissue sarcoma in children [86]. Several distinct histologic groups have prognostic significance, including embryonal rhabdomyosarcoma (ERMS), which occurs in 55% of patients; the botryoid variant of ERMS, which occurs in 5% of patients; alveolar RMS, which occurs in 20% of patients; and undifferentiated sarcoma, which occurs in 20% of patients [87]. Although RMS is believed to arise from primitive muscle cells, tumors can occur anywhere in the body except bone. The most common sites are the head and neck (28%), extremities (24%), and genitourinary (GU) tract (18%). Other notable sites include the trunk (11%), orbit (7%), and retroperitoneum (6%). Treatment responses and prognoses vary depending on tumor location and histology.

In patients with localized disease, overall 5-year survival rates have improved to more than 80% with the combined use of surgery, radiation, and chemotherapy [88]. Approximately 15% of patients will present with metastatic disease and the overall cure rate for these patients is below 30%. If metastatic disease is present, symptoms of bone pain, respiratory distress secondary to lung nodules, anemia, thrombocytopenia, and neutropenia may all be present. Currently, there is no standard role for metastasectomy [68].

EFS was found to correlate with certain risk factors: age less than 1 year or at least 10 years, unfavorable site of primary tumor (extremity), bone or bone marrow involvement, and three or more metastatic sites. EFS is 50% for patients without any of these four adverse factors and was respectively 42, 18, 12, and 5% in patients with one, two, three, or four risk factors [89].

Synovial Sarcoma

Synovial sarcomas represent 5–10% of all soft tissue sarcomas [90], which are rare tumors of connective tissue. Despite the name, synovial sarcomas are not thought to originate from the joint, but instead occur nearby. This lesion tends to affect young individuals within the age range of 15–40, and is divided into three histological types: biphasic, monophasic, and poorly differentiated [91]. Half of all patients will develop metastatic disease with the lungs the most

common location [92, 93]. In one series [91], 74% of patients had developed metastatic disease by 5 years and 81% by 10 years. The median survival following a diagnosis of metastatic disease was 22 months. Prognostic factors correlate with an age less than 35 and response to first-line chemotherapy. There was no evidence that metastasectomy improved survival.

Germ Cell Tumors

Testicular cancer is the most common neoplasm in males under the age of 40 [94]. It constitutes about 2% of all malignancies, and 95% of all testicular tumors are of germ cell origin [95]. At the time of diagnosis, it is estimated that pulmonary metastases are present in 50% of patients with retroperitoneal involvement as opposed to only 10% of patients without retroperitoneal extension (Fig. 13.12) [96]. Germ cell tumors are chemosensitive lesions with a long-term survival rate of 90% [97]. Forty percent of patients will harbor viable tumor cells within radiographically visible lesions post-therapy [97–101]. Therefore, the role of pulmonary metastasectomy is primarily to define the presence of viable tumor in lesions after chemotherapy and for determining further treatment regimens [80].

13.1.4   Pediatric Central Airway Neoplasm

Central airway tumors are rare in children and often misdiagnosed leading to a delay in definitive treatment. Patients are symptomatic due to airway obstruction and present with common complaints such as cough, stridor, wheeze, recurrent pneumonia, or persistent atelectasis. Imaging is often not performed until it becomes evident that standard therapies are ineffective. Bronchoscopy can be useful for diagnosis of central airway neoplasms as it allows for direct visualization of the tumor. A biopsy of the lesion may provide a definitive diagnosis; however, the true extent of the tumor is often hard to appreciate. Therefore, CT may be needed in conjunction with bronchoscopy.

Benign tumors occur more frequently in the larynx or upper trachea, while malignant tumors occur more distally. The most common benign tumors of the central airways are hemangiomas and papillomas. Other benign central airway tumors include granular cell tumors, hamartomas, plasma cell granulomas, leiomyomas, and mucous gland

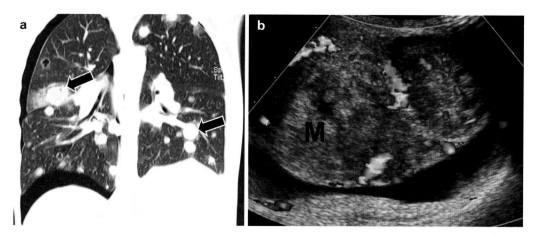

Fig. 13.12. Twelve-year-old boy presented with shortness of breath and enlarged scrotum on physical examination. Surgical pathology was consistent with testicular neoplasm. (a) Coronal lung window CT image shows multiple pulmonary masses (*arrows*). Also noted is a right-sided pneumothorax. (b) Transverse view of right testicle shows heterogeneous intratesticular mass (M)

tumors. Malignant central airway tumors in children include bronchial adenomas, a group of malignant tumors consisting of carcinoid tumor, mucoepidermoid carcinoma, and adenoid cystic carcinoma.

Benign

Hemangioma

Although airway hemangiomas are present at birth, symptoms usually develop between 1 and 6 months of age [102, 103]. Lesions are most often found in the subglottic area, and present with symptoms of obstruction or recurrent hemoptysis. Hemangiomas appear as rounded soft tissue masses on CT with marked contrast enhancement (Fig. 13.13). Symptomatic patients can be treated with laser removal.

Papilloma

Recurrent respiratory papillomatosis (RRP) is a benign lesion of the larynx and trachea caused by human papillomavirus (HPV), usually types 6 and 11. RRP is the most common benign neoplasm of the larynx among children and the second most frequent cause of hoarseness in childhood [104]. The incidence in children is estimated at 4.3 cases per 100,000 persons. It is typically acquired during delivery through the birth canal and most commonly affects the larynx and trachea. However, in some cases the distal bronchial tree and esophagus can be involved [5]. Spread into the distal trachea and the lung parenchyma rarely occurs; however, if extension does occur solid nodules or cystic air-filled cavities are

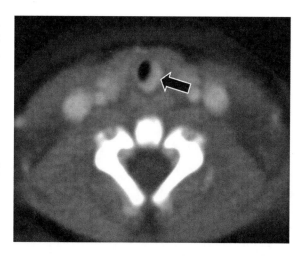

Fig. 13.13. Two-month-old girl with increasing respiratory distress. Enhanced axial CT examination shows markedly enhancing subglottic lesion (*arrow*), consistent with subglottic hemangioma

seen (Fig. 13.14) [28]. As the papilloma grows, the airway becomes more obstructed leading to changes in a patient's voice, or stridor which may progress from inspiratory to biphasic. The age of presentation is variable, but commonly occurs in patients between 2 and 3 years of age. Papillomas of the larynx do not become symptomatic prior to 6 months of age. The differential diagnosis includes asthma, croup, allergies, vocal cord nodules, and bronchitis. Diagnosis is made by flexible laryngoscopy in the office or rigid bronchoscopy in the operating room. Although considered a benign lesion, progression to squamous cell carcinoma has been reported. Therefore, it is essential to biopsy the lesion at the time of surgical excision. Treatment consists of excision by a carbon dioxide laser. Younger age at diagnosis is associated with more aggressive disease and the need for more frequent surgical procedures to decrease the airway burden. Children may require surgical excision as frequently as every 2–4 weeks due to recurrence until the disease becomes quiescent in adolescence. There is currently no known effective medical adjuvant therapy.

Granular Cell Tumor

Granular cell tumors are uncommon benign lesions, although there are case reports of these tumors behaving in a malignant fashion. This entity has been described in patients as young as 6 months of age, with a median age of 31 years [105]. Granular cell

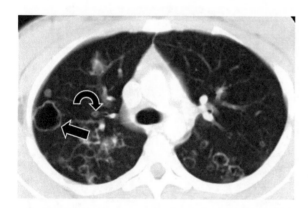

Fig. 13.14. Seventeen-year-old boy with known papillomatosis. Lung window axial CT image shows a combination of cavitary (*arrow*) and noncavitary (*curved arrow*) nodules in both lungs

tumors are often asymptomatic, thus can be present for up to 3 years before being diagnosed. Most cases are managed by bronchoscopic excision, but recurrent pneumonia has occasionally necessitated radical lobectomy or pneumonectomy (Fig. 13.15) [106].

Malignant

Bronchial Adenomas

Bronchial adenoma is a misnomer as this refers to a group of malignant lesions found in the airway. The most common tumors in this group are carcinoid tumors, mucoepidermoid carcinomas, and adenoid cystic carcinomas in decreasing order of frequency. The overall incidence is unknown, but bronchial adenomas may account for 5% of all primary pulmonary neoplasms in children [107]. However, they are the largest group (40%) of primary malignant lung lesions in the pediatric population [7, 26].

Carcinoid Tumor

Bronchial carcinoid tumors are characterized by neuroendocrine differentiation and a relatively indolent clinical course. Originally characterized as an adenoma, they are now classified as malignant tumors due to their potential to metastasize. Bronchial carcinoids are the most common primary malignant lung neoplasm in children and typically present in late adolescence. The incidence ranges from 0.2 to 2/100,000 population per year. The majority of carcinoid tumors arise in the proximal airways and patients are symptomatic at presentation. The obstructive lesion manifests as cough, wheeze, chest pain, recurrent pneumonia, atelectasis, and even

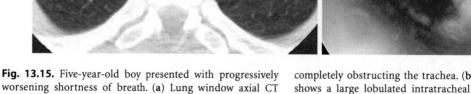

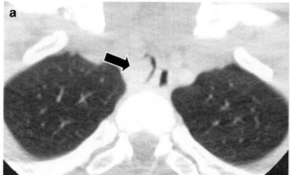

Fig. 13.15. Five-year-old boy presented with progressively worsening shortness of breath. (**a**) Lung window axial CT image demonstrates a large intratracheal mass (*arrow*) almost completely obstructing the trachea. (**b**) Bronchoscopy image shows a large lobulated intratracheal mass diagnosed as a granular cell tumor

hemoptysis due to its hypervascularity. About 25% of carcinoids originate peripherally and are detected on routine CXR. Patients with peripheral carcinoids are usually asymptomatic, which leads to a delay in diagnosis. Although bronchial carcinoids have the potential to metastasize, they rarely do so. In localized disease carcinoid syndrome rarely occurs, and only does so in tumors of larger size (>5 cm) [108]. However, carcinoid syndrome will occur in over 80% of patients with liver metastasis.

There are two types of bronchial carcinoids, and they are defined by their histological appearance. Typical carcinoids (90%) are low grade, slow growing neoplasms that rarely metastasize, and have a more favorable prognosis. Atypical carcinoids (10%) are higher-grade lesions, present more often with hilar or mediastinal nodal metastases, and have a higher recurrence rate. Between 5 and 20% of typical carcinoids metastasize to lymph nodes compared to 30–70% of atypical lesions [109].

Diagnosis of a carcinoid tumor can be suggested by CXR and CT scan and then confirmed by bronchoscopy and biopsy (Fig. 13.16). Up to 75% of patients with a bronchial carcinoid will have an abnormal CXR. CT scan is more sensitive and frequently shows marked enhancement of the lesion due to its hypervascularity. Treatment is primarily surgical; however, endoscopic resection is not recommended due to the risk of hemorrhage and incomplete resection [5]. Local invasion or distant metastases have been reported in 27% of children, but overall survival is excellent and estimated to be approximately 90% [110, 111]. The 5-year survival rates for local, regional, and disseminated disease are 81, 77, and 26%, respectively [112].

Mucoepidermoid Carcinoma

Mucoepidermoid tumor (MET) is another "bronchial adenoma." These tumors typically arise from bronchial mucous glands in the main stem bronchus or in the proximal portion of lobar bronchi as an endobronchial polypoid growth covered by normal epithelium [113]. The true incidence is unknown, but the tumor is quite rare and usually presents with signs of obstruction such as cough, dyspnea, wheeze, hemoptysis, or obstructive pneumonia. Chest films are usually abnormal showing a central mass or a nodule in 66% of cases (Fig. 13.17) [113]. Diagnosis is made most often by endobronchial biopsy. MET is classified as either low or high grade based on the histological appearance [114]. Low-grade tumors are

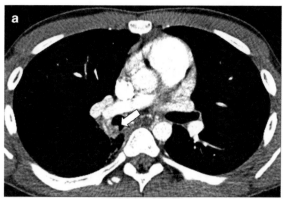

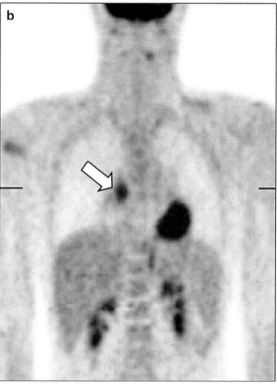

Fig. 13.16. Fifteen-year-old boy with cough and one episode of hemoptysis. (**a**) Enhanced axial CT image demonstrates a heterogeneously enhancing endoluminal mass (*arrow*) in the proximal right lower lobe bronchus. (**b**) Coronal PET image shows an abnormal focus of uptake adjacent to the mediastinum in the right chest correlating with the site of the endobronchial mass seen in (**a**). Histologic diagnosis was carcinoid tumor

mostly cystic, tend not to have local invasion into the parenchyma, and metastasis to lymph nodes is unusual. High-grade tumors have more solid areas of growth. Mitotic activity and necrosis are common in high-grade lesions as well as metastases to regional lymph nodes [115]. Low-grade tumors occur in patients younger than 30 years of age over 50% of the time whereas high-grade tumors are more common in an older population [116]. Treatment is surgical

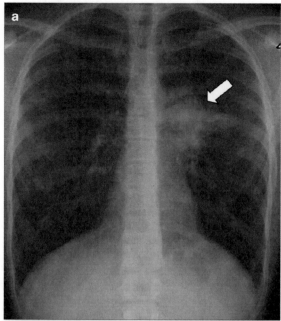

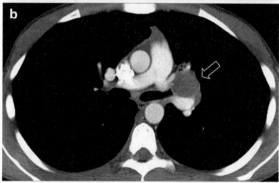

Fig. 13.17. Eleven-year-old boy with respiratory distress. Surgical pathology of left hilar mass was consistent with mucoepidermoid carcinoma. (**a**) Frontal chest radiograph shows a large mass-like opacity (*arrow*) in the left hilar region. (**b**) Enhanced axial CT image demonstrates a mildly enhancing soft tissue mass (*arrow*) located in the left hilar region

resection. Low-grade METs have an excellent prognosis with a 5-year survival rate around 80%. However, high-grade tumors carry a significantly worse prognosis with 5-year survival rates as low as 31%. Survival seems to correlate with lymph node metastasis [115].

Adenoid Cystic Carcinoma

Adenoid cystic carcinoma is the last major tumor classified as a bronchial adenoma. It is a slow growing, infiltrative, salivary gland-like tumor. It is rare in children but has been reported in adolescents. There is often a long interval between onset of symptoms and diagnosis as the CXR is often negative. One series

found a mean duration of symptoms before diagnosis to be 15 months. The most common presenting symptoms are shortness of breath, wheeze, cough, stridor, and hemoptysis [117]. This tends to be a locally invasive tumor that extends beyond the wall of the trachea and it is often difficult to safely extend the surgical resection far enough to obtain tumor-free margins at the transected ends of the airway. Local recurrence may occur years after resection.

Adenoid cystic carcinoma has a higher likelihood of distant metastasis compared with MET and has a poorer prognosis. Hematogenous metastasis occur in over half of the patients, most often to the lungs, and rarely to the lymphatics. However, most patients do not have evidence of metastasis at the time of initial diagnosis. In fact, metastasis often occur years after the diagnosis of the primary tumor. Treatment consists of both surgery and radiation. Many cases are amenable to segmental resection of the airway with removal of all gross disease and reconstruction by primary anastomosis. Most tumors will respond to radiation, which may be a reasonable adjuvant therapy to offer all patients with adenoid cystic carcinoma, and definitely in those patients with residual tumor after resection [117].

13.1.5   Pediatric Chest Wall Neoplasm

Benign chest wall tumors are uncommon lesions that originate from blood vessels, nerves, bone, cartilage, or fat. Although radiologic characteristics of benign and malignant chest wall tumors often overlap, there are certain features that can suggest a specific diagnosis. Such features include the presence of mature fat tissue with little or no septation (lipoma), phleboliths and vascular enhancement (cavernous hemangioma), evidence of neural origin combined with a target-like appearance on MRI (neurofibroma), well-defined continuity of cortical and medullary bone with the site of origin (osteochondroma), or fusiform expansion and ground-glass matrix (fibrous dysplasia) [118].

Chest wall tumors are uncommon in children, but when they do occur they are usually malignant. They present as a rapidly growing, palpable mass which may cause pain and respiratory distress. Chest films are part of the initial evaluation, but most often a CT or even an MRI is required. CT scan is more sensitive than a plain film for detecting calcification and cortical destruction. MRI can further characterize the soft tissue component of the tumor burden and help determine the extent of tumor invasion. Imaging techniques can often help to narrow the differential, but an incisional biopsy is often necessary since many of these lesions are malignant in nature. Malignant chest wall tumors are classified into eight diagnostic categories: muscular, vascular, fibrous and fibrohistiocytic, peripheral nerve, osseous and cartilaginous, adipose, hematologic, and cutaneous [61].

Osseous Tumors

Benign

Fibrous dysplasia. Fibrous dysplasia of the bone is a skeletal developmental anomaly in which mesenchymal osteoblasts fail to undergo normal morphologic differentiation and maturation [118]. Patients are most often asymptomatic but may present with pain from a pathologic fracture due to a weakened bone. Fifty percent of patients with fibrous dysplasia will have a fracture [119]. Asymptomatic patients can be observed, whereas surgery is indicated for prevention or treatment of fractures or major deformities.

Osteochondroma. Osteochondromas are the most common benign bone tumors. They are cartilage-capped bony projections on the external surface of a bone (Fig. 13.18). Whether sessile or pedunculated, the medullary canal of the stalk and the bone are in continuity by definition. Osteochondromas grow until skeletal maturity; growth generally stops once the growth plates fuse [120]. Most are diagnosed in patients younger than 20 years of age, most commonly as an incidental finding on radiographs obtained for other reasons. The second most common presentation is a mass, which may or may not be associated with

pain. Most of these lesions do not need to be treated, and asymptomatic lesions can be safely ignored. However, when painful, they need to be evaluated properly. Complications include fractures, osseous deformity, vascular injury, neural compression, and malignant transformation. Pain at the lesion site, bone erosion, irregular calcification, or thickening of the cartilage cap depicted on radiographic imaging can indicate malignant transformation [118].

Malignant

Osteosarcoma. Osteosarcomas in the thorax are rare, and are usually osseous in origin. They tend to occur in the second and third decades of life and present as a painful mass. Sites of origin include ribs, scapula, and the clavicle (Fig. 13.19). Local recurrence and metastatic spread (up to 70% of patients) to the lungs and lymph nodes occur more frequently in osteosarcomas of the chest wall compared to those in the extremities [61]. Treatment consists of preoperative chemotherapy followed by resection. Five-year survival rates are approximately 15% compared with osteosarcomas in the extremities which can reach 60–70%.

Ewing's sarcoma. Ewing sarcomas are associated with a chromosome 22 translocation and are composed of small round cells [121]. The Ewing sarcoma family of tumors includes Ewing sarcoma, peripheral primitive neuroectodermal tumor (PNET)/Askin tumor, neuroepithelioma, and atypical Ewing sarcoma. These tumors are treated similarly on the basis of their clinical presentation (e.g., metastatic or localized) rather than their histologic subtype. Tumors

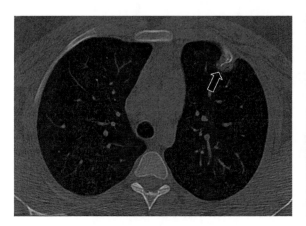

Fig. 13.18. Seventeen-year-old girl with left chest pain. Bone window axial CT image demonstrates a cartilage-capped bony projection (*arrow*) arising from the inner surface of the left rib, consistent with osteochondroma

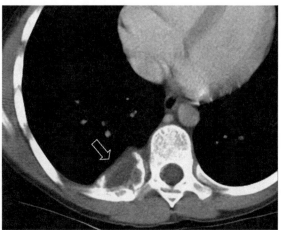

Fig. 13.19. Twelve-year-old boy with right lower thoracic pain. Enhanced axial CT image shows a mass (*arrow*) composed of both soft tissue and osseous components. Surgical pathology of this mass was consistent with osteosarcoma

that arise in the chest wall usually do so from the rib or less commonly the scapula, and account for 15% of Ewing sarcomas [122]. This is the most common tumor of the chest wall in children and young adults and usually presents as a painful chest mass. Treatment consists of chemotherapy followed by resection with or without radiation. Prognosis is determined by metastases which occur in 75% of patients. Five-year survival rates are less than 30% with metastatic involvement, but can approach 100% with localized disease [122].

Soft Tissue Tumors

Benign

Hemangioma. Cavernous hemangiomas consist of dilated, tortuous, thin-walled vessels. They are most often large cutaneous lesions which are poorly circumscribed (Fig. 13.20). These benign chest wall masses are either present at birth or appear before the age of 30.

Lipoma. Lipomas are common benign mesenchymal tumors occurring in 1% of the population, and are usually asymptomatic. They are slow-growing, benign fatty tumors that form soft, lobulated masses enclosed by a thin, fibrous capsule. Lipomas must be differentiated from other masses or tumors. In the subcutaneous location, the primary differential diagnosis is a sebaceous cyst or an abscess. When they arise from fatty tissue between the skin and deep fas-

cia, typical features include a soft, fluctuant feel, and free mobility of overlying skin. A characteristic *slippage sign* may be elicited by gently sliding the fingers off the edge of the tumor. The tumor will be felt to slip out from under your fingers, as opposed to a sebaceous cyst or an abscess that is tethered by surrounding induration. The overlying skin is typically normal. Most of these are small subcutaneous tumors that are removed for the following reasons: (1) cosmetic reasons (>5 cm in size); (2) continuous growth resulting in symptoms; and (3) evaluation of their underlying histology.

Malignant

Rhabdomyosarcoma. Primary thoracic sarcomas are rare and are classified by histological features. They occur in the lung, mediastinum, pleura, and chest wall. These tumors are large, heterogeneous masses that have a wide spectrum of radiologic appearances. Angiosarcoma, leiomyosarcoma, RMS, and mesothelioma are the most common primary intrathoracic tumors [121]. RMSs are high-grade sarcomas characterized by skeletal muscle differentiation. Pulmonary RMS is more common in pediatric patients and represents approximately 0.5% of all RMSs in children [26]. It is the most common cardiac sarcoma in children.

Rhabdomyosarcomas in the chest wall manifest as rapidly growing masses and may cause pain due to nerve compression (Fig. 13.21). Primary tumors invade the bone up to 20% of the time [61]. The alveolar

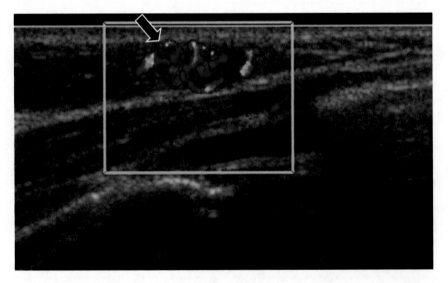

Fig. 13.20. Two-year-old girl with a palpable right-sided chest wall lesion. Ultrasound shows a subcutaneous soft tissue mass (*arrow*) with increased internal vascularity, consistent with hemangioma

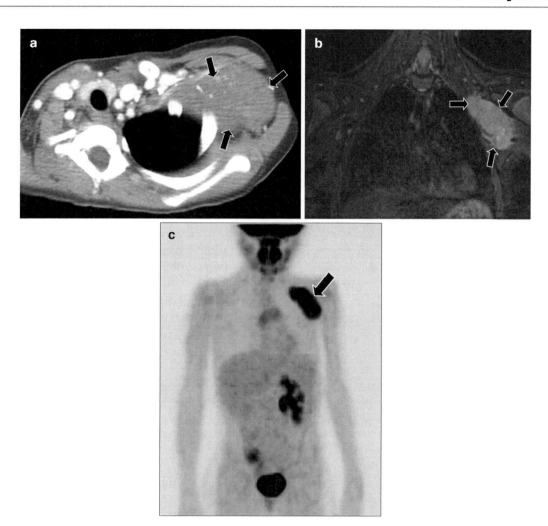

Fig. 13.21. Six-year-old girl with left chest and arm pain. Surgical pathology of the left chest wall mass was consistent with rhabdomyosarcoma (RMS). (**a**) Enhanced axial CT image shows a large heterogeneously enhancing mass (*arrows*) located in the left upper chest wall. (**b**) Coronal STIR MR image demonstrates a large left upper chest wall mass (*arrows*) with increased MR signal intensity. (**c**) Coronal PET image shows abnormally increased uptake (*arrow*) in the left chest wall area corresponding well with a large mass seen on CT (**a**) and MR (**b**) images

subtype is the most common and carries the worst prognosis, while the embryonal subtype typically occurs in children.

Pulmonary lesions tend to present with cough and dyspnea, whereas chest wall tumors present with pain. The mass is usually large on imaging studies with necrotic and cystic components. Focal invasion is common and treatment consists of chemotherapy. The prognosis is related to the histological subtype with embryonal and pleomorphic subtypes having a better prognosis than the alveolar RMS [123]. Well-differentiated tumors have the best prognosis and survival may be greater than 80% if the tumor is localized [121].

Primitive neuroectodermal tumor (Askin tumor). The Askin tumor is a rare, malignant small-cell neuroepithelioma that arises from the soft tissues of the chest wall or lung and is seen predominantly in children and young adults [124]. This neoplasm is now recognized as a type of PNET. They are undifferentiated small-round-cell sarcomas which develop from embryonal migrating cells of the neural crest. The Askin tumor must be differentiated from other tumors that have small round cells, such as undifferentiated neuroblastoma, ERMS, Ewing's sarcoma, and lymphoma [125]. Both Ewing's sarcoma and PNET carry the (11;22) translocation, but neurosecretory granules on electron microscopic examination will be seen in the latter

[124, 126, 127]. Clinically, the Askin tumor presents as a chest wall mass with or without pain. Rapid growth may result in destruction of adjacent anatomic structures [124], with bone destruction being the most common complication. Metastatic disease at presentation has been reported to range from 10% [124, 128, 129] to 38% [130]. MRI is useful in determining involvement of the chest wall muscle whereas CT is better for detecting pulmonary metastases. Treatment consists of chemotherapy, surgery, and radiation. This tumor has a tendency to recur locally with direct extension into the pleura and lung or to develop pulmonary nodules [131]. This is a sign of initial treatment failure. One series showed a disease-free survival rate of 56% after 3 years for patients with localized PNET, whereas no curative approach seems available for patients with metastatic disease [132].

13.1.6 Conclusion

Pediatric thoracic tumors are rare and present with nonspecific physical and radiographic findings. Therefore, a high index of suspicion is necessary to make the correct diagnosis when patients have persistent clinical symptoms. In general, malignant tumors are more common in children that benign lesions with the majority being metastatic in nature. Complete surgical resection is the mainstay of treatment in primary lesions and is becoming more defined in secondary malignancies. Some lesions are amenable to adjuvant therapy, and prognosis varies depending on tumor location, stage, and type.

Malignant Mediastinal Masses

SHASHI H. RANGANATH AND EDWARD Y. LEE

Malignant mediastinal masses are uncommon in children. Due to their rarity and often nonspecific clinical presentations, the correct diagnosis is unfortunately often initially missed or delayed in children. While these malignant mediastinal masses may be incidental findings in some children, they can also result in various symptoms depending on their size, location, mass effect upon adjacent mediastinal structures, and production of specific biochemical products. Imaging plays an important role for early and correct diagnosis,

which in turn can improve patient care by guiding the next appropriate step in management. In this section, we discuss malignant mediastinal masses in pediatric patients with an emphasis on reviewing (1) clinical presentation; (2) practical imaging approaches to diagnosis; and (3) radiological imaging findings.

13.2.1 Clinical Presentations of Malignant Mediastinal Masses in Pediatric Patients

Various clinical presentations may lead to the suspicion and detection of a mediastinal malignant neoplasm in pediatric patients. Often, tumors are incidentally found when a patient undergoes an imaging study for some other unrelated complaint. However, approximately one-half to two-thirds of mediastinal masses in children are symptomatic [133–136]. Clinical signs and symptoms with which patients present depend on the benignity or malignancy of the mass, its size, location, presence or absence of infection, production of specific biochemical products, and associated disease states [133–136]. When symptomatic, malignant mediastinal masses in children often present with lethargy, fever, and chest pain [133–136]. In infants and children, respiratory symptoms such as dyspnea, cough, and stridor are common, particularly when there is an associated mass effect upon adjacent airways resulting in airway compression [133, 136]. Common diagnoses of these symptoms in children such as infection, reactive small airway disease, gastroesophageal reflux, and foreign body aspiration should first be carefully considered and evaluated, since mediastinal tumors are relatively rare compared with other more common causes.

When a malignant mediastinal neoplasm is present, invasion of adjacent structures such as the chest wall, pleura, and nerves can be also seen. Specific findings of chest pain, pleural effusion, hoarseness, Horner's syndrome, superior vena cava syndrome, paraplegia, and diaphragmatic paralysis may occur. Constitutional symptoms such as weight loss and fever may also be present [133–136]. The onset of mediastinal malignancy may be slow and insidious. The initial physical finding may be enlarged lymph nodes in the neck or supraclavicular region. Although imaging evaluation is paramount in devising a diagnostic and therapeutic plan, tissue sampling is typically required for a definitive diagnosis for most malignant mediastinal masses in children.

13.2.2 Practical Imaging Approach for Diagnosing Malignant Mediastinal Masses in Pediatric Patients

For diagnosing suspected malignant mediastinal masses on imaging, the first step is to localize the mass in three artificially divided mediastinal compartments (i.e., anterior, middle, or posterior mediastinal compartment) on the lateral chest radiograph (Fig. 13.22). The anterior mediastinal compartment is defined by the space bordered anteriorly by the sternum and posteriorly by the pericardium [137–140]. The middle mediastinal compartment is located between the anterior border of the pericardium and an imaginary line drawn approximately 1 cm posterior to the anterior border of the thoracic vertebral bodies [137–140]. The posterior mediastinal compartment is defined as the space bordered anteriorly by an imaginary line drawn approximately 1 cm posterior to the anterior border of the vertebral bodies and posteriorly by the posterior paravertebral gutters [137–140]. Localizing

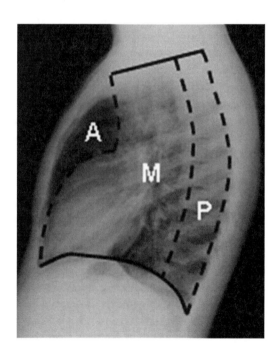

Fig. 13.22. Lateral chest radiograph depicting the three mediastinal compartments, anterior (A), middle (M), and posterior (P). The anterior mediastinal compartment is the space bordered anteriorly by the sternum and posteriorly by the pericardium. The middle mediastinal compartment is the space between the anterior border of the pericardium and an imaginary line drawn approximately 1 cm posterior to the anterior border of the thoracic vertebral bodies. The posterior mediastinal compartment is the space bordered anteriorly by an imaginary line drawn approximately 1 cm posterior to the anterior border of the vertebral bodies and posteriorly by the posterior paravertebral gutters

the mediastinal masses in these three mediastinal compartments helps to generate possible diagnostic considerations and narrow them. Furthermore, it also helps in guiding the next appropriate imaging studies for further characterization of mediastinal masses for a correct diagnosis.

Chest radiography is usually the first imaging modality used to determine the presence of a malignant mediastinal mass [136]. While chest radiographs often demonstrate mediastinal masses with a reasonably high degree of accuracy, they are limited in their capacity to establish a specific diagnosis [136]. After a mediastinal mass has been identified and localized on the lateral chest radiograph, cross-sectional imaging such as computed tomography (CT) or MRI can help confirm its location and further characterize the mass. CT is excellent for accurately diagnosing the nature, size, location, and organ involvement by mediastinal masses due to its high temporal and spatial resolution [136].

While CT is most often used in mediastinal mass assessment due to its wide availability and its ability to concomitantly assess airway and lung abnormalities, MRI can also provide important information. With its high contrast resolution and multiplanar capabilities, MR is the preferred modality in evaluating neurogenic tumors because it provides information regarding the nature and extent of intraspinal involvement from malignant mediastinal neoplasms. MRI can also help to characterize lesions as cystic or solid with more confidence than CT [136, 141, 142]. In pediatric patients with contraindications to iodinated contrast material, MR is a particularly useful alternative imaging modality to CT. The most important advantage of MR is the lack of ionizing radiation during image acquisition, an important consideration in pediatric patients. A disadvantage of MR, however, is the poor depiction of calcification, poorer spatial resolution, susceptibility to motion artifact, and longer scanning time often requiring sedation when compared to CT [135, 136, 138, 143]. For MR, general anesthesia may be required in younger or cognitively impaired children to avoid motion artifact.

Of relevance for both CT and MR, when there is a large anterior mediastinal mass, there may be accentuated compression of the trachea when the patient is supine. This may be severe enough to cause physiologically significant airway obstruction which is not present if the patient is not supine. In this instance, it may be necessary to treat the disease and shrink the mass before performing cross-sectional imaging.

13.2.3   Radiological Imaging Findings of Malignant Mediastinal Masses in Pediatric Patients

Anterior Mediastinum

Lymphoma (Hodgkin and Non-Hodgkin)

Lymphoma is the most common anterior mediastinal mass in children and is traditionally classified into two types: Hodgkin and non-Hodgkin [134–136, 142–144]. Hodgkin lymphoma represents about 5% of cases, while non-Hodgkin lymphoma (NHL) accounts for the remaining 95% of mediastinal lymphoma in pediatric patients [145, 146]. Lymphadenopathy from lymphoma may be asymptomatic or cause symptoms such as cough, chest pain, dyspnea, dysphagia, hemoptysis, or superior vena cava syndrome [133–136]. Other more nonspecific symptoms, termed B symptoms, include fever, weight loss, and night sweats, are more common in aggressive lymphomas [133–136].

Hodgkin lymphoma is histologically characterized by the presence of the Reed–Sternberg cell and has a good prognosis with an approximately 90% cure rate [134, 135, 142, 144]. It is traditionally classified into four types: (1) lymphocytic predominant; (2) nodular sclerosing; (3) mixed cellularity; and (4) lymphocyte-depleted [146]. Hodgkin lymphoma often involves the anterior mediastinum, with the thymus reportedly involved in 40–50% of patients with the nodular sclerosing subtype of Hodgkin disease [142]. The Ann Arbor classification is currently the most widely used staging system which is based on the number of nodal sites and the location of lymphoma involvement [146]. Approximately 85% of Hodgkin lymphoma demonstrates intrathoracic involvement at presentation, most commonly involving the anterior superior mediastinal lymph nodes (Fig. 13.23) [134, 135, 142–144, 147]. The lymph nodes rarely calcify before treatment; approximately 5% calcify after treatment [142]. Associated findings, in addition to enlarged lymph nodes or conglomerations of nodes, include multiple pulmonary nodules or multifocal consolidation. Pleural effusions can be seen in approximately 15% of patients of Hodgkin lymphoma [134–136, 141, 144–148]. As is true for other malignancies, lymphoma is tracer avid for ^{18}F-fluorodeoxyglucose (FDG) which is used effectively to determine anatomic extent of disease.

NHL is traditionally classified into two categories based on histology: (1) lymphoblastic and (2) nonlymphoblastic. Nonlymphoblastic is further classified into histiocytic and undifferentiated, of which there are Burkitt and non-Burkitt types [146]. Unlike its adult manifestation, NHL is primarily extranodal in distribution [146]. T-cell-derived NHL is commonly found in the thorax, while the lineage of B-cell NHL usually occurs in the abdomen [146].

While Hodgkin lymphoma typically occurs in the first decade of life, NHL is common in both the first and second decades of life [136]. NHL has multiple manifestations but depends on the bulk of disease and histopathologic diagnosis, with the possibility of low-grade tumors evolving to higher-grade tumors [134, 135, 143, 144, 147]. Approximately, 50% of NHL cases demonstrate intrathoracic involvement [134–136, 141, 145, 148]. The CT appearance of NHL is varied and may demonstrate bulky mediastinal lymphadenopathy or extranodal disease. Involvement of anterior and posterior mediastinal nodes is equally likely, except for large B-cell lymphoma and lymphoblastic, which tend to exclusively involve the anterior mediastinum (Fig. 13.24a). Associated findings of lymphoma within the thorax also include pulmonary nodules, with or without cavitation, as well as airspace consolidation and diffuse interstitial thickening. Pleural involvement may manifest by effusions or pleural masses (Fig. 13.24b) [134–136, 141, 145, 148]. The presence of a large amount of pleural fluid is suggestive of NHL rather than Hodgkin disease. Systemic involvement is typical at the time of diagnosis, obviating the need for radiographic staging. All patients receive chemotherapy, and the prognosis of children with lymphoma is worse if they have bone marrow and central nervous system involvement [146].

Plain radiographs of lymphoma usually demonstrate findings of an anterior mediastinal mass with obliteration of the retrosternal clear space and/or mediastinal widening (Fig. 13.23). Since it can be difficult to differentiate an anterior mediastinal mass from the normal thymus in children, the trachea should be carefully inspected, as the normal but prominent thymus does not usually cause mass effect on or displace the trachea. Ultrasound or airway fluoroscopy can also help differentiate the two, as the soft, pliable thymus appears distinct from a nonmobile mediastinal mass. On inspiration, the thymus will appear to shrink as its transverse diameter decreases with increasing lung volume. A pathologic mass will not change in apparent size.

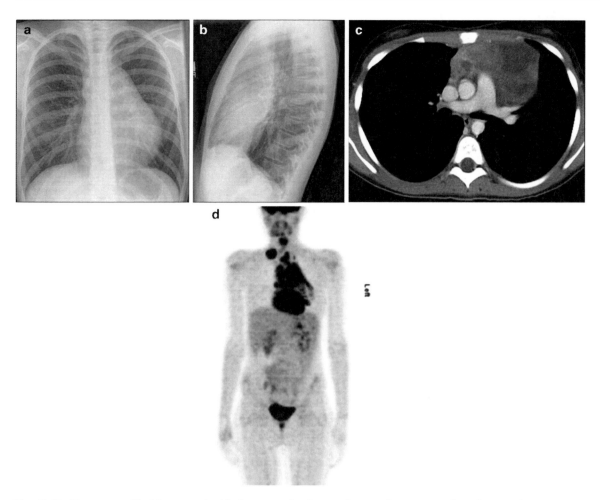

Fig. 13.23. Eleven-year-old girl presented with shortness of breath and weight loss. (**a**) Frontal chest radiograph shows a large mediastinal mass. (**b**) Lateral chest radiograph demonstrates the location of the mediastinal mass to be within the anterior mediastinal compartment. (**c**) Enhanced axial CT image shows a heterogeneously enhancing large anterior mediastinal mass. (**d**) Frontal PET image shows markedly increased FDG uptake in the anterior mediastinal mass and right supraclavicular lymph nodes in this patient with Hodgkin disease

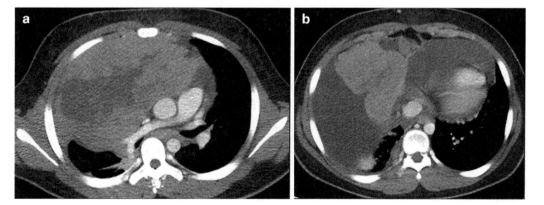

Fig. 13.24. Fifteen-year-old boy with shortness of breath. (**a**) Enhanced axial CT image demonstrates a large, heterogeneous anterior mediastinal mass with central low density regions consistent with necrosis. (**b**) Enhanced axial CT image more inferiorly in the same patient shows a pleural effusion adjacent to this large mass in this patient with NHL

Lymphoma often appears as homogeneous enlargement of the thymus from tumor infiltration on CT. However, larger nodal conglomerates often become heterogeneous from areas of necrosis or cystic change. While MRI is not typically used to evaluate mediastinal lymphoma since CT depicts anatomic extent of disease so well, PET is often used in the initial staging as well as to follow treatment response (Fig. 13.23d) [134–136, 141, 145, 148].

Eighty percent of patients with Hodgkin lymphoma have event-free survival prolonged by treatment regimens [149]. The preferred approach to treatment involves combined modalities, which limits toxicity of individual drugs and provides a synergistic effect. Currently both radiation therapy and chemotherapy are the modalities of treatment. Similar therapies are used for NHLs, in addition to bone marrow transplantation [150]. With the initial treatment of NHL, there may be a rapid, significant increase in the size of the pleural effusion.

Thymoma

The thymus is normally seen in children up to 3 years of age but may be seen in older children up to 9 [145, 146]. Rebound of the thymus, where there is unusually pronounced enlargement of the thymus following cessation of prolonged physiologic stress (such as treatment of malignancy), may be seen as late as the end of the second decade. The thymus' primary function is maturation of T-lymphocytes. A neoplasm that arises from thymic epithelium, a thymoma contains varying numbers of intermixed lymphocytes [142]. The admixture of epithelial cells and lymphocytes, which varies with each tumor, gives rise to the histologic subtyping of thymoma as predominantly lymphocytic, mixed lymphoepithelial, and predominantly epithelial types [142]. In the predominantly lymphocytic form, in which there are few interspersed epithelial tumor cells, the histologic differentiation from lymphoma may be difficult [142].

Thymomas represent approximately 20% of all mediastinal tumors. However, thymomas are quite infrequent in the pediatric population, accounting for approximately 1–2% of mediastinal tumors [141, 144–146]. Thymomas may be discovered incidentally, although approximately 25–30% cause symptoms related to local compression or invasion [135, 151–154].

Approximately 40% of patients with thymomas may present with a paraneoplastic syndrome such as hypogammaglobulinemia, red cell aplasia, or most commonly, myasthenia gravis [151–155]. Of patients with myasthenia gravis, approximately 10–30% have a thymoma. Approximately 30–35% of patients with a thymoma will develop myasthenia [142]. In patients with myasthenia gravis being evaluated for thymoma, CT can demonstrate small tumors that are invisible on radiographs [142]. However, very small thymic tumors may not be distinguishable from a normal or hyperplastic gland with CT, particularly in younger patients who have a large amount of residual thymic tissue [142].

Thymomas are typically classified into two different types: (1) noninvasive thymoma and (2) invasive thymoma. Invasive thymoma refers to a thymoma that has invaded its fibrous capsule. Such lesions tend to spread locally, with invasion of adjacent mediastinal structures, as well as the chest wall [154]. In addition, invasive thymomas tend to spread contiguously along the pleural surface, usually unilaterally. Noninvasive thymomas tend to demonstrate well-defined margins on imaging studies, since they have not extended past their fibrous capsules [154]. Since encapsulated and invasive thymomas are histologically the same, the diagnosis of invasive thymoma is based on visualizing gross or microscopic extension through the capsule. Because the capsule needs full evaluation, most thymomas require surgical excision [154, 155]. Therapy for myasthenia graves also includes thymectomy.

On plain radiographs, thymomas most often appear as an oval mass within the mediastinum, usually projecting to one side [154, 155]. They are often seen best on lateral view, obliterating the retrosternal clear space. Invasive thymomas can present with pleural nodules or masses (Fig. 13.25). CT imaging confirms an oval or lobulated enhancing mass within the anterior mediastinum, some with thin capsular calcification (Fig. 13.26). Cystic regions and necrosis are present in approximately 30%, particularly in larger tumors [142–146]. Signs of invasion include obliteration of mediastinal fat planes surrounding mediastinal vascular structures, pericardial thickening, chest wall, or diaphragmatic and pleural extension [136, 141, 145, 151–155]. MR typically demonstrates high signal intensity on T2 weighted images, but usually does not provide additional diagnostic information over CT.

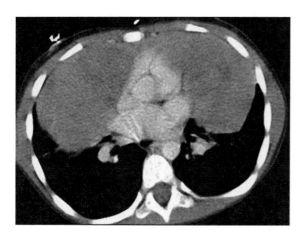

Fig. 13.25. Five-year-old boy with a large thymoma presented with persistent cough. Enhanced axial CT image demonstrates a very large, heterogeneous pleural mass draped over the heart

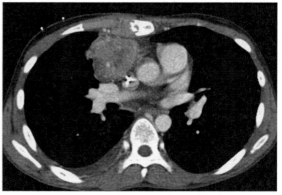

Fig. 13.27. Six-year-old girl with thymic carcinoma presented with chest pain. Enhanced axial CT image shows a heterogeneous mass in the anterior mediastinum with irregular borders and chest wall invasion, including sternal destruction

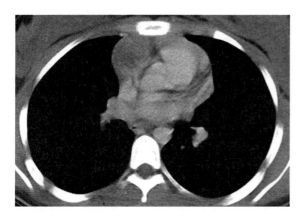

Fig. 13.26. Fourteen-year-old girl with a thymoma presented with fainting spell and abnormal chest radiographs. Enhanced axial CT image shows a relatively well-circumscribed lobulated mass in the anterior mediastinum abutting the right anterior heart

Thymic Carcinoma

Thymic carcinomas usually present in the fifth or sixth decade of life, and are exceedingly rare in the pediatric population [145, 146, 154, 155]. Thymic carcinoma is an aggressive epithelial carcinoma histologically characterized by malignant features of nuclear atypia, numerous mitotic figures, and necrosis [142]. Almost all patients are symptomatic at presentation, usually demonstrating constitutional symptoms such as weight loss, fatigue, night sweats, as well as chest pain [154, 155].

Thymic carcinomas usually present as large, irregular anterior mediastinal masses with aggressive local spread and mediastinal vascular invasion (Fig. 13.27) [134, 153, 156]. Often, these masses enhance heterogeneously with areas of necrosis, containing variable amounts of calcification. Thymic carcinoma may be indistinguishable from an invasive thymoma on imaging studies unless distant metastases are present. Unlike invasive thymomas, a thymic carcinoma tends to metastasize hematogenously [154, 155]. Prognosis is poor with progressive local growth and distant metastatic disease common [154, 155]. Treatment options include neoadjuvant chemotherapy to improve the resectability of the tumor, in addition to postoperative radiation therapy [157].

Germ Cell Tumor

Germ cell neoplasms arise from collections of primitive germ cells that arrest in the anterior mediastinum on their journey to the gonads during embryologic development [142, 151]. Because they are histologically indistinguishable from germ cell tumors arising in the testes and ovaries, the diagnosis of a primary malignant mediastinal germ cell neoplasm requires exclusion of a primary gonadal tumor as a source of mediastinal metastases [142].

Malignant germ cell tumors include immature teratomas, seminomas, and nonseminomatous germ cell tumors (NSGCT). Seminomas include germinoma and dysgerminoma, whereas NSGCT include embryonal cell, endodermal sinus/yolk sac tumors, choriocarcinoma, and mixed germ cell tumors [158, 159]. Seminoma, choriocarcinoma, and endodermal sinus/yolk sac tumors are malignant lesions seen primarily in young men [142, 151]. Seminoma is the most common malignant germ cell neoplasm, accounting for 30% of these tumors [142, 151]. Since these tumors may either be asymptomatic or present with nonspecific symptoms of dyspnea or chest pain, lab values are also useful for narrowing the diagnosis. Elevated serum alpha-fetoprotein (AFP) can be seen in NSGCTs, and human chorionic gonadotropin (hCG) is often elevated in both seminomas and NSGCTs [142, 151].

Malignant germ cell tumors usually appear as large anterior mediastinal masses arising either within or adjacent to the thymus. An immature teratoma is difficult to distinguish from its benign counterpart, the mature teratoma, as hallmarks of both include fat, fluid, and calcified components which differentiate from other mediastinal masses [145, 146]. One helpful feature is the presence of solid tissue, which is more prominent in immature teratomas [151, 159, 160]. While benign teratomas tend to displace adjacent structures, malignant teratomas tend to invade them [145, 146].

Seminomas often appear as large, lobulated masses of near homogenous soft tissue density, and sometimes show internal necrosis. They often straddle the midline and may extend into the middle and posterior mediastinum or infiltrate fat planes (Fig. 13.28). NSGCTs are often large with heterogeneous density, often showing central areas of low density, and demonstrate irregular margins with obliterated fat planes. Lymphadenopathy and lung or liver metastases may also be present [134, 136, 143, 158].

While mature teratomas may be treated by surgery alone, malignant tumors must be treated with multimodality approaches. Seminomas are usually treated with chemotherapy followed by radiation for bulky tumors and surgery for residual disease. Nonseminomatous tumors are treated with a combination of chemotherapy and surgery [160].

Middle Mediastinum

Metastatic Lymphadenopathy

Most middle mediastinal lymph node masses are malignant, representing metastases from various primary tumors or lymphoma [142]. In children, metastatic lymphadenopathy often results from primary tumors in the abdomen and pelvis, such as neuroblastoma, Wilms tumor, testicular neoplasms, and various sarcomas. Usually, these present as homogenous soft tissue masses which can be conglomerations of nodes (Fig. 13.29) [135, 136]. Lymphoma is also a common primary neoplasm that can manifest itself in any mediastinal compartment, including the middle mediastinum or as an extension from the anterior mediastinum. While it is often difficult to determine which primary tumor is responsible for metastatic lymphadenopathy, one of the more helpful characteristics is lymph node calcification, which can be often seen in treated lymphoma or osteosarcoma metastases (Fig. 13.30) [136]. Like any other mediastinal mass, metastatic lymphadenopathy may be asymptomatic or cause a variety of symptoms including dyspnea or chest pain. Management of the adenopathy includes determining the site of primary disease and its appropriate treatment.

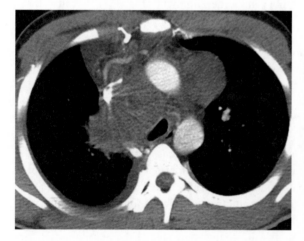

Fig. 13.28. Ten-year-old girl with chest pain and weight loss. Enhanced axial CT image shows a heterogeneously enhancing mediastinal mass with ill-defined borders and mass effect upon trachea resulting in tracheal narrowing. This mass was proven to be a seminoma

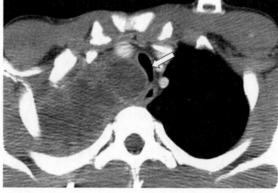

Fig. 13.29. Fourteen-year-old male with known metastatic prostate rhabdomyosarcoma. Enhanced axial CT image shows a large heterogeneously enhancing middle mediastinal mass causing tracheal narrowing (*arrow*)

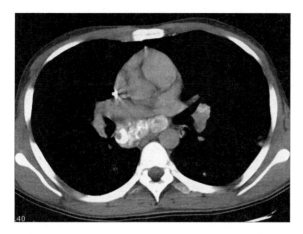

Fig. 13.30. Seventeen-year-old male with metastatic osteosarcoma. Non-enhanced axial CT image demonstrates multiple calcified mediastinal lymph nodes

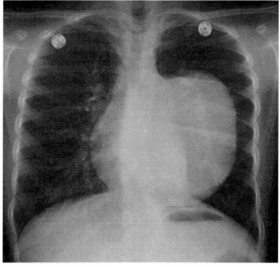

Fig. 13.31. Seven-year-old male with thoracic neuroblastoma. Note the thinning and spreading of the left seventh through ninth ribs immediately adjacent to the mass

Posterior Mediastinum

Neuroblastoma

Ninety percent of posterior mediastinal tumors are neurogenic, derived from the sympathetic chains which are located along the thoracic vertebral bodies [146, 161]. The vast majority of these neurogenic tumors are neuroblastomas in pediatric patients, while the rest are ganglioneuroblastoma or ganglioneuroma.

Neuroblastoma is a malignant tumor of primitive neural crest cells. Although it most commonly arises from the adrenal gland, it can arise from anywhere along the sympathetic chain, including the posterior mediastinum. Neuroblastoma is the third most common pediatric malignancy after leukemia and central nervous system tumors. Posterior mediastinal neuroblastoma accounts for approximately 20% of all neuroblastoma cases [162–165]. Common sites of metastases from neuroblastoma include liver and bone, with lung metastases less common. Neuroblastoma, although malignant, holds a more favorable prognosis if diagnosed under the age of 1. Typical clinical presentation includes fever, irritability, weight loss, and anemia [146, 161]. Neural symptoms from cord compression may cause paraplegia, extremity weakness, and altered bowel or bladder function [146, 161].

Plain radiographs often show soft tissue opacity in the paravertebral regions, often demonstrating erosion or destruction of the ribs and/or vertebrae or widening of intercostal spaces (Fig. 13.31). Associated calcifications are common, reportedly occurring in up to 30% on plain radiographs [162–165]. Bone metastases may also be seen and are usually permeative. CT provides further anatomic depiction of the mass and associated calcification and local extent of disease. Approximately 80% of neuroblastoma cases contain calcium on CT (Fig. 13.32a) [146, 151, 162–165]. In addition, tumor necrosis or hemorrhage can also be seen on CT.

An invasive mass that tends to surround and encase vessels, neuroblastoma also tends to invade neural foramina and the spinal canal. Neural foraminal invasion is important to recognize, as it can influence surgical planning and management [136, 141, 145, 148, 162–165]. MR often shows the tumor to be high in signal on T2 weighted sequences and low in signal on T1 weighted images, and is the best modality for detecting extension of tumor into the spinal canal, as well as local disease extent (Fig. 13.32b) [166]. Neuroblastomas on MR tend to enhance early, indicative of their high vascularity, and regions of necrosis or cystic change are well seen [136, 162–164, 166]. Imaging with metaiodobenzylguanidine (MIBG) is an excellent study for determining extent of disease, as there is avid uptake of MIBG related to catecholamine production by the tumor. Bone scan also helps stage neuroblastoma by providing information regarding local and distant osseous involvement from the tumor. The current therapy of choice for neuroblastoma in pediatric patients is surgical resection with adjuvant chemotherapy and radiation therapy for advanced disease. The prognosis of neuroblastoma in children varies depending on location

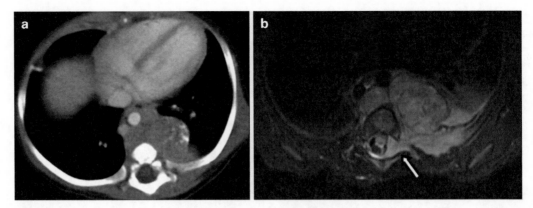

Fig. 13.32. Three-month-old male presented with vomiting. After abdominal ultrasound failed to reveal the cause of his symptoms, a CT was performed after an abnormal chest X-ray. (**a**) Enhanced axial CT image demonstrates a large left posterior mediastinal mass with regions of calcification. (**b**) MRI was also performed to evaluate for spinal involvement. Axial fluid-sensitive MRI image demonstrates extension of the neuroblastoma through the neural foramen and epidural extension (*arrow*)

of tumor. Children with thoracic neuroblastoma have more favorable prognosis than those with abdominal tumor involvement [146, 161].

Ganglioneuroblastoma

Ganglioneuroma and ganglioneuroblastoma are less aggressive counterparts along the neuroblastoma spectrum. They are also tumors of primitive neural crest cells. Ganglioneuroma and ganglioneuroblastoma may arise in the posterior mediastinum, with ganglioneuromas considered benign and ganglioneuroblastomas considered malignant, the latter because of the possibility of distant metastases [146, 162–164]. Radiologically, ganglioneuroblastomas especially are difficult to differentiate from neuroblastomas, having similar characteristics on CT and MR (Fig. 13.33). However, ganglioneuroblastoma and ganglioneuroma may have a more elongated (fusiform) configuration than usually encountered with neuroblastoma. Since the differential diagnosis for ganglioneuroblastoma includes neuroblastoma, surgical management is necessary.

Nerve Sheath Tumors

While most posterior mediastinal masses are neuroblastomas [166], benign peripheral nerve sheath tumors such as schwannomas and neurofibromas and malignant peripheral nerve sheath tumors (MPNST) may also be seen. MPNSTs are spindle cell sarcomas of nerve sheath origin, and are highly cellular with pleomorphic spindle cells. In pediatric patients, these masses most commonly arise from a preexisting plexiform neurofibroma, such as in

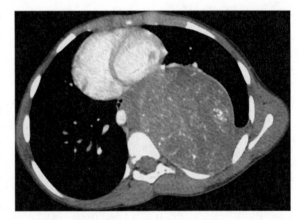

Fig. 13.33. Seven-year-old male with difficulty breathing. Enhanced axial CT image demonstrates a very large mass in the posterior mediastinum with regions of enhancement and calcification Proven to be a ganglioneuroblastoma

patients with Neurofibromatosis type 1 (NF-1). Less commonly, MPNSTs arise de novo or from preexisting schwannomas [166, 167]. Surgical removal for symptomatic or malignant lesions is the treatment of choice.

MPNSTs often appear as round or oblong posterior mediastinal masses with a widened neural foramen, following the axis of the involved nerve. On CT, these masses usually demonstrate decreased density due to lipid contents or cystic degeneration, and can have variable enhancement (Fig. 13.34). Dumbbell extension into the spinal canal can be seen on both CT and MR. Features of MPNST, whether arising de novo or from degeneration of a preexisting mass, include local invasion, osseous destruction, and pleural effusion [135, 166–168].

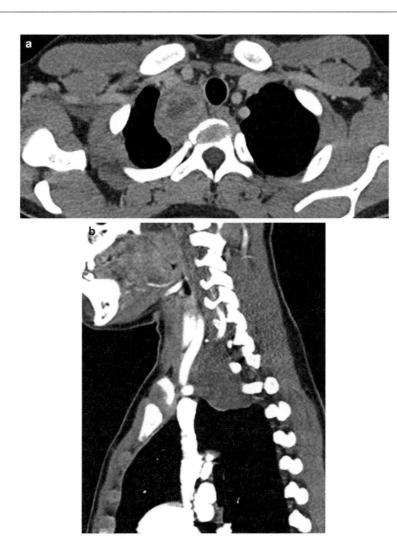

Fig. 13.34. Seventeen-year-old boy with neurofibromatosis type 1 and new Horner's syndrome. (**a**) Enhanced axial CT image demonstrates a heterogeneously enhancing mass in the mediastinum adjacent to the right lung apex which had grown substantially since a prior CT, Consistent with a MPNST (**b**) Sagittal enhanced CT image confirms that this mass is in the posterior mediastinum

13.2.4 Conclusion

Because malignant mediastinal masses are uncommon in children and often present with nonspecific clinical symptoms or with no symptoms at all, imaging plays a pivotal role in diagnosis. Once a mediastinal mass has been identified on conventional radiographs, cross-sectional imaging such as CT or MRI can be used for confirmation of findings and further characterization for generating differential diagnostic considerations. Although some malignant mediastinal tumors may have characteristic imaging appearances, definitive diagnosis relies on histopathological analysis. In regard to treatment of malignant mediastinal neoplasms in children, while some tumors respond to chemotherapy and radiation, many of them require surgical resection, often with adjuvant therapy.

References

1. Umiker Wo, Iverson L. Postinflammatory tumors of the lung; report of four cases simulating xanthoma, fibroma, or plasma cell tumor. J Thorac Surg. 1954;28(1): 55–63.
2. Griffin CA, Hawkins AL, Dvorak C, Henkle C, Ellingham T, Perlman EJ. Recurrent involvement of 2p23 in inflammatory myofibroblastic tumors. Cancer Res. 1999;59(12): 2776–80.

3. LA Bahadori M. Plasma cell granulomas of the lung. Cancer. 1973;31(1):191–208.

4. Bumber Z, Jurlina M, Manojlovic S, Jakic-Razumovic J. Inflammatory pseudotumor of the trachea. J Pediatr Surg. 2001;36(4):631–4.

5. Dishop MK, Kuruvilla S. Primary and metastatic lung tumors in the pediatric population: a review and 25-year experience at a large children's hospital. Arch Pathol Lab Med. 2008;132(7):1079–103.

6. Monzon CM, Gilchrist GS, Burgert Jr EO, O'Connell EJ, Telander RL, Hoffman AD, et al. Plasma cell granuloma of the lung in children. Pediatrics. 1982;70(2):268–74.

7. Hartman GE, Shochat SJ. Primary pulmonary neoplasms of childhood: a review. Ann Thorac Surg. 1983;36(1):108–19.

8. Berardi RS, Lee SS, Chen HP, Stines GJ. Inflammatory pseudotumors of the lung. Surg Gynecol Obstet. 1983;156(1):89–96.

9. Warter A, Satge D, Roescin N. Angio-invasive plasma cell granuloma of the lung. Cancer. 1987;59:435–43.

10. Janik JS, Janik JP, Lovell MA, Hendrickson RJ, Bensard DD, Greffe BS. Recurrent inflammatory pseudotumors in children. J Pediatr Surg. 2003;38(10):1491–5.

11. Cerfolio RJ, Allen MS, Nascimento AG, Deschamps C, Trastek VF, Miller DL, et al. Inflammatory pseudotumors of the lung. Ann Thorac Surg. 1999;67(4):933–6.

12. Vera-Roman JM, Sobonya RE, Gomez-Garcia JL, Sanz-Bondia JR, Paris-Romeu F. Leiomyoma of the lung. Literature review and case report. Cancer. 1983;52(5):936–41.

13. Lynn RB, Macfadyen DJ. Solitary primary leiomyoma of the lung. Can J Surg. 1958;2(1):93–6.

14. Sherman RS, Malone BH. A roentgen study of smooth muscle tumors primary in the lung. Radiology. 1950;54:507–15.

15. De Chadarevian JP, Wolk JH, Inniss S, Lischner HW, D'Amore F, Faerber EN, et al. A newly recognized cause of wheezing: AIDS-related bronchial leiomyomas. Pediatr Pulmonol. 1997;24(2):106–10.

16. Warren JS, Seo IS, Mirkin LD. Massive congenital mesenchymal malformation of the lung: a case report with ultrastructural study. Pediatr Pathol. 1985;3(2–4):321–8.

17. Alobeid B, Beneck D, Sreekantaiah C, Abbi RK, Slim MS. Congenital pulmonary myofibroblastic tumor: a case report with cytogenetic analysis and review of the literature. Am J Surg Pathol. 1997;21(5):610–4.

18. McGinnis M, Jacobs G, el-Naggar A, Redline RW. Congenital peribronchial myofibroblastic tumor (so-called "congenital leiomyosarcoma"). A distinct neonatal lung lesion associated with nonimmune hydrops fetalis. Mod Pathol. 1993;6(4):487–92.

19. Coffin CM. Lipoblastoma: an embryonal tumor of soft tissue related to organogenesis. Semin Diagn Pathol. 1994;11(2):98–103.

20. O'Donnell KA, Caty MG, Allen JE, Fisher JE. Lipoblastoma: better termed infantile lipoma? Pediatr Surg Int. 2000;16(5–6):458–61.

21. Chung EB, Enzinger FM. Benign lipoblastomatosis. An analysis of 35 cases. Cancer. 1973;32(2):482–92.

22. Bertana S, Parigi GP, Giuntoli M, Pelagalli M, Battisti C, Bragheri R, et al. Lipoblastoma and lipoblastomatosis in children. Minerva Pediatr. 1999;51(5):159–66.

23. Hicks J, Dilley A, Patel D, Barrish J, Zhu SH, Brandt M. Lipoblastoma and lipoblastomatosis in infancy and childhood: histopathologic, ultrastructural, and cytogenetic features. Ultrastruct Pathol. 2001;25(4):321–33.

24. Chun YS, Kim WK, Park KW, Lee SC, Jung SE. Lipoblastoma. J Pediatr Surg. 2001;36(6):905–7.

25. Dilley AV, Patel DL, Hicks MJ, Brandt ML. Lipoblastoma: pathophysiology and surgical management. J Pediatr Surg. 2001;36(1):229–31.

26. Hancock BJ, Di Lorenzo M, Youssef S, Yazbeck S, Marcotte JE, Collin PP. Childhood primary pulmonary neoplasms. J Pediatr Surg. 1993;28(9):1133–6.

27. van den Bosch JM, Wagenaar SS, Corrin B, Elbers JR, Knaepen PJ, Westermann CJ. Mesenchymoma of the lung (so called hamartoma): a review of 154 parenchymal and endobronchial cases. Thorax. 1987;42(10):790–3.

28. Eggli KD, Newman B. Nodules, masses, and pseudomasses in the pediatric lung. Radiol Clin North Am. 1993;31(3):651–66.

29. Fudge TL, Ochsner JL, Mills NL. Clinical spectrum of pulmonary hamartomas. Ann Thorac Surg. 1980;30(1):36–9.

30. Karasik A, Modan M, Jacob CO, Lieberman Y. Increased risk of lung cancer in patients with chondromatous hamartoma. J Thorac Cardiovasc Surg. 1980;80(2):217–20.

31. Fontenelle LJ. Primary adenocarcinoma of lung in a child: review of the literature. Am Surg. 1976;42(4):296–9.

32. French CA. Demystified molecular pathology of NUT midline carcinomas. J Clin Pathol. 2010;63(6):492–6.

33. French CA, Miyoshi I, Kubonishi I, Grier HE, Perez-Atayde AR, Fletcher JA. BRD4-NUT fusion oncogene: a novel mechanism in aggressive carcinoma. Cancer Res. 2003;63(2):304–7.

34. French CA, Kutok JL, Faquin WC, Toretsky JA, Antonescu CR, Griffin CA, et al. Midline carcinoma of children and young adults with NUT rearrangement. J Clin Oncol. 2004;22(20):4135–9.

35. Mertens F, Wiebe T, Adlercreutz C, Mandahl N, French CA. Successful treatment of a child with t(15;19)-positive tumor. Pediatr Blood Cancer. 2007;49(7):1015–7.

36. Engleson J, Soller M, Panagopoulos I, Dahlen A, Dictor M, Jerkeman M. Midline carcinoma with t(15;19) and BRD4-NUT fusion oncogene in a 30-year-old female with response to docetaxel and radiotherapy. BMC Cancer. 2006;6:69.

37. French CA, Ramirez CL, Kolmakova J, Hickman TT, Cameron MJ, Thyne ME, et al. BRD-NUT oncoproteins: a family of closely related nuclear proteins that block epithelial differentiation and maintain the growth of carcinoma cells. Oncogene. 2008;27(15):2237–42.

38. Stelow EB, Bellizzi AM, Taneja K, Mills SE, Legallo RD, Kutok JL, et al. NUT rearrangement in undifferentiated carcinomas of the upper aerodigestive tract. Am J Surg Pathol. 2008;32(6):828–34.

39. Vargas SO, French CA, Faul PN, Fletcher JA, Davis IJ, Dal Cin P, et al. Upper respiratory tract carcinoma with chromosomal translocation 15;19: evidence for a distinct disease entity of young patients with a rapidly fatal course. Cancer. 2001;92(5):1195–203.

40. Teixeira MR. Recurrent fusion oncogenes in carcinomas. Crit Rev Oncog. 2006;12(3–4):257–71.

41. Miniati DN, Chintagumpala M, Langston C, Dishop MK, Olutoye OO, Nuchtern JG, et al. Prenatal presentation and outcome of children with pleuropulmonary blastoma. J Pediatr Surg. 2006;41(1):66–71.

42. Manivel JC, Priest JR, Watterson J, Steiner M, Woods WG, Wick MR, et al. Pleuropulmonary blastoma. The so-called pulmonary blastoma of childhood. Cancer. 1988;62(8):1516–26.

43. Weinblatt ME, Siegel SE, Isaacs H. Pulmonary blastoma associated with cystic lung disease. Cancer. 1982;49(4): 669–71.

44. Federici S, Domenichelli V, Tani G, Sciutti R, Burnelli R, Zanetti G, et al. Pleuropulmonary blastoma in congenital cystic adenomatoid malformation: report of a case. Eur J Pediatr Surg. 2001;11(3):196–9.

45. Tagge EP, Mulvihill D, Chandler JC, Richardson M, Uflacker R, Othersen HD. Childhood pleuropulmonary blastoma: Caution against nonoperative management of congenital lung cysts. J Pediatr Surg. 1996;31(1):187–9; discussion 190.

46. Holland-Moritz RM, Heyn RM. Pulmonary blastoma associated with cystic lesions in children. Med Pediatr Oncol. 1984;12(2):85–8.

47. Pleuropulmonary blastoma registry [homepage on the Internet]; 2005. www.ppbregistry.org. Accessed 25 May 2011.

48. Priest JR, McDermott MB, Bhatia S, Watterson J, Manivel JC, Dehner LP. Pleuropulmonary blastoma: a clinico-pathologic study of 50 cases. Cancer. 1997;80(1):147–61.

49. Raz DJ, He B, Rosell R, Jablons DM. Bronchioloalveolar carcinoma: a review. Clin Lung Cancer. 2006;7(5):313–22.

50. Lee KS, Kim Y, Han J, Ko EJ, Park CK, Primack SL. Bronchioloalveolar carcinoma: clinical, histopathologic, and radiologic findings. Radiographics. 1997;17(6): 1345–57.

51. Storey CF, Knudtson KP, Lawrence BJ. Bronchiolar (alveo-lar cell) carcinoma of the lung. J Thorac Surg. 1953;26(4): 331–406.

52. Greenberg SD, Smith MN, Spjut HJ. Bronchiolo-alveolar carcinoma-cell of origin. Am J Clin Pathol. 1975;63(2): 153–67.

53. Liebow AA. Bronchiolo-alveolar carcinoma. Adv Intern Med. 1960;10:329–58.

54. Manning Jr JT, Spjut HJ, Tschen JA. Bronchioloalveolar carcinoma: the significance of two histopathologic types. Cancer. 1984;54(3):525–34.

55. Clayton F. Bronchioloalveolar carcinomas. Cell types, patterns of growth, and prognostic correlates. Cancer. 1986;57(7):1555–64.

56. Granata C, Gambini C, Balducci T, Toma P, Michelazzi A, Conte M, et al. Bronchioloalveolar carcinoma arising in congenital cystic adenomatoid malformation in a child: a case report and review on malignancies originating in congenital cystic adenomatoid malformation. Pediatr Pulmonol. 1998;25(1):62–6.

57. Lack EE. Leiomyosarcomas in childhood: a clinical and pathologic study of 10 cases. Pediatr Pathol. 1986;6(2–3): 181–97.

58. Havard CW, Hanbury WJ. Leiomyosarcoma of the lung. Lancet. 1960;2(7156):902–4.

59. Timmons CF, Dawson DB, Richards CS, Andrews WS, Katz JA. Epstein-barr virus-associated leiomyosarcomas in liver transplantation recipients. Origin from either donor or recipient tissue. Cancer. 1995;76(8):1481–9.

60. Guillan RA, Wilen CJ, Zelman S. Primary leiomyosarcoma of the lung. Dis Chest. 1969;56(5):452–4.

61. Tateishi U, Gladish GW, Kusumoto M, Hasegawa T, Yokoyama R, Tsuchiya R, et al. Chest wall tumors: radio-logic findings and pathologic correlation: Part 2. Malignant tumors. Radiographics. 2003;23(6):1491–508.

62. Pettinato G, Manivel JC, Saldana MJ, Peyser J, Dehner LP. Primary bronchopulmonary fibrosarcoma of childhood and adolescence: reassessment of a

low-grade malignancy. Clinicopathologic study of five cases and review of the literature. Hum Pathol. 1989; 20(5):463–71.

63. Guccion JG, Rosen SH. Bronchopulmonary leiomyosar-coma and fibrosarcoma. A study of 32 cases and review of the literature. Cancer. 1972;30(3):836–47.

64. Enzinger FM, Weiss SW. Soft Tissue Tumors. 2nd ed. St. Louis: CV Mosby; 1988. p. 213–20.

65. Soule EH, Pritchard DJ. Fibrosarcoma in infants and chil-dren: a review of 110 cases. Cancer. 1977;40(4):1711–21.

66. Chung EB, Enzinger FM. Infantile fibrosarcoma. Cancer. 1976;38(2):729–39.

67. Wellner LJ, Putman CE. Imaging of occult pulmonary metastases: state of the art. CA Cancer J Clin. 1986;36(1):48–58.

68. Kayton ML. Pulmonary metastasectomy in pediatric patients. Thorac Surg Clin. 2006;16(2):167–83, vi.

69. Green DM. The treatment of stages I–IV favorable histol-ogy Wilms' tumor. J Clin Oncol. 2004;22(8):1366–72.

70. Mitchell C, Jones PM, Kelsey A, Vujanic GM, Marsden B, Shannon R, et al. The treatment of Wilms' tumour: results of the united kingdom children's cancer study group (UKCCSG) second Wilms' tumour study. Br J Cancer. 2000;83(5):602–8.

71. Gatta G, Capocaccia R, Coleman MP, Ries LA, Berrino F. Childhood cancer survival in Europe and the United States. Cancer. 2002;95(8):1767–72.

72. Ehrlich PF, Hamilton TE, Grundy P, Ritchey M, Haase G, Shamberger RC, et al. The value of surgery in directing therapy for patients with Wilms' tumor with pulmonary disease. A report from the national Wilms' tumor study group (national Wilms' tumor study 5). J Pediatr Surg. 2006;41(1):162–7; discussion 162–7.

73. Schnater JM, Aronson DC, Plaschkes J, Perilongo G, Brown J, Otte JB, et al. Surgical view of the treatment of patients with hepatoblastoma: results from the first pro-spective trial of the international society of pediatric oncology liver tumor study group. Cancer. 2002;94(4): 1111–20.

74. Perilongo G, Brown J, Shafford E, Brock P, De Camargo B, Keeling JW, et al. Hepatoblastoma presenting with lung metastases: treatment results of the first cooperative, pro-spective study of the international society of paediatric oncology on childhood liver tumors. Cancer. 2000;89(8): 1845–53.

75. Young Jr JL, Ries LG, Silverberg E, Horm JW, Miller RW. Cancer incidence, survival, and mortality for children younger than age 15 years. Cancer. 1986;58(2 Suppl): 598–602.

76. Matthay KK, Villablanca JG, Seeger RC, Stram DO, Harris RE, Ramsay NK, et al. Treatment of high-risk neuroblastoma with intensive chemotherapy, radiotherapy, autologous bone marrow transplantation, and 13-cis-retinoic acid. Children's cancer group. N Engl J Med. 1999;341(16):1165–73.

77. Cowie F, Corbett R, Pinkerton CR. Lung involvement in neuroblastoma: incidence and characteristics. Med Pediatr Oncol. 1997;28(6):429–32.

78. DuBois SG, Kalika Y, Lukens JN, et al. Metastatic sites in stage IV and IVS neuroblastoma correlate with age, tumor biology, and survival. J Pediatr Hematol Oncol. 1999;21:181–9.

79. Kammen BF, Matthay KK, Pacharn P, Gerbing R, Brasch RC, Gooding CA. Pulmonary metastases at diagnosis of neuroblastoma in pediatric patients: CT findings and prognosis. AJR Am J Roentgenol. 2001;176(3):755–9.

80. Weldon CB, Shamberger RC. Pediatric pulmonary tumors: primary and metastatic. Semin Pediatr Surg. 2008;17(1): 17–29.

81. Kager L, Zoubek A, Potschger U, Kastner U, Flege S, Kempf-Bielack B, et al. Primary metastatic osteosarcoma: presentation and outcome of patients treated on neoadjuvant cooperative osteosarcoma study group protocols. J Clin Oncol. 2003;21(10):2011–8.

82. Kaste SC, Pratt CB, Cain AM, Jones-Wallace DJ, Rao BN. Metastases detected at the time of diagnosis of primary pediatric extremity osteosarcoma at diagnosis: imaging features. Cancer. 1999;86(8):1602–8.

83. Price CH, Jeffree GM. Incidence of bone sarcoma in SW England, 1946–74, in relation to age, sex, tumour site and histology. Br J Cancer. 1977;36(4):511–22.

84. Patricio MB, Vilhena M, Neves M, Raposo S, Catita J, DeSousa V, et al. Ewing's sarcoma in children: twenty-five years of experience at the instituto portuges de oncologia de francisco gentil (I.P.O.F.G.). J Surg Oncol. 1991;47(1): 37–40.

85. Sandoval C, Meyer WH, Parham DM, Kun LE, Hustu HO, Luo X, et al. Outcome in 43 children presenting with metastatic Ewing sarcoma: the St. Jude children's research hospital experience, 1962 to 1992. Med Pediatr Oncol. 1996;26(3):180–5.

86. Arndt CACW. Common musculoskeletal tumors of childhood and adolescence. N Engl J Med. 1999;341(5):342–52.

87. Pappo AS, Shapiro DN, Crist WM, Maurer HM. Biology and therapy of pediatric rhabdomyosarcoma. J Clin Oncol. 1995;13(8):2123–39.

88. Punyko JA, Mertens AC, Baker KS, Ness KK, Robison LL, Gurney JG. Long-term survival probabilities for childhood rhabdomyosarcoma. A population-based evaluation. Cancer. 2005;103(7):1475–83.

89. Oberlin O, Rey A, Lyden E, Bisogno G, Stevens MC, Meyer WH, et al. Prognostic factors in metastatic rhabdomyosarcomas: results of a pooled analysis from united states and European cooperative groups. J Clin Oncol. 2008;26(14):2384–9.

90. Enzinger W. Soft tissue tumours. 4th ed. Chicago: Mosby; 2001.

91. Spurrell EL, Fisher C, Thomas JM, Judson IR. Prognostic factors in advanced synovial sarcoma: an analysis of 104 patients treated at the royal marsden hospital. Ann Oncol. 2005;16(3):437–44.

92. Hajdu SI, Shiu MH, Fortner JG. Tendosynovial sarcoma: a clinicopathological study of 136 cases. Cancer. 1977;39(3):1201–17.

93. Cadman NL, Soule EH, Kelly PJ. Synovial sarcoma; an analysis of 34 tumors. Cancer. 1965;18:613–27.

94. Gerl A, Clemm C, Schmeller N, Hartenstein R, Lamerz R, Wilmanns W. Advances in the management of metastatic non-seminomatous germ cell tumours during the cisplatin era: a single-institution experience. Br J Cancer. 1996;74(8):1280–5.

95. Anyanwu E, Krysa S, Buelzebruck H, Vogt-Moykopf I. Pulmonary metastasectomy as secondary treatment for testicular tumors. Ann Thorac Surg. 1994;57(5):1222–8.

96. Pizzocaro G. Cancer of the testis. In: Veronesi U, Arnesjo B, Burn I, et al., editors. Surgical oncology – a European handbook. Berlin: Springer; 1989. p. 758.

97. Cagini L, Nicholson AG, Horwich A, Goldstraw P, Pastorino U. Thoracic metastasectomy for germ cell tumours: long term survival and prognostic factors. Ann Oncol. 1998;9(11):1185–91.

98. Liu D, Abolhoda A, Burt ME, Martini N, Bains MS, Downey RJ, et al. Pulmonary metastasectomy for testicular germ cell tumors: a 28-year experience. Ann Thorac Surg. 1998;66(5):1709–14.

99. Horvath LG, McCaughan BC, Stockle M, Boyer MJ. Resection of residual pulmonary masses after chemotherapy in patients with metastatic non-seminomatous germ cell tumours. Intern Med J. 2002;32(3):79–83.

100. Kesler KA, Wilson JL, Cosgrove JA, Brooks JA, Messiha A, Fineberg NS, et al. Surgical salvage therapy for malignant intrathoracic metastases from nonseminomatous germ cell cancer of testicular origin: analysis of a single-institution experience. J Thorac Cardiovasc Surg. 2005; 130(2):408–15.

101. Pfannschmidt J, Zabeck H, Muley T, Dienemann H, Hoffmann H. Pulmonary metastasectomy following chemotherapy in patients with testicular tumors: experience in 52 patients. Thorac Cardiovasc Surg. 2006;54(7): 484–8.

102. McCarthy MJ, Rosado-de-Christenson ML. Tumors of the trachea. J Thorac Imaging. 1995;10(3):180–98.

103. Pransky SM, Kang DR. Tumors of the larynx, trachea, and bronchi. In: Bluestone CD, Stool SES, Alper CM, et al., editors. Pediatric otolaryngology. 4th ed. Philadelphia: Saunders; 2002. p. 1558–72.

104. Derkay CS, Wiatrak B. Recurrent respiratory papillomatosis: a review. Laryngoscope. 2008;118(7):1236–47.

105. Khansur T, Balducci L, Tavassoli M. Granular cell tumor. Clinical spectrum of the benign and malignant entity. Cancer. 1987;60(2):220–2.

106. Majmudar B, Thomas J, Gorelkin L, Symbas PN. Respiratory obstruction caused by a multicentric granular cell tumor of the laryngotracheobronchial tree. Hum Pathol. 1981;12(3):283–6.

107. Andrassy RJ, Feldtman RW, Stanford W. Bronchial carcinoid tumors in children and adolescents. J Pediatr Surg. 1977;12(4):513–7.

108. Fischer S, Kruger M, McRae K, Merchant N, Tsao MS, Keshavjee S. Giant bronchial carcinoid tumors: a multidisciplinary approach. Ann Thorac Surg. 2001;71(1): 386–93.

109. Gustafsson BI, Kidd M, Chan A, Malfertheiner MV, Modlin IM. Bronchopulmonary neuroendocrine tumors. Cancer. 2008;113(1):5–21.

110. McCahon E. Lung tumours in children. Paediatr Respir Rev. 2006;7(3):191–6.

111. Lack EE, Harris GB, Eraklis AJ, Vawter GF. Primary bronchial tumors in childhood. A clinicopathologic study of six cases. Cancer. 1983;51(3):492–7.

112. Raut CP, Kulke MH, Glickman JN, Swanson RS, Ashley SW. Carcinoid tumors. Curr Probl Surg. 2006;43(6): 383–450.

113. Al-Qahtani AR, Di Lorenzo M, Yazbeck S. Endobronchial tumors in children: institutional experience and literature review. J Pediatr Surg. 2003;38(5):733–6.

114. DiAgostino RS, Ponn RB, Stern H. Adenoid cystic carcinoma, mucoepidermoid carcinoma, and mixed salivary gland-type tumors. In: Shields T, editor. General thoracic surgery. Philadelphia: Lea and Febiger; 1994. p. 1298–305.

115. Vadasz P, Egervary M. Mucoepidermoid bronchial tumors: a review of 34 operated cases. Eur J Cardiothorac Surg. 2000;17(5):566–9.

116. Yousem SA, Hochholzer L. Mucoepidermoid tumors of the lung. Cancer. 1987;60(6):1346–52.

117. Maziak DE, Todd TR, Keshavjee SH, Winton TL, Van Nostrand P, Pearson FG. Adenoid cystic carcinoma of the airway: thirty-two-year experience. J Thorac Cardiovasc Surg. 1996;112(6):1522–31; discussion 1531–2.

118. Tateishi U, Gladish GW, Kusumoto M, Hasegawa T, Yokoyama R, Tsuchiya R, et al. Chest wall tumors: radiologic findings and pathologic correlation: Part 1. Benign tumors. Radiographics. 2003;23(6):1477–90.

119. Ippolito E, Bray EW, Corsi A, De Maio F, Exner UG, Robey PG, et al. Natural history and treatment of fibrous dysplasia of bone: a multicenter clinicopathologic study promoted by the European pediatric orthopaedic society. J Pediatr Orthop B. 2003;12(3):155–77.

120. Nogier A, De Pinieux G, Hottya G, Anract P. Case reports: enlargement of a calcaneal osteochondroma after skeletal maturity. Clin Orthop Relat Res. 2006;447:260–6.

121. Gladish GW, Sabloff BM, Munden RF, Truong MT, Erasmus JJ, Chasen MH. Primary thoracic sarcomas. Radiographics. 2002;22(3):621–37.

122. Burt M. Primary malignant tumors of the chest wall. the memorial Sloan-Kettering cancer center experience. Chest Surg Clin N Am. 1994;4(1):137–54.

123. Rosai J, editors. Soft tissues. In: Ackerman's surgical pathology. 7th ed. St. Louis: Mosby; 1989. p. 1547–633.

124. Askin FB, Rosai J, Sibley RK, Dehner LP, McAlister WH. Malignant small cell tumor of the thoracopulmonary region in childhood: a distinctive clinicopathologic entity of uncertain histogenesis. Cancer. 1979;43(6): 2438–51.

125. Dehner LP. Peripheral and central primitive neuroectodermal tumors. A nosologic concept seeking a consensus. Arch Pathol Lab Med. 1986;110(11):997–1005.

126. Jaffe R, Santamaria M, Yunis EJ, Tannery N, Medina J, Goodman M. Neuroendocrine tumor of bone: its distinction from Ewing's sarcoma (abstr). Lab Invest. 1984;50:5P.

127. Linnoila RI, Tsokos M, Triche TJ, Marangos PJ, Chandra RS. Evidence for neural origin and PAS-positive variants of the malignant small cell tumor of thoracopulmonary region ("askin tumor"). Am J Surg Pathol. 1986;10(2): 124–33.

128. Cohen MD. Imaging of children with cancer. St. Louis: Mosby; 1992. p. 247–51.

129. Saifuddin A, Robertson RJ, Smith SE. The radiology of askin tumours. Clin Radiol. 1991;43(1):19–23.

130. Winer-Muram HT, Kauffman WM, Gronemeyer SA, Jennings SG. Primitive neuroectodermal tumors of the chest wall (askin tumors): CT and MR findings. AJR Am J Roentgenol. 1993;161(2):265–8.

131. Fink IJ, Kurtz DW, Cazenave L, Lieber MR, Miser JS, Chandra R, et al. Malignant thoracopulmonary small-cell ("askin") tumor. AJR Am J Roentgenol. 1985;145(3): 517–20.

132. Jurgens H, Bier V, Harms D, Beck J, Brandeis W, Etspuler G, et al. Malignant peripheral neuroectodermal tumors. A retrospective analysis of 42 patients. Cancer. 1988;61(2):349–57.

133. Shields TW. General thoracic surgery. 7th ed. Philadelphia: Lippincott Williams and Wilkins; 2009.

134. Grosfeld JL. Primary tumors of the chest wall and mediastinum in children. Semin Thorac Cardiovasc Surg. 1994;6:235–9.

135. Grosfeld JL, Skinner MA, Rescorla FJ, et al. Mediastinal tumors in children: experience with 196 cases. Ann Surg Oncol. 1994;1:121–7.

136. Lee EY. Evaluation of non-vascular mediastinal masses in infants and children: an evidence-based practical approach. Pediatr Radiol. 2009;39 Suppl 2:S184–90.

137. Williams PL, Warwick R, Dyson M, Bannister LH, editors. Splanchnology. In: Gray's anatomy. 37th ed. New York: Churchill Livingstone; 1989. p. 1245–475.

138. Zylak CJ, Pallie W, Jackson R. Correlative anatomy and computed tomography: a module on the mediastinum. Radiographics. 1982;2(4):555–92.

139. Felson B. The mediastinum. Semin Roentgenol. 1969;4:41–58.

140. Aquino SL, Duncan G, Taber KH, Sharma A, Hayman LA. Reconciliation of the anatomic, surgical, and radiographic classifications of the mediastinum. J Comput Assist Tomogr. 2001;25(3):489–92.

141. Laurent F, Latrabe V, Lecesne R, et al. Mediastinal masses: diagnostic approach. Eur Radiol. 1998;8:1148–59.

142. Brant W, Helms C. Fundamentals of diagnostic radiology. 2nd ed. Philadelphia: Lippincott Williams & Wilkins; 1999.

143. Whitten CR, Khan S, Munneke GJ, Grubnic S. A diagnostic approach to mediastinal abnormalities. Radiographics. 2007;27:657–71.

144. Piira T, Perkins SL, Anderson JR, et al. Primary mediastinal large cell lymphoma in children: a report from the Children's Cancer Group. Pediatr Pathol Lab Med. 1995;15:561–70.

145. Merten DF. Diagnostic imaging of mediastinal masses in children. AJR Am J Roentgenol. 1992;158:825–32.

146. Blickman JG, Parker BR, Barnes PD. Pediatric radiology: the requisites. Philadelphia: Mosby Elsevier; 2009. p. 45–54.

147. Montravers F, McNamara D, Landman-Parker J, et al. 18F FDG in childhood lymphoma: clinical utility and impact on management. Eur J Nucl Med Mol Imaging. 2002;29: 1155–65.

148. Williams HJ, Alton HM. Imaging of paediatric mediastinal abnormalities. Paediatr Respir Rev. 2003;4:55–66.

149. DeVita VT. A selective history of the therapy of Hodgkin's disease. Br J Haematol. 2003;122:718–27.

150. Ansell SM, Armitage J. Non-Hodgkin lymphoma: diagnosis and treatment. Mayo Clin Proc. 2005;80(8):1087–97.

151. Rosado-de-Christenson ML, Galobardes J, Moran CA. Thymoma: radiologic-pathologic correlation. Radiographics. 1992;12(1):151–68.

152. Morgenthaler TI, Brown LR, Colby TV, Harper Jr CM, Coles DT. Thymoma. Mayo Clin Proc. 1993;68(11):1110–23.

153. Kim DJ, Yang WI, Choi SS, Kim KD, Chung KY. Prognostic and clinical relevance of the World Health Organization schema for the classification of thymic epithelial tumors: a clinicopathologic study of 108 patients and literature review. Chest. 2005;127(3):755–61.

154. Freundlich IM, McGavaran MH. Abnormalities of the thymus. J Thorac Imaging. 1996;1:58–65.

155. McLoud TC, Boiselle PM. Thoracic radiology: the requisites. 2nd ed. Philadelphia: Mosby; 2010. p. 427–9, 452–3.

156. Yaris N, Nas Y, Cobanoglu U, Yavuz MN. Thymic carcinoma in children. Pediatr Blood Cancer. 2006;47(2): 224–7.

157. Lucchi M, Mussi A, Basolo F, Ambrogi MC, et al. The multimodality treatment of thymic carcinoma. Eur J Cardiothorac Surg. 2001;19(5):566–9.

158. Ueno T, Tanaka YO, Nagata M, et al. Spectrum of germ cell tumors: from head to toe. Radiographics. 2004;24: 387–404.

159. Khan AN. Mediastinal germ cell tumor imaging. http://emedicine.medscape.com/article/359110-overview; 2008.

160. Sakurai H, Asamura H, Suzuki K, et al. Management of primary malignant germ cell tumor of the mediastinum. Jpn J Clin Oncol. 2004;34(7):386–92.

161. Reed JC, Hallet KK, Feigin DS. Neural tumors of the thorax: subject review from the AFIP. Radiology. 1978;126:9–17.

162. Mehta K, Haller JO, Legasto AC. Imaging neuroblastoma in children. Crit Rev Comput Tomogr. 2003;44(1):47–61.

163. Lonergan GJ, Schwab CM, Suarez ES, Carlson CL. Neuroblastoma, ganglioneuroblastoma, and ganglioneuroma: radiologic-pathologic correlation. Radiographics. 2002;22(4):911–34.

164. Donnelly LF, Frush DP, Zheng JY, Bisset III GS. Differentiating normal from abnormal inferior thoracic paravertebral soft tissues on chest radiography in children. AJR Am J Roentgenol. 2000;175(2):477–83.

165. Temes R, Allen N, Chavez T. Primary mediastinal malignancies in children: report of 22 patients and comparison to 197 adults. Oncologist. 2000;5:179–84.

166. Strollo DC, Rosado-de-Christenson ML, Jett JR. Primary mediastinal tumors: part II. Tumors of the middle and posterior mediastinum. Chest. 1997;112:1344–57.

167. Levine E, Huntrakoon M, Wetzel LH. Malignant nerve-sheath neoplasms in neurofibromatosis: distinction from benign tumors by using imaging techniques. AJR Am J Roentgenol. 1987;149(5):1059–64.

168. Temes R, Allen N, Chavez T. Primary mediastinal malignancies in children: report of 22 patients and comparison to 197 adults. Oncologist. 2000;5:179–84.

Asthma

Annabelle Quizon

CONTENTS

14.1   Definition and Pathophysiology

Asthma is a chronic disorder of the airways characterized by variable and recurring symptoms of cough, wheezing and chest tightness, airflow obstruction, bronchial hyperresponsiveness, and underlying inflammation. Airway inflammation is a key feature and is associated with the basic physiologic and clinical attributes of asthma such as airway hyperresponsiveness, airflow limitation, and the chronic nature of the disease.

Airway inflammation involves the interaction of a number of cells such as mast cells, eosinophils, T lymphocytes, macrophages, neutrophils, and epithelial cells. These cells release mediators that contribute to the characteristic features of asthma. The development of chronic inflammation may result in airway remodeling which involves irreversible changes of all components of the airway. Airway remodeling has a direct role in the response to treatment and the persistent and chronic nature of the disease.

14.2   Factors Influencing Asthma Manifestations

Host factors and environmental exposures play important roles in the clinical manifestations of asthma. Predominant among these is the complex interplay of genetic factors; several genes have been linked to asthma and atopy, and aggregates in families [1–3]. Moreover, genetics also play a role in the response to drugs used in the treatment of asthma. Polymorphisms in the beta adrenergic and corticosteroid receptors determine response to these common therapies [4].

Environmental factors that are associated with disease prevalence are legion and include diet, microbial exposure and viral respiratory tract infections, airborne allergens, tobacco smoke exposure, and outdoor pollution [5–9]. Such allergen exposure may underlie the high prevalence of asthma in inner city populations. Respiratory viruses have been associated as well with the development of asthma and its

Annabelle Quizon (✉)
Division of Pediatric Pulmonology, Batchelor Children's Research Institute, University of Miami/Miller School of Medicine, Miami, FL, USA
e-mail: aquizon@med.miami.edu

R.H. Cleveland (ed.), *Imaging in Pediatric Pulmonology*,
DOI 10.1007/978-1-4419-5872-3_14, © Springer Science+Business Media, LLC 2012

recurrences or exacerbations. Respiratory syncytial virus (RSV) and rhinovirus infections have also been associated with recurrent and persistent wheezing into late childhood [10, 11]. In contrast to the above, the *hygiene hypothesis* suggests that exposure to infection early in life switches the child's immune system along a nonallergic pathway and thereby reduce the risk of asthma and other allergic diseases [12]. Obesity is gaining recognition as a risk factor for asthma. The nature of the association is complex and transcends the effect of obesity on chest wall mechanics to include complex inflammatory pathways shared by both conditions [13, 14].

14.3 Diagnosis of Asthma

14.3.1 Clinical Presentation

Typically, asthma presents with cough, wheezing, and dyspnea. Wheezing is typically expiratory and results from air movement though narrowed airways. In some patients, cough may be a more prominent symptom than wheezing such that the term cough-variant asthma has been used. These symptoms are recurrent, worse at night and may occur or worsen in the presence of known triggers such as exercise, viral infections, and exposure to airborne allergens or irritants.

Patients present with tachypnea, labored breathing with chest retractions, and use of accessory muscles of respiration during acute exacerbations. Physical exam findings include retractions and diffuse wheezing, usually expiratory. The absence of wheezing may, however, be an ominous sign of critical airway obstruction. Hypoxemia results from ventilation–perfusion mismatching; airway obstruction may progress to respiratory failure with hypercarbia.

14.3.2 Pulmonary Function Testing (Spirometry)

Objective assessment of airflow obstruction and its severity should be performed in patients with the diagnosis of asthma. Spirometry is usually applicable at ages over 4 years and measures the maximal volume of air forcibly exhaled from the point of maximal inhalation (FVC), the volume of air exhaled during the first second of the maneuver (FEV_1) and the ratio of FEV_1 to FVC. The most widely used parameter to define the severity of airflow obstruction is FEV_1 as a percentage of predicted. Reversibility of airflow obstruction is also ascertained by the improvement in FEV_1 after inhalation of a short-acting bronchodilator. Periodic monitoring of pulmonary function with the use of spirometry is recommended.

14.3.3 Additional Diagnostic Tests

Bronchial Challenge and Exercise Challenge Tests

Such tests are used to document bronchial hyperreactivity by inducing bronchospasm in asymptomatic patients. Bronchial challenge tests with inhalation of methacholine, hypertonic saline, histamine, or adenosine are utilized to elicit hyperresponsiveness. Exercise challenge tests are used in children with exercise-induced symptoms. The test involves treadmill, cycle, or other standardized exercise. In some laboratories, a cold air inhalation challenge is used in lieu of the exercise challenge and involves hyperventilation of subfreezing dry air for about 4 min. In these challenge tests, a positive result is standardized level of decline in FEV_1 from a predetermined baseline.

Exhaled Nitric Oxide

Measurement of exhaled nitric oxide utilizing commercial devices provides a rapid and noninvasive marker of airway inflammation. Elevated levels have been found to correlate with airway eosinophilia. It is useful as an adjunctive tool for the diagnosis of asthma and in the assessment of asthma control.

Radiographic Tests

Radiographic findings in asymptomatic children with intermittent asthma episodes often reveal a chronic, stable presence of bronchial wall thickening with normal lung volumes (Fig. 14.1). Or the chest radiograph may be normal. A chest radiograph is not a requisite to establish a diagnosis of asthma but is useful when complications are suspected or an alternative diagnosis, including acute bacterial pneumonia, is being considered (see section on alternative

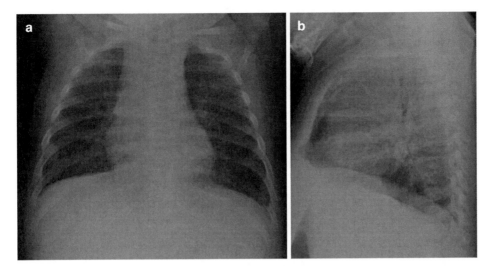

Fig. 14.1. PA (**a**) and lateral (**b**) chest radiographs show diffuse bronchial wall thickening, multifocal subsegmental atelectasis and hyperinflation. Bronchial wall thickening or peribronchial thickening (PBT) is a common manifestation of asthma and is indistinguishable from that seen in lower airway viral infections. However PBT often will be recognizable in known asthmatics who are currently asymptomatic. This is also the initial imaging manifestation in many children with cystic fibrosis. Hyperaeration is seen in asthmatics who are acutely symptomatic as is true for infants with bronchiolitis. Subsegmental atelectasis is often present in acutely ill asthmatics as well as infants with bronchiolitis

diagnoses below). Considering the variability in the severity of the disease, there are radiographic findings considered typical of asthma. Most commonly, during an acute episode, hyperinflation and peribronchial thickening are demonstrated. Peribronchial thickening refers primarily to the lobar or segmental bronchi. Hyperinflation is demonstrated by hyperlucent lungs and findings of flat or low hemidiaphragms on the frontal view. Lateral view also will show flattening of the hemidiaphragms and hyperlucency in the retrosternal and retrocardiac areas (Fig. 14.1). Subsegmental atelectasis is also encountered and may be severe enough to involve a lobe. In infants who develop viral bronchitis or bronchiolitis, it is difficult to distinguish radiographic findings consistent with viral lower respiratory tract infections and asthma, which may coexist. In both cases, atelectasis occurs and may present as ill-defined opacities which are frequently overinterpreted as representing bacterial consolidation (Fig. 14.1). Bronchial wall thickening is found in either condition and may be perceived as increased in the parahilar regions. However, the bronchial wall thickening is diffuse throughout the lungs and only seems worse centrally because of the convergence of the bronchi toward the hila. The term parahilar peribronchial thickening has been used to describe this observation but is actually a misnomer.

Intrathoracic air leaks occur as complications of asthma and in the setting of acute exacerbations. Pneumomediastinum presents as lucency adjacent to the mediastinal structures (Fig. 14.2). Patients may be asymptomatic but may complain of chest pain or dysphagia. Subcutaneous emphysema may be appreciated as gas dissects into the neck and soft tissues of the upper neck (Fig. 14.2) and sometimes even into the retroperitoneum. Pneumothoraces also occur, but a tension pneumthorax is rare in asthma.

Allergic bronchopulmonary aspergillosis (ABPA) is an uncommon complication of childhood asthma and is discussed in the section on comorbid conditions. A history of asthma is present in almost all patients. Radiographically, ABPA manifests with central bronchiectasis more prominent in the upper lobes (Fig. 14.3).

Sputum Cytology

Sputum induction by hypertonic saline inhalation has been utilized to identify the presence of eosinophils and other inflammatory cells in the sputum. Sputum cytology can provide useful information about asthma severity and response to treatment.

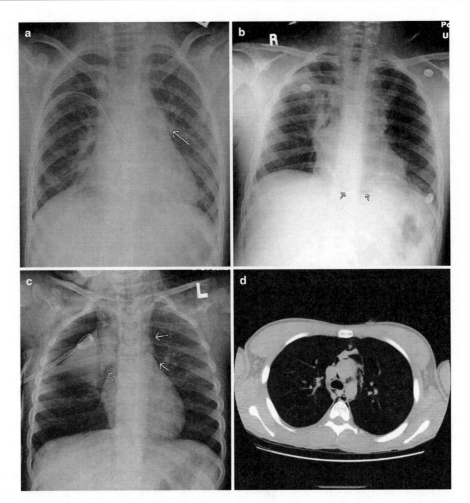

Fig. 14.2. Pneumomediastinum and subcutaneous air may be hallmarks of previously undiagnosed asthma or may be clinically suspected in children with known asthma. (**a**) There is a pneumomediastinum seen only on the left. It is distinguished from a medial pneumothorax by the small amount of air lifting the left lobe of the thymus off the mediastinum (*arrow*). (**b**) In a different patient, there is a relatively large pneumomediastinum, with a larger right component. A small amount of air is noted beneath the heart (*arrows*). Air also has extended into the neck. A small right pneumothorax is present. (**c**) Portable AP CXR reveals air within the mediastinum (*upper arrow*) with both lobes of the thymus separated from the heart by air (*lower arrows*) (air separating the thymus from the heart occurs only with pneumomediastinum or pneumopericardium). Subcutaneous air is present within the neck. There is a moderately large right pneumothorax. (**d**) In another patient, CT easily shows an extensive pneumomediastinum with small left pneumothorax

Complete Blood Cell Count

Eosinophilia usually suggests asthma or atopy, although there are other causes of peripheral eosinophilia such as parasitic infection and some malignancies.

Allergy Testing

Skin testing or in vitro serum testing for suspected allergens is usually recommended for patients in whom allergic factors are deemed by history to contribute significantly to their disease.

 14.4   Alternative Diagnosis

The diagnosis of asthma can usually be made by history, physical examination findings and response to treatment. Adjunctive tools and laboratory testing are also helpful. Because of the high prevalence of asthma worldwide, alternative diagnoses tend to be missed. Such diagnoses must be explored if there is

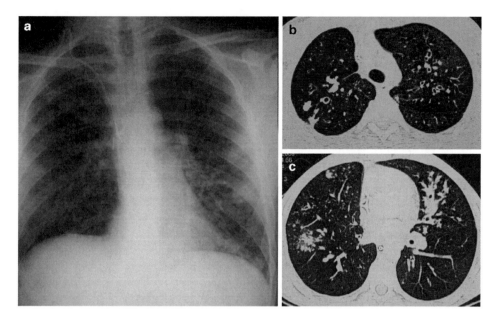

Fig. 14.3. (a–c) Allergic bronchopulmonary aspergillosis occurs in children with asthma, as well as those with cystic fibrosis (frequently those with a known asthmatic component). Sixteen-year-old boy with allergic bronchopulmonary aspergillosis (ABSA) in the setting of CF. (**a**) Chest x-ray shows ill-defined patchy opacification in the left lower and right upper lobes. (**b**) CT chest shows moderate to severe bronchial wall thickening with bronchiectasis. (**c**) On the left side there is linear branching opacification suggestive of fluid filled dilated bronchi. There are ill-defined slightly lobulated masses in the right lung

doubt about the diagnosis of asthma. Based on age, diagnoses to consider for wheezing, cough or labored breathing are detailed below.

In preschool age children, if symptoms do not respond to appropriate therapy, the following diagnoses should be considered: aspiration syndromes, bronchomalacia, bronchopulmonary dysplasia, chronic idiopathic purulent bronchitis, compression of the airway from aberrant vessels (e.g., vascular ring), cystic fibrosis, foreign body in the airway, foreign body in the esophagus (compressing airway), primary ciliary dyskinesia, pertussis, tracheal polyps or hemangioma, and tracheomalacia [15].

In older children with wheezing, the following diagnoses should be considered. With acute wheezing, they include: asthma, exercise induced asthma, angioedema and vocal cord dysfunction (adduction), infection (mycoplasma, adenovirus, RSV, metapneumovirus, parainfluenza, influenza, pertussis), inhalation of irritant substances (smoke, illicit drugs), hypersensitivity pneumonitis, aspiration/gastroesophageal reflux (GER), foreign body aspiration. For recurrent or chronic wheezing, they include asthma, angioedema, exercise induced asthma, vocal cord dysfunction, focal lesion/compression (papillomatosis, granulation tissue, carcinoid, lymphoma, enlarged lymph nodes, bronchogenic cyst, vascular ring), postinfectious (adenovirus, mycoplasma, bronchiectasis), inflammatory (cystic fibrosis, ciliary dyskinesia, immune deficiency, sarcoid, vasculitis (Wegener's, etc.), alpha 1 antitrypsin deficiency, eosinophilic bronchitis), and congestive heart failure [15].

14.5 Comorbid Conditions

When the diagnosis of asthma has been established and asthma is difficult to control with recommended therapy, morbid condition(s) that can mimic asthma and underlie airway reactivity or exacerbate veritable asthma must be considered. In the most recent recommendations of the NHLBI asthma guidelines [16], identification and treatment of the following conditions may improve asthma management: ABPA, GER, obesity, obstructive sleep apnea (OSA), rhinitis/sinusitis, and chronic stress/depression. A brief discussion of the first five conditions follows.

14.5.1 Allergic Bronchopulmonary Aspergillosis

ABPA is uncommon in childhood asthma and represents an allergic response to *Aspergillus* sp., usually *fumigatus*. The diagnosis is difficult and is based on serologic and radiologic criteria. Radiologically, patients present with transient migratory infiltrates on chest X-ray or chest CT scan; in the advanced stages, these can be complicated with bronchiectasis (Fig. 14.3).

14.5.2 Gastroesophageal Reflux

GER is one of the causes of nocturnal cough. The diagnosis is often elusive in childhood since heartburn, chest pain, sour taste in the mouth or regurgitation are frequently absent in children. Symptoms of cough and wheeze can be caused by direct aspiration of gastric contents into the airway but the symptoms can also be triggered via vagally-mediated reflexes by acid and possibly nonacid reflux of gastric contents into the distal esophagus.

14.5.3 Obesity

Obesity itself can affect pulmonary mechanics that lead to dyspnea. Adipose tissue in obese patients has been shown to express proinflammatory cytokines that affect the airway. Obesity also contributes to comorbid conditions such as GER and OSA.

14.5.4 Obstructive Sleep Apnea

Obstructive sleep apnea and nocturnal asthma may coexist. Patients with both conditions present with arousals, changes in airflow and ventilatory effort, and hypoxemia during sleep. Both conditions are also confounded by obesity. Administration of continuous positive airway pressure (CPAP) may improve symptoms of OSA in patients with unstable asthma.

14.5.5 Rhinitis and Sinusitis

Rhinitis and sinusitis contribute to asthma morbidity and invokes the concept of the upper and lower airways as a continuum. The direct mechanisms are controversial but are assumed to include postnasal drip that induces cough and wheeze. Sinus infections also trigger the release of inflammatory mediators in the bronchial mucosa. The treatment of the inflammatory processes of the upper airway often alleviates asthma symptoms.

14.6 Management

Asthma is a chronic condition and the key points of management are divided into two major categories: (1) reducing impairment via reduction of symptoms and maintenance of normal activity level, and (2) reducing risk by preventing loss of lung function and possibly lung growth as well as minimizing adverse effects of therapy.

The medical management of asthma is two-pronged and revolves around two parallel concepts: (1) chronic administration of controller medications represented predominantly by inhaled corticosteroids and leukotriene-active drugs and (2) provision of rapid-acting or short-acting reliever medications for acute exacerbations represented predominantly by beta-agonists such as albuterol. Details of these regimens are beyond the scope of this review, but they have revolutionized asthma control and the quality of life of patients. It is emerging, however, that they do not have long-term therapeutic effect in altering the predetermined course of the disease.

References

1. Cookson W, Moffatt M. Making sense of asthma genes. N Engl J Med. 2004;351(17):1794–6.
2. Daiels SE, Bhattacharrya S, James A, Leaves NI, Young A, Hill MR, et al. A genome-wide search for quantitative trait loci underlying asthma. Nature. 1996;383(6597):247–50.
3. Jenmalm MC, Bjorksten B. Cord blood levels of immunoglobulin G subclass and antibodies to food and inhalant allergens in relation to maternal atopy and the development of atopic disease during the first 8 years of life. Clin Exp Allergy. 2000;30(1):34–40.
4. Wechsler ME. Managing asthma in the 21st century: the role of pharmacogenetics. Pediatr Ann. 2006;35(9):660–9.
5. Pearce N, Pekkanen J, Beasley R. How much asthma is really attributable to atopy? Thorax. 1999;54(3):268–72.
6. Warner JO. The early life origins of asthma and related allergic disorders. Arch Dis Child. 2004;89(2):97–102.
7. Litonjua AA, Milton DJ, Celedon JC, Ryan L, Weiss ST, Gold DR. A longitudinal analysis of wheezing yin young children. The independent effects of early life exposure to house dust, endotoxin, allergens and pets. J Allergy Clin Immunol. 2002;110(5):736–42.
8. Butland BK, Strachan DP, Anderson HR. The home environment and asthma symptoms in childhood. Two population based case-control studies 13 years apart. Thorax. 1997;52(7):618–24.
9. Rosenstreich Dl. Eggleston P, Kattan M, Baker D, Slavin RG, Gergen P, et al. The role of cockroach allergy and exposure to cockroach allergen in causing morbidity among

inner-city children with asthma. N Engl J Med. 1997; 336(19):1356–63.

10. Martinez FD. Viral infections and the development of asthma. Am J Respir Crit Care Med. 1995;151(5): 1644–8.

11. Stein RT, Sherrill D, Morgan WJ, Holberg CJ, Halonen M, Taussig LM, et al. Respiratory syncytial virus in early life and risk of wheeze and allergy by age 13 years. Lancet. 1999;354(9178):541–5.

12. Strachan DP. Family size, infection and atopy. The first decade of the "hygiene hypothesis". Thorax. 2000;55 Suppl 1:2–10.

13. Romieu I, Mannino DM, Redd SC, McGeehin MA. Dietary intake, physical activity, body mass index, and childhood asthma in the Third National Health and Nutrition Survey (NHANES III). Pediatr Pulmonol. 2004;38(1):31–42.

14. Beuther DA, Sutherland ER. Overweight, obesity and incident asthma. A meta-analysis of prospective epidemiologic studies. Am J Respir Crit Care Med. 2007;175(7): 661–6.

15. Chernick V, Boat TF, Wilmott RW, Bush A, editors. Kendig's disorders of the respiratory tract in children. 7th ed. Philadelphia: WB Saunders; 2006.

16. National Heart, Lung, and Blood Institute National Asthma Education and Prevention Program. Expert Panel Report 3. Guidelines for the diagnosis and management of asthma. Bethesda: National Heart, Lung, and Blood Institute, National Institutes of Health; 2007, Sect. 3, pp. 213–39.

Cystic Fibrosis

15

Dubhfeasa Maire Slattery and Veronica Donoghue

CONTENTS

Dubhfeasa Maire Slattery, MD, PhD (✉)
Department of Respiratory Medicine, Children's University Hospital, Temple Street, Dublin 1, Ireland
e-mail: dubhfeasa.slattery@cuh.ie

Veronica Donoghue, FRCR, FFR, RCSI
Radiology Department, Children's University Hospital, Temple Street, Dublin, Ireland

R.H. Cleveland (ed.), *Imaging in Pediatric Pulmonology*,
DOI 10.1007/978-1-4419-5872-3_15, © Springer Science+Business Media, LLC 2012

15.1 Clinical Presentation

Presentation of cystic fibrosis varies according to age. The commonest presentation of cystic fibrosis is with recurrent respiratory tract infections ± associated failure to thrive, secondary to pancreatic exocrine insufficiency. Eighty-five percent of people with cystic fibrosis are pancreatic insufficient and without treatment they malabsorb fat and present with failure to gain weight, abdominal cramps, abdominal distension and steatorrhea. Ten to fifteen percent of cystic fibrosis presentations are in the neonatal period with meconium ileus which may lead to bowel obstruction, perforation and peritonitis. Older children may present with finger clubbing and respiratory symptoms, nasal polyps or acute pancreatitis.

Regarding diagnosis in the presymptomatic stage, newborn cystic fibrosis screening identifies infants in the first few days of life while chorionic villus sampling and amniocentesis in high-risk families identify cases antenatally. In countries where neonatal cystic fibrosis screening dose not occur, all siblings of a child with cystic fibrosis are screened for cystic fibrosis, whether symptomatic or asymptomatic. Clinical presentation varies according to age and is outlined in Table 15.1.

15.1.1 Causes of Cystic Fibrosis

Depletion of the periciliary liquid layer (the *low volume hypothesis*) [1], and not abnormal ion composition, is generally accepted as the explanation for airway disease in cystic fibrosis. Ineffective clearance of bacteria due to mucociliary clearance dysfunction results from reduced volume of airway surface liquid. Secondly, patients with cystic fibrosis have an exaggerated inflammatory response to infection and this in itself causes lung damage (up to 10 times more

Table 15.1. Presentations of cystic fibrosis

Age	Frequent presentation	Less frequent presentation
Antenatal	Chorionic villous sampling Amniocentesis in high risk families Fetal echogenic bowel wall	
Neonatal	Newborn Cystic Fibrosis screening Meconium ileus Fetal echogenic bowel wall	Prolonged neonatal obstructive jaundice
Infant and young child	Recurrent respiratory tract infections Failure to thrive secondary to pancreatic exocrine insufficiency	Rectal prolapse Dehydration plus electrolyte abnormality
	Screening of siblings of child with CF	Triad of anemia, edema and hypoproteinemia Deficiencies of fat soluble vitamins: vitamin K (bleeding disorder), vitamin E (hemolytic anemia), vitamin A (raised intracranial pressure)
Older children and adolescents	Recurrent respiratory tract infections Failure to thrive/fat malabsorption Finger clubbing Nasal polyps or sinusitis Screening of siblings of child with CF (in countries with no neonatal screening)	Liver disease Dehydration plus electrolyte abnormality Acute pancreatitis

inflammation than a person without CF). Thirdly, the contribution made by abnormal composition and secretion of mucus is unclear. All of this culminates in thickened secretions/sputum, ineffective clearance of bacteria, recurrent infection, bronchiectasis, fibrosis and respiratory failure. Ion and water abnormalities are likely to cause problems in other epithelial lined organs where inspissated secretions lead to obstruction, inflammation and ultimately fibrosis.

15.1.2 Genetics

This autosomal recessive disorder is caused by mutations in a single gene on the long arm of chromosome 7 that encodes the cystic fibrosis transmembrane regulator (C.F.T.R.) protein [2–4]. The gene carrier rate in North Americans is approximately 1 in 25 but varies across populations being as high as 1 in 19 in the Irish population. Heterozygotes are asymptomatic.

The C.F.T.R. protein is expressed in many cells and has many functions, not all of which have been linked with disease. C.F.T.R. protein functions mainly as an ion (Cl−) channel in the apical membrane of exocrine epithelial cells [2] that regulates liquid volume on epithelial surfaces through chloride secretion and inhibition of sodium absorption. Over 1,600 sequence variations have been identified so far along the entire CFTR gene [5]. The commonest C.F.T.R. mutation is phe508del (previously named δF508), a 3 bp deletion, causing a loss of phenylalanine at position 508 of the protein. phe508del comprises ~70% of mutations worldwide, followed by G451X and G551D at 2.4 and 1.6%, respectively [5]. However, the prevalence of different C.F.T.R. mutations varies with different populations throughout the world. There are six major classes of C.F.T.R. mutations based on their effect on C.F.T.R. function with class I, II and III being most severe with essentially no functional C.F.T.R. and class IV, V and VI less severe, with some functional C.F.T.R. [6].

15.1.3 Diagnosis

The diagnosis of cystic fibrosis traditionally has been based on clinical criteria combined with two abnormal sweat chloride results (sweat chloride >60 mmol/l) [7] or one abnormal sweat chloride and two C.F.T.R.

mutations. Cases of children with cystic fibrosis with normal sweat chlorides have been described. Currently, mutational analysis within the C.F. gene is readily available. Measurement of nasal potential difference is useful particularly in the more atypical presentations of C.F. Diagnosis pre symptoms is available with newborn screening for C.F. Antenatal diagnosis can be made with chorionic villous sampling or amniocentesis in high risk families. An echogenic fetal bowel on ultrasound, though a non-specific finding, is suggestive of cystic fibrosis [8].

15.1.4 Imaging

The imaging findings are variable and depend on the age at diagnosis and the severity of the disease. In younger infants, the chest radiograph may be normal. However, the initial imaging abnormality is diffuse bronchial wall thickening which is usually first seen in infancy [9, 10]. Occasionally, there may be some degree of hyperinflation [9, 10]. There may be areas of atelectasis, mimicking bronchiolitis or asthma. If a young child has serial Chest-x-rays (CXR) over several months with unchanging bronchial wall thickening and does not have reactive airways (asthma), this may represent early findings of cystic fibrosis and a sweat test should be performed (Fig. 15.1). As the disease progresses, the bronchial wall thickening will progress to bronchiectasis (Fig. 15.2). The latter can be suggested on radiography when the bronchus is larger than the adjacent pulmonary vessel. Areas of ill-defined opacification suggest mucous impaction or allergic bronchopulmonary aspergillosis (Fig. 15.3). Ill-defined areas of focal opacification may relate to acute pneumonia or pulmonary hemorrhage. Although cystic fibrosis has been reported as an upper lobe dominant disease, this is the case in only approximately 50% of patients [10]. Hilar lymphadenopathy is common and can occur during an episode of acute infection. Lobar pneumonia and pleural effusions are uncommon. In very severe disease, there may be evidence of right-sided cardiac failure.

The severity and extent of the various radiographic features have been scored by several methods. However, the Brasfield system is often used as it correlates closely with pulmonary function. It uses scores of 0–5 to assess air trapping, linear shadows, nodular cystic lesions, large pulmonary shadows and general

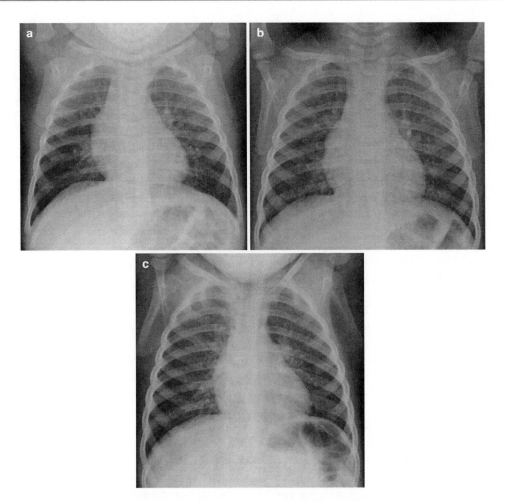

Fig. 15.1. (a) 8 months, (b) from 13 months and (c) from 21 months. All show a very similar pattern of bronchial wall thickening. The presenting symptoms at each encounter was *fever, cough and wheeze*. Two subsequent sweat tests were positive

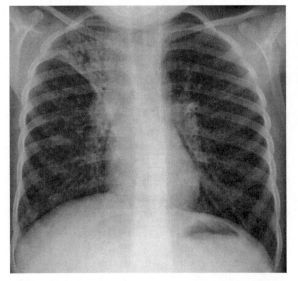

Fig. 15.2. Chest X-ray in a 7-year-old girl with cystic fibrosis. The lungs are hyperinflated. There is right upper lobe atelectasis. There is course bronchial wall thickening and the beginning of bronchiectasis. There is bilateral hilar enlargement suggesting adenopathy

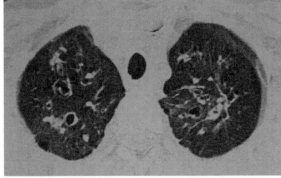

Fig. 15.3. CT chest on a 14-year-old boy showing typical findings of cystic fibrosis. There is bronchial wall thickening, bronchiectasis and areas of mucous plugging

severity. Cleveland et al. [9, 10] reported a radiography-based database which scored changes over time in patients with cystic fibrosis to provide comparison for groups undergoing new treatments such as aerosolized tobramycin [11]. Although these scoring systems have proven useful for research purposes, their use for clinical patient care is uncommon. Computed tomography (CT) studies are the most accurate method of evaluating the changes in lung disease. It is more sensitive than radiography in detecting the extent of bronchiectasis, bronchial wall thickening, mucous plugging, infiltration and hilar adenopathy. At present, however, there is no consensus on when to use CT in the various pediatric age groups with cystic fibrosis. There is also the issue of cumulative radiation dose in patients with any lifelong condition. This has become even more important since the introduction of multislice CT which has a much higher dose burden than high resolution thin slices at intervals. At present, the lowest doses required to identify lung disease on high resolution CT are still not available from the various manufacturers of CT scanners and there is still no consensus on when a volume sequence is required instead of high resolution images. In 1991, Bhalla et al. introduced a CT-based system where they scored the severity and extent of bronchiectasis, the severity of bronchial wall thickening, mucous plugging, bullous disease, emphysema, collapse and consolidation together with the involvement of the number of bronchial divisions [12]. Since then other scoring systems have been published and adopted by several clinicians.

15.1.5   Management

Management of children with cystic fibrosis is by the multidisciplinary cystic fibrosis team, including dedicated doctors, nurse specialists, dietitians, physiotherapists, psychologists and social workers. Maintenance of good nutrition is critical to maintenance of good lung function. A high calorie, high fat diet is instituted together with administration of pancreatic enzymatic supplementation and fat soluble vitamins (A, D, E and K) in those who are proven pancreatic insufficient. Prevention of respiratory illness with vaccines, e.g., influenza, pneumococcal and varicella, in countries where these are not already part of the national immunization schedule, is important. Different forms of chest physiotherapy and airway clearance techniques, a spectrum of antibiotics (nebulized and or oral) and agents such as rhDNAse and hypertonic saline, are all part of daily treatment in the life of a child with cystic fibrosis.

15.1.6   Prognosis

Although cystic fibrosis is much less common in non-Caucasians, it remains the most common, life-shortening genetic disorder in Caucasians. Life expectancy continues to improve. The Canadian C.F. Foundation patient Data Registry Report [13] showed improvements in survival from 22.8 years in 1977 to 37.0 years in 2002 (the latter without the previous pronounced gender gap where males survived longer than females). Median survival ages reported from the United States in 1993 was 28 years rising to 35.1 years by 2004 [14]. The predicted median survival for babies born in the twenty-first century is now more than 50 years [15]. Despite this improvement over time, the majority of people (approximately 90%) with cystic fibrosis still die of respiratory failure.

15.2   Respiratory Tract Disease

The respiratory tract extends from the mouth and nose to the alveoli, lined throughout with pseudostratified ciliated epithelium.

15.2.1   Respiratory Viruses

Incidence

Respiratory viruses may precipitate up to 40% of respiratory exacerbations [16–18]. The same viruses affect children with cystic fibrosis as children without, e.g., respiratory syncytial virus (R.S.V.), adenovirus, influenza A and B, para-influenza types 1, 2 and 3, rhinovirus [19] and likely metapneumovirus.

Risk Factors for Viral Infections

There is no evidence to suggest that people with cystic fibrosis have an increased risk of contracting a viral infection but they have a worse outcome because the lower respiratory tract is affected more often [16, 19–21].

Clinical Presentation of Bronchiolitis

Clinical presentation of bronchiolitis in an infant with cystic fibrosis is the same as for any infant with bronchiolitis. They present with acute respiratory distress, tachypnea, nasal flaring, accessory muscle use, intercostal and subcostal recession and scattered crackles and wheeze on auscultation. In older children and adults, presentation is similar as above.

Risk Factors for Developing R.S.V.

Risk factors for the development of R.S.V. bronchiolitis in all infants include being born during the winter R.S.V. season (October to March in the northern hemisphere), siblings at day care and smokers at home.

Investigations

Investigations include a nasopharyngeal aspirate checking for R.S.V., influenza, para-influenza, adenovirus, oxygen saturation measurement in room air and if clinically indicated a chest radiograph. Further investigations are not usually required but this decision depends on the clinical state of the infant.

Chest Radiograph

Chest radiography may not be required in patients with a typical presentation of bronchiolitis particularly if the symptoms are mild but may be necessary if there is more severe respiratory difficulty or diagnostic uncertainty in order to identify other conditions which may mimic bronchiolitis. Typically, there are varying degrees of hyperinflation with flattening of the diaphragms (Fig. 15.4). There may be associated atelectasis. Viral infections may cause localized or diffuse interstitial disease and rarely hilar lymphadenopathy. However, it may be difficult to distinguish bacterial from non-bacterial infection on chest radiography.

Treatment for Viral Infection

Inpatient hospital treatment includes supportive therapy with oxygen, fluids (either nasogastric or intravenous – the latter if vomiting) and attention to nutrition. Intravenous antibiotics may be added if there is an associated secondary bacterial infection.

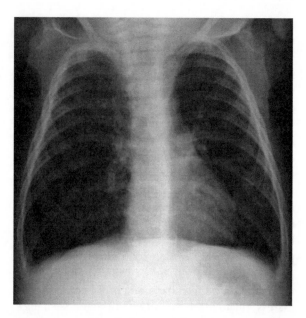

Fig. 15.4. Ten-month-old boy with bronchiolitis, subsequently diagnosed with CF. There is flattening of the diaphragms and bilateral perihilar streaky opacification and bronchial wall thickening

The first isolation of *Pseudomonas aeruginosa* in cystic fibrosis often follows a viral infection [22, 23]. Whether this is due to epithelial damage and airway inflammation caused by the virus or because the bacteria are simply isolated at the time of increased mucus production is not clear.

Prognosis

Viral infections may lead to increased frequency and duration of hospitalization for respiratory exacerbations [24] and deterioration in clinical status and lung function which may persist for several months [19, 24]. R.S.V. bronchiolitis in infants with cystic fibrosis can cause prolonged hospitalization and hypoxemia which may require mechanical ventilation. A 2-year follow-up study documented increased respiratory symptoms and worsening chest radiograph scores in infants with cystic fibrosis who had R.S.V. bronchiolitis [24]. In older children, influenza can cause a significant deterioration in lung function [25] and clinical status [26]. Annual influenza vaccine is recommended in children (>6 months of age) and adults with cystic fibrosis. Interestingly, a recent Cochrane systemic review did not find evidence that this vaccine is beneficial to patients with cystic fibrosis [27].

15.2.2 Respiratory Bacterial Infections

Incidence

Bronchoscopic studies have demonstrated that respiratory infection occurs early in life. While *Staphylococcus aureus, Haemophilus influenza and P. aeruginosa* [28, 29] predominate in the first few years of life, *P. aeruginosa* is the most common pathogen in the second decade. Other bacteria include *Stenotrophomonas maltophilia*, A. *xylosoxidans* and *Burkolderia cepacia*. Non-tuberculous mycobacteria are important pathogens to check for in patients with established lung disease. Fungi may cause infection and allergy in the airways.

Pathophysiology

A cycle of infection, inflammation and lung injury is established in cystic fibrosis. The presence of bacteria in the airways incites a host response of neutrophil inflammation and pro-inflammatory cytokines and chemokines. Inflammation is increased in the presence of infection [28, 30], but whether inflammation occurs independently of infection remains controversial [30]. Thick tenacious secretions block the airways. These secretions are particularly viscous secondary to dehydration of airway surface liquid, mucins and DNA from necrotic neutrophils and bacteria [31]. Chronic inflammation, infection and airway obstruction leads to ongoing lung injury and ultimately bronchiectasis.

Clinical Presentation

Symptoms include increased cough with increased sputum production and purulence [32], shortness of breath, dyspnea on exertion, hemoptysis, tiredness, anorexia with or without weight loss, sinus pain or change in sinus discharge. Examination varies from mild tachypnea and lethargy to hypoxia, weight loss, stigmata of acute respiratory distress and new crackles on auscultation. A decrease in baseline forced expiratory volume in one second (FEV$_1$) and new changes on chest radiography may be seen.

Risk Factors

Patients with pancreatic exocrine insufficiency have poorer lung function than those with pancreatic exocrine sufficiency [6]. The latter live an average of 10 years longer than the former.

Investigations

Sputum culture and sensitivity, pulmonary function tests, chest radiograph and blood tests are useful.

Imaging

Chest radiography findings are non-specific and bacterial infection must be considered in patients who have an acute increase in pulmonary opacification. Lobar consolidation is uncommon.

Treatment

The vast majority of patients have their intravenous antibiotic treatment at home. Chest physiotherapy, airway clearance techniques, nebulized rhDNAse (*pulmozyme*), hypertonic saline, nebulized salbutamol and attention to nutrition are all critical components of treatment of a pulmonary exacerbation of cystic fibrosis. Protection with vaccines is important including pneumococcal vaccines, annual influenza vaccine and varicella vaccines in countries where these are not part of the national immunization schedule. Lung transplantation is the final treatment option for all patients with end-stage lung disease resulting in respiratory failure (see Chap. 17, Lung Transplant in Pediatric Patients).

15.2.3 *Pseudomonas aeruginosa*

P. aeruginosa is the most common organism causing chronic lung disease in patients with cystic fibrosis. It is the most important cause of morbidity [33, 34] and an important predictor of survival. Chronic *Pseudomonal* infection with the mucoid form is impossible to permanently eradicate and is associated with a decline in lung function and poorer prognosis [34, 35]. The formation by *P. aeruginosa* of a biofilm is associated with increased resistance [33–36]. Neutrophils become *frustrated* and release damaging proteases and free radicals [37] into the airway when they become apoptotic or necrotic. The first isolation of *P. aeruginosa* (usually non-mucoid) in a patient is treated aggressively with dual antibiotic therapy in an attempt to eradicate it. Patients with cystic fibrosis are segregated in clinics based on the bacteria they culture e.g., *Pseudomonas* clinics or *S. aureus* clinics and each patient has an individual clinic room. Patient-to-patient spread can occur in clinics [38–42] and in camps [42] and for this reason the latter have been discontinued in the cystic fibrosis community. Once a patient is chronically colonized with mucoid *P.aeruginosa*, prophylactic nebulized antibiotics are used. *Pseudomonas* has a propensity to develop resistance, so dual antibiotic therapy [43] is employed to treat a pulmonary exacerbation when oral antibiotics fail.

Prognosis

Pseudomonas is associated with poorer lung function than other organisms.

Staphylococcus aureus

Methicillin-sensitive *S. aureus* (MSSA) is the most common pathogen isolated in sputum of children with cystic fibrosis during the first decade [44, 45]. Flexible bronchoscopy studies demonstrate up to 40% of children aged <3 years cultured *S. aureus* on broncho-alveolar lavage. It often co-infects in patients chronically infected with *P. aeruginosa, B cepacia* complex and other gram-negative organisms [46, 47].

Treatment

Treatment is usually with oral antibiotics. If the patient is deteriorating despite oral antibiotics, then intravenous antibiotics may be effective [46]. Eradication of *S. aureus was achieved* in 74% of patients after a 14-day course of anti-staphylococcal antibiotics and in almost all after a 3-month treatment [48].

Prophylaxis

Oral prophylaxis for *S. aureus is recommended* by the United Kingdom CF Trust *for all* children with C.F. up to the age of 2 years. This has been associated with a reduction in cough, antibiotic requirements and number of hospital admissions [32] without a benefit in pulmonary function tests in this age group [49]. In other countries, treatment is based on symptoms and positive sputum cultures [45, 50, 51].

Prognosis

Patients who culture *S. aureus* have a slower decline in lung function than those chronically colonized with *P. aeruginosa*.

15.2.4 Methicillin-Resistant *S. aureus*

Methicillin-resistant *S. aureus* (M.R.S.A) may be healthcare or community acquired. Patient-to-patient spread is well documented [52, 53]. A prevalence of up to 23% has been reported in some North American centres [54]. Controversy exists in the literature regarding whether M.R.S.A. is associated with significant deterioration in lung function [55] or not [53]. These patients require isolation. Eradication should be attempted. Skin or nasal carriage should be treated. Dual antibiotic therapy, based on sensitivity, is required to eradicate M.R.S.A. from sputum. Three clear sputums are required over a 6- to 12-month period before these patients are deemed *clear*.

15.2.5 *Burkholderia cepacia* Complex Group

There are nine members of the *Burkholderia cepacia* complex group and all cause infection in cystic fibrosis. The majority of infections are caused by *B. cenocepacia* (previously genomovar III) and *B. multivorans* (genomovar II). *B. vietnamiensis* is the next most common.

Accurate identification is crucial. Appropriate selective medium is required [56]. If identified, the organism should be sent to a specialized laboratory for confirmation because high false-positive (10%) and false-negative rates (30%) [57] have been reported. *B cenocepacia* is the most highly transmissible of the group, in particular the *B. cenocepacia* related to electrophoresis type 12 (ET 12) [58, 59].

Treatment

Infection control is hugely important. *B cepacia* is multiply resistant and frequently pan-resistant [44].

Prognosis

Infection with *B. cepacia* complex is associated with increased morbidity and reduced survival in cystic fibrosis [58, 59]. *B. cepacia* is associated with a rapid deterioration and early death in up to one third of patients who acquire the organism (*cepacia syndrome*). Other patients experience a more rapid decline in lung function than documented with *P. aeruginosa* [59, 60]. The remainder of patients remain stable despite chronic infection [61]. The outcome from lung transplantation is significantly worse in patients with *B cepacia* than *P. aeruginosa* [62, 63]. Infection with *B multivorans* is less severe and a significant proportion subsequently clear it [64].

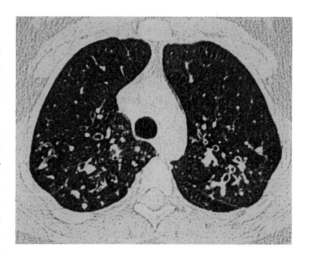

Fig. 15.5. Fifteen-year-old girl with Non-TB Mycobacteria. There is bronchiectasis with ill-defined densities. *Tree in bud* opacification is seen in the left lower lobe

15.2.6   Non-Tuberculous Mycobacterial Infection

Incidence

Mycobacterium avium complex (M.A.C.) is the most common non-tuberculous mycobacterial (N.T.M.) infection in patients with cystic fibrosis, accounting for approximately 70% of isolates while *Mycobacterium abscessus* accounts for 16% [65]. Patients who develop N.T.M. infection tend to be older, have better lung function and lower incidence of *P. aeruginosa*.

Clinical Presentation

Clinical presentation may be as for any exacerbation or N.T.M. may be found on annual sputum screen.

Diagnosis

Diagnosis can be difficult despite the American Thoracic Society guidelines for diagnosis of N.T.M. [66] which are limited due to the overlap of symptoms and radiology findings in cystic fibrosis. Systemic symptoms, three or more sequential positive sputum cultures, a reduction in lung function, new changes on high resolution CT and persistence of symptoms and CT changes despite *P. aerugonisa* treatment is indicative of active N.T.M. infection.

Investigations

Investigations include multiple sputum for acid fast bacilli stain and N.T.M. culture and sensitivity, mantou test, chest radiograph, C.T. and lung function testing.

Imaging

The chest radiographic features in N.T.M. may be indistinguishable from those in tuberculosis. There may be cavitation which tends to be more thin walled than the cavitation seen in tuberculosis. There may also be peribronchial or nodular opacification. The nodules may be single or in clusters and they may occur bilaterally. Computed tomography can better delineate cavity formation and demonstrate bronchiectasis with *tree in bud* opacification, centrilobular nodules and pleural thickening [67] (Fig. 15.5).

Prognosis

Patients with N.T.M. infection do not demonstrate a faster decline in lung function over those that do not [68]. *Mycobacterium abscessus* is more virulent than other types of N.T.M. and only one case report in the literature has demonstrated eradication [69].

15.3 **Non-infectious Complications of Cystic Fibrosis Respiratory Disease**

15.3.1 Hemoptysis

Incidence

Hemoptysis is seen in established lung disease and more common in older patients. The Cystic Fibrosis Foundation (C.F.F.) Patient Registry over a 10-year period demonstrated that the annual incidence of massive hemoptysis was 0.87%. Overall 4.1% of patients experienced hemoptysis over a two-year period [70].

Physiology

Bleeding is usually from the bronchial arteries. Other vessels, which form collaterals with these, may also be a source of hemorrhage. Hemoptysis is due to chronic infection culminating in the formation of small blood vessels which rupture with coughing.

Clinical Presentation

Clinical presentation varies from mild blood streaked sputum (usually of no great significance) to large volumes of fresh blood with clots. Severe hemoptysis is defined as 250 mL in 1 day or 100 mL daily for a 3- to 7-day period [70]. This volume is arbitrary and significant bleeding less than this should be treated seriously. Identify whether the bleed is fresh i.e., bright red blood or old i.e., coffee ground. The presence or absence of clots and identification from which lung the patient feels he is bleeding is important. Epistaxis and hematemesis need to be excluded. Non-steroidal anti-inflammatory drugs and penicillin derivatives should be discontinued.

Risk Factors

Risk factors include *S. aureus* culture and diabetes [14].

Investigations

Investigations include a full blood count to rule out anemia and thrombocytopenia, a coagulation screen

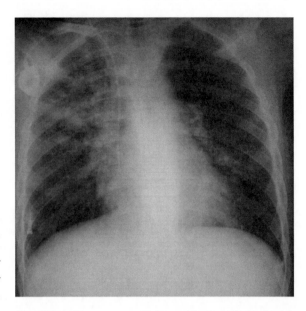
Fig. 15.6. Thirteen-year-old boy with CF. Admitted with hemoptysis. There is ill-defined right upper lobe and lingular opacifications

looking for a prolonged prothrombin time, blood group and cross match, liver function tests, venous blood gas, chest radiograph and sputum for culture and sensitivity.

Chest Radiograph

Chest radiograph may not reveal any specific abnormality or non-specific ill-defined airspace opacification may be evident (Fig. 15.6).

Treatment

Moderate hemoptysis is treated in hospital with oxygen where required, antibiotics to treat infection and gentle chest physiotherapy. Treatment of severe hemoptysis involves stabilization of the patient, ensuring good intravenous access (two large bore cannulas), fluids for resuscitation, oxygen, placing the patient in the lateral position with affected side down (to prevent aspiration into upper lobe) and vitamin K administration (onset of action is days). Intravenous vasopressin and more recently terlipressin has been found useful by some clinicians in the United Kingdom. Fluid retention may occur and a diuretic and glycerine trinitrate patch may be useful. Embolization with gelatin pledgets, steel coils (less common) or polyvinyl alcohol may be used. Potential complications include paralysis, if the spinal arteries are occluded, organ infarction or death. In the acute situation, embolization may be life saving [71–74] but it may need to be repeated. In one study, over half of 23 children required repeat embolization within 5 days to 21 months [75]. Intubation with endobronchial tamponade with balloon catheters, ligation of the bronchial artery or lobectomy are options if embolization fails.

Prognosis

Massive hemoptysis is a poor prognostic indicator because it occurs with significant established lung disease and is life threatening. The C.F.F. patient registry demonstrated that patients with massive hemoptysis were older (mean age 24 years), with more severe lung disease, had an increased morbidity and mortality after massive hemoptysis and that >1/3 died within 1 year [76].

15.3.2 Pneumothorax

Pneumothoraces occur in patients with cystic fibrosis who have established lung disease and the incidence increases in adolescent and adult life [77].

Physiology

A pneumothorax is caused by the rupture of a subpleural bleb in the visceral pleura or may be iatrogenic secondary to central line placement.

Clinical Presentation

While small pneumothoraces may be asymptomatic, larger pneumothoraces may present with pleuritic chest pain, sudden onset shortness of breath, hemoptysis, pallor, cyanosis and tachypnea. It is important to have a high index of clinical suspicion in patients with established lung disease or a previous pneumothorax.

Diagnosis

Diagnosis may be made clinically with tachypnea, tracheal and mediastinal deviation (as seen with a large tension pneumothorax), hypoxia, increased resonance to percussion and reduced breath sounds.

Investigations

Initial investigations include oxygen saturations in room air, blood gas and chest radiograph.

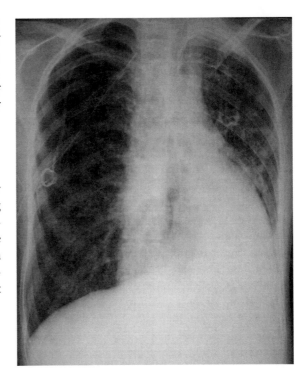

Fig. 15.7. Sixteen-year-old boy with extensive changes of CF with left lower lobe atelectasis. He developed a right apical pneumothorax requiring drainage. The chest X-ray demonstrates a residual pneumothorax. The chest drain tip is projected over the apex of the lung medially

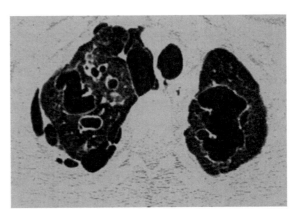

Fig. 15.8. CT post drainage of right apical pneumothorax in patient in Fig. 15.7. There are large bullae in both lung apices

Imaging

A chest radiograph confirms the diagnosis (Fig. 15.7). Air in the pleural space is evident and the degree of mediastinal shift is related to the size of the pneumothorax. Following drainage, a CT of the thorax is useful to identify the presence of subpleural bullae as a cause (Fig. 15.8).

Treatment

Small and asymptomatic pneumothoraces are observed in hospital for 24 h to ensure they do not increase in size and there is no associated hemothorax. Medium to large pneumothoraces require the insertion of a chest tube connected to underwater drainage. If there is no re-expansion after 24 h, suction should be applied. Surgical advice regarding a pleurodesis should be sought if there is no re-expansion after 4–5 days. Limited mechanical abrasion pleurodesis is a good option because extensive pleurectomy or talc pleurodesis may complicate the field if lung transplant is required later. Prolonged chest tube insertion runs the risk of bronchopleural fistula.

High-dose oxygen (up to 10 L) via a non-rebreather mask may promote resolution but many of these patients with cystic fibrosis retain CO_2, so the $PaCO_2$ must be carefully monitored. By reducing the total pressure of gas (particularly nitrogen) in the capillaries, high-flow oxygen creates a higher gradient between the pleural capillaries and pleural cavity and therefore air is resorbed: up to four times faster than without oxygen therapy [78]. In a patient unfit for general anesthetic, a blood or betadine pleurodesis may be used. Temporary use of a Heimlich valve may be an option particularly in a patient with end-stage lung disease, who is too unwell for general anesthetic and where pleurodesis under local anesthetic has failed repeatedly.

Prognosis

Pneumothoraces in cystic fibrosis carry a poor prognosis. The median survival after pneumothorax is 30 months [79]. Post pneumothorax, an increased rate and duration of hospital admissions was documented in the U.S.A. together with an increased 2-year mortality: 49 vs. 12% when compared to patients who never had a pneumothorax [80]. Pneumothoraces carry a recurrence risk in patients with cystic fibrosis.

15.3.3 Allergic Bronchopulmonary Aspergillosis

Allergic bronchopulmonary aspergillosis (A.B.P.A) is a hypersensitivity disorder of the lung due to an immune response to *Aspergillus fumigatus* antigens. *Aspergillus* is found in damp buildings, moldy hay and construction sites. The prevalence of A.B.P.A. in cystic fibrosis in Europe has been reported at 7.8% [81], while in North America it is reported as 2% [82]. This variation may be partly explained by the different diagnostic criteria used which are more strict in Europe than North America.

Physiology

The inhaled spores are trapped in airway mucus; they germinate and form mycelia which release allergens. A type I and III immune response follow with production of specific IgG and IgE antibodies and an exaggerated T helper type-2 lymphocyte response leading to release of interleukin (IL) 4, IL-5 and IL-13, all associated with allergy. Secondly, the aspergillus bound to the epithelial cells, grows on them, chronic airway inflammation occurs, extending to the alveoli and small airways resembling an eosinophilic pneumonia.

Risk Factors

Risk factors include male gender, adolescence, poor lung function, *P. aeruginosa* [82] and poor nutritional status [82]. Atopy is a significant risk factor: A.B.P.A. occurs in 22% of atopic cystic fibrosis patients versus 2% of non-atopic cystic fibrosis patients. A.B.P.A. is less common in young children (<6 years of age).

Clinical Presentation

Presentation may be acute or chronic. In an acute presentation, patients may present with wheeze, shortness of breath, increased production of sputum which contains brown/blacks specks, chest pain, mild fever and myalgia similar to an *influenza-like* illness. Alternatively, patients may present as if for a sub-acute infective pulmonary exacerbation but not respond to intravenous antibiotics.

Diagnosis and Investigations

Diagnosis in patients with cystic fibrosis may be difficult because there is an overlap between some symptoms and signs of A.B.P.A. and cystic fibrosis. The triad of clinical symptoms, serological and radiological evidence is required for the diagnosis as outlined in the C.F. Foundation consensus statement [83] and the United Kingdom C.F. Trust [84]. A classic presentation would include clinical deterioration,

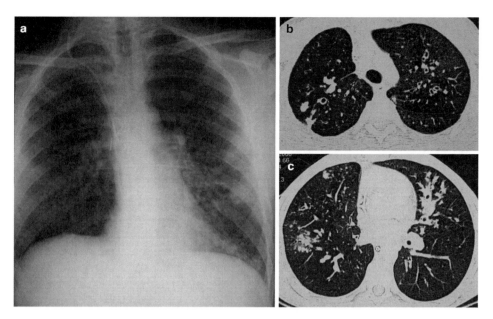

Fig. 15.9. Sixteen-year-old boy with allergic bronchopulmonary aspergillosis (ABPA). (a) Chest X-ray shows ill-defined patchy opacification in the left lower and right upper lobes. (b) CT chest shows moderate to severe bronchial wall thickening with bronchiectasis. (c) On the left side there is linear branching opacification suggestive of fluid filled dilated bronchi. There are ill-defined slightly lobulated masses in the right lung

plus or minus wheeze, an elevated total IgE > 1000 IU/mL, precipitating antibodies to *A. fumigatus* or serum IgG to *A. fumigatus*, elevated serum IgE antibody to *A. fumigatus* or immediate cutaneous reactivity to *Aspergillus* together with new changes on chest radiography or CT which does not clear with antibiotics and physiotherapy. For more minor cases, a total IgE of >500 I.U./mL is accepted.

Imaging

The chest radiographic features tend to be non-specific. There may be evidence of bronchiectasis with patchy opacification, compatible with mucous plugging (Fig. 15.9a). The opacification may involve the perihilar regions and extend towards the lung periphery. On CT, there is evidence of central bronchiectasis of a moderate to severe degree, bronchial wall thickening and lobulated opacification (Figs. 15.9b, c).

Screening

A total IgE should be performed annually on all patients over 6 years of age (C.F. Foundation) and if >500 I.U./mL other markers should be measured and if 200–500 I.U./mL repeat total IgE in 3 months.

Treatment

Non-enteric coated oral corticosteroids are the main stay of treatment and are employed for their ability to attenuate the inflammatory and immunological reaction [83]. However, their effect on long-term progression of the disease is unclear [85]. Recurrence occurs. Oral antifungal agents, studied in asthmatics with A.B.P.A., lead to clinical improvement in addition to reduction in corticosteroid dose and eosinophilic inflammation [86, 87]. Anti-IgE therapy has been used with some success.

Prognosis

A.B.P.A. recurs and may require repeated treatment. While untreated, A.B.P.A. can progress to central bronchiectasis, Epidemiologic Registry For Cystic Fibrosis data have shown that it has no effect on longitudinal decline in FEV_1 [81] when divided into severity subgroups.

15.3.4 Sinus Disease

Incidence

Nasal polyposis is a feature of cystic fibrosis. This has probably been underreported in the past with a reported incidence of 10–15% in teenagers. More recent studies report 50% of pediatric [88] and 32–45% of adult cystic fibrosis patients have nasal polyposis [89–91]. Of the children reported, less than two thirds were symptomatic. Children presenting with nasal polyposis should be referred to a respiratory pediatrician to rule out cystic fibrosis.

Pathophysiology

The pathophysiology is unclear but felt to be a combination of failure to clear thickened secretions leading to chronic inflammation and sinus ostial obstruction with superimposed infection usually with the same bacteria that have colonized the lower airway i.e., *S. aureus, H. influenza* and later *P. aeruginosa.*

Clinical Presentation

Clinical presentation of chronic sinusitis includes, most commonly, headache and peri-orbital pain [92]. Other symptoms include *pressure symptoms* across the forehead (frontal sinuses), below the eyes (maxillary sinuses), nasal obstruction, rhinorrhea, snoring and voice change. Anosmia is the commonest symptom in those with polyposis [92].

Physical Examination

Physical examination may reveal that the patient is a *mouth breather.* Widening of the nasal bridge can be appreciated in some children with massive polyposis giving rise to the impression of hypertelorism. Tenderness over the affected sinuses is present in one-third of patients with acute sinusitis. Polyps may cause obstruction of the nasal airway. Large polyps may be visible on direct examination of the nose but up to 25% may be missed [93]. Referral to an Ear, Nose and Throat (E.N.T.) specialist for complete E.N.T. examination with flexible endoscopy is recommended if polyps are suspected.

Risk Factors

Patients with nasal polyps are more likely to have *P. aeruginosa* in their lower airways than those who do not [94]. *Aspergillus* allergy is more common in patients with cystic fibrosis who have polyps than those who do not [95].

Imaging

Imaging of the sinuses is recommended only in patients with cystic fibrosis who have symptomatic sinusitis and polyposis because pan sinusitis is almost universal in cystic fibrosis whether symptomatic or not. Sinus radiographs may show sinus opacification (Fig. 15.10) and may show an air fluid level. If imaging is indicated, sinus CT is the investigation of choice to identify the extent of mucosal thickening, polyposis, sinus wall displacement and obstruction of the osteomeatal complex (Fig. 15.11). It provides a clear picture for the surgeon. Classically, the frontal and sphenoidal sinuses are hypoplastic in CF.

Treatment

Mild to moderate cases are treated with medical management reserving surgical approaches for severe, symptomatic cases only. Chronic rhinosinusitis may

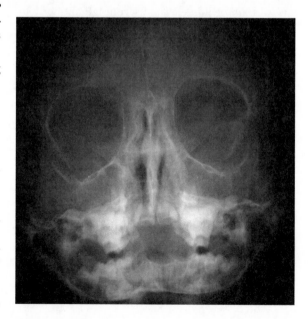

Fig. 15.10. Sinus radiograph in a 7-year-old girl demonstrating complete opacification of the maxillary sinuses, compatable with sinusitis

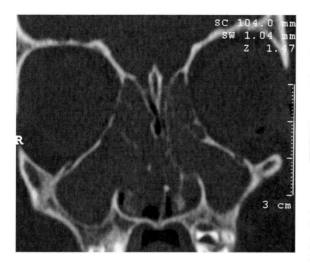

Fig. 15.11. Coronal CT of sinuses in a 4-year-old girl. There is complete opacification of both maxillary sinuses and ethmoid sinuses compatible with sinusitis. The medial wall of the right antrum is thinned and displaced. On endoscopic examination polyps were identified requiring functional endoscopic sinus surgery (FESS)

be treated with antibiotics, anti-inflammatory agents and nasal irrigations, e.g., nasal saline irrigations either hyper or hypotonic. This disease is incurable but symptoms can be controlled. Single polyps causing mild symptoms can be treated conservatively with intranasal steroid sprays. Betamethasone drops may reduce polyp size versus placebo but should be used for short periods only because of risk of systemic side effects, e.g., adrenal suppression [96].

Surgical intervention ranges from simple nasal polypectomy to extensive removal of all diseased mucosa, removal of ethmoid labyrinth and opening of the maxillary (and if present frontal and sphenoid) sinuses. Symptoms recur. While 50% of a pediatric patient group had on average a symptom-free period of 11.3 years post sinus surgery, endoscopic review demonstrated a 50% chance of reverting to preoperative state within 18–24 months [97]. There may be some role for functional endoscopic sinus surgery and wide antrostomy with postoperative saline and antibiotic irrigation in prelung transplant patients with reported rare recurrence of polyposis and fewer *P. aeruginosa* infections [98].

15.3.5 Lung Transplant

Lung transplantation is indicated for children with cystic fibrosis when they develop end-stage lung disease despite maximal therapy. It is important to refer a child for transplant assessment early enough that there is an optimal time for assessment and listing. For further detail, please refer to Chap. 17, Lung Transplant in Pediatric Patients.

15.4 Non-Respiratory Conditions of Cystic Fibrosis

A detailed discussion of non-respiratory CF conditions is beyond the scope of this book. However, CF patients are often affected by one or more of the following conditions which may be serendipitously recognized during imaging of the chest.

15.4.1 Gastrointestinal System

Eighty-five percent of people with cystic fibrosis are pancreatic insufficient and approximately 15% are pancreatic sufficient. Between 6 and 20% of patients with cystic fibrosis present with meconium ileus and approximately 16% experience distal intestinal obstruction syndrome (D.I.O.S.).

Meconium Ileus

Meconium ileus occurs in neonates with cystic fibrosis. Forty percent of patients present with complications such as intestinal atresia, volvulus or antenatal perforation with meconium peritonitis (Figs. 15.12–15.14). *If treatment with a gastrografin enema fails, the patient proceeds to surgery.*

Distal Intestinal Obstruction Syndrome

D.I.O.S. refers to distal intestinal obstruction after the neonatal period and has replaced the term *meconium ileus equivalent.* It is when the distal small bowel, i.e., terminal ileum, cecum and possibly the right colon become impacted and obstructed with inspissated, fecal material. D.I.O.S. is more common in adolescents and adults. Prevalence ranges from 2% of patients with C.F. <5 years to 27% of those >30 years [99] (Fig. 15.15). Treatment includes rehydration, adjustment of pancreatic enzyme dose, dietary fiber, gastrografin enemas [100] and occasionally surgery.

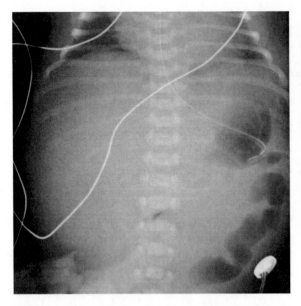

Fig. 15.12. Newborn with meconium ileus. Abdominal radiograph shows abdominal distension. There is a curvilinear area of calcification on the right side indicating antenatal bowel perforation and meconium peritonitis

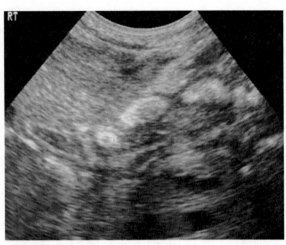

Fig. 15.13. Newborn with meconium ileus. Abdominal ultrasound scan shows multiple echogenic areas in the peritoneum indicating calcification as a result of antenatal bowel perforation

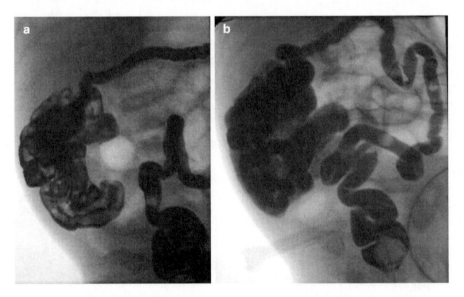

Fig. 15.14. Newborn with meconium ileus. (a) There is a microcolon and the ileal loops are filled with meconium. (b) Contrast has refluxed into the dilated loops proximal to the meconium

Gastroesophageal Reflux

Gastroesophageal reflux (G.E.R.) is very common in cystic fibrosis. In children aged 5 years or less, increased esophageal acid exposure has been demonstrated in 76% [101] and 80% [102] of patients. In older children, abnormal results were demonstrated in 55% [103] and 60% [104]. Thickened feeds, elevation of head of the bed, proton pump inhibitors and

prokinetic agents e.g., low dose antibiotics or surgical fundoplication are treatment options.

Fibrosing Colonopathy

Fibrosing colonopathy is very rare now but was noticed as a new disease when there was a switch from conventional to high strength pancreatic enzymes and in patients receiving typically more

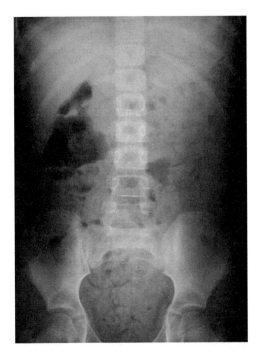

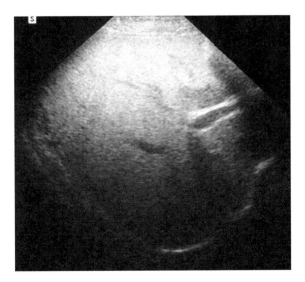

Fig. 15.16. Ultrasound scan through the right lobe of the liver in a 7-year-old girl showing significant increased echogenicity in keeping with fatty infiltration

Fig. 15.15. Abdominal radiograph in a 13 year old girl with distal intestinal obstruction syndrome (DIOS). The entire colon is impacted with fecal material

than 24,000 international units (I.U.) of lipase/kg body weight per day. The majority of cases were children with a mean age 5 years [105]. Most cases occurred 7–15 months after starting high strength preparations. No cases in children have been reported since 1995 when the dose was restricted to 10,000 I.U. lipase/kg/day and enzymes with Eudragit L coatings have been avoided [106]. *If symptomatic surgical resection of strictured bowel is required.*

Enteric Infections

Patients with cystic fibrosis may have some resistance to certain enteric infections or enterotoxins. Jejunal mucosa from patients with cystic fibrosis is unresponsive to various enterotoxins in vitro [107]. It has been postulated that cystic fibrosis confers some protection against *Clostridium difficile* either by exposure early in life promoting immunity or due to C.F.T.R.-related abnormalities of electrolyte transport across the intestinal epithelium. Once confirmed, treatment is directed towards management of *C. difficile* enterocolotis.

Hepatobiliary Disease

Hepatobiliary involvement in cystic fibrosis is well recognized and occasionally dominates the clinical picture. Recent prospective studies report that approximately 20–25% of patients with cystic fibrosis will develop liver disease, 6–8% have evidence of cirrhosis and 2–3% will progress to liver decompensation. The majority of patients present in childhood or early teens, so liver disease is an early complication [108, 109]. Generally, liver disease has little impact on clinical condition until the late stages.

Focal biliary cirrhosis is the pathognomonic lesion in cystic fibrosis. Clinical features of liver disease in cystic fibrosis include cholestasis in the neonatal period which usually self-resolves. The most common hepatic association with cystic fibrosis is fatty infiltration of the liver. Cirrhosis is usually an asymptomatic diagnosis on routine screening by ultrasound.

Extrahepatic biliary disease: structural abnormalities of the extrahepatic biliary system are commonly observed in cystic fibrosis. Patients with cystic fibrosis have a four- to fivefold increased risk of gallstones over their age-matched controls giving a prevalence of approximately 20–25% in cystic fibrosis. This prevalence increases with age. Complications of gallstones, which are usually radiolucent, occur in 4% of cystic fibrosis patients and include biliary colic, acute cholecystitis, empyema of the gall bladder, bile duct obstruction, cholangitis and gallstone pancreatitis.

Imaging studies of patients with cystic fibrosis have shown a wide spectrum of biliary abnormalities [110–113] (Figs. 15.16 and 15.17). An undetectable or micro-gallbladder has been documented in up to 30% of cases. Stenosis or atresia of the cystic duct is also a common finding. Ursodeoxycholic acid, a hydrophilic bile acid is used to treat liver disease. End-stage liver failure requires a liver transplant.

Pancreatic Disease

Pancreatic exocrine insufficiency is present in 85% or patients with CF while the remaining are pancreatic sufficient. Ultrasound of the pancreas is frequently echogenic (Fig. 15.18) and may be small. On CT, the pancreas is frequently profoundly lucent.

The mean age of presentation with pancreatitis in cystic fibrosis is in the late teens [114, 115]. Most patients who develop symptomatic pancreatitis are pancreatic sufficient. For almost 30% of patients with symptomatic pancreatitis, this is the presenting feature leading to a diagnosis of cystic fibrosis [114, 115]. Occasionally in cystic fibrosis, the pancreas can be completely replaced by cysts (Fig. 15.19).

Cystic fibrosis-related diabetes (C.F.R.D.) is an age-related phenomenon. Initially, exocrine function is lost in the pancreas, followed years later, by loss of endocrine function. *Insulin is the treatment of choice.*

15.4.2   Skeletal System

Approximately 25% of young adults with cystic fibrosis have low bone mineral density (B.M.D.). Treatment includes adequate vitamins D and K, calcium supple-

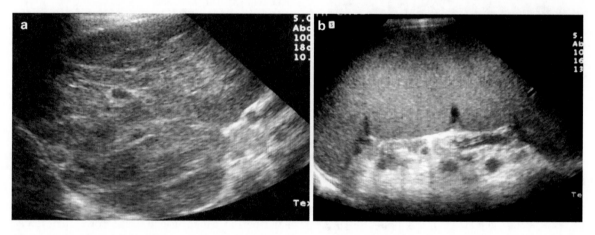

Fig. 15.17. (a, b) Liver ultrasound scan in a 16-year-old boy. The echogenicity of the liver tissue is not uniform and the liver margin is slightly lobulated suggesting cirrhosis

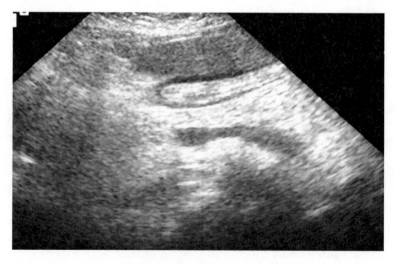

Fig. 15.18. There is uniform increased echogenicity of the pancreas

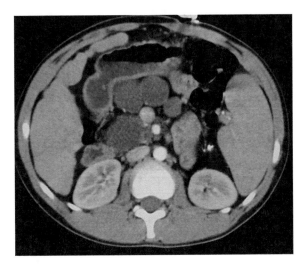

Fig. 15.19. Patient with cystic fibrosis with multiple pancreatic cysts

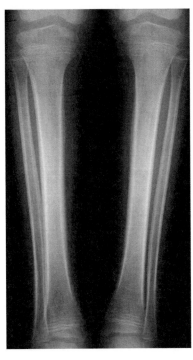

Fig. 15.20. Fourteen-year old boy with hypertrophic pulmonary osteoarthropathy. There is regular periosteal new bone formation at the diaphyses of the tibia and fibula bilaterally

ments and exercise and avoidance of oral corticosteroids if possible.

Twelve percent of patients with cystic fibrosis have symptoms related to joints: related to cystic fibrosis directly, related to drug treatment or related to the presence of coincidental disease. The most common form of arthritis in cystic fibrosis is episodic arthritis occurring in 2–8% of adults. It may be monoarticular or polyarticular affecting large joints e.g., knees, ankles, hips, shoulders and wrists. Episodes may be associated with a high fever, vasculitic rash, erythema nodosum and are typically transient lasting 7–10 days [70, 116, 117]. Treatment is symptomatic with non-steroidal anti-inflammatory agents and occasionally oral corticosteroids.

Hypertrophic pulmonary osteoarthropathy (H.P.O.A.) occurs in 2–7% of cystic fibrosis patients, predominately younger adults and rarely affects children less than 10 years of age (Fig. 15.20). The median onset is 20 years. There is a consistent relationship between H.P.O.A. and severity of lung disease or infective exacerbations [118].

15.4.3 Reproductive Tract Disorders

Congenital bilateral absence of the vas deferens results in infertility in males with cystic fibrosis. Seminal vesicles are often hypoplastic. C.F.T.R. is expressed in the epididymis and vas deferens [119]. In infertile males who do not have cystic fibrosis, mutations in C.F.T.R. are frequent. Women with cystic

fibrosis successfully conceive but fertility may be reduced [120]. C.F.T.R. is expressed in the uterus and cervix [119].

References

1. Matsui H, Grub BR, Tarran R, Randell SH, Gatzy JT, Davis CW, et al. Evidence for periciliary liquid layer depletion, not abnormal ion composition, in the pathogenesis of cystic fibrosis airways disease. Cell. 1998;95: 1005–15.
2. Riordan JR, Rommens JM, Kerem B, et al. Identification of the cystic fibrosis gene: cloning and characterization of complementary DNA. Science. 1989;245:1066–73.
3. Kerem B, Rommens JM, Buchanan JA, et al. Identification of the cystic fibrosis gene: genetic analysis. Science. 1989; 245:1073–80.
4. Rommens JM, Iannuzzi MC, Kerem B, et al. Identification of the cystic fibrosis gene: chromosome walking and jumping. Science. 1989;245:1059–65.
5. Cystic fibrosis genetic analysis consortium. Cystic fibrosis mutation data base. www.genet.sickkids.on.ca/cftr/ Published (1989). Updated 2 March 2007. Accessed 29 May 2011
6. Cleveland RH, Zurakowski D, Slattery D, Colin AA. Cystic fibrosis genotype and assessing rates of decline in pulmonary status. Radiology. 2009;253:813–21.
7. Le Grys VA. Sweat testing for the diagnosis of cystic fibrosis: practical considerations. J Pediatr. 1996;129:892–7.

8. Monaghan KG, Feldman GL. The risk of cystic fibrosis with prenatally detected echogenic bowel in an ethnically and socially diverse North American population. Prenat Diagn. 1999;19:604–9.

9. Cleveland RH, Neish AS, Zurakowski D, Nichols DP, Wohl ME, Colin AA. Cystic fibrosis: a system for assessing and predicting progression. Am J Roentgenol. 1998;170: 1067–72.

10. Cleveland RH, Neish AS, Zurakowski D, Nichols DP, Wohl ME, Colin AA. Cystic fibrosis: predictors of accelerated decline and distribution of disease in 230 patients. Am J Roentgenol. 1998;171:1311–5.

11. Slattery DM, Zurakowski D, Colin AA, Cleveland RH. CF: an X-ray database to assess effect of aerosolized tobramycin. Pediatr Pulmonol. 2004;38(1):23–30.

12. Bhalla M et al. Cystic fibrosis: scoring system with thin section. CT Radiology. 1991;179:783–8.

13. Canadian Cystic Fibrosis Foundation. Report of the Canadian Patient Data registry 2002. Toronto, Ontario, 2002

14. Cystic fibrosis foundation. Patient Registry 2004 Annual Report. Bethesda, Maryland, 2005

15. Dodge JA, Lewis PA, Stanton M, Wilsher J. Cystic fibrosis mortality and survival in the UK: 1947–2003. Eur Respir J. 2007;29:522–6.

16. Wang EE, Prober CG, Manson B, et al. Association of respiratory viral infection with pulmonary deterioration in patients with cystic fibrosis. N Engl J Med. 1984;311: 1653–8.

17. Abman SH, Ogle JW, Butler-Somin N, et al. Role of respiratory syncytial virus in early hospitalization for respiratory distress of young infants with cystic fibrosis. J Pediatr. 1988;113:826–30.

18. Smyth AR, Smyth RL, Tong CY, et al. Effect of respiratory virus infections, including rhinovirus on clinical status in cystic fibrosis. Arch Dis Child. 1995;73:117–20.

19. Wat D, Doull I. Respiratory virus infections in cystic fibrosis. Pediatr Respir Rev. 2003;4:172–7.

20. Ramsey BW, Gore EJ, Smith AL, et al. The effect of respiratory viral infections on patients with cystic fibrosis. Am J Dis Child. 1989;143:662–8.

21. Hiatt PW, Grace SC, Kozinetz CA, et al. Effects of viral lower respiratory infection on lung function in infants with cystic fibrosis. Pediatrics. 1999;103:619–26.

22. Peterson NT, Hoiby N, Mordhorst CH, et al. Respiratory infections in cystic fibrosis patients caused by virus, Chlamydia and mycoplasma: possible synergism with *Pseudomonas aeruginosa*. Acta Paediatr Scand. 1981;70: 623–8.

23. Collinson J, Nicholson KG, Cancio JB, et al. Effects of upper respiratory tract infections in patients with cystic fibrosis. Thorax. 1996;51:1115–22.

24. Abman SH, Ogle JW, Harbeck RJ, et al. Early bacteriologic, immunologic and clinical courses of young infants with cystic fibrosis identified by neonatal screening. J Pediatr. 1991;119:211–7.

25. Pribble CG, Black PG, Bosso A, et al. Clinical manifestations of exacerbations of cystic fibrosis associated with nonbacterial infections. Pediatrics. 1990;117:200–4.

26. Conway SP, Simmonds EJ, Littlewood JM. Acute severe deterioration in cystic fibrosis associated with influenza A virus infection. Thorax. 1991;47:112–4.

27. Bhalla P, Tan A, Smyth R. Vaccines for preventing influenza in people with cystic fibrosis. The cochrane database of systemic reviews 2000. Issue 1. Art. no. CD001753

28. Armstrong DS, Grimwood K, Carlin JB, et al. Lower airway inflammation in infants and young children with cystic fibrosis. Am J Respir Crit Care Med. 1997;156: 1197–204.

29. Rosenfeld M, Gibson RL, McNamara S, et al. Early pulmonary infection, inflammation and clinical outcomes in infants with cystic fibrosis. Pediatr Pulmonol. 2001;32:356–66.

30. Balough K, McCubbin M, Weinberger M, et al. The relationship between infection and inflammation in the early stages of lung disease from cystic fibrosis. Pediatr Pulmonol. 1995;20:63–70.

31. Chimiel JF, Berger M, Konstan MW. The role of inflammation in the pathophysiology of C.F. lung disease. Clin Rev Allergy Immunol. 2002;23:5–27.

32. Bradley J, McAlister O, Elborn JS. Pulmonary function, inflammation, exercise capacity and quality of life in cystic fibrosis. Eur Resp J. 2001;17:712–5.

33. Lyczak JB, Cannon CL, Peir GM. Lung infections associated with cystic fibrosis. Clin Microbiol Rev. 2002;15: 194–222.

34. Demko CA, Byard PJ, Davis PB. Gender differences in cystic fibrosis: *Pseudomonas aeruginosa* infection. J Clin Epidemiol. 1995;48:1041–9.

35. Parad RJ, Gerard CJ, Zurakowski D, et al. Pulmonary outcome in cystic fibrosis in influenced primarily by mucoid *Pseudomonas aeruginosa* infection and immune status and only modestly by genotype. Infec Immun. 1999;67: 4744–50.

36. Courtney JM, Ennis M, Elborn JS. Cytokines and inflammatory mediators in cystic fibrosis. J Cyst Fibros. 2004;3:223–31.

37. Watt AP, Courtney J, Moore J, et al. Neutrophil cell death, activation and bacterial infection in Cystic Fibrosis. Thorax. 2005;60:659–64.

38. Cheng K, Smyth RL, Govan JR, et al. Spread of a beta-lactam resistant *Pseudomonas aeruginosa* in a cystic fibrosis clinic. Lancet. 1996;348:639–42.

39. Jones AM, Webb AK, Govan JR, et al. *Pseudomonas aeruginosa* cross-infection in cystic fibrosis. Lancet. 2002;359:527–8.

40. O'Carroll MR, Syrmis MW, Wainwright CE, et al. Clonal strains of *pseudomonas aeruginosa* in pediatric and adult cystic fibrosis units. Eur Resp J. 2004;24:101–6.

41. Jones AM, Dodd ME, Govan JR, et al. Prospective surveillance for *Pseudomonas* aeruginosa cross-infection at a cystic fibrosis center. Am J Respir Crit Care Med. 2005;171:257–60.

42. Ojeniyi B, Frederiksen B, Hoiby N. Pseudomonas aeruginosa cross-infection among patients with cystic fibrosis during a winter camp. Pediatr Pulmonol. 2000;29: 177–81.

43. Stutman HR, Lieberman JM, Nussbaum E, Marks MI. Antibiotic prophylaxis in infants and young children with cystic fibrosis: a randomized controlled trial. J Pediatrics. 2002;140:299–305.

44. Gibson RL, Burns J, Ramsey BW. Pathophysiology and management of pulmonary infections in cystic fibrosis. Am J Resp Crit Care Med. 2003;168:918–51.

45. Elborn JS. Treatment of *Staphylococcus aureus* in cystic fibrosis. Thorax. 1999;54:377–8.

46. Conway S, Denton M. Staphylococcus aureus and MRSA. Prog Respir Res. 2006;34:153–9.

47. Mc Manus TE, Moore JE, Crowe M, et al. A comparison of pulmonary exacerbations with single and multiple

organisms in patients with cystic fibrosis and chronic Burkholderia cepacia infection. J Infect. 2003;46:56–9.

48. Koch C, Hoiby N. Diagnosis and treatment of cystic fibrosis. Respiration. 2000;67:239–47.

49. Beardsmore CS, Thompson JR, Williams A, et al. Pulmonary function in infants with cystic fibrosis: the effect of antibiotic treatment. Arch Dis Child. 1994;71: 133–7.

50. Marshall BC. Pulmonary exacerbations in cystic fibrosis: it's time to be explicit! Am J Respir Crit Care Med. 2004;169:781–2.

51. Weaver LT, Green MR, Nicholson K, et al. Prognosis in cystic fibrosis treated with continuous flucloxacillin from the neonatal period. Arch Dis Child. 1994;70:84–9.

52. Miall LS, McKinley NT, Brownlee KG, Conway SP. Methicillin-resistant *Staphylococcus aureus* (MRSA) infection in cystic fibrosis. Arch Dis Child. 2001;84: 160–2.

53. Thomas SR, Gyi KM, Gaya H, Hodson ME. Methicillin-resistant Staphylococcus aureus: impact at a national cystic fibrosis centre. J Hosp Infect. 1998;40:203–9.

54. Palvecino E. Community acquired MRSA infections. Clin Lab Med. 2004;24:403–18.

55. Garske LA, Kid TJ, Gan R, et al. Rifampicin and sodium fusidate reduces the frequency of methicillin-resistant Staphylococcus aureus (MRSA) isolation in adults with cystic fibrosis and chronic MRSA infection. J Hosp Infect. 2004;56:208–14.

56. Henry DA, Campbell MR, LiPuma JJ, Speert DP. Identification of Burkholderia cepacia isolates from patients with cystic fibrosis and use of a simple new selective medium. J Clin Microbiol. 1997;35:614–9.

57. McMenamin JD, Zaccone TM, Coenye T, et al. Misidentification of Burkholderia cepacia in US cystic fibrosis treatment centres: an analysis of 1051 recent sputum isolates. Chest. 2000;117:1661–5.

58. Govan JR, Brown PH, Maddison J, et al. Evidence for transmission of Pseudomonas cepacia by social contact in cystic fibrosis. Lancet. 1993;342:15–9.

59. McCloskey M, McCaughern J, Redmond AOB, Elborn JS. Clinical outcome after acquisition of Burkholderia cepacia in patients with cystic fibrosis. Irish J Med Sci. 2001;170:28–31.

60. Courtney JM, Dunbar KEA, McDowell A, et al. Clinical outcome of Burkholderia cepacia complex infection in cystic fibrosis adults. J Cys Fibros. 2004;3:93–8.

61. Frangolias DD, Mahenthiralingam E, Rae S, et al. Burkholderia cepacia in cystic fibrosis: variable disease course. Am J Respir Crit Care Med. 1999;160:1572–7.

62. DeSoyza A, McDowell A, Archer L, et al. Burkholderia cepacia complex genomovars and pulmonary transplantation outcomes in patients with cystic fibrosis. Lancet. 2001;358:1780–1.

63. Aris RM, Routh JC, LiPuma JJ, et al. Lung transplantation for cystic fibrosis patients with Burkholderia cepacia complex: survival linked to genomovar type. Am J Respir Crit Care Med. 2001;164:2102–6.

64. Jones AM, Dodd ME, Govan JRW, et al. Burkholderia cenocepacia and Burkholderia multivorans: influence on survival in cystic fibrosis. Thorax. 2004;59:948–51.

65. Olivier KN, Weber DJ, Wallace RJ, et al. Non-tuberculous mycobacteria :I: Mulitcenter prevalence study in cystic fibrosis. Am J Respir Crit Care Med. 2003;167:828–34.

66. American Thoracic Society. Diagnosis and treatment of disease caused by non- tuberculous mycobacteria.

[This official statement of the American Thoracic Society was approved by the board of directors, March1997.]. Am J Respir Crit Care Med. 1997;156:S1–25.

67. Martinez S, Page McAdams H, Batchu CS. The many faces of pulmonary nontuberculous mycobacterial infection. Am J Roentgenol. 2007;199:177–86.

68. Olivier KN, Weber DJ, Lee JH, et al. Non-tuberculous mycobacteria.II: nested– cohort study of impact on cystic fibrosis lung disease. Am J Respir Crit Care Med. 2003;167:835–40.

69. Cullen A, Cannon CL, Mark EJ, Colin AA. Mycobacteria abscessus infection in cystic fibrosis. Colonization or infection? Am J Resp Crit Care Med. 2000;161((2 pt 1)):641–5.

70. Schidlow DV, Taussig LM, Knowles MR. Cystic fibrosis foundation consensus conference report on pulmonary complications of cystic fibrosis. Pediatr Pulmonol. 1993;15:187–98.

71. Fairfax AJ, Ball J, Batten JC, et al. A pathological study following bronchial artery embolisation for haemoptysis in cystic fibrosis. Br J Dis Chest. 1980;74:345–52.

72. Sweezey NB, Fellows KE, Boat TF, et al. Treatment and prognosis of massive haemoptysis in cystic fibrosis. Am Rev Respir Dis. 1978;117:825–8.

73. Stern RC, Wood RE, Boat TF, et al. Treatment and prognosis of massive severe hemoptysis in cystic fibrosis. Am Rev Respir Dis. 1978;117:825–8.

74. Cohen AM. Haemoptysis: role of angiography and embolisation. Pediatr Pulmonol. 1992;8(Suppl):85–6.

75. Barben J, Robertson D, Olinsky A, et al. Bronchial artery embolisation in young patients with cystic fibrosis. Radiology. 2002;224:124–30.

76. Flume PA, Yankaskas JR, Ebeling M, et al. Massive hemoptysis in cystic fibrosis. Chest. 2005;128:729–38.

77. Penketh AR, Knight RK, Hodson ME, et al. Management of pneumothorax in adults with cystic fibrosis. Thorax. 1982;37:850–3. otic-associated.

78. Northfield TC. Oxygen therapy for spontaneous pneumothorax. Br Med J. 1971;4(5779):86–8.

79. Spector ML, Stern RC. Pneumothorax in cystic fibrosis: a 26-year experience. Ann Thorac Surg. 1989;47:204–7.

80. Flume PA, Strnage C, Ye X, et al. Pneumothorax in cystic fibrosis. Chest. 2005;128:720–8.

81. Mastella G, Rainisio M, Harms HK, et al. For the epidemiologic registry of cystic fibrosis. allergic broncho-pulmonary aspergillosis in cystic fibrosis: a european epidemiological study. Eur Resp J. 2000;16:464–71.

82. Geller DE, Kaplowitz H, Light MJ, Colin AA. For the scientific advisory group, investigators and coordinators of the epidemiologic study of cystic fibrosis. allergic broncho-pulmonary aspergillosis in cystic fibrosis: reported prevalence, regional distribution and patient characteristics. Chest. 1999;116:639–46.

83. Stevens DA, Moss RB, Kurup VP, et al. Allergic broncho-pulmonary aspergillosis in cystic fibrosis: state of the art: cystic Fibrosis Consensus Conference. Clin Infect Dis. 2003;37 Suppl 3:S225–64.

84. Cystic Fibrosis Trust. 2002. http://www.cftrust.org.uk/ aboutcf/publications/consensusdoc/accessed 2010

85. Wark P. Pathogenesis of allergic broncho-pulmonary aspergillosis and an evidence- based review of azoles in treatment. Respir Med. 2004;98:915–23.

86. Stevens DA, Schwartz HJ, Lee JY, et al. A randomized trial of itraconazole in allergic broncho-pulmonary aspergillosis. N Eng J Med. 2000;342:756–62.

87. Wark PA, Hensley MJ, Saltos N, et al. Anti-inflammatory effect of itraconazole in stable allergic bronchopulmonary aspergillosis: a randomized controlled trial. J Allergy Clin Immunol. 2003;111:952–7.

88. Slieker MG, Schilder AG, Uiterwaal CS, Van der Ent CK. Children with cystic fibrosis: who should visit the otorhinolaryngologist? Arch Otolaryngol Head Neck Surg. 2002;128:1245–8.

89. Brihaye P, Jorissen M, Clement PA. Chronic rhinosinusitis in cystic fibrosis (mucoviscidosis). Acta Otorhinolaryngol Belg. 1997;51:323–37.

90. Hadfield PJ, Rowe-Jones JM, Mackay IS. The prevalence of nasal polyps in adults with cystic fibrosis. Clin Otolaryngol Allied Sci. 2000;25:19–22.

91. Coste A, Gilain L, Roger G, et al. Endoscopic and CT-scan evaluation of rhinosinusitis in cystic fibrosis. Rhinology. 1995;33:152–6.

92. Gentile VG IG. Paranasal sinus disease in patients with cystic fibrosis. Otolaryngol Clin N Am. 1996;29:193–205.

93. Brihaye P, Clement PA, Dab I, Desprechin B. Pathological changes of the lateral nasal wall in patients with cystic fibrosis (mucoviscidosis). Int J Pediatr Otorhinolaryngol. 1994;28(2–3):141–7.

94. Henriksson G, Westrin KM, Karpati F, et al. Nasal polyps in cystic fibrosis: clinical endoscopic study with nasal lavage fluid analysis. Chest. 2002;121:40–7.

95. Cimmino M, Cavaliere M, Nardone M, et al. Clinical characteristics and genotype analysis of patients with cystic fibrosis and nasal polyposis. Clin Ololaryngol Allied Sci. 2003;28:125–32.

96. Hadfield PJ, Rowe-Jones JM, Mackay IS. A prospective treatment trial of nasal polyps in adults with cystic fibrosis. Rhinology. 2000;38(2):63–5.

97. Rowe-Jones JM, Mackay IS. Endoscopic sinus surgery in the treatment of cystic fibrosis with nasal polyposis. Laryngoscope. 1996;106(12 Pt 1):1540–4.

98. Davidson TM, Murphy C, Mitchell M, et al. Management of chronic sinusitis in cystic fibrosis. Laryngoscope. 1995;105(4 Pt 1):354–8.

99. Rubinstein S, Moss R, Lewiston N. Constipation and meconium ileus equivalent in patients with cystic fibrosis. Pediatrics. 1986;78:473–9.

100. O'Halloran SM, Gilbert J, Mckendrick OM, et al. Gastrografin in acute meconium ileus equivalent. Arch Dis Child. 1986;61:1128–30.

101. Vic P, Tassin E, Turck D, et al. Frequency of gastro-oesophageal reflux in infants and in young children with cystic fibrosis. Arch Pediatr. 1995;2:742–6 [in French].

102. Malfoot A, Dab I. New insights on gastro-oesophageal reflux in cystic fibrosis by longitudinal follow up. Arch Dis Child. 1991;66:1339–45.

103. Brodzicki J, Trawinska-Bartnicka M, Korzon M. Frequency, consequences and pharmacological treatment of gastro-oesophageal reflux in children with cystic fibrosis. Med Sci Monit. 2002;8:CR529–37.

104. Gustafsson PM, Fransson SG, Kjellman NI, et al. Gastro-oesophageal reflux and severity of pulmonary disease in cystic fibrosis. Scand J Gastroenterol. 1991;26:449–56.

105. Fitzsimmons SC, Burkhart GA, Borowitz D, et al. High-dose pancreatic-enzyme supplements and fibrosing colonopathy in children with cystic fibrosis. N Engl J Med. 1997;336:1283–9.

106. Breckenridghe A, Raine J. Concern about records of fibrosing colonopathy study. Lancet. 2001;357:1527.

107. Baxter PS, Goldhill J, Hardcastle J. Accounting for cystic fibrosis. Nature. 1988;335:211.

108. Corbett K, Kelleher S, Rowland M, et al. Cystic fibrosis associated liver disease: a population-based study. J Pediatr. 2004;145:327–32.

109. Lamireau T, Monnereau S, Martin S, et al. Epidemiology of liver disease in cystic fibrosis: a longtitudinal study. J Hepatol. 2004;41:920–5.

110. McHugo JM, McKeown C, Brown MT, et al. Ultrasound findings in children with cystic fibrosis. Br J Radiol. 1987;60:137–41.

111. King LJ, Scurr ED, Murugan N, et al. Hepatobiliary and pancreatic manifestations of cystic fibrosis: MR imaging appearances. Radiographics. 2000;20:767–77.

112. Angelico M, Gandin C, Canuzzi P, et al. Gallstones in cystic fibrosis: a critical appraisal. Hepatology. 1991;14:768–75.

113. Yang Y, Raper SE, Cohn JA, et al. An approach for treating the hepatobiliary disease of cystic fibrosis by somatic gene transfer. Proc Natl Acad Sci USA. 1993;90:4601–5.

114. De Boeck K, Wilschanski M, Castellani C, et al. Cystic fibrosis: terminology and diagnostic algorithms. Thorax. 2006;61:627–35.

115. Durno C, Corey M, Zielenski J, et al. Genotype and phenotype correlations in patients with cystic fibrosis and pancreatitis. Gastroenterology. 2002;123:1857–64.

116. Bourke S, Rooney M, Fitzgerald M, et al. Episodic arthropathy in adult cystic fibrosis. Quart J Med. 1987;64:651–9.

117. Rush PJ, Shore A, Coblentz C, et al. The musculoskeletal manifestations of cystic fibrosis. Semin Arthritis Rheum. 1986;15:213–25.

118. Braude S, Kennedy H, Hodson M, et al. Hypertrophic osteoarthropathy in cystic fibrosis. Br Med J. 1984;288:822–3.

119. Tizzano EF, Silver MM, Chitayat D, et al. Differential cellular expression of cystic fibrosis transmembrane regulator in human reproductive tissues: clues for the infertility in patients with cystic fibrosis. Am J Pathol. 1994;144:906–14.

120. Phillipson G. Cystic fibrosis and reproduction. Reprod Fertil Dev. 1998;10:113–9.

Percutaneous Chest Intervention

16

Pradeep Govender, Meguru Watanabe, and Ahmad I. Alomari

CONTENTS

Pradeep Govender, LRCP & SI, MB, BCh, BAO, FFRRCSI (✉) •
Ahmad I. Alomari, MD, MSc, FSIR
Division of Vascular and Interventional Radiology,
Children's Hospital Boston, Harvard Medical School,
Boston, MA 02115, USA
e-mail: Pradeep.Govender@childrens.harvard.edu

Meguru Watanabe, MD, PhD
Department of Radiology, Children's Hospital Boston,
Boston, MA, USA

R.H. Cleveland (ed.), *Imaging in Pediatric Pulmonology*,
DOI 10.1007/978-1-4419-5872-3_16, © Springer Science+Business Media, LLC 2012

16.1   Pneumothorax

A pneumothorax refers to the presence of air or gas in the pleural cavity (Fig. 16.1a). It may be spontaneous or secondary to a wide variety of etiologies. Common causes of a pneumothorax are spontaneous, pneumonia, bronchopleural fistula (BPF), chest trauma, and iatrogenic. Tension pneumothorax refers to progressive accumulation of air under pressure in the pleural space resulting in serious cardiopulmonary compromise. Regardless of the etiology, a symptomatic pneumothorax can be effectively drained with a chest tube.

16.1.1   Indications

There are several therapeutic options for managing a pneumothorax including observation, oxygen therapy, thoracentesis, image-guided tube thoracostomy, or open thoracostomy. The type of therapy employed depends on the severity of the symptoms, the degree of lung collapse, and the presence of underlying lung

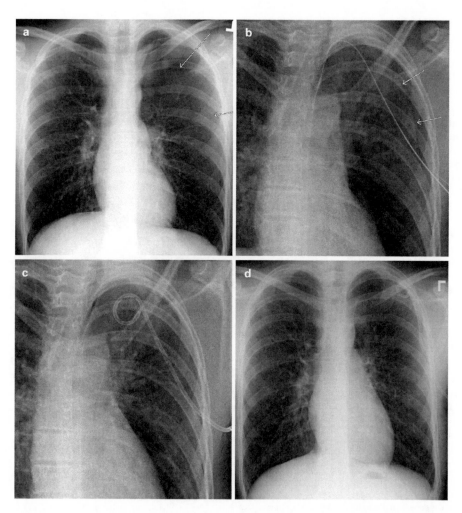

Fig. 16.1. (a) A 17-year-old male presented with acute severe left pleuritic chest pain and mild shortness of breath. Frontal chest radiograph demonstrated moderate-sized left pneumothorax. *Arrows* point to the edge of the retracted lung. (b) Fluoroscopic-guided tube thoracostomy – collimated fluoroscopic guidance was used to advance 5 French Yueh needle attached to an empty syringe above the rib and through the intercostal space into the pleural space while gentle aspiration is applied with the syringe. Once air is withdrawn into the syringe, a guide wire is advanced through the needle into the pleural space. (c) Fluoroscopic-guided tube thoracostomy – a pigtail drainage catheter is placed over the wire under fluoroscopic guidance. The catheter is appropriately secured to the skin and connected to continuous Pleurovac underwater seal suction device at −20 cm water. (d) After air was no longer aspirated on continuous underwater seal suction device, the drainage catheter is switched to underwater seal drainage, and a frontal chest radiograph confirmed complete re-expansion of the left. The drainage catheter may be removed

disease. A small pneumothorax, not infrequently seen post-lung biopsy, typically resolves spontaneously. A tension pneumothorax requires immediate decompression with supplement and placement of a chest tube.

16.1.2 Technique: Tube Thoracostomy

Tube thoracostomy (or chest tube placement) in pediatric patients is often performed under sedation or general anesthesia. A guiding imaging modality needs to be selected for the procedure. Fluoroscopy is used for the treatment of a pneumothorax while sonographic guidance is used for treating a fluid collection in the pleural space and, at times, computed tomography (CT) for loculated lung abscesses. In selected patients, chest tubes can be inserted using local anesthetic injections without sedation.

Blood workup including basic coagulation parameters (platelet count, PT, INR, PTT) is necessary before the procedure particularly in patients with known coagulopathy. Cardiopulmonary monitoring is routinely utilized. The site and size of drainage catheter are determined before the procedure; guided by the imaging finding. Typically, an 8–12 Fr drainage catheter is sufficient to treat a pneumothorax.

An initial fluoroscopic examination in supine position is initially performed and an entry site is chosen and marked. Under sterile conditions, local anesthetic agent (e.g., buffered 1% Lidocaine) is administered to the skin and chest wall. A small skin incision is made with a scalpel. Under collimated fluoroscopic guidance, a needle (e.g., 5 French Yueh) attached to an empty syringe is advanced above the rib and through the intercostal space into the pleural space while gentle aspiration is applied with the syringe. Once air is withdrawn into the syringe, a guide wire is advanced through the needle into the pleural space. Over the wire, the tract is dilated sequentially to the desired diameter (Fig. 16.1b). A pigtail drainage catheter is placed over the wire under fluoroscopic guidance (Fig. 16.1c). The catheter is appropriately secured to the skin and connected to continuous underwater seal suction device (e.g., Atrium or Pleurovac drainage system) at −20 cm water. The patient is usually observed in the recovery room. After the patient is discharged from the recovery room, the drainage catheter is flushed with 5–15 mL of sterile saline twice per day and monitored for air leakage.

16.1.3 PostProcedure Management

The patient is usually observed in a postprocedure recovery room on bed rest for 2–4 h. Vital signs should be monitored every 15 min for 1 h, every 30 min for another 1 h, and then every 60 min for 2 h. The drainage catheter may be connected to continuous suction at −20 cm water. After the patient is discharged from the recovery room, the drainage catheter is flushed with 5–15 mL of sterile saline solution twice per day, and monitored for air leakage. When air is no longer aspirated, the drainage catheter is switched to underwater seal drainage, and a chest radiograph is obtained. The drainage catheter may be removed unless there is a recurrent pneumothorax that occurs while on underwater seal for 24 h.

16.1.4 Results and Complications

When air leak ceases, the tube is switched from suction to water seal. The chest tube is then removed once the lung expands and pneumothorax ceases, as depicted on serial chest radiographs. Premature removal of the chest tube should be avoided, particularly in children with secondary or recurrent pneumothorax.

For recurrent or persistent pneumothorax, pleurodesis and/or bullectomy might be considered. With proper imaging guidance, complications of chest tube placement are quite infrequent and include malfunction of the tube (due to malposition, occlusion, kinking), bleeding from the access site and skin infection.

16.1.5 Removal of the Chest Tube

A chest radiograph should be taken and assessed before removing the chest tube, to confirm the expansion of the lung (Fig. 16.1d). The chest tube can be removed at the patient's bedside; typically without any sedation.

The operator should cut the end of the pigtail drainage catheter in order to release the locking loop before removing the catheter. When the catheter is removed, the patient is asked to hold breath at maximum inspiration, if possible, to avoid inadvertent aspiration of air into the pleural cavity. Gentle pressure should be applied immediately to the skin insertion site upon removal of the chest tube, which then is sterilely dressed. A chest radiograph is typically obtained after removal of the chest tube.

16.2 Pleural Effusion: Hydrothorax, Empyema, Hemothorax, Chylothorax, and Malignant Pleural Effusion

A pleural effusion refers to the presence of a fluid collection in the pleural space (Fig. 16.2a). Among the many causes of pleural effusion, bacterial pneumonia is still the most common culprit (Table 16.1). It can be divided into two main types: transudate or exudate based on several biochemical and physical characters of the fluid (Table 16.2).

Hydrothorax (transudative, noninflammatory fluid) is often associated with an accumulation of fluid in the peritoneal cavity or in the subcutaneous tissues, caused mostly by cardiac, renal, or hepatic diseases. An exudate typically results from a local aggressive, inflammatory etiology, has a specific gravity >1.020, and contains more cells and proteins than a transudate. Thoracentesis can elucidate the type of effusion, thereby directing treatment to the underlying etiology. Large compressive effusions with symptoms should be drained to provide symptomatic relief.

16.2.1 Thoracentesis and Tube Thoracostomy

Sonographic guidance is typically the preferred guidance for thoracentesis and tube thoracostomy (see tube thoracostomy for pneumothorax) for pleural effusions (Fig. 16.2b). An adjuvant fluoroscopic guidance can also be used; though it is difficult to differentiate between fluid and consolidated or collapsed lung tissue on fluoroscopy. A pigtail drainage

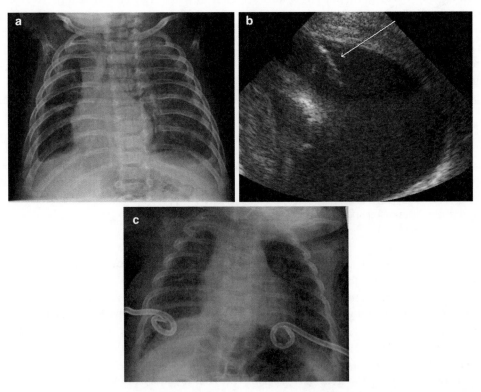

Fig. 16.2. (a) Two-month old with bilateral pleural effusions, worsening respiratory distress, and congenital chylothoraces. Frontal chest radiograph demonstrated bilateral pleural effusions, moderate-sized on the right and large-sized on the left. There was mediastinal shift to the right. (b) Sonographic-guided tube thoracostomy – sonographic guidance was used to advance a needle (*arrow*) (e.g., 5 French Yueh) above the rib and through the intercostal space into the pleural effusion. (c) Postprocedural frontal chest radiograph demonstrated bilateral pigtail pleural drainage catheter projected over the lung bases with complete resolution of the pleural effusions and return of mediastinum to the midline

Table 16.1. Various causes of transudate and exudate

Transudate	Exudate
Congestive heart failure	Hemothorax
Cirrhosis	Lung infection
Nephritic syndrome	Neoplasm
Iatrogenic hydrothorax (central catheters, VP shunts)	Chylothorax
Pulmonary embolism	
Peritoneal dialysis	
Pericardial disease	
Collagen vascular disease	

Table 16.2. Characteristic laboratory findings of transudative and exudative fluids

Fluid type	Transudate	Exudate
Specific gravity	<1.020	>1.020
pH	>7.2	<7.2
Protein: pleural/serum	<0.5	≥0.5
LDH (IU)	<200	>200
LDH: pleural/serum	<0.6	>0.6
Amylase: pleural/serum	<1	>1
Glucose (mg/dL)	>40	<40
RBC	<5,000	>5,000
WBC	<1,000 (monos)	>10,000 (polys)

catheter is the most frequently used. Larger pigtail catheters are preferred for thick, exudative fluids (Fig. 16.2c). Continuous drainage of the effusion is aided by treatment of the primary etiology (e.g., intravenous antibiotics).

16.2.2 Empyema

Empyema refers to the presence of pus in the pleural space. Three stages of empyema formation are classically described:

- Exudative: Accumulation of free-flowing protein-rich fluid with rapidly increasing neutrophils. Glucose and pH levels are normal.
- Fibropurulent: the viscosity of the pleural fluid increases the appearance of pus and coating of the pleural membrane with an adhesive meshwork of fibrin. Glucose and pH levels are lower than normal. Fluid loculation may be seen.
- Organizing: Fluid loculation and formation of fibrous inelastic membrane (pleural peel) encasing the lung occurs [1].

If untreated, an empyema in the last stage could spontaneously drain into the lung through a BPF or out through the chest wall (empyema necessitans). Multiloculated collections are often seen in empyemas in the fibropurulent and organizing stages. Treatment options include tube thoracostomy with or without the instillation of fibrinolytics, video-assisted thorascopic surgery (VATS) or open thoracotomy and decortication. Fibrinolytic agents can be used to optimize the drainage of loculated pleural collections [2].

Fibrinolytic Therapy for Empyema

Empyema is associated with fibrinous, hemorrhagic, and suppurative processes, leading to fibrous organization, adhesions, and fibrous pleural thickening. The rationale to instill fibrinolytic agents (such as tissue plasminogen activator [t-PA], streptokinase, and urokinase) into the pleural cavity is based on the idea that these agents break down fibrinous tissues thereby promoting drainage [3]. The fibrinolytic agent can be infused via the chest tube into the pleural space. There are several formulas to prepare the fibrinolytic solution. Examples are:

1. t-PA (2–6 mg in a 50–250 mL, depending on the size of the effusion).
2. Streptokinase (250,000 U in 100 mL normal saline once per day for 1–3 days).
3. Urokinase (80,000 U units every 8 h for 1–3 days).

After instillation, the chest tube is closed for 2 h to allow the fibrinolytic agent to spread throughout the pleural space. After 2 h, the tube is then opened for drainage.

Results of fibrinolytic therapy in children have demonstrated high successful rates (as high as 99%) [4]. Although retrospective studies showed efficacious results of these agents, only urokinase has been evaluated in a randomized controlled trial in children and more controlled randomized studies are needed [3, 4].

16.2.3 Hemothorax

Hemothorax (blood in the pleural space) in children is often associated with chest trauma and surgical procedures. It may occur from erosion of a blood vessel associated with inflammatory processes in the lungs or rarely from rupture of a pulmonary arteriovenous malformation (PAVM). Thoracentesis is the gold standard to make a diagnosis of hemothorax.

16.2.4 Chylothorax

A chylothorax refers to chyle (milky lymph rich in fat and nutrients absorbed from the intestines) in the pleural space. In children, it is usually a sequela of injury of the thoracic duct during cardiothoracic surgery with a reported incidence of 0.89–6.6% [5,6]. Chylothorax may also occur due to malformation of the central conducting lymphatic channels. Management of chylothorax is challenging and may require progressive escalation of therapy if it is not resolving [7, 8]. If suspected, thoracentesis should be performed to confirm the presence of chylous fluid in the thoracic cavity. Conservative treatment includes low-fat, high protein diets with medium chain triglycerides supplemented with fat-soluble vitamins A, D, E, and K, total parenteral nutrition or somatostatins. Spontaneous recovery has been reported in infants less than 1 year old [9]. Thoracentesis or tube thoracostomy may be required in cases of significant respiratory distress or persistent chylous effusions. Repeated drainage of large volumes of chyle can lead to protein loss, lymphopenia, hypogammaglobulinemia, and abnormal lymphocyte function [8]. Iatrogenic chylothoraces refractory to medical therapy may require alternate interventions such as pleurodesis, a pleuroperitoneal shunt, embolization, or surgical ligation of the thoracic duct.

16.2.5 Malignant Effusion

Management of malignant pleural effusions in pediatric oncology patients is not well established. Respiratory benefit from pleurodesis using doxycycline for terminal pediatric oncology patients with malignant effusions has been reported [10].

16.2.6 Pleurodesis

Pleurodesis refers to obliteration of the pleural space by the administration of sclerosing agents via a chest tube. The resulting fibrosis and adhesion prevent the accumulation of fluid or air between the pleural layers. It can be performed to treat persistent or recurrent pneumothoraces or pleural effusions. In pediatric oncology patients, the use of pleurodesis should be preceded by a multidisciplinary discussion as the long-term effect of pleurodesis on lung development is still unclear. The procedure can be quite painful and typically performed under general anesthesia.

Technique

Prior to chemical pleurodesis, a large chest tube should already be in place. In cases of pleural effusions, the fluid in the pleural space should be aspirated via the indwelling drainage catheter as much as possible. Next, a sclerosing agent is injected into the pleural space via the chest tube. A specimen of the pleural fluid should be obtained to confirm or exclude evidence of malignancy. The chest tube can be removed when the pleural drainage is persistently minimal. Several sclerosing agents can be used, with the most experience in adults: talc, doxycycline, and Bleomycin.

16.3 Bronchopleural Fistula

A BPF refers to an abnormal communication between the bronchial tree and the pleural space. The most common cause by far is a postoperative complication following a pulmonary resection. The reported incidence is between 1.5 and 28% after pulmonary resection [11–14]. Other recognized etiologies include lung necrosis complicating a pulmonary infection, spontaneous pneumothorax, chemotherapy, or radiotherapy for lung cancer and tuberculosis [11]. A BPF is a rare entity that carries a high morbidity and mortality. Therapeutic options include various medical, surgical and now gaining more acceptance, endoscopic procedures to deliver various embolic agents to occlude the fistulous communication. However, there are only a few reports describing bronchoscopic or fluoroscopically guided embolization of a BPF in pediatric patients. Therefore, the various procedures should be seen as complementary and treatment should be individualized.

16.3.1 Indication

The location and size of the BPF will guide whether surgery or an endoscopic procedure is performed. Bronchoscopic or fluoroscopically guided embolization has typically been performed on patients who are too high-risk for surgery. A distal small fistula is more suitable for bronchoscopic or fluoroscopic therapy, while a large or central fistula is best managed with surgery or stent placement.

16.3.2   Technique

The patients with a BPF typically have a pneumothorax, with or without pleural effusion, usually empyema. A chest tube has been typically already placed. The presence of BPF can be suspected when air leakage is prolonged via a chest tube for more than 4 days. CT scan, instillation of nontoxic dye (e.g., methylene blue), bronchography, and inhalation of 133 Xe gas may also be used to identify the fistula.

The American College of Chest Physicians recommendations for the management of patients with persistent pneumothorax is helpful for further management: continue observation for 4 days. If an air leak persists longer than 4 days, intervention may be considered. Thoracoscopy is the preferred management procedure. If surgery is contraindicated, chemical pleurodesis is an alternative [15]. The use of several sealing or sclerosing agents has been reported including ethanol, polyethylene glycol, cyanoacrylate glue, fibrin glue, blood clot, antibiotics, albumin-glutaraldehyde tissue adhesive, cellulose, gel foam, coils, balloon catheter occlusion, silver nitrate, among others. Successful embolization of BPF under fluoroscopic guidance using a microcatheter has also been reported. Postprocedural evaluation includes observation of air leakage via the chest tube and serial chest radiographs.

16.4   Local Tumor Therapy: Thermal Ablation

Thermal ablative therapy is a minimally invasive technique used to treat focal tumors, either through hyperthermic injury – radiofrequency, microwave, and laser ablation – or through hypothermic injury – cryoablation. Radiofrequency ablation (RFA) is the most commonly used thermal ablative therapy. It was initially established as an effective therapy to treat primary and metastatic malignancies of the liver; then, it was rapidly used to treat focal tumors in other organs. The liver and the lung are the most common sites for metastases. Following the initial experience by Dupuy et al. in 2000, there have been several studies demonstrating the effectiveness of RFA in treating primary and metastatic malignancies in the lung [16]. One such large study demonstrated that it has low morbidity, negligible mortality, and improved quality of life [17, 18].

In children, primary lung malignancies are rare, accounting for only 0.19% of all pediatric malignancies. However, metastatic pulmonary tumors are approximately 12 times more common than primary lung malignancies [19]. Several studies report survival benefit in excision of osteosarcoma pulmonary metastases [19–22]. Metastasectomy can play a role in other tumors resistant to chemotherapy and radiotherapy such as adrenocortical carcinoma and chondrosarcoma.

The use of RFA in children is not a novel therapy as it is commonly used to treat cardiac conduction abnormalities and osteoid osteomas. While RFA performed in adults can be potentially extended to children, the currently available experience is limited with no definite evidence of efficacy of RFA in treating pediatric lung tumors. The major potential use of RFA in children is as an adjunct to radiotherapy or systemic therapy, especially in palliation.

16.5   Airway Obstruction

In both adults and children, airway obstruction causes significant morbidity and mortality. However, the underlying etiologies are quite different. In adults, malignant diseases predominate while in children, airway obstructions are attributed mainly to benign stenoses or malacia [23, 24]. In general, tracheobronchomalacia occurring in infancy have a good long-term prognosis as most resolve at about 18 months to 2 years of age [25].

Management of airway obstruction in children is challenging due to the small and soft airways and the required long-term tolerance and adaption to growth [24]. Treatment options include surgical and endoscopic procedures; operative management is the first line therapy for treating congenital abnormalities of the airway including cardiac anomalies causing airway narrowing [25]. However, there is a cohort of patients that may benefit from balloon dilatation or stenting of airway stenoses. There have been several reports describing the role of endoscopic procedures, such as balloon tracheobronchoplasty and airway stenting, in treating airway obstruction in children [24–31].

16.5.1 Indications

Balloon tracheobronchoplasty refers to balloon dilatation of an airway narrowing with an angioplasty balloon under bronchoscopic or fluoroscopic guidance. A stent refers to an artificial hollow structure inserted into tracheobronchial tree with the goal to maintain airway patency. Treatment is guided by the location and etiology of the airway narrowing. Children with focal malacia, unlike diffuse disease, will benefit from the surgical intervention or even external airway splint. Diffuse malacia usually respond to long-term CPAP delivered via a tracheostomy [32]. Balloon dilatation is often used to treat recurrent stenoses following surgery or airway stenting [25]. In cases of resistant stenoses, the use of cutting balloons may decrease the rate of re-stenosis [33].

The types of airway stents available are plastic (silicon or silastic), metallic (balloon-expandable or self expanding), and bioabsorbable stents. The main indications for airway stenting in children are recurrent stenoses after surgery and/or stenoses that do not respond to balloon dilatation. In addition, stents have been used to treat incompletely surgically treated focal malacia and extrinsic compression, not correctable by surgery. Stents should only be considered when conservative and surgical options have been exhausted. In children with malignant disease or severe congenital anomalies, stents may be used with palliative intent to improve quality of life [24, 25].

16.5.2 Results and Complications

There have been no randomized trials evaluating balloon dilatation or airway stenting in children, but the success rates in pediatric patients have been reported in several case series. Analysis of published case series demonstrated the calculated initial success rate of 92.6% (112 patients among 121), and mortality rate of 11.6% (14 patients among 121). Most of these 121 children were in critical situation before stent placement, had no other therapeutic choices.

Complications during balloon dilatation and airway stenting are uncommon. Minor complications seen are migration and tissue granulation formation. Major complications reported to date include death from bleeding, erosion into aorta, stent fracture, erosion into adjacent tissues, and mucous retention. Lethal complications have been reported with an estimated mortality from these case series of 12.9% [24].

16.6 Percutaneous Needle Biopsy of Pulmonary and Mediastinal Lesions

Management of pulmonary, mediastinal, pleural, and chest wall lesions is similar to that of adults. In the past, particularly in children, surgeons obtained tissue through open or transthoracic procedures but more recently, through video-assisted thorascopic biopsies (VATS). Less invasive methods such as image-guided percutaneous or transbronchial approaches have gained favor due to the decreased procedural morbidity. The safety and efficacy of percutaneous image-guided biopsy in children have been reported in the literature [34–42]. The various methods used to obtain tissue should be considered complementary with preference for more minimally invasive procedures.

16.6.1 Indications

There are similar indications [34, 37, 43] as in adult patients. They include:

- Focal pulmonary lesion, or multiple pulmonary focal opacities [41]
- Focal infectious lung lesion, particularly when bronchoscopy is unsuccessful [37].
- Mediastinal masses or lymphadenopathy.
- Focal or diffuse pleural thickening.
- Chest wall masses or fluid collections.
- Staging of tumors (lung cancer and extrathoracic malignancy).
- Needle localization for small pulmonary lesions [40, 42].

Suitability for transbronchial vs. percutaneous biopsy depends on the size and location of the lesion. Central lesions adjacent to major bronchi may be more amenable to a transbronchial approach. However, the size of the airway in children may preclude a transbronchial biopsy. Imaging modalities used to guide percutaneous biopsies include computed tomography (CT), ultrasonography, and fluoroscopy.

16.6.2 Contraindications

There are similar contraindications [43] as in adult patients. They include:

- Severe underlying pulmonary disease.
- Contralateral pneumonectomy or severely limited function in the contralateral lung.
- Patients on positive pressure ventilation.
- Bleeding diathesis (INR >1.5 or platelet counts <50,000/mm^3).
- Pulmonary arterial hypertension in those who are at higher risk of hemorrhage.

16.6.3 Technique

Pre-procedural imaging studies including chest radiographs and contrast-enhanced chest CT scan should be reviewed to determine the safest approach – transbronchial vs. image-guided percutaneous biopsy. Coagulopathy should be corrected. Depending on the clinical status and technical difficulty, the procedure may be performed with local anesthesia, intravenous sedation, or general anesthesia. The latter is preferred when respiratory control is required to stabilize the lesion during the biopsy [34, 38]. In selected cooperative children, biopsies may be performed with local anesthesia, especially for superficial lesions in the chest wall, large peripheral lung, or mediastinal lesions.

For deeper lung lesions with intervening aerated tissue, CT guidance is the most often used imaging modality. It clearly delineates structures such as lung tissue, fissures, large vessels, bullae, and vital cardiovascular structures to avoid during the biopsy (Fig. 16.3a–c). Ultrasound guidance may be suitable for chest wall, pleural, superior mediastinal, and peripheral lung lesions [36] (Fig. 16.4a,b). Fluoroscopy can be used if the lesion can be visualized in two projections. The main advantages of fluoroscopic and ultrasound guidance are real-time imaging and less radiation exposure. The most direct route to the lesion should be used. Avoiding traversing other structures such as pulmonary vessels, fissures, and major bronchi decreases the risk of complications.

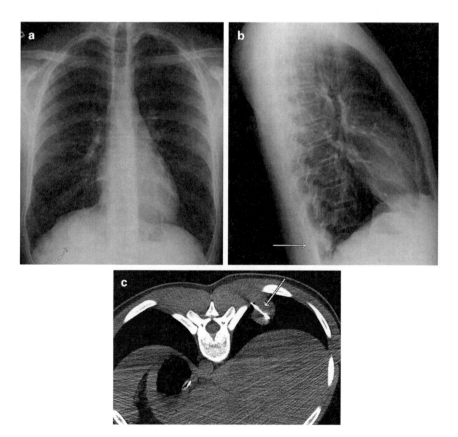

Fig. 16.3. (a, b) Seventeen-year-old young man with incidental finding right lower lobe lesion on frontal and lateral chest radiograph (*arrow*). (c) CT-guided core biopsy (*arrow*) was performed using a coaxial technique with the patient positioned prone

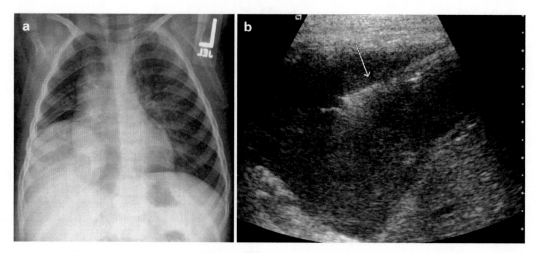

Fig. 16.4. (a) Twenty-one-month-old boy with neurofibromatosis type I and large right lung mass seen on routine frontal chest radiograph. (b) Sonographic-guided core biopsy (*arrow*) was performed through the intercostal space using a core axial technique

The patient is positioned prone or supine. The lesion is re-imaged for proper localization. For CT guidance, a radio-opaque skin marker can be placed over the area of interest and thin axial sections are obtained through the lesion and skin marker. The appropriate lesion, size, depth, safest trajectory, and skin entry site are determined. After a sterile preparation and applying local anesthetics, the biopsy needle is advanced incrementally to its predetermined position. The position of the needle is confirmed with CT imaging before a biopsy is taken. A coaxial biopsy system is used if multiple biopsies are to be taken. Temporary suspension of breathing is valuable for lesions that move with respiration. The lung is then re-imaged after needle placement and following the biopsy. An occlusive patch can be placed over the puncture site [34].

The sample type (needle aspiration or core biopsy) is often dictated by the type, size, and location of the lesion.

Samples are obtained using either an aspiration or core biopsy needle via a single-needle (Chiba, Franseen or Westcott needle), coaxial needle, or tandem needle technique. When a single-needle technique is used, multiple pleural punctures are required to obtain multiple samples. A coaxial needle system can be used to obtain multiple samples using a single pleural puncture. Core samples are usually obtained from 18 to 20 gauge core biopsy needles but a large bore needle, such as 14 gauge needle, has been shown to be safe and effective in children [39].

Large pleural-based lesions or parenchymal lesions with no intervening aerated lung can be biopsied with a large bore needle with direct puncture. A single pass technique is recommended for parenchymal lesions with intervening aerated lung, with or without the formation of a saline window [34]. A 1 cm throw should be used for small <2 cm lesion and a 2 cm throw for >2 cm lesions. For smaller lesion, <1 cm, wire localization can assist a thoracoscopic resection of small pulmonary nodules in children [40, 42].

16.6.4   Postoperative Management

An immediate postbiopsy scan is typically obtained to evaluate for a pneumothorax. Recovery is typically done with cardiopulmonary monitoring and special attention to signs of pneumothorax and hemothorax. A small, stable pneumothorax in an asymptomatic patient may not need any treatment. However, a pneumothorax should be drained (see Sect. 16.1) if the child develops a large (or enlarging) pneumothorax or symptoms (dyspnea or chest pain). The rare tension pneumothorax requires immediate needle decompression followed by chest tube placement under image guidance.

16.6.5   Results and Complications

The safety and efficacy of percutaneous lung biopsy in children have been reported only in retrospective case series of small numbers of patients. Diagnostic yields of CT-guided or US-guided percutaneous lung biopsy in children have been reported between 85 and 95% [34, 36, 41]. Percutaneous biopsies are less time-consuming, less invasive, require shorter post-procedural stay and are less costly than transthoracic procedures [35].

The most common complication is pneumothorax (12–30%) and hemoptysis (4%). The risk is higher in small (<2 cm) and deep lesions [44]. Significant pneumothoraces requiring treatment usually occur within 1 h after the biopsy. Fungal lesions seem to have a higher incidence of hemorrhage spontaneously and at the time of biopsy [34]. Fatal pericardial tamponade, tension pneumothorax, air embolism, and pulmonary hemorrhage have been reported in the literature, but the risk is quite low.

16.7 Pulmonary Angiography and Hemodynamic Assessment in Children

Recent advances in noninvasive CT and MR pulmonary angiography has made the need for invasive pulmonary angiography less frequent. However, conventional pulmonary angiography is still considered the definitive test in evaluating some of the diseases involving the pulmonary vasculature. In addition, it allows for hemodynamic measurements and therapeutic intervention.

16.7.1 Indications

In pediatric patients, similar to adult patients, recognized indications for pulmonary angiography include [45]:

- Evaluation of pulmonary hypertension [46].
- Evaluation and treatment of PAVMs [47].
- Cardiopulmonary disorders pre- or postcardiac surgery.
- Assessment and intervention for congenital cardiac anomalies.
- Pre-retrieval foreign body in the pulmonary arterial tree.

- Evaluation of clinically suspected pulmonary embolism or foreign body.
- Evaluation of massive hemoptysis and hemothorax, especially with a negative bronchial angiogram.

Acute pulmonary embolism is uncommon in pediatric patients. Despite recent advances in CT imaging of the pulmonary artery vasculature, in selected cases, pulmonary angiography is still a gold standard to evaluate patients with suspected pulmonary embolism. In many children, pulmonary angiograms are performed under general anesthesia in order to minimize the effect of respiratory and cardiac motion on the digitally subtracted images. Prolonged breath-holding needed for diagnostic quality images is not possible in infants and small children, especially if they have underlying cardiopulmonary disease.

16.7.2 Relative Contraindications

Relative contraindications [45] include:
- Coexisting severe pulmonary hypertension. Echocardiography may be helpful.
- Left bundle-branch block on 12-lead electrocardiogram (ECG). Placement of a temporary transvenous pacing catheter will break complete heart block that may occur due to catheter-induced right bundle-branch block.
- Ventricular irritability.
- Other concomitant life-threatening illness (e.g., decompensated congestive heart failure).
- Severe contrast allergy.

16.7.3 Preoperative Management

Coagulation system and renal function should be evaluated. The patient's ECG and echocardiography studies should be evaluated prior to pulmonary angiography to exclude a left bundle-branch block. A temporary prophylactic pacemaker can be inserted before the catheter is introduced into the right atrium and ventricle for the patients with a left bundle-branch block.

16.7.4   Techniques

Procedures were usually performed under general anesthesia with continuous cardiac monitoring. Evaluation of the pulmonary vasculature requires venous access with the femoral vein being most frequently used. Alternate accesses include the jugular or brachial veins.

Pressure measurement is performed with simultaneous tracing of the ECG prior to contrast injections. The commonly recorded pressures are those of the central veins, right atrium, right ventricle, pulmonary artery, and pulmonary capillary wedge pressure. The latter usually requires a Swan-Ganz catheter. Continuous ECG monitoring should be performed while introducing a catheter into the right atrium and right ventricle.

Different types of catheters can be used to select the main pulmonary artery. A pigtail or angled-tip catheter is advanced into the main pulmonary artery under fluoroscopic guidance (Fig. 16.5a). Larger special catheters (such as Grollman catheter of 7 Fr or wider diameter) are unlikely to be needed in smaller children. Digital subtraction angiography is performed with breath holding. Nonionic low osmolality contrast agents are used. Pulmonary arteriography should be performed with extreme caution in patients with PAVM and pulmonary hypertension.

16.7.5   Results and Complications

There has been no evaluation of the safety and efficacy of pulmonary angiography in children. The reported mortality of pulmonary angiography is between 0.1 and 0.5% [48, 49]. Retrospective studies have shown that mortality due to acute cor

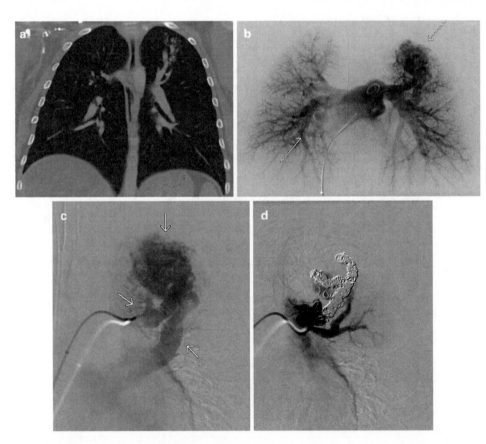

Fig. 16.5. A 14-year-old boy with hereditary hemorrhagic telangiectasia (HHT), bilateral pulmonary arteriovenous malformation (PAVM)s and shortness of breath. (**a**) There is a large, complex PAVM in the left upper lobe with enlarged feeding arteries and draining veins. (**b**) Pulmonary angiogram demonstrates the complex left upper lobe PAVM (*left upper arrow*). A smaller pulmonary AVM is seen in the right lower lobe (*left lower arrow*). (c) Selective angiogram of the left upper lobe demonstrated the pulmonary AVM (*upper arrow*) with a large complex, branching feeding artery (*middle arrow*) and dominant draining pulmonary vein (*lower left arrows*). (**d**) Postcoil embolization angiogram. There is cessation of shunting through the two dominant feeding artery. However, the malformation is still fed by another branch of the left pulmonary artery (*arrow*)

pulmonale was associated with severely elevated pulmonary artery and right ventricular end-diastolic pressures [49, 50]. Nonfatal major and minor complications are 1 and 5%, respectively. They include right ventricular perforation (1%), significant arrhythmia (0.8%), contrast reaction (0.8%), and renal dysfunction (1%) [48, 50].

16.8   Pulmonary Artery Embolization and Pulmonary Arteriovenous Malformations

PAVMs refers to an abnormal direct communication between a pulmonary artery and vein resulting in a high-flow, low pressure right-to-left shunt and subsequently hypoxemia, cyanosis, dyspnea, platypnea, or orthodeoxia. The lack of a capillary plexus can result in paradoxical embolization with neurological complications such as stroke or cerebral abscess [51]. They may result in serious hemoptysis or hemothorax due to spontaneous rupture. Patients may have symptoms of dizziness, syncope, or polycythemia and may eventually develop symptoms of congestive heart failure and/or respiratory failure [52].

Idiopathic congenital PAVMs are congenital arteriovenous malformations (AVMs) that are not associated with hereditary hemorrhagic telangiectasia (HHT). These PAVMs tend to be single with fewer associated physical findings. However, approximately 70% of PAVMs are associated with HHT and 15–30% of individuals with HHT have a PAVM [51–53]. PAVMs may be acquired due to trauma, occurring in patients with hepatopulmonary syndrome – 47% patients with end-stage liver disease acquire abnormal arterial venous communications – or following surgery for congenital cyanotic heart disease such as Glenn or modified Fontan procedures.

16.8.1   Hereditary Hemorrhagic Telangiectasia

HHT, also known as Osler-Weber-Rendu syndrome, is an autosomal dominant disorder manifested by mucocutaneous telangiectases and AVMs that can affect the nasopharynx, CNS, lung, liver, spleen, including the urinary and GI tracts. Majority of patients, up to 90%, manifest by the fourth decade of life with epistaxis being the most frequent clinical manifestation. HHT is diagnosed clinically based on the Curaçao criteria, established in 2000 by the HHT Foundation's Scientific Advisory Board (Table 16.3) [54]. Due to delayed manifestation of the typical features of HHT, the use of Curaçao criteria to establish the diagnosis of HHT in children is less reliable than in adults.

There are at least four gene defects implicated in HHT that affect the signaling of transforming growth factor beta (TGF-b), an important pathway in vascular formation and repair [52]. However, genetic abnormalities may be present in patients with PAVMs who do not have HHT. The first two genetic mutations linked to HHT were mutation in endoglin (ENG) protein (chromosome 9, 9q33-34) called HHT type 1 and mutation for encoding activin receptor-like kinase (ALK1; also called ACVRL1, activin A receptor kinase, type II like 1) called HHT type 2 [55, 56]. PAVMs are more frequently seen in patients with HHT type 1 mutation. In the last few years, two other gene mutations have been implicated – HHT type 3, a mutation of chromosome 5 (5q31.1-32) and HHT-juvenile polyposis overlap syndrome (JPHT), a mutation in MADH4 of chromosome 18 (encoding SMAD4). JHPT is autosomal dominant with clinical features of HHT and juvenile polyposis [57, 58].

The vast majority of PAVMs are simple (single feeding pulmonary branch and single draining vein), located in the lower lobes and have a fusiform aneurysm of the immediate draining vein. Around one fifth of PAVMs are complex (two or more feeding arteries or draining veins). The size of the PAVMs may vary from microscopic to the typical size of 1–5 cm [47]. Multiple lesions occur in more than one third of the patients and bilateral disease in one half.

Table 16.3. Curacao criteria: diagnosis is classified as definite if three criteria are present, possible or suspected if two criteria are present, and unlikely if fewer than 2 criteria are present

Criterion	Description
Epistaxis	Spontaneous, recurrent nosebleeds
Telangiectases	Multiple at characteristic sites such as lips, oral cavity, fingers, and nose
Visceral lesions	Such as gastrointestinal (GI) telangiectasia (with or without bleeding), pulmonary, hepatic, cerebral, or spinal AVM
Family history	A first-degree relative with HHT

From Shovlin et al. [54], with permission.

16.8.2 Indication

Several retrospective series have demonstrated the severe disabling and life-threatening complications of PAVMs, such as stroke, TIA, cerebral abscess, massive hemoptysis, and spontaneous hemothorax [47, 59–61]. These complications have also been reported in the pediatric literature [47, 61, 62]. The rationale for treatment is to prevent any potential complications especially in cases of diffuse PAVMs [63]. Likewise, screening of asymptomatic patients including children and family members with PAVM or HHT should be performed to determine individuals requiring treatment.

Treatment should commence if there is evidence of:

- History of paradoxical embolization
- Signs and symptoms: hypoxemia, dyspnea, fatigue, poor growth, etc.
- The presence of large or enlarging feeding artery [61–64]

Noteworthy, the standard recommendation for embolotherapy for PAVMs with feeding artery >3 mm may not be relevant in children with multiple small symptomatic PAVMs. For asymptomatic children, the decision to treat smaller shunts should be made on a case-by-case basis [62].

Transarterial catheter-directed embolization, rather than lung resection, is the preferred choice for treating PAVMs, especially in patients with multiple or bilateral PAVMs or poor candidates for surgery. The safety and efficacy of embolization has been demonstrated in several large series in adults and one series in children [60, 61, 64–66].

Confirm prophylactic antibiotic use. Since patients with pulmonary AVMs are at higher risk of brain abscess due to the pulmonary right-to-left shunt, life-long prophylactic antibiotic treatment is advised [62]. Compared with techniques in adult patients, diagnostic angiography and embolization should be performed on the same day in children.

16.8.3 Techniques

General anesthesia is preferred to intravenous sedation for children as it allows for better quality digital subtraction images during pulmonary angiography and for continuous monitoring for potentially protracted procedures. Imaging studies (chest radiograph, contrast-enhanced CT studies, and prior pulmonary angiograms) are reviewed (Fig. 16.5a). The use of prophylactic antibiotics and air filters for all vascular accesses is essential. Pulmonary hemodynamic measurements and angiography via a femoral vein route are initially preformed. Selective pulmonary angiography helps illustrate the feeding artery and determine the size of the embolic tools needed for complete permanent occlusion (Fig. 16.5b, c). Coils are the commonly used embolic agent. For smaller shunts, a coaxial system with a microcatheter can be used to deploy microcoils under fluoroscopic guidance.

Embolization should be performed as close to the fistulous communication as possible. The distal segment of the feeding artery is selectively cannulated and carefully embolized avoiding obliteration of normal branches or venous aneurysm. For smaller shunts, the use of microcatheters facilitates the procedure. This is especially important in multiple complex PAVMs in symptomatic children. Embolization is performed with either pushable or detachable coils. Other alternative embolic tools, such as detachable balloons or Amplatzer vascular plugs, can also be used [47, 53]. Techniques such as anchoring, scaffolding or balloon-assisted embolization can help prevent coil paradoxical embolization, especially in large PAVMs [47]. Postembolization angiography is subsequently performed to confirm the occlusion of the feeding arteries.

16.8.4 Postoperative Management

The patient is observed in the recovery room. Chest radiograph and arterial blood gas are obtained within 24 h. Antibiotic is given intravenously. The patient should be monitored for hemorrhage, vascular disruption due to balloon dilatation, chest pain due to pulmonary infarction, and arterial or venous obstruction due to thrombosis or vasospasm.

Follow-up assessment in pediatric patients is not standardized. A follow-up CT scan can be obtained within 6–12 months. CT is used to detect reperfusion by noninvolution of aneurysmal sac/fistulous communication. Transthoracic contrast echocardiography has been shown to not be useful postembolization, given that it remains positive in approximately 90% of patients postembolization [67]. Follow-up patients with small untreated PAVMs or with suspected microscopic PAVMs should be determined on a case-by-case basis (approximately every 1–5 years) with CT thorax [62]. If canalization is suspected, pulmonary angiography should be performed.

16.8.5 Results and Complications

Several case series have shown transarterial catheter-directed embolization to be efficacious and safe with complications being rare in long-term follow-up [60, 64–66]. Faughnan et al. reviewed several case series and demonstrated high rates of PAVM involution (85–97%) and improved oxygen saturation. Long-term reperfusion was seen in 15% of treated PAVMs and growth of small PAVMs in up to 18% [62]. Recurrences occurred due to incompletely occluded arteries or accessory arteries. Recurrent lesions can be treated with re-embolization. There have been a few case reports and case series of PAVM embolization in pediatric populations. Faughnan et al. evaluated transarterial catheter-directed embolization in 42 pediatric patients (aged 4–18 years) with 172 PAVMs – 71% with focal and 21% with diffuse PAVMs. There was improved oxygen saturation and absence of complications was noted 100 and 83%, respectively [61]. There is little experience with embolization of PAVMs in children under the age of 4 years.

Potential complications of blood vessel rupture, tachyarrhythmias, bradyarrhythmias, and vascular occlusion have been reported but are uncommon. Likewise, long-term complications were rare. The most common complication was self-limiting pleuritic chest pain, observed in up to 12% of patients. Also, reported was paradoxical air embolization in up to 5% of patients and paradoxical device embolization, in less than 1–4% .Complication rates in children were similar to adults [61].

16.9 Acute Pulmonary Embolism

Acute pulmonary embolism (PE) is uncommon in the pediatric population. The exact incidence is unknown but pediatric autopsy studies have estimated an incidence of 0.73–4.2% [68, 69]. Children may be protected from thromboembolism due to decreased capacity to generate thrombin, increased capacity of alpha-2 macroglobulin to inhibit thrombin and enhanced antithrombotic potential by the vessel wall [70, 71]. Despite this, pulmonary embolism can be potentially life-threatening when it occurs.

Multiple etiologic and risk factors have been implicated in the pathogenesis of pulmonary embolism – burns, central venous line and catheters, deep vein thrombosis, dehydration, heart disease, hematologic disorders, immunosuppression, neoplasia, obesity, renal disease, sepsis, shock, stem cell transplantation, surgery, thrombophilia/hypercoagulable, trauma or vascular malformation (such as, Klippel-Trenaunay syndrome) [72]. However, the most important acquired risk factor in children is central venous lines [73]. With advances in pediatric care, the incidence of pulmonary embolism is likely to increase.

Clinical presentation is variable depending on the degree of pulmonary artery occlusion, amount of liberated vasoactive amines, and underlying cardiopulmonary studies of the child [72]. Pulmonary embolism is often silent in children with dyspnea and tachycardia being less common reflecting the better physiological reserve in children. With large degree of pulmonary artery obstruction, clinical symptoms and signs may be similar to adults. Although not validated in children, diagnostic algorithms for the evaluation of pulmonary embolism are similar to adults.

16.9.1 Treatment of Acute Pulmonary Embolism

Large clinical trials evaluating the safety and efficacy of thrombolysis for acute PE in children have not been done. Therefore, children are treated according to recommendations based on small pediatric studies and clinical trials in adult populations [74]. Treatment should be guided by the risk associated with pulmonary embolism in the setting of other comorbid conditions. Treatment options for children with pulmonary embolism include supportive care, anticoagulant therapy with heparin or low molecular weight heparin and warfarin, thrombolysis, IVC filtration, and surgical or interventional thrombectomy [72]. Anticoagulation therapy should be considered in patients with stable hemodynamics in order to prevent thrombus extension and development of late complications. However, hemodynamically unstable patients, such as those in shock, need more aggressive therapy to reduce thrombus burden to improve right ventricular function [74]. More aggressive therapy includes thrombolysis or thrombectomy.

Systemic or catheter-directed pharmacologic thrombolysis can be considered in cases of massive pulmonary embolism or thrombus not responding to anticoagulants; however, the latter is infrequently used. When thrombolysis is contraindicated, surgical or interventional thrombectomy may be considered. There are several catheter-directed thrombectomy techniques: aspiration thrombectomy, fragmentation thrombectomy, and rheolytic thrombectomy [75, 76]. Effective fragmentation and rheolytic thrombectomy have been reported in infants and children [76–80]. Combined thrombolysis and thrombectomy technique has been reported. It involves fragmentation of central thrombus and dislodging of the fragments to the periphery resulting in relative gain of nonobstructed cross-sectional artery area and increased surface area of the thrombus fragments accessible for thrombolysis [74, 76]. The decision to treat pulmonary embolism with catheter-directed thrombolysis should be made by a multidisciplinary team familiar with the treatment alternatives and risks. Among thrombolytic agents, tPA is the most widely used.

Contraindication to pharmacologic thrombolysis includes active bleeding, history of internal or intracranial bleeding, recent intracranial or intraspinal surgery or trauma, intracranial neoplasm, AVM, or aneurysm, known coagulation disorders or severe, uncontrolled hypertension. Many of these contraindications are relative and the potential risk of treatment should be evaluated with respect to the risk of not treating the thrombosis.

16.9.2 Preoperative Management

Documentation of the site and extent of thrombosis with imaging modalities deemed satisfactory by the experienced interventional radiologists. The risk and time window should be assessed between the interventionalists, referring service, intensivists, and hematologists. Baseline clinical and laboratory documentation is required, which includes complete blood cell counts and disseminated intravascular coagulopathy (DIC) panel (including fibrinogen and D-dimer), kidney and liver function tests. Clinical signs of PE must be documented. For prolonged infusion of lytic agents, the patients stay in the ICU with adequate hydration and monitoring of the vital signs, coagulation parameters, and access sites.

16.9.3 Technique

Appropriate informed consents with detailed discussion of the benefits and serious bleeding risk are mandatory. If indicated, an inferior vena cava (IVC) filter is placed under the same setting. Initially, venography and IVC filter placement are performed. If the patient has a lower extremity DVT, a jugular approach is preferable. Pulmonary arteriography and pressure measurements are performed before thrombolysis. A catheter is placed within the thrombus with fluoroscopic guidance. The thrombolytic agent is directly infused into the thrombus. Heparin can be concomitantly used. Mechanical thrombectomy is an adjuvant tool in selected patients. With large residual embolus, prolonged transcatheter infusion of lytic agents can be considered. If so, the patient is transferred to the ICU and monitored per ICU protocol. Coagulation parameters are obtained as follows:

- CBC, fibrinogen, and D-dimer every 4–6 h.
- Maintain fibrinogen >100, and platelet count >100,000, neonates fibrinogen >150.
- Check stool for occult blood and urine dipstick with each void and for 8 h after the infusion.

If major bleeding occurs, lytic agent and heparin must be discontinued immediately. Appropriate consults and imaging are obtained. Aminocaproic acid (Amicar®), cryoprecipitate, and Packed Red Blood Cells can be administered. In case of moderate bleeding, i.e., bleeding without significant homodynamic changes, the tPA and heparin doses should be lowered. Minor bleeding, i.e., oozing of blood around arterial sheaths, is frequent and does not constitute an indication for treatment change. Gentle manual or/and compression dressing can be administered around the puncture site.

16.9.4 Results

Mortality rate of acute pulmonary embolism in pediatric patients is lower than that in adults. Mortality rates in children with pulmonary embolism have been reported up to 10% [74]. In adult patients, mortality of PE in the high-risk population is 65% if untreated, and 10–40% when treated with catheter-directed thrombolysis. Limited numbers of cases have been reported in pediatric patients for whom rheolytic or pharmacomechanical thrombectomy was successful in removing a pulmonary thrombosis.

16.9.5 Complications

Complications of thrombolysis include bleeding within the lungs or GI tract or within the intracranial ventricular system. Complications of rheolytic thrombectomy include vessel perforation, particularly <6 mm, and transient bradycardia and hypotension, presumably by stretching the vessel wall, have been reported in adult patients who received pharmacomechanical thrombectomy [77]. No complications have been reported in children.

16.10 Hemoptysis and Bronchial Artery Embolization

Hemoptysis refers to the expectoration of blood from the respiratory tract. It poses a potentially life-threatening respiratory emergency with major hemoptysis warranting prompt investigation and intervention. Conservative management of massive hemoptysis has a 50–100% mortality rate [81–83]. The most common etiology in children is tuberculosis and other chronic lung infections or cystic fibrosis. Episodes of major hemoptysis occur in 1% of all patients with cystic fibrosis, more frequently with severe lung disease and rarely seen in children less than 10 years old [84]. Other recognized potential causes of life-threatening hemoptysis in children are summarized in Table 16.4 [85].

There is no consensus for grading the severity of hemoptysis. A commonly used definition of major

Table 16.4. Causes of life-threatening hemoptysis in children

- Cystic fibrosis
- Inflammatory conditions
    o Tuberculosis
    o Other causes of bronchiectasis
    o Other infections (necrotic lung, lung abscess, fungal)
- Tumors and tumor-like conditions
- Congenital heart disease and pulmonary artery interruption
- Iatrogenic causes
    o Tracheostomy and other airway surgery
    o Airway stenting
    o Lung biopsy (percutaneous, transbronchial)
- Pulmonary arteriovenous malformations
- Vasculitis
- Foreign body aspiration

From Najarian and Morris [83], with permission.

hemoptysis is acute massive bleeding of greater than 240 mL/day, recurrent bleeding of substantial volume (>100 mL/day) for a few days or weeks or chronic recurrent small-volume hemoptysis (<100 mL/day) that interferes with a person's lifestyle and/or prevents effective physical therapy [86]. The cause of death is due to asphyxiation rather than exsanguination – approximately 400 mL of blood in the alveolar space is sufficient to significantly prevent gaseous exchange [81, 82]. In children, hemoptysis tends to be mild and self-limiting. Life-threatening hemoptysis in a child can be defined as >8 mL/kg in a 24 h period [87]. Nevertheless, the decision to intervene does not rely solely on these numbers and the overall clinical picture must likewise be taken into consideration.

Bronchial artery embolization is now considered the initial intervention for major refractory hemoptysis, either as first line or as an adjunct to surgery. In addition, a large portion of patients are not suitable for surgery due to preexisting comorbidity, poor pulmonary reserve, and high mortality rates (up to 40%) following emergency surgery [88]. It is a safe procedure but requires knowledge of the anatomy, pathophysiology, and procedural pitfalls in order to minimize the risks and improve the outcome.

16.10.1 Bronchial Artery Anatomy and Pathophysiology

The bronchial arteries have variable origins, branching patterns, and course. They typically originate between the superior margin of T5 and the inferior margin of T6 in 70–83% [89]. Nonorthotopic bronchial feeders originating outside this zone are frequent. They may originate from the aortic arch, brachiocephalic artery, subclavian artery, internal mammary artery, thyrocervical trunk, costocervical trunk, inferior phrenic artery, or abdominal aorta. These variants extend along the course of the major bronchi which distinguish them from nonbronchial systemic arteries that do not course in parallel to the major bronchi and enter the lung parenchyma through adherent pleura or pulmonary ligaments [89, 90]. Four common branching patterns have been described based on a large cadaveric study (Fig. 16.6) [89].

There is a dual arterial supply to the lungs from the pulmonary and bronchial arteries that are connected by numerous anastomoses at the level of the bronchi and pulmonary lobules [91]. The pulmonary

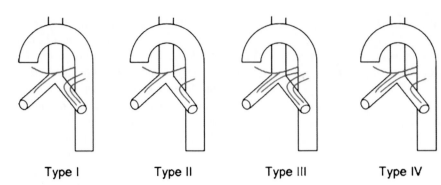

Type I   Type II   Type III   Type IV

Fig. 16.6. Four main types of bronchial artery anatomy. Type I: one right bronchial artery from right bronchointercostal trunk, two left bronchial arteries (40.6%). Type II: one on the right from bronchointercostal trunk, one on the left (21.3%). Type III: two on the right (one from bronchointer- costal trunk and one bronchial artery), two on the left (20.6%). Type IV: two on the right (one from bronchointercostal trunk and one bronchial artery), one on the left (9.7%) (from Chun et al. [92], with kind permission of Springer Science + Business Media)

arteries account for 99% of the arterial supply and are responsible for gaseous exchange. The bronchial arteries account for the remaining 1% and supply nutrient branches to the bronchi, vasa vasorum to the pulmonary arteries and veins, and smaller bronchopulmonary branches to the lung parenchyma [92]. There is a physiological right-to-left shunt in the anastomoses that accounts for approximately 5% of the total cardiac output [93].

Pulmonary circulation compromise, such as in hypoxic vasoconstriction or chronic inflammation, the bronchial arteries proliferate and enlarge to replace the pulmonary circulation. The inflammatory process causes the release of angiogenic growth factors that stimulate neovascularization and recruitment of collateral vessel from the systemic circulation. These new vessels are prone to rupture into the airways as they are thin-walled and fragile and exposed to the high systemic arterial pressure or eroded by an infective process [88, 94]. While the bronchial arteries are the most common source for major hemoptysis (>90%), in a minority of cases, the pulmonary arteries (5%) or nonbronchial systemic arteries (5%) may be the source of the hemorrhage [88].

16.10.2 Indication

In children, mild hemoptysis tends to be mild and self-limiting. Life-threatening hemoptysis in a child has been defined as >8 mL/kg volume in a 24 h period [87]. While bleeding often stops spontaneously within a few days, other conservative treatments may control symptoms such as bed rest, intensive intravenous

antibiotic treatment, vitamin K therapy, blood transfusion, and temporary discontinuation of physical therapy [85]. Pharmacologic treatment has not been proven. However, there is consideration for vasopressin, an intravenous octreotide infusion (a selective bronchial vasoconstrictor) or oral or intravenous tranexamic acid, an antifibrinolytic agent. In general, bronchial artery embolization is recommended when other measures have failed to control a major or life-threatening hemoptysis episode. Recurrent hemoptysis, even postbronchial artery embolization, warrants a repeat procedure to evaluate for recanalization and bleeding from a nonbronchial artery.

16.10.3 Preoperative Management

Initial evaluation should be focused on identifying the source of bleeding and determine the underlying cause. Diagnostic evaluation includes sputum examination, chest radiograph, contrast-enhanced CT scan, and bronchoscopy. A chest radiograph may lateralize the bleeding and underlying parenchymal abnormality; however, the reported diagnostic yield is only 50% [95]. Multidetector CT has increased the localization of hemorrhage and demonstrated 100% of bronchial and 62% of nonbronchial artery hemoptysis [96]. In adults, according to the American College of Physicians, clinicians favored early bronchoscopy within the first 24 h [97]. However, bronchoscopy detected the site of hemorrhage in only 50% of the cases and less likely to determine the underlying cause [98, 99]. Due to the smaller airways in children, routine bronchoscopic examination prior to bronchial artery embolization is controversial. The advantage of bronchoscopy is that it may treat bleeding from larger airways with cautery, laser, topical adrenaline, or rarely an occlusion balloon in severe cases [85].

16.10.4 Technique

Sedation or general anesthesia is typically required in children. General anesthesia has some advantages such as respiratory control for better imaging quality, particularly in younger children and lengthy procedures. However, there are some concerns about effects of intubation itself on hemoptysis and respiratory efforts in advanced lung disease. Arterial access is usually via the common femoral artery. A selective catheter (such as a Cobra, Sos or Michelson) is used to evaluate the bronchial arteries, intercostal arteries, and nonbronchial arteries. Spinal arteries arising from the bronchointercostal trunks should be identified. A microcatheter is often used to catheterize as distal as possible in the bronchial artery to avoid nontarget embolization. A target bronchial artery is embolized using polyvinyl alcohol particles (350–500 μm in diameter), and optionally nBCA. Coil embolization is contraindicated, because coils in the proximal portion of the artery allow the development of collateral flow in the distal area, and make subsequent embolization difficult when the patient needs repeated endovascular occlusion for recurrent hemoptysis in the future, which is commonly encountered. If a bleeding vessel and a spinal artery arising from bronchial arteries are identified, a microcatheter should be advanced distal to the spinal artery.

16.10.5 Results and Complications

Immediate success rate, defined as no bleeding within 24 h, has been reported as high as 95% in some reports for cystic fibrosis patients with hemoptysis. However, 55% of the patients required repeat embolization during the long-term follow-up [85]. Early rebleed can be attributed to incomplete embolization which may be due in part to the extensive underlying pulmonary disease or incomplete evaluation of nonbronchial

vessels. Late rebleed can be attributed to recanalization of previously embolized vessels or revascularization of collateral vessels secondary to progression of the underlying pulmonary disease [92].

Several complications have been reported in the literature. Minor complications such as chest pain, fever, and dysphagia have been reported. Severe hemoptysis during a procedure is thought to be related to the positive pressure during general anesthesia; however, it may be fatal. Neurological complications have been reported. Phrenic nerve palsy has been attributed to embolization of the internal thoracic artery pericardiophrenic branch. Spinal cord ischemia has been reported to occur in <1% of bronchial artery embolization procedures but it is often temporary with only a small risk of permanent paraplegia [85]. Brain injury may occur because embolic agents inadvertently communicate to the left circulation through a shunt or aberrant communication with the vertebral arteries. Other reported complications include myocardial injury, fingertip ischemia, bowel ischemia, and bronchoesophageal fistula [85]. Although severe complications of bronchial artery embolization have been reported, bronchial artery embolization, as performed by experienced interventional physicians, is a safe treatment.

16.11 Venous and Lymphatic Malformations

Vascular malformations and tumors of the thorax are frequently encountered. These lesions can impact the development of chest wall, spinal column, and lungs with potential effect on respiratory function. Management of children with vascular anomalies requires interdisciplinary expertise at specialized centers.

The widely accepted classification of vascular anomalies distinguishes two types of vascular lesions: tumors and malformations [100]. Infantile hemangiomas are the prototype of the former while vascular malformations are represented by the slow-flow (lymphatic, capillary, and venous), high-flow (arteriovenous) and combined types. In addition, some of the overgrowth syndromes with complex vascular anomalies may present with peculiar thoracic involvement.

16.11.1   Slow-Flow Malformations

Venous Malformations

Venous malformations (VMs) are slow-flow vascular anomalies that result from faulty development of the venosus system. The anomalous venous spaces progressively expand with stagnant blood, predisposing to clot formation and pain. Superficial lesions are bluish, compressible and may contain palpable phleboliths. Deeper lesions of the chest wall may involve the skin, subcutaneous fat, muscles, and bones or extend into the thoracic cavity. Larger VMs of the chest wall may be associated with scoliosis. Phlebectasia refers to dilated orthotopic or accessory veins which can be associated with altered flow dynamics and thromboembolism. Central and thoracic phlebectasia in CLOVES syndrome (Congenital Lipomatous Overgrowth, Vascular malformations, Epidermal nevi, and Skeletal/Scoliosis/Spinal anomalies) is common and increases the risk of pulmonary embolism [101].

Lymphatic Malformations

Lymphatic Malformations (LMs) can be divided into two major types: macrocystic (identifiable fluid-containing cysts) and microcystic. In addition, a combination of both types frequently exists. Macrocystic LMs manifest as cystic masses, microcystic lesions as diffuse tissue swelling and overgrowth. LMs are prone to recurrent flare-ups due to infections and intralesional bleeding. Less common manifestations include deformity of the chest wall, cutaneous vesicles and, with the rare involvement of the conducting lymphatic channels, chylothorax, chylous reflux, and interstitial lung disease.

Thoracic involvement can be isolated or more commonly, part of an extensive cervicofacial or axillary disease. Large cervical LMs frequently extend into the superior mediastinum via the thoracic inlet. Chest wall and mediastinal lymphatic malformations are common in CLOVES syndrome [102].

16.11.2   Sclerotherapy

Sclerotherapy refers to instillation of a toxic agent into an abnormal cavity with the goal of inducing intralesional fibrosis and shrinkage. Sclerotherapy has been documented in the literature as an effective primary treatment modality of lymphatic and venous malformations. MRI is superior to other imaging modalities to assess the soft tissue extension of the malformation. For VMs, the most common indications for treatment are pain and size of the lesion. Small, painless lesions can be observed though many will eventually become symptomatic. A combination of sclerotherapy and surgical resection is often used with large lesions. Treatment, when indicated, is preferably initiated early in life. For LMs, the major indications for treatment are size of lesion and recurrent infections. Skin vesicles may cause leakage, bleeding, and hygienic problems.

Sclerotherapy is typically performed under anesthesia with the access planned based on the imaging studies. Sonographic (with high-resolution probes) or fluoroscopic guidance directs the access into the malformation. Multiple needles are carefully placed within the lesion. For VMs, venography is performed after intralesional placement is confirmed by free blood return. Sclerosants with or without contrast opacification are then injected into the malformation. Other portions of the malformation can be treated similarly.

For LMs, the macrocysts are cannulated with small gauge needles, lymph is aspirated and the sclerosant is then injected.

Postsclerotherapy swelling is maximal within the first 24 h after the procedure. Appropriate analgesics are used when needed. Hemoglobinuria secondary to hemolysis is a frequent complication of sclerotherapy for VMs and is managed by hydration and alkalization of urine. Clinical assessment is scheduled 2 months after the procedure (Fig. 16.7). The procedure can be repeated if the residual lesion is significant.

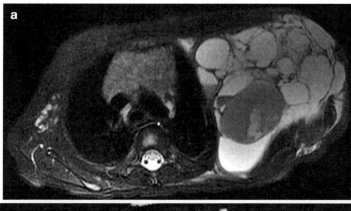

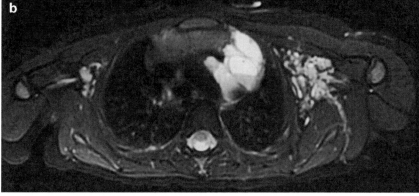

Fig. 16.7. (a) Axial fat-saturated T2-W MR image shows extensive macrocystic lymphatic malformation of the right chest wall and axilla. Note evidence of intralesional bleeding (darker T2 signal in one of the large macrocysts). (b) The size of the malformation markedly shrunk following sclerotherapy

References

1. Balfour-Lynn IM, Abrahamson E, Cohen G, et al. BTS guidelines for the management of pleural infection in children. Thorax. 2005;60 Suppl 1:i1–21.
2. Sahn SA. Diagnosis and management of parapneumonic effusions and empyema. Clin Infect Dis. 2007;45:1480–6.
3. Thomson AH, Hull J, Kumar MR, Wallis C, Balfour Lynn IM. Randomised trial of intrapleural urokinase in the treatment of childhood empyema. Thorax. 2002;57: 343–7.
4. Wells RG, Havens PL. Intrapleural fibrinolysis for parapneumonic effusion and empyema in children. Radiology. 2003;228:370–8.
5. Milonakis M, Chatzis AC, Giannopoulos NM, et al. Etiology and management of chylothorax following pediatric heart surgery. J Card Surg. 2009;24:369–73.
6. Nath DS, Savla J, Khemani RG, Nussbaum DP, Greene CL, Wells WJ. Thoracic duct ligation for persistent chylothorax after pediatric cardiothoracic surgery. Ann Thorac Surg. 2009;88:246–51. discussion 242–51.
7. Soto-Martinez M, Massie J. Chylothorax: diagnosis and management in children. Paediatr Respir Rev. 2009;10:199–207.
8. Epaud R, Dubern B, Larroquet M, et al. Therapeutic strategies for idiopathic chylothorax. J Pediatr Surg. 2008; 43:461–5.
9. Jernite M, Donato L, Favre R, Haddad J, Esposito M, Messer J. Medical treatment of chylous effusions in newborn infants. Apropos of 3 cases. Arch Fr Pediatr. 1992;49:811–4.
10. Hoffer FA, Hancock ML, Hinds PS, Oigbokie N, Rai SN, Rao B. Pleurodesis for effusions in pediatric oncology patients at end of life. Pediatr Radiol. 2007;37:269–73.
11. Lois M, Noppen M. Bronchopleural fistulas: an overview of the problem with special focus on endoscopic management. Chest. 2005;128:3955–65.
12. McManigle JE, Fletcher GL, Tenholder MF. Bronchoscopy in the management of bronchopleural fistula. Chest. 1990;97:1235–8.
13. Cerfolio RJ. The incidence, etiology, and prevention of postresectional bronchopleural fistula. Semin Thorac Cardiovasc Surg. 2001;13:3–7.
14. Sirbu H, Busch T, Aleksic I, Schreiner W, Oster O, Dalichau H. Bronchopleural fistula in the surgery of non-small cell lung cancer: incidence, risk factors, and management. Ann Thorac Cardiovasc Surg. 2001;7:330–6.
15. Park J, Bae I, Park K, Kim S, Jeon M, Hong J. Fluoroscopy-guided treatment of a bronchopleural fistula with a platinum vascular occlusion coil and N-butyl-2-cyanoacrylate (NBCA): a case report. J Korean Soc Radiol. 2009;61:375–8.
16. Dupuy DE, Zagoria RJ, Akerley W, Mayo-Smith WW, Kavanagh PV, Safran H. Percutaneous radiofrequency ablation of malignancies in the lung. AJR Am J Roentgenol. 2000;174:57–9.

17. Steinke K, Sewell PE, Dupuy D, et al. Pulmonary radiofrequency ablation – an international study survey. Anticancer Res. 2004;24:339–43.

18. Sano Y, Kanazawa S, Gobara H, et al. Feasibility of percutaneous radiofrequency ablation for intrathoracic malignancies: a large single-center experience. Cancer. 2007;109:1397–405.

19. Dishop MK, Kuruvilla S. Primary and metastatic lung tumors in the pediatric population: a review and 25-year experience at a large children's hospital. Arch Pathol Lab Med. 2008;132:1079–103.

20. Tronc F, Conter C, Marec-Berard P, et al. Prognostic factors and long-term results of pulmonary metastasectomy for pediatric histologies. Eur J Cardiothorac Surg. 2008;34:1240–6.

21. Chen F, Miyahara R, Bando T, et al. Repeat resection of pulmonary metastasis is beneficial for patients with osteosarcoma of the extremities. Interact Cardiovasc Thorac Surg. 2009;9:649–53.

22. Hacker FM, von Schweinitz D, Gambazzi F. The relevance of surgical therapy for bilateral and/or multiple pulmonary metastases in children. Eur J Pediatr Surg. 2007;17:84–9.

23. Chin CS, Litle V, Yun J, Weiser T, Swanson SJ. Airway stents. Ann Thorac Surg. 2008;85:S792–6.

24. Nicolai T. Airway stents in children. Pediatr Pulmonol. 2008;43:330–44.

25. McLaren CA, Elliott MJ, Roebuck DJ. Tracheobronchial intervention in children. Eur J Radiol. 2005;53:22–34.

26. Pillai JB, Smith J, Hasan A, Spencer D. Review of pediatric airway malacia and its management, with emphasis on stenting. Eur J Cardiothorac Surg. 2005;27:35–44.

27. Anton-Pacheco JL, Cabezali D, Tejedor R, et al. The role of airway stenting in pediatric tracheobronchial obstruction. Eur J Cardiothorac Surg. 2008;33:1069–75.

28. Filler RM, Forte V, Chait P. Tracheobronchial stenting for the treatment of airway obstruction. J Pediatr Surg. 1998;33:304–11.

29. Hebra A, Powell DD, Smith CD, Othersen Jr HB. Balloon tracheoplasty in children: results of a 15-year experience. J Pediatr Surg. 1991;26:957–61.

30. Kumar P, Bush AP, Ladas GP, Goldstraw P. Tracheobronchial obstruction in children: experience with endoscopic airway stenting. Ann Thorac Surg. 2003;75:1579–86.

31. Maeda K, Yasufuku M, Yamamoto T. A new approach to the treatment of congenital tracheal stenosis: balloon tracheoplasty and expandable metallic stenting. J Pediatr Surg. 2001;36:1646–9.

32. Jacobs IN, Wetmore RF, Tom LW, Handler SD, Potsic WP. Tracheobronchomalacia in children. Arch Otolaryngol Head Neck Surg. 1994;120:154–8.

33. Watters K, Russell J. The cutting balloon for endoscopic dilatation of pediatric subglottic stenosis. Int J Pediatr Otorhinolaryngol. 2008;3:39–43.

34. Cahill AM, Baskin KM, Kaye RD, Fitz CR, Towbin RB. CT-guided percutaneous lung biopsy in children. J Vasc Interv Radiol. 2004;15:955–60.

35. Hayes-Jordan A, Connolly B, Temple M, et al. Image-guided percutaneous approach is superior to the thoracoscopic approach in the diagnosis of pulmonary nodules in children. J Pediatr Surg. 2003;38:745–8.

36. Fontalvo LF, Amaral JG, Temple M, et al. Percutaneous US-guided biopsies of peripheral pulmonary lesions in children. Pediatr Radiol. 2006;36:491–7.

37. Heyer CM, Lemburg SP, Kagel T, et al. Evaluation of chronic infectious interstitial pulmonary disease in children by low-dose CT-guided transthoracic lung biopsy. Eur Radiol. 2005;15:1289–95.

38. Bendon AA, Krishnan BS, Korula G. CT-guided lung biopsies in children: anesthesia management and complications. Paediatr Anaesth. 2005;15:321–4.

39. Wilkinson AG, Paton JY, Gibson N, Howatson AG. CT-guided 14-G cutting needle lung biopsy in children: safe and effective. Pediatr Radiol. 1999;29:514–6.

40. Waldhausen JH, Shaw DW, Hall DG, Sawin RS. Needle localization for thoracoscopic resection of small pulmonary nodules in children. J Pediatr Surg. 1997;32:1624–5.

41. Connolly BL, Chait PG, Duncan DS, Taylor G. CT-guided percutaneous needle biopsy of small lung nodules in children. Pediatr Radiol. 1999;29:342–6.

42. Partrick DA, Bensard DD, Teitelbaum DH, Geiger JD, Strouse P, Harned RK. Successful thoracoscopic lung biopsy in children utilizing preoperative CT-guided localization. J Pediatr Surg. 2002;37:970–3. discussion 970–3.

43. Yankelevitz D, Shaham D, Goitein O. Biopsy procedures of the lung, mediastinum and chest wall. In: Kandarpa K, Aruny J, editors. Handbook of interventional radiologic procedures. Philadelphia: Lippincott Williams & Wilkins; 2002. p. 144–53.

44. Yeow KM, Su IH, Pan KT, et al. Risk factors of pneumothorax and bleeding: multivariate analysis of 660 CT-guided coaxial cutting needle lung biopsies. Chest. 2004;126: 748–54.

45. Kandarpa K, Hagspiel K. Pulmonary arteriography. In: Kandarpa K, Aruny J, editors. Handbook of interventional radiologic procedures. Philadelphia: Lippincott Wiliams & Wilkins; 2002. p. 35–42.

46. Hofmann LV, Lee DS, Gupta A, et al. Safety and hemodynamic effects of pulmonary angiography in patients with pulmonary hypertension: 10-year single-center experience. AJR Am J Roentgenol. 2004;183:779–86.

47. White Jr RI, Pollak JS, Wirth JA. Pulmonary arteriovenous malformations: diagnosis and transcatheter embolotherapy. J Vasc Interv Radiol. 1996;7:787–804.

48. Stein PD, Athanasoulis C, Alavi A, et al. Complications and validity of pulmonary angiography in acute pulmonary embolism. Circulation. 1992;85:462–8.

49. Perlmutt LM, Braun SD, Newman GE, Oke EJ, Dunnick NR. Pulmonary arteriography in the high-risk patient. Radiology. 1987;162:187–9.

50. Mills SR, Jackson DC, Older RA, Heaston DK, Moore AV. The incidence, etiologies, and avoidance of complications of pulmonary angiography in a large series. Radiology. 1980;136:295–9.

51. Kjeldsen AD, Oxhoj H, Andersen PE, Elle B, Jacobsen JP, Vase P. Pulmonary arteriovenous malformations: screening procedures and pulmonary angiography in patients with hereditary hemorrhagic telangiectasia. Chest. 1999;116:432–9.

52. Shovlin CL, Letarte M. Hereditary haemorrhagic telangiectasia and pulmonary arteriovenous malformations: issues in clinical management and review of pathogenic mechanisms. Thorax. 1999;54:714–29.

53. De Cillis E, Burdi N, Bortone AS, et al. Endovascular treatment of pulmonary and cerebral arteriovenous malformations in patients affected by hereditary haemorrhagic teleangiectasia. Curr Pharm Des. 2006;12:1243–8.

54. Shovlin CL, Guttmacher AE, Buscarini E, et al. Diagnostic criteria for hereditary hemorrhagic telangiectasia (Rendu-Osler-Weber syndrome). Am J Med Genet. 2000;91:66–7.

55. McAllister KA, Grogg KM, Johnson DW, et al. Endoglin, a TGF-beta binding protein of endothelial cells, is the gene for hereditary haemorrhagic telangiectasia type 1. Nat Genet. 1994;8:345–51.

56. Johnson DW, Berg JN, Baldwin MA, et al. Mutations in the activin receptor-like kinase 1 gene in hereditary haemorrhagic telangiectasia type 2. Nat Genet. 1996;13:189–95.

57. Cole SG, Begbie ME, Wallace GM, Shovlin CL. A new locus for hereditary haemorrhagic telangiectasia (HHT3) maps to chromosome 5. J Med Genet. 2005;42:577–82.

58. Gallione CJ, Repetto GM, Legius E, et al. A combined syndrome of juvenile polyposis and hereditary haemorrhagic telangiectasia associated with mutations in MADH4 (SMAD4). Lancet. 2004;363:852–9.

59. Moussouttas M, Fayad P, Rosenblatt M, et al. Pulmonary arteriovenous malformations: cerebral ischemia and neurologic manifestations. Neurology. 2000;55:959–64.

60. Pollak JS, Saluja S, Thabet A, Henderson KJ, Denbow N, White Jr RI. Clinical and anatomic outcomes after embolotherapy of pulmonary arteriovenous malformations. J Vasc Interv Radiol. 2006;17:35–44. quiz 45.

61. Faughnan ME, Thabet A, Mei-Zahav M, et al. Pulmonary arteriovenous malformations in children: outcomes of transcatheter embolotherapy. J Pediatr. 2004;145:826–31.

62. Faughnan ME, Palda VA, Garcia-Tsao G, et al. International guidelines for the diagnosis and management of hereditary hemorrhagic telangiectasia. J Med Genet. 2011;48(2):73–87.

63. Lacombe P, Lagrange C, Beauchet A, El Hajjam M, Chinet T, Pelage JP. Diffuse pulmonary arteriovenous malformations in hereditary hemorrhagic telangiectasia: long-term results of embolization according to the extent of lung involvement. Chest. 2009;135:1031–7.

64. Gupta P, Mordin C, Curtis J, Hughes JM, Shovlin CL, Jackson JE. Pulmonary arteriovenous malformations: effect of embolization on right-to-left shunt, hypoxemia, and exercise tolerance in 66 patients. AJR Am J Roentgenol. 2002;179:347–55.

65. Prasad V, Chan RP, Faughnan ME. Embolotherapy of pulmonary arteriovenous malformations: efficacy of platinum versus stainless steel coils. J Vasc Interv Radiol. 2004;15:153–60.

66. Mager JJ, Overtoom TT, Blauw H, Lammers JW, Westermann CJ. Embolotherapy of pulmonary arteriovenous malformations: long-term results in 112 patients. J Vasc Interv Radiol. 2004;15:451–6.

67. Lee WL, Graham AF, Pugash RA, et al. Contrast echocardiography remains positive after treatment of pulmonary arteriovenous malformations. Chest. 2003;123:351–8.

68. Byard RW, Cutz E. Sudden and unexpected death in infancy and childhood due to pulmonary thromboembolism. An autopsy study. Arch Pathol Lab Med. 1990;114:142–4.

69. Buck JR, Connors RH, Coon WW, et al. Pulmonary embolism in children. J Pediatr Surg. 1981;16:385–91.

70. Chan AK, Deveber G, Monagle P, et al. Venous thrombosis in children. J Thromb Haemost. 2003;1:1443–55.

71. Anton N, Massicotte MP. Venous thromboembolism in pediatrics. Semin Vasc Surg. 2001;1:111–22.

72. Babyn PS, Gahunia HK, Massicotte P. Pulmonary thromboembolism in children. Pediatr Radiol. 2005;35:258–74.

73. Andrew M, David M, Adams M, et al. Venous thromboembolic complications (VTE) in children: first analyses of the Canadian Registry of VTE. Blood. 1994;83:1251–7.

74. Van Ommen CH, Peters M. Acute pulmonary embolism in childhood. Thromb Res. 2006;118:13–25.

75. Uflacker R. Interventional therapy for pulmonary embolism. J Vasc Interv Radiol. 2001;12:147–64.

76. Robinson A, Fellows KE, Bridges ND, Rome JJ. Effectiveness of pharmacomechanical thrombolysis in infants and children. Am J Cardiol. 2001;87:496–9.

77. Sur JP, Garg RK, Jolly N. Rheolytic percutaneous thrombectomy for acute pulmonary embolism in a pediatric patient. Catheter Cardiovasc Interv. 2007;70:450–3.

78. Peuster M, Bertram H, Windhagen-Mahnert B, et al. Mechanical recanalization of venous thrombosis and pulmonary embolism with the Clotbuster thrombectomy system in a 12-year-old boy. Z Kardiol. 1998;87:283–7.

79. Feldman JP, Feinstein JA, Lamberti JJ, Perry SB. Angiojet catheter-based thrombectomy in a neonate with postoperative pulmonary embolism. Catheter Cardiovasc Interv. 2005;66:442–5.

80. Vincent RN, Dinkins J, Dobbs MC. Mechanical thrombectomy using the Angioject in a child with congenital heart disease. Catheter Cardiovasc Interv. 2004;64:253–5.

81. Crocco JA, Rooney JJ, Fankushen DS, DiBenedetto RJ, Lyons HA. Massive hemoptysis. Arch Intern Med. 1968;121:495–8.

82. Jean-Baptiste E. Clinical assessment and management of massive hemoptysis. Crit Care Med. 2000;28:1642–7.

83. Najarian KE, Morris CS. Arterial embolization in the chest. J Thorac Imaging. 1998;13:93–104.

84. FitzSimmons SC. The changing epidemiology of cystic fibrosis. J Pediatr. 1993;122:1–9.

85. Roebuck DJ, Barnacle AM. Haemoptysis and bronchial artery embolization in children. Paediatr Respir Rev. 2008;9:95–104.

86. Barben J, Robertson D, Olinsky A, Ditchfield M. Bronchial artery embolization for hemoptysis in young patients with cystic fibrosis. Radiology. 2002;224:124–30.

87. Batra PS, Holinger LD. Etiology and management of pediatric hemoptysis. Arch Otolaryngol Head Neck Surg. 2001;127:377–82.

88. Yoon W, Kim JK, Kim YH, Chung TW, Kang HK. Bronchial and nonbronchial systemic artery embolization for life-threatening hemoptysis: a comprehensive review. Radiographics. 2002;22:1395–409.

89. Cauldwell EW, Siekert RG, et al. The bronchial arteries; an anatomic study of 150 human cadavers. Surg Gynecol Obstet. 1948;86:395–412.

90. Botenga AS. The role of bronchopulmonary anastomoses in chronic inflammatory processes of the lung. Selective arteriographic investigation. Am J Roentgenol Radium Ther Nucl Med. 1968;104:829–37.

91. Pump KK. Distribution of bronchial arteries in the human lung. Chest. 1972;62:447–51.

92. Chun JY, Morgan R, Belli AM. Radiological management of hemoptysis: a comprehensive review of diagnostic imaging and bronchial arterial embolization. Cardiovasc Intervent Radiol. 2010;33:240–50.

93. Deffebach ME, Charan NB, Lakshminarayan S, Butler J. The bronchial circulation. Small, but a vital attribute of the lung. Am Rev Respir Dis. 1987;135:463–81.

94. McDonald DM. Angiogenesis and remodeling of airway vasculature in chronic inflammation. Am J Respir Crit Care Med. 2001;164:S39–45.

95. Hirshberg B, Biran I, Glazer M, et al. Hemoptysis: etiology, evaluation and outcome in a tertiary referral hospital. Chest. 1997;112:440–4.

96. Khalil A, Fartoukh M, Tassart M, et al. Role of MDCT in identification of the bleeding site and the vessels causing hemoptysis. AJR Am J Roentgenol. 2007;188:W117–25.

97. Haponik EF, Fein A, Chin R. Managing life-threatening hemoptysis: has anything really changed? Chest. 2000;118:1431–5.

98. Yoon W, Kim JK, Kim YH, et al. Bronchial and nonbronchial systemic artery embolization for life-threatening hemoptysis: a comprehensive review. Radiographics. 2002;22:1395–409.

99. Hsiao EI, Kirsch CM, Kagawa FT, et al. Utility of fibreoptic bronchoscopy before bronchial artery embolization for massive hemoptysis. AJR Am J Roentgenol. 2001;177:861–86.

100. Mulliken JB, Glowacki J. Haemangiomas and vascular malformations in infants and children: a classification based on endothelial characteristics. Plast Reconstr Surg. 1982;69:412–22.

101. Alomari AI, Burrows PE, Lee EY, Hedequist DJ, Mulliken JB, Fishman SJ. CLOVES syndrome with thoracic and central phlebectasia: increased risk of pulmonary embolism. Thorac Cardiovasc Surg. 2010;140(2):459–63.

102. Alomari AI. Characterization of a distinct syndrome that associates complex truncal overgrowth, vascular, and acral anomalies: a descriptive study of 18 cases of CLOVES syndrome. Clin Dysmorphol. 2009;18:1–7.

Lung Transplant

17

GARY VISNER, DEBRA BOYER, AND EDWARD Y. LEE

CONTENTS

Lung and heart–lung transplantation are established therapies for children with end-stage lung or congenital heart disease (CHD)/pulmonary vascular disease (PVD) in which there are no other therapeutic options. Lung transplantation was first successfully performed in 1983. Since 1986, there have been more than 1,500 procedures performed in children worldwide [1]. Based on the current age definition of UNOS and ISHLT for transplantation, *children* are identified as being under 18 years of age. The majority of lung or heart–lung transplants in children are from age 12 to 17. As of April 2009, there are more than 100 children on the lung transplant waiting list in the USA (OPTN).

The most common indications for transplantation differ by age group (Table 17.1). Cystic fibrosis is the most common overall indication at approximately 55% and is the diagnosis for nearly 70% of the lung recipients for the 12–17 years age group. In children younger than 1 year, the most common indications are CHD/PVD and diffuse lung disease from surfactant abnormalities. Additional diagnoses include transplant and nontransplant bronchiolitis obliterans and pulmonary fibrosis/interstitial pneumonitis.

Survival in pediatric patients following lung transplantation is approximately 80% after 1 year and approximately 50% after 5 years. Primary graft failure is the major cause of early mortality (<1 month), while infection is the most common cause of death within the first year. Infection remains a significant complication throughout the life of the pediatric lung transplant patient. The major complication for long-term survival in lung transplantation in both adult and pediatric patients is bronchiolitis obliterans, which is believed to be the manifestation of chronic lung rejection.

In children, bilateral lung transplantation is the most common surgical technique. Fewer than 10% of the procedures have been single lung transplants. In the USA, heart–lung transplantation is primarily for patients with complex CHD or pulmonary vascular abnormalities or a small number of patients with primary pulmonary hypertension. From 1995 to 2005, living lobar donor surgeries made up approximately 10% of pediatric lung transplantation mostly in older children who had a better size match with the two lower lobes from adult donors. With the new lung allocation system in 2005 in which lung allocation is based on a number of factors such as lung function rather than time on the list, there has been a decrease in the number of living lobar donor transplantations.

17.1   Pretransplant Evaluation

Imaging evaluation plays a crucial role in all phases of the lung transplant process from evaluation of the recipient and donor lungs, to early and late posttransplant management. Imaging studies in the

GARY VISNER (✉) • DEBRA BOYER, MD
Department of Medicine, Pulmonary Division,
Children's Hospital Boston and Harvard Medical School,
Boston, MA, USA
e-mail: gary.visner@childrens.harvard.edu

EDWARD Y. LEE, MD, MPH
Division of Thoracic Imaging, Department of Radiology and
Medicine, Pulmonary Division, Children's Hospital Boston,
Harvard Medical School, Boston, MA, USA
e-mail: Edward.Lee@childrens.harvard.edu

R.H. Cleveland (ed.), *Imaging in Pediatric Pulmonology*,
DOI 10.1007/978-1-4419-5872-3_17, © Springer Science+Business Media, LLC 2012

Table 17.1. Indications for pediatric lung transplantation

Diagnosis	Age: <1 year		Age: 1–5 years		Age: 6–11 years		Age: 12–17 years	
Cystic fibrosis			3	3.7%	107	54.9%	441	69%
Primary pulmonary hypertension	10	16.1%	18	22.2%	23	11.8%	53	8.3%
Retransplant: obliterative bronchiolitis			6	7.4%	8	4.1%	22	3.4%
Congenital heart disease	19	30.6%	8	9.9%	2	1.0%	5	0.8%
Idiopathic pulmonary fibrosis			7	8.6%	6	3.1%	23	3.6%
Obliterative bronchiolitis (not re-TX)			5	6.2%	9	4.6%	21	3.3%
Retransplant: not OB	3	4.8%	1	1.2%	7	3.6%	16	2.5%
Interstitial pneumonitis	6	9.7%	11	13.6%	1	0.5%	5	0.8%
Pulmonary vascular disease	7	11.3%	4	4.9%	6	3.1%	1	0.2%
Eisenmenger's syndrome	1	1.6%	5	6.2%	5	2.6%	6	0.9%
Pulmonary fibrosis, other	1	1.6%	1	1.2%	4	2.1%	11	1.7%
Surfactant protein B deficiency	9	14.5%	2	2.5%				
COPD/emphysema			1	1.2%	2	1.0%	5	0.8%
Bronchopulmonary dysplasia	1	1.6%	2	2.5%	6	3.1%		
Bronchiectasis					3	1.5%	4	0.6%
Other	5	8.1%	7	8.6%	6	3.1%	26	4.1%

Modified from Aurora et al. [1], with permission

evaluation process is usually dependent upon the disease indication; however, all patients will have some form of lung imaging. Chest radiographs and computed tomography (CT) of the chest are typically performed to assess lung pathology as to the extent of the disease process and assessment of chest and lung size in virtually all patients undergoing lung transplant evaluation. With the development and widespread availability of multidetector CT (MDCT), CT has assumed a greater role in the prelung transplant evaluation in children. MDCT provides high-resolution images, faster scan times, and high-quality multiplanar (MPR) and three-dimensional (3D) images of the airways and vascular structures. The high-quality MPR and 3D images have enhanced the display of airways and vascular structures which improves communication among patients, patients' parents, clinicians, and surgeons before and after lung transplantation. In older adult patients, chest CT scans are also useful to screen for occult lung cancer, which is less of an issue in the pediatric population. Ventilation–perfusion (V/Q) scans can give some indication of lung function and assist in deciding which lung to transplant for single lung transplantation. The vast majority of pediatric patients receive bilateral lung transplants, and a V/Q scan may help decide which lung to transplant first if the procedure is not performed using cardiopulmonary bypass. V/Q scans may also be indicated in evaluating underlying pulmonary hypertension and chronic thromboembolic pulmonary hypertension.

Additional studies may include sinus CT scans especially for patients with cystic fibrosis to assess severity of chronic sinusitis and possible need for intervention. Imaging the abdomen most commonly by ultrasound is valuable to evaluate for abdominal organ pathology. Most patients with cystic fibrosis will have an abdominal ultrasound. Echocardiography and/or cardiac catheterization is used to assess cardiac function and for pulmonary vascular disease. Bone densitometry may be performed especially in patients with chronic steroid use or limited physical activity. Patients will receive chronic steroid therapy post transplantation, which may aggravate their bone disease and increase the risk for fractures.

17.2 Donor Evaluation

A chest radiograph is standard evaluation of donor lungs to assess lung size and potential pulmonary pathology. The ideal donor will have a clear CXR with no evidence of lung pathology along with other parameters such as PaO_2 of >300 mmHg on and FiO_2 1.0 and a normal bronchoscopy. Although a normal CXR is considered ideal for the donor lung, there is no data in regard to the use of abnormal CXRs. It is common to find atelectasis in donors and CXR is valuable in identifying atelectasis which may clear with increased airway clearance and/or bronchoscopy to clear mucus plugging thereby potentially salvaging an otherwise unusable lung. On occasion, chest CT scan may help in delineating lung pathology and the feasibility of the lung for organ donation.

Posttransplant Imaging

Early complications of post lung transplantation include hyperacute rejection and primary graft dysfunction. Hyperacute rejection is an uncommon complication occurring minutes to hours after transplantation as a result of recipient antibody response to donor vascular endothelium [2]. This results in respiratory failure with CXR showing severe pulmonary edema and diffuse consolidation. This has a very poor survival. Primary graft dysfunction (PGD) has recently been classified as PGD 1, 2, or 3 based on CXR abnormalities and oxygenation index (PaO_2/FiO_2) within the first 72 h [3]. Contributing factors that may need to be excluded include hyperacute rejection, cardiogenic pulmonary edema, pulmonary venous obstruction, pneumonia, and possibly transfusion related acute lung injury. Based on this new classification, the incidence of severe PGD (PGD3 with P/F <200 after 48 h posttransplant) appears to be ~15% and more importantly PGD3 is associated with an increase in both early and late graft failure and mortality [4]. CXR typically shows bilateral pulmonary edema and basal air-space consolidation (Fig. 17.1) [5].

Mechanical complications may occur when there is a size mismatch between donor lungs and recipients thoracic cavity. Lungs that are too large may result in distortion of the airways and atelectasis, which may progress to scarring. Lungs that are too small may result in hemodynamic compromise, exercise limitations, and pulmonary hypertension from an inadequate pulmonary vascular circulation. There may also be delayed filling of the entire thoracic cavity with persistent pleural air. Another possible complication is injury to the phrenic nerve resulting in diaphragmatic dysfunction.

As a result of the transplant procedure, pleural abnormalities are seen which include pneumothorax and pleural effusions, and chest tubes are routinely placed upon completion of the lung transplant surgery. With increased capillary permeability and impaired lymphatic clearance, pleural effusions are commonly seen and usually self limiting within approximately 2 weeks. Persistent or delayed effusions may result from complications such as empyema, rejection, or vascular abnomalities.

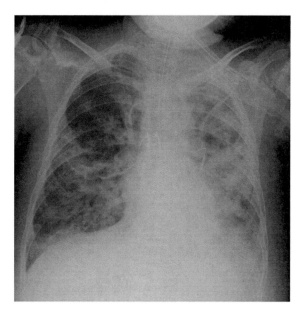

Fig. 17.1. A fourteen-year-old girl with bilateral lung transplantation for cystic fibrosis. Chest radiograph shows pulmonary edema associated with patchy air-space opacities in both lungs immediately after lung transplantation, compatible with primary graft dysfunction

In the early period of lung transplantation, bronchial complications were frequent and limited the utility of this procedure. With improved donor preservation, surgical techniques, and immunosuppression, these are much less frequent; however, the incidence of airway complications is still estimated to be 10% [6]. Since the bronchial circulation is not reconnected with the transplant procedure, the airway circulation is dependent upon retrograde perfusion through the pulmonary circulation. Bronchial dehiscence is an early complication which is best detected by CT scan with the presence of extraluminal air around the anastomosis site. New or persistent pneumothorax or pneumomediastinum may be indirect evidence of a bronchial air leak. Bronchial stenosis, which is a complication of surgical anastomotic healing or dehiscence, is a serious complication that can occur after lung transplantation [5]. Although diagnosis of bronchial stenosis can be made with bronchoscopy, MDCT with 3D imaging of the central airways is a useful noninvasive imaging modality. On CT, focal or diffuse narrowing of the airway, typically at the site of surgical anastomosis is seen (Fig. 17.2). Vascular complications are less common and can be evaluated by perfusion scan and visualized by angiographic studies. However, MDCT with 3D imaging can also be used as an alternative

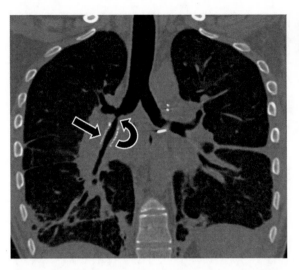

Fig. 17.2. A eighteen-year-old girl with bilateral lung transplantation for cystic fibrosis. Coronal reformatted CT demonstrates right sided bronchial narrowing (*curved arrow*). Also noted is a metallic stent (*straight arrow*) located in the right lower lobe bronchus

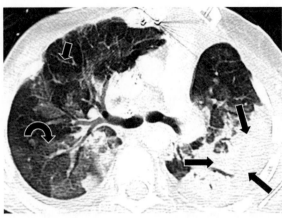

Fig. 17.3. A fifteen-year-old girl with bilateral lung transplantation for cystic fibrosis. Axial lung window CT image shows ground-glass opacification (*curved arrow*), septal thickening (*short arrow*), and air-space consolidation (*long arrows*) compatible with acute cellular rejection

noninvasive imaging modality to detect vascular complications in children after lung transplantation.

Infections and acute cellular rejection (ACR) are common complications in lung transplant patients and difficult to differentiate based on clinical or radiographic parameters. Bronchoscopy with bronchoalveolar lavage and transbronchial biopsy is currently the procedure to differentiate infection and rejection. ACR may occur without CXR changes or the CXR may show new or persistent infiltrates or pleural effusion. CT findings of ACR include areas of ground-glass attenuation, interlobular septal thickening, small nodules (<1 mm), decreased vascularity, and air-space disease (Fig. 17.3) [5]. In addition to detecting ACR, CT may be useful for localizing the site of disease for biopsy to confirm the diagnosis.

Because of immunosuppression, lung denervation, loss of cough reflex, and impaired lymphatic drainage, lung transplant patients are at increased risk for infections and may not present with the usual clinical signs and symptoms. Bacterial infections are most frequent within the first month, but in pediatric patients, this is one of the more common complications of morbidity and mortality. The common bacterial pathogens which affect children with lung transplantation include *Enterobacter*, *Pseudomonas*, and *Streptococcus pneumoniae* [5]. Radiologic presentation may include lobar or multifocal infiltrates, consolidation, ground glass opacities, cavitation, or lung nodules (Fig. 17.4) [5]. Rarely, pulmonary or

mediastinal abscess can be also seen. Fungal infections, which can occur within the first few postoperative weeks or as late as several years after transplantation, are less common, although there is a higher mortality associated with invasive fungal infections. *Candida albicans* and *Aspergillus* are the two most common causes of fungal infection in children with lung transplantation [5]. Radiographic findings may include consolidation, ground glass or cavitary opacities, and ill-defined nodules. CT typically shows nodular air-space disease, cavitary lesions, and mediastinal adenopathy (Fig. 17.5) [5].

Viral infections are also a frequent complication in the pediatric transplant population. Cytomegalovirus (CMV) pneumonitis is the most common viral infection in children with lung transplantation, followed in frequency by herpes simplex and Epstein-Barr virus infections. CMV infection previously was a common cause of pneumonia in the post transplant period and highest incidence in donor (+)/recipient (−) CMV exposure in lung transplant patients. With the use of CMV prophylaxis in patients that are donor or recipient (+), CMV pneumonia is much less frequent. CXR may show diffuse parenchymal haziness or reticulonodular interstitial opacities, and CT scan may show ground glass attenuation, interlobular septal thickening, micronodules, or consolidation [5]. Diagnosis of CMV infection can be definitively made when CMV inclusion bodies are detected within pneumocytes microscopically.

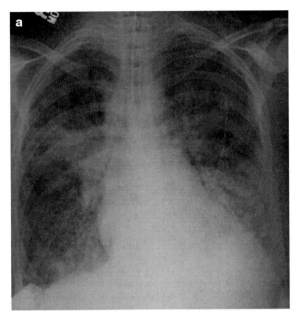

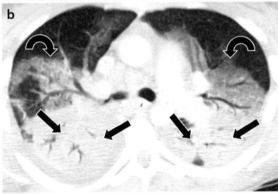

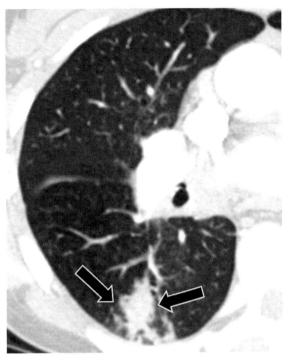

Fig. 17.5. A fifteen-year-old girl with bilateral lung transplantation for cystic fibrosis. Axial CT lung window image shows nodular air-space opacity (*arrows*), which was found to be aspergillous infection

Fig. 17.4. A seventeen-year-old girl with bilateral lung transplantation for cystic fibrosis who presents with fever and elevated white blood cell counts. *Staphylococcus aureus* pneumonia was confirmed on bronchoalveolar lavage. (a) Chest radiograph shows multifocal air-space consolidations in both lungs. (b) Axial lung window CT image demonstrates groundglass opacifications (*curved arrows*) and air-space consolidations (*straight arrows*) in both lungs. Also noted are several air bronchograms within the consolidated portions of lungs

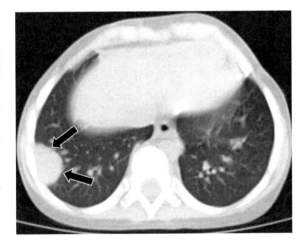

Fig. 17.6. A six-year-old boy who is status post bilateral lung transplant approximately 8 months ago. Follow-up chest radiographs showed an opacity in the right lung base and CT was subsequently obtained for confirmation and further characterization. Axial lung window CT image showed round pleural based mass (*arrows*) located in the right lower lobe. Biopsy of this mass confirmed PTLD

Posttransplant lymphoproliferative disorder (PTLD) typically occurs within the first year after transplantation [7]. However, it can also manifest months to years post transplantation. In the majority of patients, it is associated with EBV infection/reactivation and is thought to be secondary to B-cell proliferation although there are EBV negative cases and even reports of T cell abnormalities. PTLD can vary from polyclonal lymphoid proliferation to aggressive high grade lymphoma. Early detection of PTLD is paramount because most cases of PTLD are reversible with reduction of the immunosuppressants. The incidence in pediatric lung transplant recipients is ~15% and most commonly seen as solitary or multiple pulmonary nodules or masses in addition to often necrotic mediastinal lymphadenopathy (Fig. 17.6) [8]. However, it also occurs in extrapulmonary sites especially of the head and neck region as well as abdomen and pelvis with a relatively high rate (34%) of abdominal involvement by PTLD in children with allograft lung transplantation [7].

Bronchiolitis obliterans (BO) is the major limitation for long-term survival and a frequent complication in both adult and pediatric patients. It is a histologic diagnosis, although transbronchial biopsy is not a very sensitive study and frequently misses the diagnosis since it is initially a heterogeneous lesion. The clinical correlate is bronchiolitis obliterans syndrome which is an unexplained drop in lung function after infection, ACR, and airway complications have been ruled out. Early in the course, the CXR may be normal and later may show attenuated vessels, bronchial cuffing, subsegmental atelectasis, and irregular linear opacities. CT scan is a more sensitive imaging modality showing mosaic attenuation, bronchial dilatation, and bronchial wall thickening, and the most sensitive study may be with the addition of an expiratory CT scan showing air trapping [9]. It has been reported that the sensitivity of inspiratory CT for enabling diagnosis of BO was 71%; the specificity, 78%; the positive predictive value, 62%; and the negative predictive value, 84% [10]. By contrast, the sensitivity of expiratory CT for enabling diagnosis of BO was 100%; the specificity, 71%; the positive predictive value, 64%; and the negative predictive value, 100% [10]. Furthermore, it has been shown that expiratory CT scores correlated more strongly with pulmonary function test-based scores than did inspiratory CT scores in children diagnosed with BO after lung transplantation [10].

Imaging study plays an important role in managing all phases of the pediatric lung transplant patient. It is useful in defining the severity of the disease process of the lung transplant candidate, assessing donor quality and size, and in monitoring the post lung transplant process. Our program has established protocols for both the evaluation and posttransplant monitoring as outlined in Table 17.2.

Table 17.2. Lung transplant imaging protocol

Prelung transplant imaging evaluation
Plain chest radiographs (PA and lateral views)
CT angiogram (with 2D and 3D reconstruction of airway and vascular structures)
Postlung transplant imaging evaluation
Plain chest radiographs (AP view of the chest) – everyday during hospitalization
Plain chest radiographs (PA and lateral views) – on the day of discharge from the hospital
Plain chest radiographs (PA and lateral views) – 1 month F/U clinic visit
CT angiogram (with 2D and 3D reconstruction of airway and vascular structures) – 1 month F/U clinic visit
Chest CT with expiratory cuts – 3 month F/U and 6 month F/U clinic visit
Chest CT with expiratory cuts – yearly F/U

References

1. Aurora P, Edwards LB, Christie J, Dobbels F, Kirk R, Kucheryavaya AY, et al. Registry of the International Society for Heart and Lung Transplantation: eleventh official pediatric lung and heart/lung transplantation report–2008. J Heart Lung Transplant. 2008;27:978–83.
2. Zander DS, Baz MA, Visner GA, Staples ED, Donnelly WH, Faro A, et al. Analysis of early deaths after isolated lung transplantation. Chest. 2001;120:225–32.
3. Christie JD, Carby M, Bag R, Corris P, Hertz M, Weill D. Report of the ISHLT Working Group on Primary Lung Graft Dysfunction part II: definition. A consensus statement of the International Society for Heart and Lung Transplantation. J Heart Lung Transplant. 2005;24:1454–9.
4. Prekker ME, Nath DS, Walker AR, Johnson AC, Hertz MI, Herrington CS, et al. Validation of the proposed International Society for Heart and Lung Transplantation grading system for primary graft dysfunction after lung transplantation. J Heart Lung Transplant. 2006;25:371–8.
5. Medina LS, Siegel MJ. CT of complications in pediatric lung transplantation. Radiographics. 1994;14:1341–9.
6. Choong CK, Sweet SC, Zoole JB, Guthrie TJ, Mendeloff EN, Haddad FJ, et al. Bronchial airway anastomotic complications after pediatric lung transplantation: incidence, cause, management, and outcome. J Thorac Cardiovasc Surg. 2006;131:198–203.
7. Siegel MJ, Lee EY, Sweet SC, Hildebolt C. CT of posttransplantation lymphoproliferative disorder in pediatric recipients of lung allograft. AJR Am J Roentgenol. 2003; 181:1125–31.
8. Boyle GJ, Michaels MG, Webber SA, Knisely AS, Kurland G, Cipriani LA, et al. Posttransplantation lymphoproliferative disorders in pediatric thoracic organ recipients. J Pediatr. 1997;131:309–13.
9. Lau DM, Siegel MJ, Hildebolt CF, Cohen AH. Bronchiolitis obliterans syndrome: thin-section CT diagnosis of obstructive changes in infants and young children after lung transplantation. Radiology. 1998;208:783–8.
10. Siegel MJ, Bhalla S, Gutierrez FR, Hildebolt C, Sweet S. Post-lung transplantation bronchiolitis obliterans syndrome: usefulness of expiratory thin-section CT for diagnosis. Radiology. 2001;220:455–62.

Fetal Imaging of the Chest

Dorothy Bulas and Alexia Egloff

CONTENTS

Ultrasonography (US) is the screening method of choice for the evaluation of the fetal airway and chest. It is safe, inexpensive and easily performed. Advances in US technique including higher resolution transducers, Doppler and 3D/4D imaging have allowed for

improved assessment of the congenital thoracic masses. The assessment of the fetal chest by US, however, is operator dependent and evaluation may be limited due to fetal position, maternal obesity, overlying bone, and/or oligohydramnios. Ultrasound evaluation is sensitive in the diagnosis of many prenatal lung lesions but has low specificity [1].

Magnetic Resonance Imaging (MRI) is an alternative modality that uses no ionizing radiation, has excellent tissue contrast, a large field of view, is not limited by obesity or overlying bone and can image the fetus in multiple planes regardless of fetal lie. Faster scanning techniques allow studies to be performed without sedation in the second and third trimester with minimal motion artifact. Fetal MRI helps confirm the presence of masses identified by US, can delineate anatomy such as the trachea not visualized by US and may demonstrate additional subtle anomalies. Experts in fields such as pediatric surgery and neonatology not comfortable interpreting US imaging can provide additional expertise when reviewing MR images. This multidisciplinary approach is crucial for the success of handling these complex cases [2–5].

Thus, advances in US and MRI have improved our ability to accurately diagnose fetal airway and chest anomalies and furthered our understanding of the evolution of fetal lung lesions.

The prenatal and postnatal prognosis for fetuses with chest anomalies is quite variable. Fetal imaging not only is important for the initial diagnosis of the lesion but is also useful for follow-up in case nonimmune hydrops develops. Preparation for delivery at a tertiary institution is critical for the fetus with a large airway or chest mass. The decision to perform in utero intervention or an Ex Utero Intrapartum Treatment (EXIT) delivery places both the mother and fetus at risk and thus benefits from precise evaluation and accurate assessment of the situation.

Dorothy Bulas, MD (✉)
Department of Diagnostic Imaging and Radiology,
George Washington University Medical Center,
Children's National Medical Center, Washington, DC, USA
e-mail: dbulas@cnmc.org

Alexia Egloff, MD
Department of Radiology, Pediatric Radiologist, Children's
National Medical Center, Washington, DC, USA

R.H. Cleveland (ed.), *Imaging in Pediatric Pulmonology*,
DOI 10.1007/978-1-4419-5872-3_18, © Springer Science+Business Media, LLC 2012

Prenatal evaluation not only allows for the planning of in utero therapy but can optimize postnatal therapeutic planning with reduction in neonatal imaging, useful when caring for the unstable infant [2–4].

Prenatal diagnosis does not always result in improved outcome as some cases are associated with lethal pulmonary hypoplasia. A small chest mass can be associated with severe chromosomal anomalies or other lethal anatomic abnormalities. Thus, accurate chromosomal and structural assessment of the entire fetus is also important for appropriate counseling and planning of in utero interventional procedures, delivery and postnatal management.

18.1 Ultrasonography Imaging of the Fetal Neck and Chest

18.1.1 Ultrasonography of the Fetal Chest

Ultrasound is the initial imaging modality in the detection of fetal chest masses. On axial images, the normal fetal chest is oval or round. The heart is positioned within the anterior half of the left chest and bordered on both sides by lung tissue. The apex of the heart touches the wall of the left anterior chest while the intersection of the atrial septum with the posterior heart border lies just to the right of center. The lungs, thorax and heart grow proportionally, so the normal cardiothoracic ratio is constant throughout the pregnancy and the cardiac position and axis should not change over time. The fetal ribs are echogenic and encompass more than half the chest circumference on either side. The ultrasound appearance of normal fetal lungs is typically homogeneous and echogenic. In early pregnancy, the lungs are less echogenic than the liver but echogenicity increases through gestation as the lungs become more fluid filled. At times, the echogenicity of the lung may appear similar to the adjacent liver and bowel making it difficult to differentiate sonographically from surrounding organs. Inferiorly, the diaphragms border the lungs and are dome shaped and hypoechoic. It is important to remember that visualization of a seemingly intact diaphragm does not exclude a diaphragmatic hernia as a small defect may be missed. The thymus, a homogeneous anterior mediastinal structure, is often not well seen because of overlying rib shadowing.

Three-dimensional US can provide lung volumetry measurements [6]. Obtaining volume measurements, however, can be difficult in all three planes as oligohydramnios, maternal obesity or fetal lie may make differentiation of lung and surrounding structures difficult.

Sonographically, congenital lung masses can appear hypoechoic/cystic or hyperechoic/microcystic/solid, small or large (Fig. 18.1). When a solid lung mass is present, the echogenicity may be similar to adjacent liver and lung and thus, difficult to identify. Shift of the heart and flattening of the diaphragms may be the first clue that a lung mass or diaphragmatic hernia is present (Fig. 18.2). Echogenic masses may become less visible later in gestation as the surrounding lung tissue becomes more echogenic and rib shadowing increases. The differential for lung masses includes congenital diaphragmatic hernia (CDH), congenital pulmonary airway malformation (CPAM/CCAM), bronchopulmonary sequestration (BPS), congenital lobar emphysema (CLE)/bronchial atresia, hybrid lesions and congenital hydrothorax [7–9]. Ultrasound while sensitive in the identification of many lung lesions due to their abnormal echogenicity and/or mass affect has a low specificity [1].

18.1.2 Ultrasonography of the Fetal Neck

Ultrasound imaging the fetal neck is also important in the assessment of the fetal airway and lungs. Axial images of the neck may demonstrate the larynx and pharynx sonographically if they are fluid filled but the trachea is typically not visualized. Axial images of the posterior neck are important for the identification of nuchal translucency at 11–14 weeks and nuchal thickening at 16–20 weeks both of which are markers for aneuploidy. The jugular vein and carotid artery can be identified by color Doppler and may be deviated if a mass is present. A detailed exam of the neck is not always possible by ultrasound when oligohydramnios, maternal obesity or fetal lie prevents adequate visualization. If the neck is in fixed extension, there should be concern that a neck mass is present.

When a neck mass is identified, internal characteristics may help determine the diagnosis. There are a wide variety of neck masses which can be cystic (lymphatic malformation (lymangioma/cystic hygroma), branchial cleft cyst, thyroglossal duct

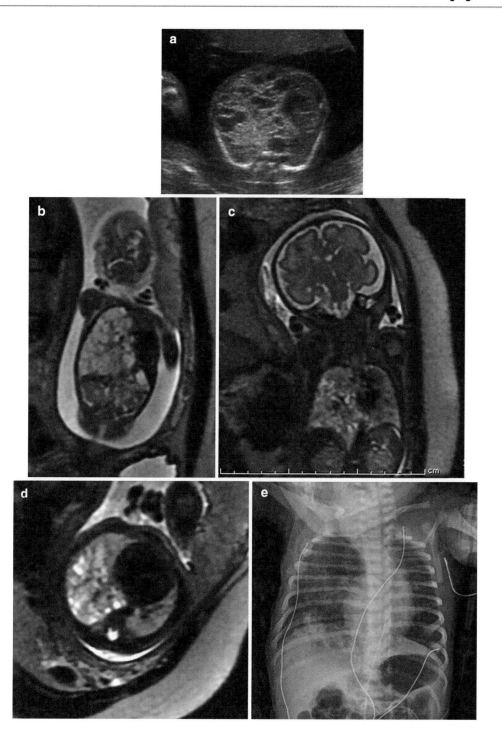

Fig. 18.1. Congenital pulmonary airway malformation. (a) Axial US at 21 weeks gestation demonstrates a large mixed macrocystic and microcystic mass in the right hemithorax with compression of normal left lung. (b) Coronal SSFSE T2w MR image also at 21 weeks confirms the presence of a large multicystic mass in the right hemithorax everting the diaphragm inferiorly and deviating the heart to the left. The CVR measures 2.4 high risk for developing hydrops. Follow up coronal (c) and axial (d) MR images at 30 weeks gestation demonstrates growth of the fetus with stable size of the right lung mass. The mass no longer everts the diaphragm nor deviates the heart to the left. The CVR has improved and now measures 1.4 low risk for developing hydrops. (e) At delivery the infant had minimal respiratory distress. Chest radiograph demonstrates minimally heterogeneous right lower lobe

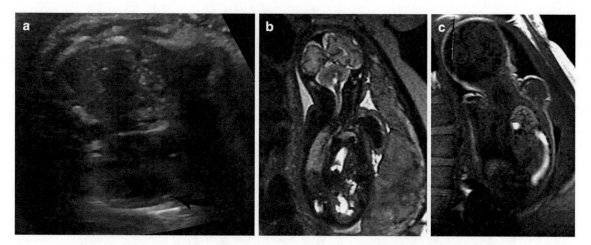

Fig. 18.2. Congenital diaphragmatic hernia. (a) Axial US of a fetal chest demonstrates a heterogeneous mass in the left hemithorax deviating the heart (*curved arrow*) to the right. (b) Coronal SSFSE T2w image of the fetal chest demonstrates that small and large bowel is herniated into the left hemithorax consistent with a diaphragmatic hernia rather than CPAM. (c) Coronal T1w image confirms that high signal meconium filled bowel is herniated into the left hemithorax

cyst, laryngocele, cervical meningomyelocele), solid (goiter, neuroblastoma, fibroma) or complex (teratoma, hemangioma, goiter). The two most common causes for neck masses are lymphangioma and teratomas [10].

The prognosis of a cervical mass is dependent on the amount of airway compression, presence of other anomalies and development of hydrops. As the airway is not directly seen by US, secondary signs of airway compression such as polyhydramnios or a small stomach may suggest severity of airway compromise.

18.2 Magnetic Resonance Imaging of the Fetal Neck and Chest

18.2.1 Fetal Magnetic Resonance Technique

Advances in MR including single shot rapid acquisition with relaxation enhancement sequences has significantly decreased movement artifact on 1.5 T magnets. Slices are acquired individually with each slice obtained by a single excitation pulse taking less than 400 ms. A series can be obtained in less than 30–40 s with slices as thin as 2–3 mm. These T2-weighted images have excellent contrast and spatial resolution and good signal to noise ratios.

Sequences available include single slice fast spin echo, ssFSE (GE, Milwaukee, WI) and half-Fourier acquisition single shot turbo spin echo, HASTE (Siemens, Erlangen, Germany) [11, 12]. Additional MR sequences include heavy T2w hydrography, fast T1w sequences including fast multiplanar spoiled gradient-echo, diffusion weighted sequences and 2-dimensional fast low angle shot. These sequences take longer, may require breath holding and thicker slices for sufficient signal/noise ratios.

Total study time can average 20–40 min, depending on fetal movement which is particularly problematic in cases of polyhydramnios and younger gestations. Studies may be limited due to maternal size, claustrophobia and maternal discomfort in the supine position. Left lateral decubitus position can be helpful in patients with back pain or with supine hypotension. A fast multiplanar spoiled gradient echo sequence or large field of view (48 cm; section thickness 8 mm; intersection gap 2 mm) coronal ssFSE localizer is first performed to evaluate fetal position and select future imaging planes. Each subsequent plane is placed orthogonal to the previous sequence to account for fetal movement. Axial, sagittal and coronal T2w images angled to the fetal chest are obtained at 3–5 mm thickness, 0 mm section gap. Planes angled to the fetal brain and abdomen are important for complete assessment of the fetus. Quiet maternal breathing is adequate for T2w images, with breath hold T1w, echoplanar and angiographic sequences added as needed. Fetal MRI provides improved anatomic evaluation of the airway and lungs, helps corroborate the diagnosis and often provides additional information useful for management planning including fetal intervention [2, 3]. More specific diagnosis prenatally provides improved counseling, decreasing the level of stress that could result when a thoracic anomaly is diagnosed [5].

18.2.2 Fetal Magnetic Resonance Safety

There is no definitive evidence that MRI produces harmful effects on human embryos or fetuses using current clinical parameters with a 1.5-T magnet. The long-term safety of MRI exposure to the fetus, however, has not been definitively demonstrated [13, 14]. There has been concern that prolonged exposure to high-field MRI may affect embryogenesis, chromosomal structure or fetal development [3]. Animal studies on embryos have not demonstrated any growth abnormalities or genetic damage at clinical levels of exposure so far [15, 16]. There is concern that with higher strength units and prolonged scanning times, biological effects may occur if applied at sensitive stages of fetal development [17, 18].

Compliance with the United States Food and Drug Administration (FDA) and International Commission on Nonionizing Radiation Protection (ICNIRP) guidelines requires control of specific absorption rate (SAR) values [19, 20]. Medical Device Agency (MDA) guidelines require control of the maximum SAR (10 g) within the fetus. The most frequently used sequences do operate at the SAR limit recommendations. These limits need to be carefully followed with higher field systems as well [21]. MR is not routinely recommended during the first trimester due to concerns regarding the developing embryo's susceptibility to injury. The small fetal size and significant fetal motion limit imaging at this gestation as well.

Gadolinium should not be used with fetal imaging as it has been shown to cross the placenta. The fetus excretes then swallows gadolinium which gets reabsorbed from the gastrointestinal tract. In animal studies, growth retardation has been reported after high doses of gadolinium (Magnevist product information, Berlex Labs, Wayne, NJ). Thus, gadolinium contrast is not recommended for usage in pregnant patients.

18.2.3 MRI of the Fetal Chest

Fetal MRI is a useful adjunct in the assessment of the fetal airway and chest. Fluid in the trachea and larynx is high T2w and thus well delineated [22]. Fetal lungs are homogeneously brighter than muscle and increase in signal after 24 weeks' gestation due to the development of alveoli and production of alveolar fluid [23] in the third trimester. Normal lung when compressed by a mass may be slightly hypointense compared to noncompressed normal lung. Normal lung parenchyma is easily separated from abnormal lung masses which tend to be higher in signal.

The mediastinal structures, liver and lung are easily differentiated by MR. The liver and spleen are low in signal on T2w with liver higher in signal on T1w than normal lung. On T2w, meconium is low in signal while fluid-filled small bowel is high in signal. This reverses on T1w when meconium is bright and fluid-filled small bowel is low in signal and is easily distinguished from adjacent lung and liver in cases of CDH (Fig. 18.2). The thymus is homogenous and of higher signal than heart which appears as a flow void on T2w.

The ability to image in any plane and large field of view aids in the delineation of fetal lung masses. Lung volumes can be measured in any plane and normative data are being accumulated for various gestational ages. Volumetric lung measurements appear to be reproducible and increase with gestational age. The right lung measures approximately 56% of the total lung volume. When oligohydramnios limits visualization of the fetus sonographically, MR can still demonstrate many anomalies and lung volumes can be measured to assess for pulmonary hypoplasia. In complex cases, such as thoracopagus conjoined twins, the large field of view can be particularly helpful. Thus, while US is the initial modality in detecting chest masses, MRI is useful in confirming the presence of a mass, providing assessment of residual lung volume and further characterizing the lesion increasing specificity.

18.2.4 MRI of the Fetal Airway

Prenatal evaluation of the fetal neck is difficult with complex embryology involving the development of vascular, lymphatic, musculoskeletal and digestive systems. Masses such as teratomas and lymphangiomas can share both cystic and solid components, with precise histologic diagnosis difficult prenatally. If the neck mass is large and compresses the airway, death may occur at delivery if a patent airway is not established quickly. Thus, detection of a neck mass prenatally is important to prepare for the timing, location and mode of delivery.

Fetal MRI is a useful adjunct in the evaluation of neck and thoracic masses which compress the fetal airway. The normal fetal airway can be visualized on T2w due to high signal fluid within the larynx, trachea and bronchi. The esophagus is not typically visualized but may be identified when distended by a distal obstruction. T1w images are useful for the diagnosis of a goiter which is of high signal on T1w.

When a neck mass is identified, MRI can delineate if the mass extends into the oropharynx. The amount of tracheal deviation and compression can be directly visualized. MRI is also useful for the evaluation of tracheal compression from thoracic masses. Mediastinal masses are rare and include foregut cysts, teratomas, esophageal duplication cysts and bronchogenic cysts. Foregut cysts including bronchogenic, enteric and neurenteric are typically fluid filled with high T2w homogeneous signal. Mediastinal teratomas have a complex heterogenous appearance due to fat and fluid. These masses may compress the great vessels and result in hydrops and/or compress the esophagus and result in polyhydramnios [23].

The location of cystic and solid components of neck and mediastinal masses can be evaluated in three dimensions allowing the surgeon to plan for in utero intervention or post delivery cyst aspiration or resection. In the fetus greater than 32 weeks' gestation with a large lesion expected to have difficulty breathing at delivery, EXIT may be considered. This partial delivery followed by intubation and intravenous access prior to clamping the umbilical cord can improve the survival of these difficult cases [24].

18.3 Prenatal Diagnosis and Management of Chest Anomalies

When an airway or chest abnormality is identified prenatally, several questions need to be answered.

- Are additional anomalies or hydrops present?
- Will there be pulmonary hypoplasia at delivery?
- Will there be airway obstruction at delivery?
- Can in utero intervention help?

The most common congenital thoracic lesions include CDH, congenital pulmonary airway malformation (CPAM/CCAM), BPS, CLE/bronchial atresia, hybrid lesions and congenital hydrothorax [25]. Pulmonary hypoplasia, agenesis and aplasia are less common. A definitive diagnosis of a chest mass is usually possible only after surgical resection and histopathological evaluation [7–9].

In the fetus, the clinical importance of these lesions lies primarily in the mass effect on surrounding structures. This can result in compression of the airway, blood vessels, lymphatics and normal lung with development of pleural effusions, polyhydramnios, hydrops and pulmonary hypoplasia. Outcome depends on the timing of secondary effects and severity of pulmonary hypoplasia. With improvement in fetal imaging, more aggressive fetal interventions have advanced. While the majority of cases with lung masses survive, masses that result in hydrops in the past were typically lethal. Now these masses may be amenable to fetal interventions such as maternal steroids, fetal thorocentesis, laser therapy and in utero surgery [26–31].

18.3.1 Congenital Pulmonary Airway Malformation

Congenital pulmonary airway malformation (CPAM/CCAM) have varying appearances sonographically dependent on subtype. The pathologic classifications by Stocker et al. have no real prognostic value prenatally [32]. A simpler fetal classification by Adzick et al. [28] based on gross anatomy and imaging appearance has been recommended for prenatal assessment.

- Macrocystic – One or more macrocysts measuring >5 mm. These cysts are hypoechoic by ultrasound and high signal by MR. This subtype has a more favorable prognosis, grow less rapidly but may develop hydrops and can require prenatal intervention (Fig. 18.3).
- Microcystic – Multiple microcysts <5 mm that appear homogeneously echogenic/solid by ultrasound and are high signal by MR. When large, they may be associated with mediastinal shift, pulmonary hypoplasia, polyhydramnios and non-immune hydrops requiring in utero intervention.

By ultrasound, macrocysts are well delineated from adjacent echogenic normal parenchyma.

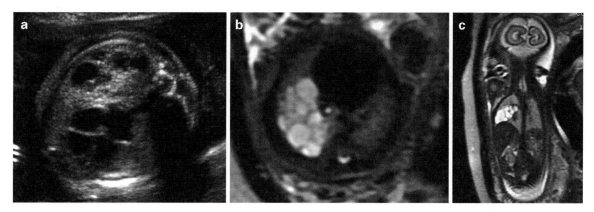

Fig. 18.3. Macrocystic CPAM. (**a**) Axial US image of the fetal chest demonstrates multiple macrocysts within the right hemithorax. Axial (**b**) and coronal (**c**) SSFSE T2w MR images confirms that the high signal macrocysts are limited to the right middle lobe with normal intermediate signal right upper and lower lobe parenchyma

The microcystic subtype is echogenic as compared to normal lung, but may become more difficult to visualize as gestational age advances due to the normal increase in echogenicity of surrounding normal lung as alveoli develop (Fig. 18.4). Shadowing from overlying ribs becomes more problematic in the third trimester limiting lung parenchymal visualization. When the mass is large, mediastinal shift can be identified by rotation and deviation of the heart axis.

When severe, vena cava and cardiac compression may result in hydrops, with pleural effusions, pericardial effusions, skin thickening and ascites developing. Esophageal compression can result in a small stomach and polyhydramnios. Color and power Doppler imaging are useful in looking for a systemic feeding vessel [5] while 3D/4D imaging can be used to measure lung volumes [6].

By MR, CPAM are typically higher in signal than adjacent normal lung with mediastinal shift easily demonstrated. MR is particularly valuable when a rare bilateral CPAM is present. Lung volumes are easily measured in any plane by MR.

Prognosis does not depend on the type of lesion [28], rather, it is dependent on the size of the mass, amount of mediastinal shift and pulmonary hypoplasia, fetal hemodynamics, associated anomalies and gestational age at delivery [25, 28].

CPAM is rarely associated with chromosomal anomalies but associated anomalies should still be searched for [29]. Karyotyping is not necessary if no other anomalies or risk factors are identified [29]. In the absence of hydrops, early survival without any intervention is higher than 95% [30].

Follow-up ultrasounds are critical to assess stability of mass size and the potential development of hydrops. Up to 33% of fetuses with CPAM can develop hydrops [33]. The presence of hydrops is the most important indicator of poor outcome and can result in perinatal death approaching 100% without intervention [28].

A CPAM volume ratio (CVR) has been described as a predictor of hydrops and outcome [33]. It is obtained by calculating the volume of the lung mass and normalizing it by gestational age using the head circumference [33].

$$CVR = \frac{\text{height} \times \text{anteroposterior diameter} \times \text{transverse diameter} \times 0.52 \, (\text{constant})}{\text{Head circumference}}.$$

If the CVR is less than 1.6, the risk of developing hydrops is low [33]. If the ratio is more than 1.6, the fetus is at high risk for developing hydrops and intervention should be considered to increase survival.

CPAM typically show progressive growth between weeks 20 and 26 of gestation and at 26–28 weeks, growth begins to plateau. Usually, no hydrops develops after reaching the 28 weeks' growth plateau [33].

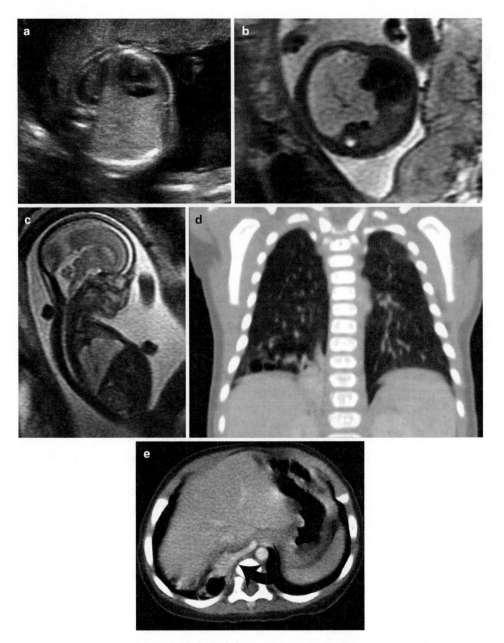

Fig. 18.4. Microcystic hybrid lung mass. (a) Axial US image of the fetal chest demonstrates a homogeneous echogenic mass deviating the heart to the left. Axial (b) and sagittal (c) SSFSE T2w MR confirm the presence of a high signal right lower lobe mass. (d) Coronal reformatted image of a chest CT at 5 months of age demonstrates a small residual mixed cystic and solid mass in the right lower lobe. (e) Axial CT with intravenous contrast demonstrates the presence of a feeding systemic vessel (*curved arrow*) consistent with a hybrid sequestration

If hydrops develops and gestation is less than 32 weeks, various interventions have been attempted with the objective of decreasing fetal compromise and preventing lung hypoplasia [8]. Best approach is selected for each individual case depending on the presence of hydrops and the type of anomaly. Interventions include maternal steroids, fetal thoracentesis, cyst aspiration, thoracoamniotic shunt, laser therapy, sclerotherapy and in utero surgical resection [33–41].

Successful fetal surgery depends on surgical experience as well as optimal maternal anesthesia and uterine relaxation, hysterotomy and fetal exposure techniques: intraoperative fetal monitoring, reliable amniotic membrane and uterine closure. Close postoperative follow-up and early detection and treatment of preterm labor are fundamental. To undergo fetal surgery, maternal health needs to be considered to decrease the risk of complications [28].

Up to 50% of CPAM actually resolve prenatally [31]. Of the lesions that resolve in utero, 60% show no abnormality on postnatal imaging; [31]. The remaining 40% with apparent prenatal resolution are still present postnatally but not well seen by follow-up prenatal imaging due to increase in normal lung echogenicity and difficulty in differentiating normal from abnormal lung [33]. When a persistent mass is seen, it is confirmed by postnatal imaging in over 95% of cases.

Persistent masses can decrease in size during the late second trimester [28], or have a relative decrease in size due to normal fetal growth. Some do actually increase in size. Implications for delivery and postnatal management include size of mass at delivery and the presence of hydrops. If small with no hydrops, the obstetrician and neonatologist need to be aware of the potential need for respiratory support. However, the majority of these infants do well, can be delivered vaginally with no additional support required [42]. Following delivery, these infants should be assessed for respiratory stability and feeding tolerance. If stable, the infant can be discharged home. Follow-up may include radiographs and CT scans, the timing of which should be dependent on whether the infant is symptomatic or not.

For large masses that cause mediastinal shift and/ or hydrops, delivery at a tertiary care center with an intensive care nursery capable of resuscitation of a neonate with respiratory difficulties, including capability of ECMO, needs to be planned [34, 40].

In the fetus is greater than 32 weeks' gestation with hydrops, delivery by EXIT should be prepared for with likely need of the mass to be resected at birth [40].

18.3.2 Bronchopulmonary Sequestration

BPS typically have the appearance of a homogeneous triangular echogenic mass with well-defined borders by ultrasound. By definition, BPS have systemic feeding and draining vessels and consist of lung parenchyma without communication to the bronchial tree. The mass is often in the lower hemithorax adjacent to the diaphragm. Hybrid lesions can have a cystic component with feeding systemic vessels and typically have a better prognosis than patients with CPAM without systemic feeding vessels. Careful color and power Doppler assessment are critical to identify the vessel branching from the aorta below the diaphragm (Fig. 18.5). Even with careful assessment, the vascular supply may be difficult to demonstrate prenatally [27, 43].

MRI appearance is typically of a hyperintense T2w mass in the lower lobe [25, 27] The feeding vessel may be a low signal line coursing from the aorta

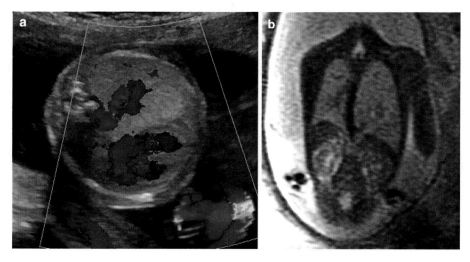

Fig. 18.5. Bronchopulmonary sequestration. (a) Axial US image of the fetal chest with power Doppler documents an echogenic mass in the left lung with systemic vessels coursing into the mass. (b) Coronal SSFSE T2w image confirms the presence of a low signal line coursing to the high signal mass consistent with a sequestration

into the mass. MRI does not always demonstrate the abnormal vessels but is helpful in delineating the mass, evaluating the contralateral lung and assessing for other congenital abnormalities [27, 44]. It is particularly useful in assessing if the mass is thoracic, in the diaphragm or infradiaphragmatic. When infradiaphragmatic in location, BPS tend to be suprarenal and can mimic a neuroblastoma [27, 45].

Prognosis is favorable with only rare reports of associated hydrops. If hydrops develops after 32 weeks' gestation, early delivery is recommended. Prior to 32 weeks, in utero surgical resection may be considered or limited to thoracentesis [46–49]. Lesions may appear to resolve in utero but are usually present on postnatal CT. Postnatal CT with contrast or MRI are useful in identifying the feeding vessel.

18.3.3 Congenital Lobar Hyperinflation/ Congenital Lobar Emphysema/ Bronchial Atresia

Criteria for the diagnosis of congenital lobar hyperinflation (CLH) include hyperlucent lung with normal lung architecture and absence of macroscopic cysts. This diagnosis may be difficult to differentiate from microcystic CPAM prenatally (Fig. 18.6). The presence of normal pulmonary vascularity and lack of cysts can help suggest the diagnosis. Diagnosis is confirmed with postnatal CT [50, 51].

By ultrasound, CLH is characterized as a homogeneous echogenic lung mass, thought to be secondary to accumulation of the pulmonary fluids within the lung [51]. MRI images demonstrate a homogeneous

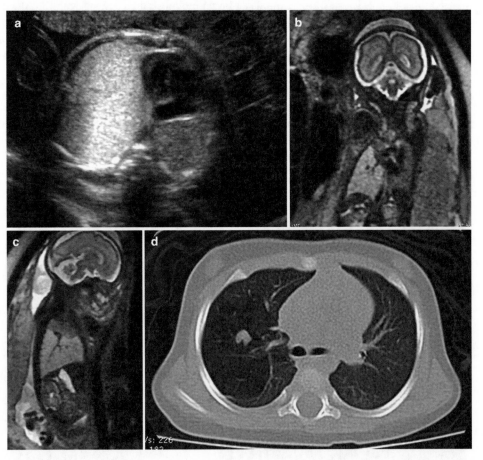

Fig. 18.6. Congenital lobar hyperinflation (CLH). (**a**) Axial US at 27 weeks gestation demonstrates a large echogenic mass in the right hemithorax deviating the heart to the left. No systemic feeding vessel was identified. (**b**) Coronal and (**c**) sagittal SSFSE T2w MR image at 27 weeks gestation confirms the presence of a high signal mass in the right lower lobe. (**d**) Axial chest CT scan at 5 months of age demonstrate an emphysematous lobe consistent with CLH

thoracic mass with increased T2 signal. CLE is usually located in the apical and posterior segments of the left upper lobe and can occur in segmental or lobar bronchi. Displacement of the mediastinum to the contralateral side, polyhydramnios and hydrops have been described especially secondary to bronchial atresia of lobar bronchi [50–52].

18.3.4 Diaphragmatic Hernia

Herniated bowel loops into the hemithorax can mimic a multicystic, heterogeneous lung mass by US (Fig. 18.2). Mediastinal and cardiac deviation may be the first hint that a CDH is present if the stomach remains infradiaphragmatic. When the stomach is herniated into the hemithorax, nonvisualization of stomach bubble within the abdomen is helpful for suggesting the diagnosis [27, 30]. Peristalsis of bowel loops in the thorax can sometimes be seen by ultrasound [27]. MRI is particularly useful in confirming the diagnosis and assessing amount of liver herniation and delineation of small and large meconium-filled bowel in the chest.

MR is most helpful in the evaluation of right and bilateral CDH. In these cases, with the stomach often in the abdomen, it may be difficult by US to differentiate a CPAM from a CDH. MRI can easily distinguish abdominal contents within the chest from cystic lesions. MRI can provide specific information on hernia content, size of diaphragmatic defect and volume of ipsilateral and contralateral lung.

18.3.5 Congenital Hydrothorax

Pleural fluid may develop with or without an associated mass. It is considered abnormal at any gestational age and can be unilateral or bilateral.

Chylothorax is the most common cause of congenital hydrothorax and can be due to thoracic duct anomalies (Fig. 18.7). Lesions associated with pleural effusions include entities such as CPAM, BPS, lymphagiectasia, cardiac anomalies, Turners syndrome, trisomy 21, cystic hygroma and TORCH infection. Thus, careful assessment is required to identify associated anomalies and karyotyping is recommended [53].

Ultrasound will demonstrate anechoic fluid in the pleural space. MRI demonstrates high signal fluid surrounding lung parenchyma and may help identify a cause for the hydrothorax such as an underlying CPAM.

Overall mortality can be as high as 50%. Outcome is best if the effusion is unilateral. Primary chylothorax may resolve spontaneously. If effusions progress to hydrops, mortality increases to 75%. If the effusion is small, conservative observation is appropriate. If the effusion is large and the infant is less than 32 weeks' gestation, fetal thoracentesis and thoracoamniotic shunting are potential prenatal treatment options, although reaccumulation of fluid is frequently described [53].

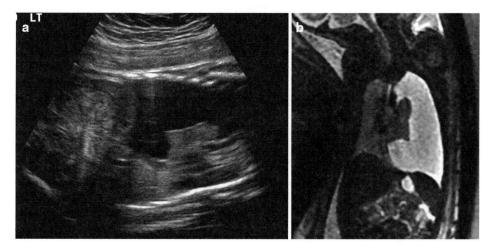

Fig. 18.7. Chylous effusion. (**a**) Coronal US of the chest demonstrate a large fluid collection in the left hemithorax compressing the left lung. (**b**) SSFSE coronal MR image confirms the presence of a large left pleural effusion with compressed lung parenchyma and no underlying lung mass

18.3.6 Congenital High Airway Obstruction

Congenital high airway obstruction (CHAOS) should be included in the differential when bilateral large echogenic lung masses are identified. [30]. This rare entity can be due to laryngotracheal atresia, tracheal stenosis or a thick web. Aberrant pulmonary budding off the foregut is present. Most cases have a connection with the esophagus. By ultrasound, both lungs are symmetrically enlarged and echogenic due to fluid trapping. The heart is compressed and the diaphragms inverted. Hydrops may develop with ascites. There can be increased or decreased amniotic fluid.

MRI demonstrates abnormally large high signal lungs on T2w that are enlarged causing eversion of the diaphragms. Identification of dilated fluid-filled trachea and bronchi help to confirm the diagnosis and differentiate this diagnosis from bilateral CPAM. EXIT delivery with airway control is recommended but with prognosis poor [30].

18.3.7 Pulmonary Hypoplasia

Pulmonary hypoplasia is a wide spectrum which includes agenesis, aplasia as well as hypoplasia. Agenesis is the actual absence of lung parenchyma and bronchi (Fig. 18.8). Aplasia is the absence of lung tissue with rudimentary bronchi. Hypoplasia is the presence of alveoli and bronchi that are underdeveloped with a decreased number of airways and alveoli resulting in a decrease in size and weight of the lungs. Alveoli and pulmonary vascularity develop concomitantly, so associated anomalies of pulmonary vessels are common.

Pulmonary hypoplasia causes severe respiratory failure at birth often resulting in rapid death. Hypoplasia is often secondary to premature rupture of membranes, renal anomalies, lung masses or a skeletal dysplasia. Severity of the hypoplasia is dependent of gestation age at onset.

Prenatal US diagnosis of pulmonary hypoplasia is often limited. Various measurements have been proposed to predict pulmonary hypoplasia including lung area, ratio of lung to thoracic area, thoracic to abdominal circumference and 3D volumetric measurements. High resistance patterns in peripheral pulmonary arteries have been reported in fetuses with pulmonary hypoplasia [54]. Oligohydramnios and maternal obesity, however, limit US evaluation, so prognosis is often difficult to predict.

Fetal lung volume by MR is also being used to assess pulmonary hypoplasia [55–62] (Fig. 18.9). Relative lung volume based on gestational age and lung volume to body weight ratios have been evaluated. Normal lungs are progressively hyperintense on T2w with maturation. Decreased signal has been described in hypoplastic lungs. Relative lung signal intensity and spectroscopy are potential methods for the further assessing severity of hypoplasia [60, 61].

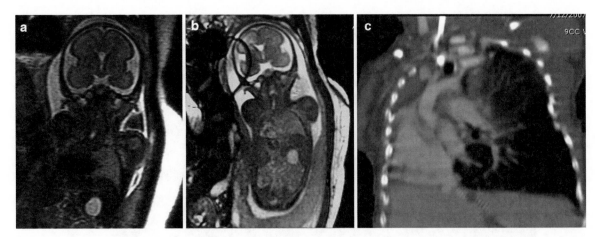

Fig. 18.8. Right lung agenesis. (a) Coronal SSFSE and (b) FIESTA T2w images at 21 weeks gestation demonstrates shift of the heart to the right with no right lung parenchyma or right mainstem bronchus identified. (c) Contrast chest CT after delivery confirms the diagnosis of agenesis of the right lung

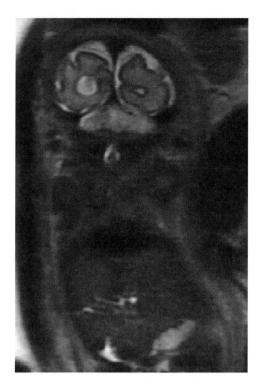

Fig. 18.9. Pulmonary hypoplasia. Coronal SSFSE MR image of the fetal chest demonstrates small low signal pulmonary parenchyma in this fetus with renal anomalies resulting in oligohydramnios

18.4 Conclusion

Congenital lung malformations are rare, often involute prenatally with a small percentage developing hydrops in utero. A majority have no respiratory symptoms at delivery. Ultrasound is the initial study to identify a congenital lung malformation which can be cystic, solid or mixed. Fetal MRI can be a useful adjunct in the assessment of large lung masses for improved counseling and management planning. While rare, hydrops can develop with congenital pulmonary masses, is a sign of impending demise and may be an indication for fetal intervention.

References

1. Kline-Fath BM. Is prenatal sonography accurate in identification of Congenital lung lesions? Scientific paper presented at SPR, Boston, MA. April 15; 2010.
2. Breysem L, Bosmans H, Dymarkowski S, et al. The value of fast MR imaging as an adjunct to ultrasound in prenatal diagnosis. Eur Radiol. 2003;13:1538–48.
3. Quinn TM, Hubbard AM, Adzick NS. Prenatal MRI enhance fetal diagnosis. J Pediatr Surg. 1998;33: 553–8.
4. Bulas DI. Fetal magnetic resonance imaging as a complement to fetal ultrasonography. Ultrasound Q. 2007;23(1): 3–22.
5. Aite L, Zaccara A, Trucchi A, et al. When uncertainty generates more anxiety than severity: the prenatal experience with cystic adenomatoid malformation of the lung. J Perinat Med. 2009;37:539–42.
6. Ruano R, Joubin L, Abry MC, et al. Anomogram of fetal lung volumes estimated by 3D US using the roataional technique (virtual organ computer aided analysis). J Ultrasound Med. 2006;35:701–9.
7. Harmath A, Csaba A, Hauzman E, et al. Congenital lung malformations in the second trimester: prenatal ultrasound diagnosis and pathologic findings. J Clin Ultrasound. 2007;35(5):250–5.
8. Lecompte B, Hadden H, Coste K, et al. Hyperechoic congenital lung lesions in a non-selected population: from prenatal detection till perinatal management. Prenat Diagn. 2009;29:1222–30.
9. Ankerman T, Oppermann HC, Engler S, et al. Congenital masses of the lung, cystic adenomatoid malformation versus congenital lobar emphysema: prenatal diagnosis and implications for postnatal treatment. J Ultrasound Med. 2004;23:1379–84.
10. Johnson AM, Hubbard AM. Congenital anomalies of the fetal/neonatal chest. Semin Roentgenol. 2004;39: 197–214.
11. Coakley FV, Glenn OA, Qayyam A, et al. Fetal MRI: a developing technique for the developing patient. AJR. 2004;182:243–52.
12. Prayer D, Brugger PC, Prayer L. Fetal MRI: techniques and protocols. Pediatr Radiol. 2004;34:685–93.
13. Baker PN, Johnson IR, Harvey PR, et al. A three year follow up children imaged in utero with echoplanar magnetic resonance. Am J Obstet Gynecol. 1994;170:32–3.
14. De Wilde JP, Rivers AW, Price DU, et al. A review of the current use of magnetic resonance imaging in pregnancy and safety implications for the fetus. Prog Biophys Mol Biol. 2005;87:335.
15. Yip YP, Capriotti C, Tlagala SL, et al. Effects of MR exposure at 1.5 T on early embryonic development of the chick. J Magn Reson Imaging. 1994;4:742–8.
16. Yip YP, Capriotti C, Yip JW. Effects of MR exposure on axonal outgrowth in the sympathetic nervous system of the chick. J Magn Reson Imaging. 1995;5:457–62.
17. Vadeyar SH, Moore RJ, Strachan BK, et al. Effect of fetal magnetic resonance imaging on fetal heart rate patterns. Am J Obstet Gynecol. 2000;182:666–9.
18. Mevissen M, Buntenkotter S, Loscher W. Effect of static and time varying magnetic field on reproduction and fetal development in rats. Teratology. 1994;50:229–37.
19. Shellock FG, Kanal E. Policies, guidelines and recommendations for MR imaging safety and patient management. JMRI. 1991;1:97–101.
20. United Nations Scientific Committee on the effects of atomic radiation. Ionizing radiation levels and effects. 1972 report to the General Assembly Vol 2 Effects New York, NY; 1972
21. Hand JW, Li Y, Thomas EL, et al. Prediction of specific absorption rate in mother and fetus associated with MRI examinations during pregnancy. Magn Reson Med. 2006;55:883–93.

22. Frates MC, Kumar AJ, Benson CB, et al. Fetal anomalies: comparison of MR imaging and US for diagnosis. Radiology. 2004;232:398–404.

23. Levine D, Barnewolt CE, Mehta TS, et al. Fetal thoracic abnormalities: MR imaging. Radiology. 2003;228:379–88.

24. Kunisaki SM, Fauza DO, Barnewolt CE, et al. Exutero intrapartum treatment with placement of extracorporeal membrane oxygenation for fetal thoracic masses. J Pediatr Surg. 2007;42(2):420–5.

25. Daltro P, Werner H, Gasparetto TD, et al. Congenital chest malformations: a multimodality approach with emphasis on fetal MR Imaging. Radiographics. 2010;30:385–95.

26. Curran PF, Jelin EB, Rand L, et al. Prenatal steroids for microcystic congenital cystic adenomatoid malformations. J Pediatr Surg. 2010;45:145–50.

27. Azizkhan RG, Crombleholme TM. Congenital cystic lung disease: contemporary antenatal and postnatal management. Pediatr Surg Int. 2008;24:643–57.

28. Adzick NS. Management of fetal lung lesions. Clin Perinatol. 2009;36:363–76.

29. Kumar AN. Perinatal management of common neonatal thoracic lesions. Indian J Pediatr. 2008;75:931–7.

30. Bush A, Hogg J, Chitty LS. Cystic lung lesions – prenatal diagnosis and management. Prenat Diagn. 2008;28:604–11.

31. Cavoretto P, Molina F, Poggi S, et al. Prenatal diagnosis and outcome of echogenic fetal lung lesions. Ultrasound Obstet Gynecol. 2008;32:769–83.

32. Stocker TJ, Manewell JE, Drake RM. Congenital cystic adenomatoid malformation of the lung: classification and morphologic spectrum. Hum Pathol. 1977;8:155–71.

33. Crombleholme TM, Coleman B, Hedrick H, et al. Cystic adenomatoid malformation volume ratio predicts outcome in prenatally diagnosed cystic adenomatoid malformation of the lung. J Pediatr Surg. 2002;37(3):331–8.

34. Mann S, Wilson RD, Bebbington MW, et al. Antenatal diagnosis and management of congenital cystic adenomatoid malformation. Semin Fetal Neonatal Med. 2007;12:477–81.

35. Coleman BG, Adzick NS, Crombleholme TM, et al. Fetal therapy: state of the art. J Ultrasound Med. 2002;21:1257–88.

36. Morris LM, Lim FY, Livingston JC, et al. High-risk fetal congenital pulmonary airway malformations have a variable response to steroids. J Pediatr Surg. 2009;2004:60–5.

37. Kunisaki SM, Barnewolt CE, Estroff JA, et al. Large fetal congenital cystic adenomatoid malformations: growth trends and patient survival. J Pediatr Surg. 2007;42(2):404–10.

38. Knox EM, Kilby MD, Martin WL, et al. In-utero pulmonary drainage in the management of primary hydrothorax and congenital cystic lung lesion: a systematic review. Ultrasound Obstet Gynecol. 2006;28:726–34.

39. Fortunato S, Lombardo S, Dantrell J. Intrauterine laser ablation of a fetal cystic adenomatoid malformation with hydrops: the application of minimally invasive surgical techniques to fetal surgery. Am J Obstet Gynecol. 1997;177:S84.

40. Adzick NS. Open fetal surgery for life-threatening fetal anomalies. Semin Fetal Neonatal Med. 2009; (epub ahead of print).

41. Bermudez C, Perez-Wulff J, Arcadipane M, et al. Percutaneous fetal sclerotherapy for congenital cystic adenomatoid malformation of the lung. Fetal Diagn Ther. 2008;24:237–40.

42. Marshall KW, Blane CE, Teitelbaum DH, et al. Congenital cystic adenomatoid malformation: impact of prenatal diagnosis and changing strategies in the treatment of the asymptomatic patient. AJR. 2000;175:1551–4.

43. Vijayaraghavan SB, Rao PS, Selvarasu CD, et al. Prenatal sonographic features of intralobar bronchopulmonary sequestration. J Ultrasound Med. 2003;22:541–4.

44. Sepulveda W. Perinatal imaging in bronchopulmonary sequestration. J Ultrasound Med. 2009;28:89–94.

45. Zeidan S, Gorincour G, Potier A, et al. Congenital lung malformation: evaluation of prenatal and postnatal radiologic findings. Respirology. 2009;14:1005–11.

46. Witlox RS, Lopriore E, Rikkers-Mutsaerts ER, et al. Single-needle laser treatment with drainage of hydrothorax in fetal bronchopulmonary sequestration with hydrops. Ultrasound Obstet Gynecol. 2009;34:355–7.

47. Oepkes D, Devlieger R, Lopriore E, et al. Successful ultrasound-guided laser treatment of fetal hydrops caused by pulmonary sequestration. Ultrasound Obstet Gynecol. 2007;29:457–9.

48. Ruano R, de A Pimenta EJ, Marques da Silva M, et al. Percutaneous intrauterine laser ablation of the abnormal vessel in pulmonary sequestration with hydrops at 29 weeks' gestation. J Ultrasound Med. 2007;26:1235–41.

49. Becmeur F, Horta-Geraud P, Donato L, et al. Pulmonary sequestrations: prenatal ultrasound diagnosis, treatment and outcome. J Pediatr Surg. 1998;33:492–6.

50. Seo T, Ando H, Kaneko K, et al. Two cases of prenatally diagnosed congenital lobar emphysema caused by lobar bronchial atresia. J Pediatr Surg. 2006;41:E17–20.

51. Pariente G, Aviram M, Landau D, et al. Prenatal diagnosis of congenital lobar emphysema: case report and review of the literature. J Ultrasound Med. 2009;28:1081–4.

52. Peranteau WH, Merchant AM, Hedrick HL, et al. Prenatal Course and postnatal management of peripheral bronchial atresia: association with congenital cystic adenomatoid malformation of the lung. Fetal Diagn Ther. 2008;24:190–6.

53. Aubard Y, Derouineau I, Aubard V, et al. Primary fetal hydrothorax: a literature review and proposed antenatal clinical strategy. Fetal Diagn Ther. 1998;13:325–33.

54. Chaoui R, Kalache K, Tennstedt C, et al. Pulmonary arterial Doppler velocimetry in fetuses with lung hypoplasia. Eur J Obstet Gynecol Repord Biol. 1999;84:179–85.

55. Keller TM, Rake A, Michel SC, Seifert B, et al. MR assessment of fetal lung development using lung volumes and signal intensities. Eur Radiol. 2004;14(6):984–9.

56. Osada H, Kaku K, Masuda K, Iitsuka Y, Seki K, Sekiya S. Quantitative and qualitative evaluations of fetal lung with MR imaging. Radiology. 2004;231:887–92.

57. Tanigaki S, Miyakoshi K, Tanaka M, et al. Pulmonary hypoplasia: prediction with use of ratio of MRI measured fetal lung volume to US estimated fetal body weight. Radiology. 2004;232:767–72.

58. Ward VL, Nishino M, Hatabu H, et al. Fetal lung volume measurements: determination with MR imaging – effect of various factors. Radiology. 2006;240(1):187–93.

59. Williams G, Coakley FV, Qayyum A, et al. Fetal relative lung volume: quantification by using prenatal MR imaging lung volumetry. Radiology. 2004;233:457–62.

60. Keller TM, Rake A, Michel SC, Seifert B, Wisser J, et al. MR assessment of fetal lung development using lung volumes and signal intensities. Eur Radiol. 2004;14(6):984–9.

61. Kuwashima S, Nishimura G, Limura F, et al. Low intensity fetal lungs on MRI may suggest the diagnosis of pulmonary hypoplasia. Pediatr Radiol. 2001;31:669–72.

62. Zaretsky M, Ramus R, McIntire D, et al. MR calculation of lung volumes to predict outcome in fetuses with genitourinary abnormalities. Am J Roentgenol. 2005;185(5):1328–34.

Pulmonary Incidentalomas

Anne Cameron Coates and Robert G. Zwerdling

CONTENTS

19.1 Case Presentation

A 1.5-cm nodule (Fig. 19.1) was discovered at the base of the right lung in an otherwise healthy 17-year-old girl during an emergency room evaluation of abdominal pain. The radiologist recommended a follow-up chest CT be performed. This was completed 4 months later and was found to be normal. The abdominal pain resolved spontaneously while she was in the emergency room.

19.2 Discussion

An *incidentaloma* is an unexpected finding unrelated to the patient's primary problem or an expected finding that requires additional evaluation but is eventually found to be irrelevant to the management of the patient [1]. Widespread use of advanced imaging techniques increases the risk of discovering such findings. As a result, clinicians face the dual problems of deciding on the best course of action with respect to these findings in asymptomatic patients [2] and how to lessen the chance of finding them in the first place. Currently there is a paucity of data or guidelines addressing this situation in the young. We should accomplish this in as safe, nontraumatic, and cost-effective manner as possible.

The occurrence of incidental findings and normal variants is not new. In 1973, Dr. Benjamin Felson reported his experience cataloging over 30,000 US Military Induction Chest Roentgenograms reviewed systematically, published in his classic textbook, *Chest Roentgenology*. Included among his numerous findings were 1,350 cases of calcifications noted in the hilum, mediastinum, lymph nodes, or lungs which ranged in size from less than 5 mm up to 10 mm in diameter [3]. Dr. Felson's work highlighted the presence of multiple unexpected findings in apparently normal individuals and raised the question of their diagnostic significance and how to manage them.

Since Felson's observations, computerized imaging, and other advanced imaging techniques have revolutionized radiology and the practice of medicine. It is estimated that more than 62 million CT scans per year are currently obtained in the United States, including at least four million for children [4] representing a sevenfold increase in CT use over the past 10 years [5]. Decreasing image acquisition time eliminates the need for anesthesia further tempting the clinician to utilize the technique [6]. While faster acquisition times decrease misregistration artifacts, the thinner slice sections enable the depiction of more and smaller lung lesions [7]. Detection of focal rounded pulmonary opacities as small as 1–2 mm in diameter has become routine [8].

Anne Cameron Coates, MD
Lucille Packard Children's Hospital at Stanford,
770 Welch Road, Suite 350, Palo Alto, CA 94304, USA

Robert G. Zwerdling, MD (✉)
UMass Memorial Medical Center, 55 Lake Avenue North,
Worcester, MA 01655, USA
e-mail: robert.zwerdling@umassmemorial.org

R.H. Cleveland (ed.), *Imaging in Pediatric Pulmonology*,
DOI 10.1007/978-1-4419-5872-3_19, © Springer Science+Business Media, LLC 2012

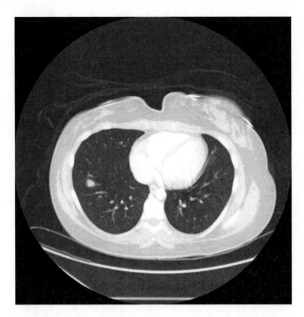

Fig. 19.1. Imaging of the lung bases, obtained as part of an abdominal CT, reveal an approximately 1.5 cm nodule in the right lower lobe

These previously unseen findings are reported and therefore must be addressed.

Since the detection incidentalomas is, for the most part, a phenomenon relating to CT imaging, an assessment of CT use in pediatrics becomes relevant to the discussion. In recent years, there has been a growing awareness that the irradiation doses from some CT studies may lead to a statistical increase in the risk of cancer [4]. This has lead to an awareness of the need to decrease the CT dose as much as possible. This is reflected in a commitment of the radiologic community to the adherence of the As Low As Reasonably Achievable (ALARA) concept for radiation dose [1]. As is emphasized in the ALARA concept, avoiding unnecessary CT is optimal. As diagnostic imaging has proliferated, there has been a recognition that much of the imaging does not provide contributory information [9]. To some degree this may relate to current practice patterns with a high degree of reliance on ancillary studies [10] and proliferation of new technology before clinical outcome data is developed or available [11, 12]. In addition, the practice of recommending follow-up studies for indeterminate opacities may be partly related to perceived liability if a cancer should develop [13]. This process has been termed the cascade effect: "A chain of events (which) tends to proceed with increasing momentum, so that the further it progresses the more difficult it is to stop" [14]. This unfortunate cycle is established where children are subjected to CT, placed at increased risk of the discovery of an incidentaloma for which, if it is found, there are no guidelines as to the management of it, thus potentially subjecting them to further radiation from follow-up studies out of perceived liability. Once this chain of events is initiated, as a result of an incidental finding, follow-up radiographic studies, biopsies, and other invasive procedures often result. Furthermore there is the anxiety of patients and families created by the discovery of incidentalomas and a lack of data as to how to proceed regarding further investigation and other interventions that in most cases end up demonstrating that the finding is of no clinical significance [1]. Adding to the pressure is the concern for the importance of early detection of cancer. This makes it particularly difficult to convince patients and families that follow-up CT of every nodule in every patient is unnecessary [8]. Inconsistent messages from the medical community may add to the stress and frustration patients and families may feel in this setting.

19.3   Role of the Radiologist

Radiologists should play a crucial role in educating other physicians about the appropriate imaging approach to a given diagnostic problem. A straw poll of pediatric radiologists suggests that one third of CT studies could be replaced by alternative approaches or not performed at all thus reducing the risk of incidentalomas, unnecessary radiation, and decreasing medical care costs [15]. Data is emerging demonstrating the diagnostic limitation of this imaging modality for certain types of pediatric lung problems [16, 17].

Furthermore, there is a commitment of the radiologic community to the adherence of the ALARA concept for radiation dose [1]. Where CT is a primary modality of choice in the imaging of children, it is of paramount importance that all care is taken to minimize radiation dose, while maintaining useful diagnostic image information [18]. Communication between radiologists and clinicians should enhance the process.

19.4 Role of Professional Societies

Professional societies have a responsibility to guide the evaluation of patients with pulmonary incidentalomas and to deter their discovery. To date, The Fleischner Society, an international, multidisciplinary medical society for thoracic radiology, is the only professional society to have guidelines for the management of small, incidentally found pulmonary nodules detected on CT scans for *young patients*. (The exact definition of young patients was not provided but implied to be <35 years of age). They state that primary lung cancer is rare in persons under 35 years of age (<1% of all cases), and the risks from radiation exposure are greater than in the older population. Therefore, unless there is a known primary cancer, multiple follow-up CT studies for small incidentally detected nodules should be avoided in young patients. In such cases, the Fleischner Society recommendation is that a single low-dose follow-up CT scan in 6–12 months should be considered [8]. The yield and cost-effectiveness of repeated imaging at these intervals are uncertain.

In contrast to the lack of literature in the pediatric population, there are ample professional societies' recommendations for the adult population, such as the American College of Chest Physicians (ACCP) Evidence-Based Clinical Practice Guidelines [19] in the evaluation of patients with pulmonary nodules. This is not surprising given the increased risk of malignancy with age but as the discovery of incidentalomas rises with the prolific use of CT in children, pediatric professional societies have an obligation to establish clinical guidelines on the evaluation of these findings.

At the time of this writing, the Society for Pediatric Radiology (the largest North American pediatric radiology society) is forming a working committee to establish these guidelines for pediatric imaging.

19.5 Suggestions

Until definitive guidance is provided from professional organizations and the public sector, the following may help in reducing the consequences of incidentalomas. Table 19.1 lists potential ways to lessen the performance of unneeded imaging studies. Table 19.2 lists circumstances to help determine if *watchful waiting* may be appropriate.

Table 19.1. Potential methods to reduce incidentalomas

- For otherwise healthy children, patients should be assessed with targeted evaluation of their presenting illness rather than a "complete" radiographic evaluation
- *Watchful waiting* should be utilized whenever possible
- Discourage physicians from refusing to see the patient before a CT scan is performed unless there is a specific indication for doing CT
- Plain films should be evaluated by radiologists before automatically progressing to CT scans unless specific indication exists for doing CT
- Alternative imaging, rather than CT, should be employed unless specific indications exist for doing CT
- Professional Societies must develop guidelines for dealing with incidental findings to provide both guidance and protection against potential litigation for clinicians who otherwise feel certain follow-up studies should not be performed

Table 19.2. Clinical aids for determining if *watchful waiting* may be appropriate

- Otherwise healthy – growing and developing well. No significant weight loss, hemoptysis, respiratory distress, or lymphadenopathy after the acute illness or trauma
- Unremarkable physical examination other than what would be expected from the chief complaint and known medical history
- Low pretest probability – i.e., patients who have no known history of aspiration, immunodeficiency, or an oncological process
- No unusual travel, exposure, or inhalation history
- Availability and reliability for follow-up

References

1. Reed M. Imaging utilization commentary: a radiology perspective. Pediatr Radiol. 2008;38:660.
2. van Klaveren RJ et al. Management of lung nodules detected by volume CT scanning. N Engl J Med. 2009;361(23):2221–9.
3. Felson B. Chest roentgenology. Philadelphia: W. B. Saunders Co; 1973.
4. Brenner DJ, Hall EJ. Computed tomography – an increasing source of radiation exposure. N Engl J Med. 2007;357(22):2277–84.
5. Forghani N, Cohen RA, Abbott MB. Radiation risks of CT scans. Pediatr Rev. 2006;27(2):79.
6. White K. Helical/spiral CT scanning: a pediatric radiology perspective. Pediatr Radiol. 1996;26:5–14.
7. Silva CT et al. CT characteristics of lung nodules present at diagnosis of extrapulmonary malignancy in children. Am J Roentgenol. 2010;194(3):772–8.
8. MacMahon H et al. Guidelines for management of small pulmonary nodules detected on CT scans: a statement from the Fleischner society. Radiology. 2005;237(2): 395–400.
9. Picano E. Sustainability of medical imaging. BMJ. 2004;328(7439):578–80.

10. Weinstein MC, Skinner JA. Comparative effectiveness and health care spending – implications for reform. N Engl J Med. 2010;362(5):460–5.

11. Baldwin J. New study questions marketing of spiral CT scanning to consumers. J Natl Cancer Inst. 2003;95(7):507–9.

12. Sorgen C. Local hospitals tout new technology. Washington: The Washington Post; 2010. http://www.washingtonpost.com/wp-dyn/content/article/2010/08/30/AR2010083002079.html.

13. Berlin L. Failure to diagnose lung cancer: anatomy of a malpractice trial. Am J Roentgenol. 2003;180(1):37–45.

14. Mold J, Stein HF. The cascade effect in the clinical care of patients. N Engl J Med. 1986;314:512–4.

15. Bleyer A. Helical CT and cancer resk. Panel discussion. Pediatr Radiol. 2002;32:242–4.

16. Schneebaum N et al. Use and yield of chest computed tomography in the diagnostic evaluation of pediatric lung disease. Pediatrics. 2009;124(2):472–9.

17. Vrielynck S et al. Diagnostic value of high-resolution CT in the evaluation of chronic infiltrative lung disease in children. Am J Roentgenol. 2008;191(3):914–20.

18. Punwani S et al. Paediatric CT: the effects of increasing image noise on pulmonary nodule detection. Pediatr Radiol. 2008;38(2):192.

19. Gould MK et al. Evaluation of patients with pulmonary nodules: when is it lung cancer? ACCP evidence-based clinical practice guidelines (2nd Edition). Chest. 2007;132 (3 suppl):108S–30.

Index

R.H. Cleveland (ed.), *Imaging in Pediatric Pulmonology*,
DOI 10.1007/978-1-4419-5872-3, © Springer Science+Business Media, LLC 2012

Printed by Publishers' Graphics LLC USA
MO20120417-013
2012